Liquid-Liquid Interfaces

Theory and Methods

Liquid-Liquid Interfaces

Theory and Methods

Edited by

Alexander G. Volkov, Ph.D.
David W. Deamer, Ph.D.

Department of Chemistry and Biochemistry
University of California
Santa Cruz, California

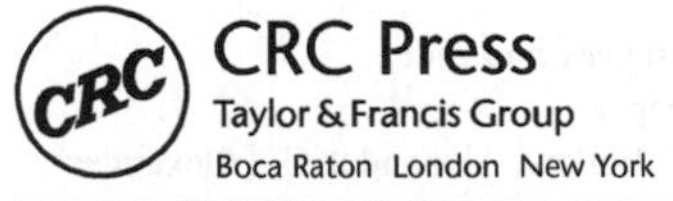
CRC Press
Taylor & Francis Group
Boca Raton London New York

CRC Press is an imprint of the
Taylor & Francis Group, an **informa** business

Published 1996 by CRC Press
Taylor & Francis Group
6000 Broken Sound Parkway NW, Suite 300
Boca Raton, FL 33487-2742

First issued in paperback 2019

ISBN-13: 978-0-367-44869-1 (pbk)
ISBN-13: 978-0-8493-7694-8 (hbk)

Visit the Taylor & Francis Web site at
http://www.taylorandfrancis.com

and the CRC Press Web site at
http://www.crcpress.com

Library of Congress Cataloging-in-Publication Data

Liquid-liquid interfaces : theory and methods / edited by Alexander G.
Volkov, David W. Deamer.
p. cm.
Includes bibliographical references and index.
ISBN 0-8493-7694-7 (alk. paper)
1. Liquid-liquid interfaces. I. Volkov, Alexander G. (Alexander George). II. Deamer, D. W.
QD509.L54L57 1996
541.3'3—dc20 95-53983
CIP

Library of Congress Card Number 95-53983

INTRODUCTION

"Liquid-Liquid Interfaces: Theory and Methods" presents contemporary reviews by world leaders in research related to electrochemical, biological and photochemical effects in interfacial phenomena. The chemical and physical properties of liquid-liquid interfaces represent a significant interdisciplinary research area for a broad range of investigators. Our aim is to provide a broadly based, modern account of research on liquid-liquid interfaces, with particular emphasis on charge transfer effects.

This topic incorporates such diverse themes as interfacial and phase transfer catalysis, electrochemistry and colloidal chemistry, ion and electron transport processes, molecular dynamics, electroanalysis, liquid membranes, emulsions, pharmacology and artificial photosynthesis. Discussions include applications in biotechnology such as drug delivery, purification of nuclear waste, catalysis, mineral extraction processes and the manufacture of biosensors and ion-selective electrodes.

The text is organized so that it can serve both as a reference book and for teaching a course on surface science, separation and extraction. We expect that electrochemists, biophysicists, colloid and physical chemists, biochemists, and their students will find this collection of contemporary research reviews to be informative and valuable.

Alexander G. Volkov and David W. Deamer
Santa Cruz, California, August 1995

THE EDITORS

Alexander George Volkov, Ph.D. received his doctoral degree in 1982 from the A. N. Frumkin Institute of Electrochemistry of the USSR Academy of Sciences, and afterwards served at the Institute as Head of the Group "Liquid-Liquid Interfaces" in the Department of Bioelectrochemistry. He is now associated with the Department of Chemistry and Biochemistry at the University of California, Santa Cruz.

Dr. Volkov is a member of the American Chemical Society, the Electrochemical Society, the Biophysical Society and the International Bioelectrochemical Society. He has presented over 70 invited lectures at international meetings and seminars, and has published over 120 research papers and 19 reviews. His current major research interests include bioelectrochemical phenomena at liquid interfaces, artificial photosynthesis, electroanalytical and surface chemistry.

David W. Deamer, Ph.D. received his doctoral degree in 1965 from the Department of Physiological Chemistry at the Ohio State University School of Medicine. He taught and carried out research in cell and molecular biology at thc University of California, Davis, from 1967 to 1993, and joined the Department of Chemistry and Biochemistry at the University of California, Santa Cruz in 1994.

Dr. Deamer is a member of the Biophysical Society and the American Society for Biochemistry and Molecular Biology. His primary research interest is in the field of membrane biophysics, particularly molecular self-assembly processes and proton transport in membranes. He has published over 130 research papers and reviews, and has edited or written eight books.

CONTRIBUTORS

Kensuke Arai
School of Pharmacy,
Tokyo University of Pharmacy
and Life Science,
1432-1 Horinouchi, Hachioji,
Tokyo 192-03, Japan

Ilan Benjamin
Department of Chemistry,
University of California,
Santa Cruz, CA 95064, USA

Pierre-Francois Brevet
Laboratory of Electrochemistry,
Swiss Federal Institute of
Technology, ICP-3, Lausanne,
Switzerland CH-1015

Vincent J. Cunnane
Advanced Sensors
Research Unit,
Department of Chemical and
Environmental Sciences,
University of Limerick,
Limerick, Ireland

David W. Deamer
Department of Chemistry
and Biochemistry,
University of California,
Santa Cruz, CA 95064, USA

Anna H. DeArmond
Department of Chemistry
and Biochemistry,
New Mexico State University,
Las Cruses,
NM 88003, USA

M. Keith Dearmond
Department of Chemistry
and Biochemistry,
New Mexico State University,
Las Cruses, NM 88003, USA

Hubert H. Girault
Laboratory of Electrochemistry,
Swiss Federal Institute of Technology,
ICP-3, Lausanne,
Switzerland CH-1015

Takashi Kakiuchi
Yokohama National University,
Laboratory of Electrochemistry,
Tokiwadai 156,
240 Yokohama, Japan

Yurij I. Kharkats
The A. N. Frumkin Institute of
Electrochemistry,
Russian Academy of Sciences,
31 Leninsky Prospect,
Moscow 117071, Russia

Zbigniew Koczorowski
Department of Chemistry,
University of Warsaw,
Ul. Pastera 1,
Warsaw, Poland 02-093

Nicolas Kotov
Department of Chemistry,
Syracuse University,
Syracuse, N.Y., 13244, USA

Fumiyo Kusu
School of Pharmacy,
Tokyo University of Pharmacy
and Life Science,
1432-1 Horinouchi,
Hachioji,
Tokyo 192-03, Japan

Michael G. Kuzmin
Department of Chemistry,
Moscow State University,
Moscow, 119899,
Russia

Alexander M. Kuznetsov
The A. N. Frumkin Institute of Electrochemistry, Russian Academy of Sciences, 31 Leninsky Prospect, Moscow, 117071, Russia

Yizhak Marcus
Department of Inorganic and Analytical Chemistry, Hebrew University, Jerusalem IL-91904, Israel

Vladislav S. Markin
Department of Cell Biology Southwestern Medical Center, University of Texas, 5233 H. Hines, Dallas, Texas 75235-9039

Lasse Murtomäki
Laboratory of Physical Chemistry and Electrochemistry Helsinki University of Technology Kemistintie 1A 02150 Espoo, Finland

Alexander N. Popov
The Institute of Inorganic Chemistry, the Latvian Academy of Sciences, 34 Miera St., Salaspils, LV-2169, Latvia

Zdeněk Samec
J. Heyrovský Institute of Physical Chemistry, Academy of Sciences of the Czech Republic, Dolejškova 3, Prague 8, Czech Republic, 182 23

Mitsugi Senda
Department Bioscience, Fukui Prefectural University, Kenjojima 4-1-1, Matsuika-cho, Yoshida-gun, Fukui, 910-11 Japan

Yury Shchipunov
Institute of Chemistry, Far East Department, Russian Academy of Sciences, 690022 Vladivostok, Russia

Kiyoko Takamura
School of Pharmacy, Tokyo University of Pharmacy and Life Science, 1432-1 Horinouchi, Hachioji, Tokyo 192-03, Japan

T. J. VanderNoot
Chemistry Department, Queen Mary & Westfield College,Mile End Road, London E1 4NS, England

Alexander G. Volkov
Department of Chemistry and Biochemistry, University of California, Santa Cruz, CA 95064, USA

Aaron Watts
Chemistry Department, Queen Mary & Westfield College, Mile End Road, London E1 4NS, England

Yukitaka Yamamoto
Department Bioscience, Fukui Prefectural University, Kenjojima 4-1-1, Matsuika-cho Yoshida-gun, Fukui, 910-11, Japan

CONTENTS

Chapter 1

PARTITION EQUILIBRIUM OF IONIC COMPONENTS IN TWO IMMISCIBLE ELECTROLYTE SOLUTIONS

Takashi Kakiuchi

The distribution potential is a concept of fundamental importance in electrochemistry at the interface between two immiscible electrolyte solutions (ITIES). All equilibrium properties of the system, such as the partition of ions and electrocapillarity, are functions of the distribution potential. From an experimental point of view, this concept is indispensable in understanding the polarizability of the ITIES and in designing reference electrodes for accurately controlling the potential drop across ITIES. Historical development of the understanding of this potential has been surveyed by Davies and Rideal[1] and more recently by Koczorowski,[2] Girault and Schiffrin,[3] and in detail by Markin and Volkov.[4] This chapter introduces the concept of the distribution potential at ITIES and then describes its use for characterizing polarized and non-polarized ITIES. The final part deals with the coupling of electron transfer and ion transfer processes in determining the phase-boundary potential.

I. DISTRIBUTION POTENTIAL

A. PHASE-BOUNDARY POTENTIAL

Any interface between two immiscible phases is electrified in that there is always a potential difference between the two phases,[5] unless the potential difference is fortuitously null. The presence of the potential across the interface has been recognized since the early days of surface physical chemistry [6,7] and its existence can be easily experienced through various surface phenomena, e.g. the stability of colloidal particles[8] or a Lippmann's beating heart.[6,9]

This potential has been ascribed to two physically distinguishable origins: the potential due to the orientation of dipoles in the vicinity of the interface and the potential due to the presence of excess free charges separated by the interface.[10] The former potential is called the surface potential, χ, and the latter, the outer potential, ψ. The sum of the two potentials is the inner potential, $\phi = \chi + \psi$.[10] The magnitude of ϕ as well as the relative contributions of χ and ψ to ϕ are determined by the conditions of the equilibrium established over the two phases in contact.

At constant temperature and pressure, the condition for the thermodynamic equilibrium is expressed by the equality of the chemical potential for each component commonly distributed in the two phases, designated hereafter as the organic phase O and the aqueous phase W,

0-8493-7694-7/96/$0.00+$.50

$$\bar{\mu}_i^O = \bar{\mu}_i^W \tag{1}$$

where $\bar{\mu}_i^\alpha$ is the chemical potential of the component i in the phase α (α = O or W). When i is a charged component, the electrostatic part of the electrochemical potential is separated to highlight the importance of electrostatic interactions on energetics and is written as

$$\bar{\mu}_i^\alpha = \mu_i^\alpha + \mu_i^{\alpha,el} \tag{2}$$

where μ_i^α and $\mu_i^{\alpha,el}$ express "chemical" energy and "electrical" energy terms of the chemical potential, respectively. The term "electrochemical potential" has been used for $\bar{\mu}_i^\alpha$ to explicitly indicate that the chemical potential of ionic components is strongly affected by the electrical state of the phase.

An intrinsic ambiguity exists in eq. (2) is that there is no unique way to divide $\bar{\mu}_i^\alpha$ into chemical and electrical terms.[5] Usually, $\mu_i^{\alpha,el}$ is identified with $z_iF\phi^\alpha$, which is the work to bring a test particle having the charge z_ie from infinity in vacuum to the inside of the phase α, where z_ie is the charge on the test particle with the unit of electronic charge e. This test charge is assumed to exercise no "chemical" interaction with its environment. Then, eq. (2) is

$$\bar{\mu}_i^\alpha = \mu_i^\alpha + zF\phi \tag{3}$$

From eqs. (1) and (3), the potential difference between the two phases can be expressed in terms of the difference in the chemical part of the electrochemical potential of i in O and W,

$$\Delta_O^W\phi = \frac{1}{z_iF}(\mu_i^O - \mu_i^W) \tag{4}$$

where $\Delta_O^W\phi = \phi^W - \phi^O$, i.e. the difference in the inner potential between the two phases, which is also called Galvani potential difference. The difference in chemical energy is thus counterbalanced by the difference in electrostatic potential at equilibrium. In other words, the inner potential difference $\Delta_O^W\phi$ can be seen as a measure of chemical affinity of the species i in the two phases.

The potential difference is a direct consequence of the presence of two distinct phases at equilibrium and at least one common charged species which establishes eq. (1). Moreover, as elementary electrostatics shows, the variation of the potential occurs only in the narrowly limited interfacial region. Therefore the potential difference thus formed is generally called the phase-boundary potential. The actual profile of the potential distribution will be discussed in I.B.5.

B. DISTRIBUTION POTENTIAL AT ITIES

Suppose that two electrolyte solutions which are not completely miscible with each other are brought into contact. Ionic components in one phase more or less dissolve into the other phase upon contact, depending on the hydrophilic-lipophilic balance of ions. At thermodynamic equilibrium, an electrical potential difference between the two phases develops, so that further dissolution of ions in both phases is suppressed.

The potential drop across the interface between the two phases in this case is determined by the inhomogeneous distribution of ionic components over the two phases in the vicinity of the interface, which leads to this particular type of the phase-boundary potential being called the distribution potential.

1. Nernst equation

By taking account of the concentration dependence of the chemical potential of ion i, eq. (4) is written as

$$\Delta_O^W\phi = \frac{1}{z_iF}(\mu_i^{O,\circ} - \mu_i^{W,\circ}) + \frac{RT}{z_iF}ln\frac{\gamma_i^O c_i^O}{\gamma_i^W c_i^W} \tag{5}$$

where $\mu_i^{O,\circ}$ is the standard chemical potential of i in α, R is the gas constant, T is the absolute temperature, γ_i^O and c_i^O are the activity coefficient and concentration of i in α. The difference $\mu_i^{O,\circ} - \mu_i^{W,\circ}$ is the standard molar Gibbs energy of transfer of ion i from O to W, $\Delta G_i^{O\to W,\circ}$. Here, we introduce the standard ion-transfer potential $\Delta_O^W\phi_i^\circ$ defined by

$$\Delta_O^W\phi_i^\circ = -\frac{1}{z_iF}\Delta G_i^{O\to W,\circ} \tag{6}$$

Then, eq. (5) is further written as

$$\Delta_O^W\phi = \Delta_O^W\phi_i^\circ + \frac{RT}{z_iF} ln \frac{\gamma_i^O c_i^O}{\gamma_i^W c_i^W} \tag{7}$$

This form is similar to the Nernst equation for redox reactions[11] and is also given the same name. In fact, Nernst used eq. (7) to describe the phase-boundary potential at liquid/solid-solution and liquid/liquid systems.[12]

The similarity between the two Nernst equations goes far beyond the formal expressions and suggests that the energetics at ITIES is dictated by the same laws as those in redox processes, for the later of which detailed knowledge has been compiled in electrochemistry. In this sense, eq. (6) first proposed by Koryta[13] in the context of voltammetry is not simply a convenient method to convert units but has played a key role in understanding of the electrochemistry of ITIES.[3,14-19]

2. Standard ion-transfer potential

The standard ion-transfer potential is a fundamental parameter which quantifies the relative affinity of an ion in the two phases where both solvents are in mutual saturation. The standard state is usually taken to be a hypothetical 1 mol dm^{-3} solution or 1 mol kg^{-1} where the activity coefficient is assumed to be unity. This is a property associated with a single ionic component and hence is not measurable with thermodynamic reliability.[20,21] There are several ways, however, to estimate the value of this quantity using extrathermodynamic assumptions (See Chapter 2).

Values of $\Delta G_i^{O\rightarrow W,\circ}$ and $\Delta_O^W\phi_i^\circ$ of interest for the study of ITIES have been compiled for certain solvent systems. Representative values are listed in Table 1. It is noted that $\Delta G_i^{O\rightarrow W,\circ}$ should be distinguished from the transfer Gibbs energy from one pure solvent to another pure solvent.

If we know the value of $\Delta G_i^{O\rightarrow W,\circ}$ or $\Delta_O^W\phi_i^\circ$, we can calculate from eq. (7) the value of $\Delta_O^W\phi_{eq}$ by knowing the concentrations of an ionic species in the two phases and their activity coefficients.

3. Calculation of distribution potential

We often need to estimate the final distribution equilibrium of the system from an initial nonequilibrium state. In an example illustrated in Fig. 1, an aqueous phase containing 0.1 mol dm^{-3} LiCl is in contact with a nitrobenzene (NB) phase containing 0.1 mol dm^{-3} tetrabutylammonium tetraphenylborate (TBATPB), an electrolyte frequently used as a supporting electrolyte in the organic phase. After the contact of two phases. Li^+ and Cl^- ions tend to dissolve into the O phase while TBA^+ and TPB^- ions tend to dissolve into the W phase.

The method of calculating a value of $\Delta_O^W\phi$ and concentrations of ions at equilibrium was first thoroughly studied by Hung, [22,23] who proposed a general method of predicting the equilibrium partition of ions from the initial concentrations of electrolytes, the values of $\Delta_O^W\phi_i^\circ$ for all ionic components, and the volumes of the two phases.

Table 1. Standard ion transfer potentials $\Delta_O^W\phi_i^\circ$ (V) for mutually saturated water-organic solvent systems at 25°C.

Ion	Nitrobenzene	1,2-Dichloroethane	Dichloromethane
Li^+	0.298	0.493	
Na^+	0.355	0.490	
H^+	0.337		
NH_4^+	0.284		
K^+	0.241	0.499	
Rb^+	0.201	0.445	
Cs^+	0.159	0.36	
Acetylcholine	0.052		
$(CH_3)_4N^+$	0.037	0.182	0.195
$(C_2H_5)_4N^+$	-0.063	0.044	0.044
$(C_3H_7)_4N^+$	-0.160	-0.091	-0.091
$(C_4H_9)_4N^+$	-0.270	-0.225	-0.230
$(C_5H_{11})_4N^+$		-0.360	-0.377
$(C_6H_5)_4As^+$	-0.372	-0.364	
Crystal violet	-0.410		
$(C_6H_{13})_4N^+$	-0.472	-0.494	-0.455
Mg^{2+}	0.370		
Ca^{2+}	0.354		
Sr^{2+}	0.348		
Ba^{2+}	0.328		
Cl^-	-0.395	-0.481	-0.481
Br^-	-0.335	-0.408	-0.408
NO_3^-	-0.270		
I^-	-0.195	-0.273	-0.273
SCN^-	-0.161		
BF_4^-	-0.091		
ClO_4^-	-0.091	-0.178	-0.221
2,4-dinitrophenolate	-0.077		
PF_6^-	0.012		
Picrate	0.047	-0.069	-0.069
$(C_6H_5)_4B^-$	0.372	0.364	
Dipicrylaminate	0.414		
Dicarbolylcobaltate	0.520		

When the O and W phases at equilibrium contain β different ionic components that can partition in the two phases, the number of unknown parameters is $2\beta + 1$ at constant temperature and pressure, i.e. β different concentrations in each phase and the equilibrium distribution potential $\Delta_O^W\phi_{eq}$. On the other hand, there are $2\beta + 1$ relationships which constitute simultaneous equations for predicting the final equilibrium conditions from the initial conditions.

When all electrolytes are completely dissociated in both phases, the conservation of mass for each component is given by

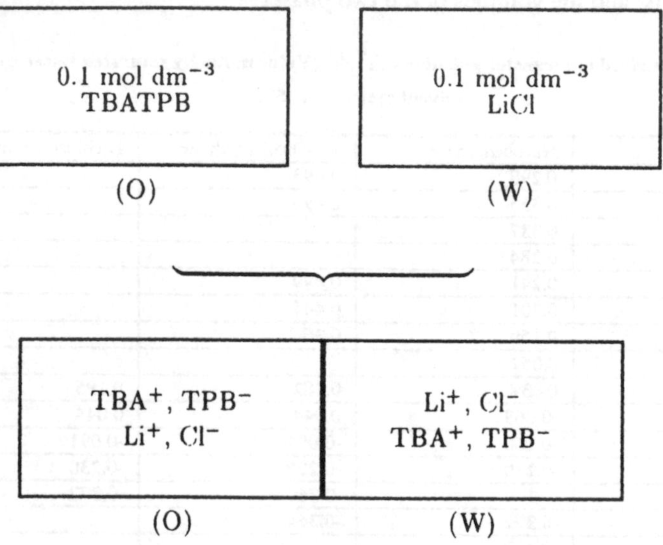

Figure 1. Partition of ions between two immiscible electrolyte solutions.

$$V^W c_i^W + V^O c_i^O = V^W c_i^{W,0} + V^O c_i^{O,0} \qquad 1, 2,\ldots\beta \tag{8}$$

where $c_i^{\alpha,0}$ is the initial concentration of i in α (α = W or O). Further, there are β different Nernst equations for all ionic components, i.e. eq. (7) for i = 1, 2 ... β. In addition, Hung assumed that the electroneutrality condition holds in each phase:

$$\sum_{i=1}^{\beta} z_i c_i^\alpha = 0 \qquad \alpha = \text{W or O} \tag{9}$$

These 2b + 1 simultaneous equations reduce to

$$\sum_{i=1}^{\beta} \frac{z_i c_i^{W,0}}{1 + r(\gamma_i^W / \gamma_i^O)e_i} + \sum_{i=1}^{\beta} \frac{r z_i c_i^{O,0}}{1 + r(\gamma_i^W / \gamma_i^O)e_i} = 0 \tag{10}$$

where

$r = V^O/V^W$ and

$$e_i = \exp[(z_i F / RT)(\Delta_O^W \phi_{eq} - \Delta_O^W \phi_i^\circ)] \tag{11}$$

Equation (10), contains one unknown, $\Delta_O^W \phi_{eq}$, and can be solved numerically. It is noted that the value of $\Delta_O^W \phi_{eq}$ generally depends on the volume ratio of the two phases. For a particular case when the system contains only one electrolyte composed of a cation K and an anion A, eq. (10) is solved for $\Delta_O^W \phi_{eq}$ to give a well known expression for the distribution potential,[1]

$$\Delta_O^W \phi_{eq} = \frac{1}{z_K + |z_A|}(z_K \Delta_O^W \phi_K^\circ - |z_A| \Delta_O^W \phi_A^\circ) + \frac{\gamma_K^O \gamma_A^W}{\gamma_K^W \gamma_A^O} \tag{12}$$

Once the value of $\Delta_O^W \phi_{eq}$ is known, the equilibrium concentration of each component is calculated through

$$c_i^W = \frac{c_i^{W,0} + r c_i^{O,0}}{1 + r(\gamma_i^W / \gamma_i^O) e_i} \tag{13}$$

and $c^O_i = e_i c^W_i$.

In the case of the example in Fig. 1 at r = 1, eq. (10) is simplified to[22]

$$\Delta_O^W \phi_{eq} = \frac{RT}{2F} \ln \frac{c_{LiCl}^{W,0} e_{Cl} + c_{TBATPB}^{O,0} e_{TBA}}{c_{LiCl}^{W,0} e_{Li} + c_{TBATPB}^{O,0} e_{TPB}} \tag{14}$$

where for γ_i^α (a = O or W) is unity for all ionic components. If the values for the NB-W system in Table 1 are used for $\Delta_O^W \phi_i^\circ$ (i = Li^+, Cl-, TBA+, and TPB^-), $\Delta_O^W \phi_{eq}$ is calculated to be 0.0575 V at the partition equilibrium. The ratios of equilibrium concentrations, c^O_i/c^W_i, are $1.76 \bullet 10^{-6}$, $4.86 \bullet 10^{-7}$, $1.64 \bullet 10^5$, and $2.07 \bullet 10^5$, for Li^+, Cl^-, TBA^+, and TPB^-, respectively. Thus, the degree of partition of hydrophilic (lipophilic) ions into the organic (water) phase is very small in this system. The minute dissolution of TBA^+ in W, however, brings about the positive value for the distribution potential. The electroneutrality of each phase is maintained mainly by the co-transport of TPB^- ion and, to the lesser degree, by the counter-dissolution of Li^+ in the NB phase.

4. Distribution potential in the presence of ion pair-formation and complex formation reactions

The above treatment has assumed the complete dissociation of electrolytes in both phases.. However, the ion-pair formation becomes significant when the dielectric constant is as low as 10, e.g. 1,2 dichloroethane. In this case, the ion association should be taken into account in calculating the distribution potential.

When a cation K and an anion A forms an ion pair KA in phase α,

$$K + A \xleftrightarrow{K^{\alpha}} KA \tag{15}$$

where K^{α} is the association constant of KA in ª defined by

$$K^{\alpha} = \frac{c_{KA}^{\alpha}}{c_K^{\alpha} c_A^{\alpha}} \tag{16}$$

the equation for the conservation of mass is modified to accommodate the formation of KA. For the cation K,

$$V^W c_K^W + V^O c_K^O + V^W c_{KA}^W + V^O c_{KA}^O = V^W c_K^{W,0} + V^O c_K^{O,0} + V^W c_{KA}^{W,0} + V^O c_{KA}^{O,0} \tag{17}$$

where the partition of ion pair KA has been taken into account. A similar modification applies for the conservation of A. This equation is combined with eq. (16) to obtain a set of nonlinear equations, which may be solved numerically. Several important limiting cases have been treated by Hung.[22]

Further generalization to include the cases of concurrent interactions of the type

$$I_1 + I_2 \xleftrightarrow{K_{121}} I_1 I_2 \tag{18}$$

$$I_1 + I_3 \xleftrightarrow{K_{131}} I_1 I_3 \tag{19}$$

where I_1, I_2, and I_3 are charged components in the phase, has been made by Hung.[23]

The complex formation of ions with neutral or charged ligands can also be treated similarly.[22] In this case, A in eq. (15) is taken as a ligand. The treatments of partition equilibria in the presence of ion pair or complex formation provide a theoretical basis for ion-pair extraction.[24]

5. Distribution of potential

In the derivation of eq. (10), we have assumed that both phases are electrically neutral. However, the presence of the distribution potential appears to imply certain deviation from electrical neutrality in each of the phases. Indeed, the distribution potential builds up the electrical double layer which consists of the two diffuse double layers at both sides of the interface and the inner part of the double layer.[25] In other words, the potential drop takes place within this double layer region.[26] The condition of electro-neutrality of the W or O phase is not applicable in this double layer region. It is therefore necessary to examine the applicability of eq. (9) for deriving the expression for distribution potential.

The magnitude of the distribution potential is usually of the order of a few hundred mV,[25] while the double layer capacitance is a few tens μF cm^{-2}.[27] The excess charge density in the double layer region is then of the order of 10 μC cm^{-2}, which corresponds to 100 pmol cm^{-2} for $z_i = 1$. On the other hand, the structure of the double layers at ITIES is well described by the Gouy-Chapman theory, no matter how the potential drop across the interface is determined:[26,28] either by the distribution potential or the externally applied potential in the case of polarized ITIES. The thickness of the double layer in which 99.99 % of the potential drop takes place is 89 nm and 8.8 nm in the W phase when the concentration of a 1:1 electrolyte is 0.1 mmol dm^{-3} and 0.1 mol dm^{-3}, respectively.[29] Unless the thickness of the solution phase is much thinner than μm or the total concentration of electrolytes is less than nmol dm^{-3}, the use of the electroneutrality condition for the solution phase is justified as a very good approximation.

6. Distribution potential in small systems

The general equation for the distribution potential, eq. (10), shows that the value of $\Delta_O^W\phi_{eq}$ depends on the volume ratio of the two phases. In many liquid-liquid systems of practical importance, the volume of one of the phases is much smaller than the other. Some examples are a solution containing microemulsion particles, a planar lipid membrane in a bathing solution, milk, and oil particles contaminating the sea. For these systems, it is useful to consider the behavior of $\Delta_O^W\phi_{eq}$ at this extreme, when $r \to 0$ or ∞.

When all ions are initially dissolved only in the W phase, eq. (10) takes a simpler form:

$$\sum_i z_i c_i^{W,0} \prod_{j \neq i} [1 + r(\gamma_j^W / \gamma_j^O) e_j] = 0 \tag{20}$$

where j ≠ k under the product Π means that the product is taken over all ionic species except *i*. When $r \to 0$, eq. (20) further simplifies to[30]

$$\sum_i z_i c_i^{W,0} \left[\sum_{j \neq i} (\gamma_j^W / \gamma_j^O) e_j \right] = 0 \tag{21}$$

In this limiting case, the distribution potential, and hence, the equilibrium concentrations of ionic species, do not depend on the volume of the two phases. Eq. (21) is useful in calculating the distribution equilibrium for systems, such as emulsions and thin membranes, as long as the assumption of the electroneutrality is valid in the smaller phase. A similar limiting case is obtained from eq. (10) for $r \to \infty$.

The importance of eq. (21) is illustrated by an example of the system in which the aqueous phase initially contains NaCl and sodium tetraphenylborate (NaTPB). It can be shown from eq. (21) that $\Delta^W_O \phi_{eq}$ is given by[30]

$$\Delta^W_O \phi_{eq} = \frac{\Delta^W_O \phi^\circ_{Na} + \Delta^W_O \phi^\circ_{TPB}}{2} + \frac{RT}{2F} \ln \left[1 - \frac{c^{W,0}_{Cl}}{c^{W,0}_{Na}} \right] \tag{22}$$

and the concentration of TPB^- ion in the O phase at partition equilibrium is

$$c^O_{TPB} = c^{W,0}_{TPB} \frac{\exp\left[(F/2RT)\left(\Delta^W_O \phi^\circ_{TPB} - \Delta^W_O \phi^\circ_{Na}\right)\right]}{[1 - c^{W,0}_{Cl} / c^{W,0}_{Na}]^{1/2}} \tag{23}$$

where we have neglected the activity coefficient term. When the W phase initially contains 1 mol dm^{-3} NaCl and 1 μmol dm^{-3} NaTPB, the concentration of NaTPB in the O phase at partition equilibrium is 1.39 mmol dm^{-3}, where the values of $\Delta^W_O \phi^\circ_i$ for the W-NB system have been employed.[30] In this limiting range of r, NaTPB is three orders of magnitude more concentrated in the O phase. This concentration effect should be taken into account in understanding the behavior of small liquid-liquid systems, e.g. ion-selective electrodes of liquid-membrane type and a planar bilayer membrane having an annulus, Plateau region, whose volume is large enough to apply the electroneutrality condition.

When the size of the smaller phase is less than of the order of μm, the electroneutrality condition cannot be employed as described above. In this case, the Poisson equation should be employed, instead, to correlate the local concentration with the potential, both of which vary with the distance from the interface and also depend on the detailed shape of the interface as well we those of the two adjacent phases.

II. POLARIZABILITY OF THE LIQUID-LIQUID INTERFACE

The importance of the polarized interface in studying electrochemical or interfacial properties is that it provides us with an additional degree of freedom, in comparison with nonpolarized interfaces, i.e. external control of the potential drop across the interface. Thermodynamically, the ideally polarized interface means that there is no common ionic species between the two phases.[4,31] However, any ions in real systems have certain solubility in both organic and aqueous phases. Hence, a more practical classification of ITIES is based on the controllability of $\Delta^W_O\phi$ externally.[32,33] Although the latter definition implies nonequilibrium properties of ITIES,[32] knowledge of the equilibrium concentrations of ions is useful to classify ITIES in terms of practical polarizability.[22,34]

Table 2. Concentration ratio of ions c_i^{NB} / c_i^W after equilibration of 0.1 mol dm^{-3} LiCl (W) and 0.1 mol dm^{-3} TBATPB (NB) at 25oC.

$\Delta^W_{NB}\phi^\circ / V$	Li^+	Cl^-	TBA^+	TPB^-
0.200	4.22×10^{-3}	2.03×10^{-10}	3.93×10^{8}	8.62×10
0.100	8.60×10^{-5}	9.93×10^{-9}	8.03×10^{6}	4.23×10^{3}
0.000	1.76×10^{-6}	4.86×10^{-7}	1.64×10^{5}	2.07×10^{5}
-0.100	3.58×10^{-8}	2.38×10^{-5}	3.34×10^{3}	1.02×10^{7}
-0.200	7.31×10^{-10}	1.17×10^{-3}	6.82×10	4.97×10^{8}

Table 2 lists the ratios of the equilibrium concentrations of each ion in W and NB with r=1 for the system in Fig. 1. In this example, the dissolution of TBA^+ in W and of Cl^- in NB is less than 0.1 mmol dm^{-3} when $\Delta^W_O\phi_{eq} > -0.1$ V, while the dissolution of Li^+ in NB and of TPB^- in W is also less than 0.1 mmol dm^{-3} when $\Delta^W_O\phi_{eq} < 0.1$ V. If the ionic current due to the presence of this amount of common ions does not significantly affect electrochemical properties under investigation or control of a potentiostat, this ITIES can be seen having polarized range of 0.2 - 0.4 V.

III. NONPOLARIZED ITIES AND REFERENCE POTENTIALS IN ORGANIC PHASES

When the both O and W phases contain substantial amounts of common ions, e.g. of the order of tens mmol dm^{-3}, slight deviation of $\Delta^W_O\phi$ from $\Delta^W_O\phi_{eq}$ would induce large currents passing through the interface. ITIES having this extreme property are called nonpolarized ITIES. The most important application of this type of interface is a reference liquid-liquid interface which is reversible to one of the ions in the O phase and, hence, works as a reference electrode in conjunction with a conventional reference electrode dipped in the aqueous side of the nonpolarized ITIES.

If only one common ionic species is present, the $\Delta^W_O\phi_{eq}$ is simply expressed by eq.(7). However, the partition of other ionic species can be significant, depending on their concentrations, $\Delta^W_O\phi_i^\circ$, and also r. A typical example is the system: tetrabutylammonium chloride (W)/TBATPB(NB).

| Ag | AgCl | TBACl (W) | TBATPB (O) |

In this case, the primary common ion is TBA^+. However, when the concentration of TBACl is high, the partition of Cl^- becomes appreciable, while the partition of TPB^- ion whose $\Delta_O^W\phi_{TPB}^\circ$ value is away from $\Delta_O^W\phi_{eq}$ is insignificant. Equation (10) then reduces to[22]

$$\Delta_O^W\phi_{eq} = \frac{RT}{F}\ln\frac{1}{2}\left\{\frac{c_{TBATPB}^{NB}}{c_{TBACl}^{W}}\exp\left[\frac{F}{RT}\right]\Delta_O^W\phi_{TBA}^\circ\right\} +$$

$$+\left\{\left(\frac{c_{TBATPB}^{NB}}{c_{TBACl}^{W}}\right)^2\exp\left[\frac{2F}{RT}\Delta\phi_{TBA}^\circ\right]+4\left(1+\frac{c_{TBATPB}^{NB}}{c_{TBACl}^{W}}\right)\exp\left[\frac{F}{RT}\left(\Delta\phi_{TBA}^\circ-\right)\left(\Delta\phi_{Cl}^\circ\right)\right]\right\} \quad (24)$$

when $r = 1$ and $\gamma_i = 1$ for all ions. When the condition

$$\Delta_O^W\phi_{TBA}^\circ - \Delta_O^W\phi_{Cl}^\circ >> \frac{RT}{F}\ln 4\frac{c_{TBATPB}^{NB}}{c_{TBACl}^{W}}\left(1+\frac{c_{TBATPB}^{NB}}{c_{TBACl}^{W}}\right) \quad (25)$$

is fulfilled, eq (24) simplifies to

$$\Delta_O^W\phi_{eq} = \Delta_O^W\phi_{TBA}^\circ + \frac{RT}{F}\ln\frac{c_{TBATPB}^{NB}}{c_{TBACl}^{W}} \quad (26)$$

that is, the interface is reversible to TBA^+ ion. In actual systems, it is noted that this type of reference ITIES is always used in nonequilibrium conditions[35] and the diffusion of ions must be considered to predict the actual behavior.

The importance of this type of ITIES in understanding the mechanism of liquid-membrane type ion-selective electrodes was first pointed out by Koryta.[36] Theoretical treatments taking account of the nonequilibrium conditions for this type of ion selective electrodes have been developed[37,38] and confirmed experimentally.[39]

IV. FREE-ENERGY COUPLING OF ION TRANSFER AND ELECTRON TRANSFER

We consider the system in which the W phase contains a redox couple, Ox1(W)/Rd1(W), while the O phase contains a redox couple, Ox2(O)/Rd2(O). If none of ionic components are transferable across the interface, the only common charged component is e^- and the phase-boundary potential is given by[40]

$$\Delta_O^W \phi_{eq} = E_{Ox2/Rd2}^{O,\circ} - E_{Ox1/Rd1}^{W,\circ} + \frac{RT}{nF} \ln \frac{c_{Ox2}^O c_{Rd1}^W}{c_{Rd2}^O c_{Ox1}^W} \tag{27}$$

where $E_{Ox2/Rd2}^{O,\circ}$ and $E_{Ox1/Rd1}^{W,\circ}$ are the standard electrode potentials of the redox couple Ox2/Rd2 in O and of Ox1/Rd1 in W and n is the number of electron transferred in the redox reaction. The value of $\Delta_O^W \phi_{eq}$ is completely determined by the redox properties.

However, some of the redox species are necessarily charged components, and counterions of redox couples also exist in the two phases. All of these ionic components can essentially distribute over the two phases, depending on its $\Delta_O^W \phi_i^\circ$ value. In this case, the equilibrium point is affected by the partition of ionic components and the value of $\Delta_O^W \phi_{eq}$ is determined by two physically different properties of the system.[41,42] The presence of supporting electrolytes also influences the point of equilibrium through the redistribution of constituent ions. This special type of mixed potential is important not only for defining the initial state of the electrochemical studies of electron transfer reactions but also for understanding other phenomena which involve free-energy coupling of electron and ion transfer reactions, e.g. energy transduction in biological systems and redox-reaction-driven uphill transport of ions across a liquid membrane.

1. Mixed potential determined by electron transfer and ion transfer at ITIES

For simplicity, we assume that none of the components in O (W) are in common with the components in W (O) before contact.

When α redox species ($0 \le \alpha \le 4$) in the redox couples and β other ionic species are transferable across the interface, the number of unknowns at final ET-IT coupling equilibrium are $4 + \alpha + 2\beta$ concentrations in addition to the inner potential difference at equilibrium, $\Delta_O^W \phi_{eq}$.

The conservation of mass for the total redox species of redox couple Ox1/Rd1 leads to,

$$^{O}c_{Rd1}^{O} + V^O c_{Ox1}^O + V^W c_{Rd1}^W + V^W c_{Ox1}^W = V^W (c_{Ox1}^{W,0} + c_{Rd1}^{W,0}) \tag{28}$$

and for Ox2/Rd2

$$^{O}c_{Rd2}^{O} + V^O c_{Ox2}^O + V^W c_{Rd2}^W + V^W c_{Ox2}^W = V^O (c_{Ox2}^{O,0} + c_{Rd2}^{O,0}) \tag{29}$$

where $c_i^{\alpha,0}$ is the initial concentration of i (i = Ox1, Rd1, Ox2, or Rd2) in the phase α (α = O or W).

The conditions for the conservation of mass and partition equilibrium for other common ionic components are given by eqs. (8) and (7), respectively. The condition of electroneutrality, eq. (9), should be applied for both phases in this case, because the two physically distinct processes take place in both phases and the neutrality of one phase does not assure the neutrality of the other.

Eqs. (7), (8), (9), (27)-(29) then constitute simultaneous equations for $5 + \alpha + 2\beta$ unknowns.

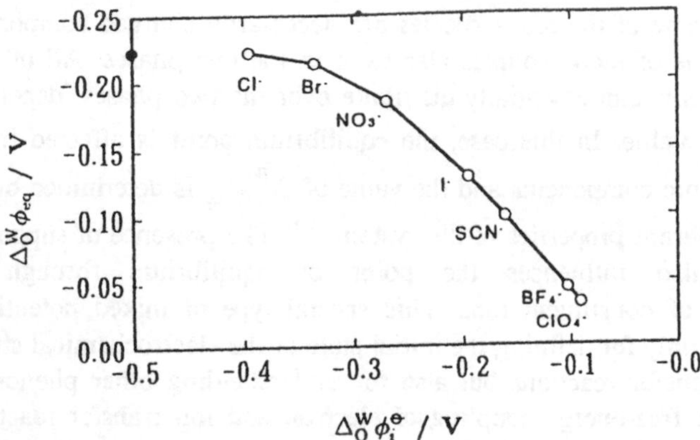

Figure 2. Change in the equilibrium inner potential difference with the lipophilicity of the counterion. The filled circle indicates the potential in the absence of counterion transfer. (From T. Kakiuchi, Electrochim. Acta, in press, 1995. With permission).

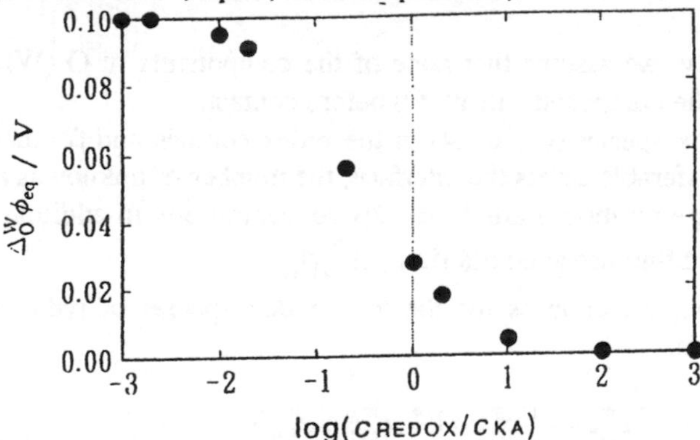

Figure 3. Variation of equilibrium potential with the ratio of the concentrations of redox species and of indifferent electrolytes. (From T. Kakiuchi, Electrochim. Acta, in press, 1995. With permission).

2. Partition of indifferent-electrolyte ions

The case when indifferent electrolyte KA is added to one of the phases is of practical importance in electrochemical studies of electron transfer reactions at the ITIES. We consider the system characterized by the parameters: $i_{c^W_{Ox1}} = i_{c^W_{Rd1}} = i_{c^O_{Ox2}} = i_{c^W_{Rd2}} = 1mM$, $z_{Ox1} = 3$, $z_{Rd1} = 2$, $z_{Ox2} = 2$, $z_{Rd2} = 1$, and

$n = 1$, $z_{A1} = z_{A2} = -1$, $E^{W,\circ}_{Ox1/Rd1} = 0.530$ V, $E^{W,\circ}_{Ox2/Rd2} = 0.307$ V. Only K and A are allowed to redistribute over the two phases, aside from electron transfer. This requirement is fulfilled when the counterions of Ox1/Rd1 couples are very hydrophilic and those of Ox2/Rd2 are very lipophilic.

The value of $\Delta^W_O\phi^\circ_K$ is taken to be 0.241 V, a value K^+ at the NB-W interface. The 17 simultaneous equations can be reduced to a nonlinear equation for $\Delta^W_O\phi_{eq}$, which can be solved numerically. When no redistribution of KA takes place, the value of $\Delta^W_O\phi_{eq}$ would be -0.223 V (cf. eq. (27).

Figure 2 shows the effect of the addition of 10 mM KA in W at $r = 1$. The shift of $\Delta^W_O\phi_{eq}$ from -0.223 V is caused by the dissolution of relatively lipophilic anions from W to O. This ion transfer drives the reduction reaction in W and oxidation reaction in O, resulting in the electron transfer from O to W across the interface. The magnitude of the shift in $\Delta^W_O\phi_{eq}$ becomes greater with the increasing lipophilicity of A.

On the other hand, the dissolution of K^+ into O in this example is negligible because the value of $\Delta^W_O\phi^\circ_K$ is relatively away from the redox potential in the absence of ion transfer in comparison with $\Delta^W_O\phi^\circ_A$ in this case. For example, in the case of KNO_3, $c^O_K / c^W_K = c^O_A / c^W_A = 2.039\ 10^{-2}$ in the absence of redox couples. When $c_{redox} = c_{KA}$, c^O_K / c^W_K changes to 1.193 10^{-3} and $c^O_A / c^W_A = 2.039\ 10^{-2}$ changes to 3.488 10^{-1}. The presence of the interfacial redox process thus enhances the transfer of A into O, and suppresses the transfer of K.

3. Relative strength of ion transfer and electron transfer

To illustrate the relative contributions of ion partition and electron transfer to $\Delta^W_O\phi_{eq}$, we consider another example of the ET-IT coupling : $E^{W,\circ}_{Ox1/Rd1} = E^{W,\circ}_{Ox2/Rd2} = 0$ V, $\Delta^W_O\phi^\circ_K = 0.2$ V, $\Delta^W_O\phi^\circ_A = 0$ V, $\Delta^W_O\phi^\circ_{A1} = -0.5$ V, and $\Delta^W_O\phi^\circ_{A2} = 0.372$ V. In this system, the difference between the value of the contact redox potential and that of the distribution potential is much smaller than that in above two cases. The values of $\Delta^W_O\phi^\circ_{A1}$ and $\Delta^W_O\phi^\circ_{A2}$ were chosen so that the transfer of A1 and A2 across the interface becomes negligible. The values of other parameters are the same as those above. Calculated values of $\Delta^W_O\phi_{eq}$ at several different values of $\log_{10}(c_{redox}/c_{KA})$, keeping constant the concentration of the two redox couples at c_{redox}. The results are shown in Fig. 3.

In this case, $\Delta^W_O\phi_{eq} = 0.1$ V in the absence of ion transfer and $\Delta^W_O\phi_{eq} = 0$ V in the absence of electron transfer. Depending on the relative magnitude of the concentrations of the redox couples and of the indifferent electrolyte, $\Delta^W_O\phi_{eq}$ takes a value between the two extreme values. In this example, the redox couples should be 100 times in excess of the indifferent electrolyte in order that $\Delta^W_O\phi_{eq}$ can be regarded to be determined solely by the interfacial redox reaction equilibrium, while the indifferent electrolyte should be 1000 times in excess of the redox couples in order that $\Delta^W_O\phi_{eq}$ can be regarded to be solely determined by the distribution potential. The value of $\Delta^W_O\phi_{eq}$ is 0.027 V at $c_{redox} = c_{KA}$. This is significantly lower than the midpoint of the two extreme values. This disparity in contribution of ion partition and interfacial redox reaction to $\Delta^W_O\phi_{eq}$ arises from the fact that in the former the change in potential is first order with respect to the concentration change, whereas the latter is second order (cf. eqs. (7) and (27).

In the absence of redox couples, $c^O_K / c^W_K = c^O_A / c^W_A = 2.039\ 10^{-2}$. When $c_{redox}=c_{KA}$, c^O_K / c^W_K changes to 1.193 10^{-3} and $c^O_A / c^W_A = 2.039\ 10^{-2}$ changes to 3.488 10^{-1}. The presence of the interfacial redox process thus enhances the transfer of A into O and suppresses the transfer of K+. Therefore, it can be equally said that the ion transfer of A is driven by the interfacial redox reaction.

The importance of the ET-IT coupling in designing experimental systems for the study of electron transfer reactions at ITIES has also been elucidated.[41]

VI. CONCLUSIONS

Problems associated with equilibrium partition of ionic components between two immiscible phases have long stimulated the thoughts of scientists in a variety of fields, deepening our understanding of not only interfacial phenomena but other bulk properties such as transfer Gibbs energy of charged components. Recent trends of research have increasingly focused on the dynamics of interfacial phenomena. However, the understanding of the equilibrium properties of ITIES and related systems continues to be indispensable for all who are involved with this intriguing field of science. It is rather surprising that new aspects of energetics at ITIES as introduced above have been revealed even more than one hundred years after Nernst's seminal work.

REFERENCES

1. **Davies, J. T. and Rideal, E. K.,** *Interfacial Phenomena*, Academic Press, New York. 2 ed, 1963, chap. 37.
2. **Koczorowski, Z.**, Galvani and Volta potentials at the interface separating immiscible electrolyte solutions, in *The Interface Structure and Electrochemical Processes at the Boundary Between Two Immiscible Liquids*, Kazarinov, V. E., Ed., Springer-Verlag, Berlin, 1987, p. 77.
3. **Girault, H. H. and Schiffrin, D. J.,** Electrochemistry of liquid-liquid interfaces, in *Electroanalytical Chemistry*, Vol. 15, Bard, A. J., Ed., Marcel Dekker, New York, 1989, chap. 1.
4. **Markin, V. S. and Volkov, A. G.,** Potentials at the interface between two immiscible electrolyte solutions, *Adv. Colloid Interface Sci.*, 31, 111, 1990.
5. **Parsons, R.**, Equilibrium properties of electrified interfaces, in *Modern aspects of Electrochemistry*, Vol. 1, Bockris, J. O'M. and Conway, B. E., Eds., Butterworths, London, 1954, p.103.
6. **Lippmann, G.**, Relation entre les phénomènes électriques et capillaires, *Compt. Rend.*, 76, 1407, 1873.
7. **Krouchkoll, M.**, Etude surles couches électriques doubles, *Ann. Chim. Phys.*, 6, 17, 129, 1889.
8. **Overbeek, J. Th. G.,** Phenomenology of lyophobic systems, in *Colloid Science. I. Irreversible Systems*, Kruyt, H. R., Ed., Elsevier, Amsterdam, 1952, chap. 2.
9. **Lin, S.-W., Keizer, J., Rock, P. R. and Stenschke, H.,** On the mechanism of oscillations in the beating mercury heart, *Proc. Nat. Acad. Sci. U.S.A.*, 71, 4477, 1974.
10. **Lange, E. and Miščenko, K. P.**, Zur Thermodynamik der Ionensolvatation, *Z. phys. Chem.*, 149, 1, 1930.
11. **Nernst, W.,** Die elektromotorische Wirksamkeit der Ionen, *Z. phys. Chem.*, 8, 129, 1891.
12. **Nernst, W.,** Über die Löslichkeit von Mischkrystallen, *Z. phys. Chem.*, 9, 137, 1892.
13. **Koryta, J., Vanýsek, P. and Březina, M.,** Electrolysis with electrolyte dropping electrode. II. Basic properties of the system, *J. Electroanal. Chem.*, 75, 211, 1977.
14. **Koryta, J., and Vanýsek, P.,** Electrochemical phenomena at the interface of two immiscible electrolyte solutions, in *Advances in Electrochemistry and Electrochemical Engineering*, Gerischer, H. and Tobias, C. W., Eds., Vol. 12, John Wiley & Sons, New York, 1981, p.131.
15. *The Interface Structure and Electrochemical Processes at the Boundary Between Two Immiscible Liquids*, Kazarinov, V. E., Ed., Springer-Verlag, Berlin, 1987.
16. **Samec, Z.,** Electrical double layer at the interface between two immiscible electrolyte solutions, *Chem. Rev.*, 88, 617, 1988.
17. **Senda, M., Kakiuchi, T. and Osakai, T.,** Electrochemistry at the interface between two immiscible electrolyte solutions, *Electrochim. Acta*, 36, 253, 1991.
18. **Girault, H. H.,** Charge transfer across liquid-liquid interfaces, in *Modern Aspects of Electrochemistry*, White, R, E., Conway, B. E. and Bockris, J. O'M., Eds., Vol. 25, Plenum Press, New York, 1993, p. 1.
19. **Samec, Z. and Kakiuchi, T.** Charge transfer kinetics at water/organic solvent phase, in *Advances in Electrochemistry and Electrochemical Science*, Gerischer, H. and Tobias, C. W., Eds., Vol. 5, VCH, Weinheim, 1995.
20. **Guggenheim, E. A.,** The conceptions of electrical potential difference between two phases and the individual activities of ions, *J. Phys. Chem.*, 33, 842, 1929.
21. **Guggenheim, E. A.,** On THE CONCEPTION OF ELECTRICAL POTENTIAL DIFFERENCE BETWEEN TWO PHASES, *J. Phys. Chem.*, 34, 1540, 1930.
22. **Hung, L. Q.,** Electrochemical properties of the interface between two immiscible electrolyte solutions. Part I. Equilibrium situation and Galvani potential difference, *J. Electroanal. Chem.*, 115, 159, 1980.

23. **Hung, L. Q.**, Electrochemical properties of the interface between two immiscible electrolyte solutions. Part III. The general case of the Galvani potential difference at the interface of the distribution of an arbitrary number of components interacting in both phases, *J. Electroanal. Chem.*, 149, 1, 1983.
24. **Kakutani, T., Nishiwaki, Y. and Senda, M.**, Theory of ion-pair extraction in terms of standard ion-transfer potentials of individual ions, *Bunseki Kagaku*, 33, E175, 1984.
25. **Gavach, C., Seta, P. and d'Epenoux, B.**, The double layer and ion adsorption at the interface between two non-miscible solutions Part I. Interfacial tension measurements for the water-nitrobenzene tetraalkylammonium bromide systems, *J. Electroanal. Chem.*, 83, 225, 1977.
26. **Kakiuchi, T. and Senda, M.**, Structure of the electrical double layer at the interface between nitrobenzene solution of tetrabutylammonium tetraphenylborate and aqueous solution of lithium chloride, *Bull. Chem. Soc. Jpn.*, 56, 1753, 1983.
27. **Samec, Z., Mareček, V. and Homolka, D.**, Double layer at liquid/liquid interfaces, *Faraday Discuss. Chem. Soc.*, 77, 197, 1984.
28. **Gros, M., Gromb, S. and Gavach, C.**, The double layer and ion adsorption at the interface between two non-miscible solutions. Part II. Electrocapillary behavior of some water nitrobenzene systems, *J. Electroanal. Chem.*, 89, 29, 1978.
29. **Mohilner, D. M.**, The electrical double layer, in *Electroanalytical Chemistry*, Vol. 1, Bard, A. J., Ed., Marcel Dekker. New York, 1966, p. 331.
30. **Kakiuchi,T.**, in preparation.
31. **Kakiuchi.T. and Senda, M.**, Thermodynamics of the electrocapillarity of oil-water interface. *Bull. Chem. Soc. Jpn.*, 56, 2912, 1983.
32. **Kakiuchi.T. and Senda, M.**, Polarizability and the electrocapillary measurements of the nitrobenzene-water interface, *Bull. Chem. Soc. Jpn.*, 56, 1322, 1983.
33. **Kakiuchi.T. and Senda, M.**, Polarizability and nonpolarizability of oil-water interface with relevance to a.c. impedance measurements, *Collect. Czech. Chem. Commun.*, 56, 112, 1991.
34. **Koryta, J.**, Electrochemical polarization phenomena at the interface of two immiscible electrolyte solution, *Electrochim. Acta*, 24, 293, 1979.
35. **Kakiuchi.T. and Senda, M.**, The liquid junction potential at the contact of two immiscible electrolyte solutions. Reference electrode reversible to alkylammonium ions and tetraphenylborate ion in nitrobenzene, *Bull. Chem. Soc. Jpn.*, 60, 3099, 1987.
36. **Koryta, J** Electrolysis at the interface of two immiscible electrolyte solutions, and its analytical aspects, *Hung. Sci. Instr.*, 49. 25, 1980.
37. **Kakiuchi.T. and Senda, M.**, The theory of liquid-ion exchange membrane ion-selective electrode based on the concept of the mixed ion-transfer potential, *Bull. Chem. Soc. Jpn.*, 57, 1801, 1984.
38. **Kihara, S. and Yoshida, Z.**, Voltammetric interpretation of the potential at an ion-selective electrode, based on current-scan polarograms observed at the aqueous/organic solution interface, *Talanta*, 31, 789, 1984.
39. **Kakiuchi, T., Obi, I. and Senda, M.**, Tetraalkylammonium ion selective electrodes with supporting electrolytes. An experimental test of the theory of liquid ion-exchange membrane type ion-selective electrodes based on the concept of the mixed ion-transfer potential, *Bull. Chem. Soc. Jpn.*, 57, 1636, 1985.
40. **Samec, Z.**, Charge transfer between two immiscible electrolyte solutions. Part I. basic equation for the rate of the charge transfer across the interface, *J. Electronal. Chem.*, 99, 197, 1979.
41. **Kakiuchi, T.**, Free energy coupling of electron transfer and ion transfer in two-immiscible fluid systems, *Electrochim. Acta*, in press, 1995.
42. **Markin, V. S. and Volkov, A. G.**, Interfacial potential at the interface between two immiscible electrolyte solutions: Some problems in definitions and interpretation, *J. Colloid Interface Sci.*, 131, 382, 1989.

Chapter 2

VOLTA AND SURFACE POTENTIALS AT LIQUID/LIQUID INTERFACES

Z. Koczorowski

I. INTRODUCTION

The Volta potential is defined as the difference between electrostatic outer potentials of two condensed phases in the equilibrium state. The measurement of this and related quantities, using the voltaic cell or surface potential technique, is one of the oldest and most frequently used experimental methods for studying free solid and liquid surfaces. When combined with a surface or interface sensitive method, it can provide important physico-chemical information.

Typical measurements of Volta potentials concern metal/metal and metal/liquid electrolyte solution phase boundaries. The results provide estimates of the electron work function of metals[1] and immersed electrodes,[2] real hydration[3] and solvation energies of ions,[4,5] as well as real potentials of ions in solid electrolytes[6]. Modern studies of the interfaces between immiscible electrolyte solutions began in the 1970s,[7] but the first Volta potential measurements of similar systems were performed in the early 1960s.[8,9]

Widely used applications of the voltaic cell method deal with surface potential changes at the metal/vacuum-, water/air- and water/hydrocarbon interface when a monolayer film is formed by an adsorbed substance.[10-17] Phospholipid monolayers on such interfaces have been extensively used to study the surface properties of the monolayers, which represent, to some extent, the surface properties of bilayers and biological as well as various artificial membranes.[10-18] Liquid/liquid interfaces, including water/polar solvent (e.g. nitrobenzene) systems,[7-10,20-26] are equally important to biomembrane and micellar studies, solvent extraction, ion transfer and liquid chromatography, but have not been so extensively examined as liquid/air interfaces. Applications of ordered thin organic films prepared by the Langmuir and Blodgett method have dominated research activity during the last decade.

Many results of Volta potential measurements at liquid/liquid interfaces have been presented in the books and reviews cited above. Therefore this presentation is restricted to clarification of the fundamentals and discussion of the most important features of voltaic cells with liquid/liquid interfaces, and to current and future applications.

0-8493-7694-7/96/$0.00+$.50

II. ELECTRIFIED LIQUID/LIQUID INTERFACES AND THEIR ELECTRICAL POTENTIALS

The presence of an electric potential drop across the boundary between two dissimilar phases, as well as at their surfaces exposed to a neutral gas phase, is a characteristic feature of every interface and surface electrified by ion separation and dipole orientation. This charge separation is usually described as the formation of an ionic double layer.

The terminology of thermodynamic and electric potentials introduced by Lange is still very useful and recommended for description of all electrified phases and interfaces.[1,27] Therefore, these potentials can be assigned to liquid/liquid boundaries,[21,22,24,28] such as the interfaces of two immiscible electrolyte solutions: water (w), and an organic solvent (s).

The Volta potential, $\Delta_s^w \psi$, sometimes called the contact potential, is the difference of the outer potentials of the phases, that are in electrochemical equilibrium in regard to charged species. Each two-phase electrochemical system, including any w/s system, may be characterised by the relation:

$$\Delta_s^w \psi = -z_i F \left(\alpha_i^w - \alpha_i^s\right) \qquad (1)$$

where α_i^w and α_i^s are the real potentials of the charged species i, defined as the sum of its chemical potential and the electrical term containing the surface potential of the phase

$$\alpha_i^s = \mu_i^s + z_i F \chi^s \qquad (2)$$

Relationships (1) and (2) together with

$$\Delta_s^w \psi = \Delta_s^w \varphi - \Delta_s^w \chi \qquad (3)$$

where $\Delta_s^w \varphi$ is the difference of the inner potentials, i.e. the Galvani potential of a two - phase system, provide important electrochemical information. This system, as illustrated in Fig. 1, is actually a three phase system, since it includes the inert gas atmosphere of the environment.

The Volta potential, in contradiction to the Galvani potential, has the advantage of being measurable, but also the disadvantage that it is determined not only by the chemical nature of the phases which create the interface, but also by the state at their surfaces, represented by the surface potentials, Eqn.(1).

In principle, the distribution of ions and dipoles at the w/s interface is different from that at the free w and s surfaces. Therefore the Galvani potential may be also written, in the absence of specific adsorption, as the sum of the charge and dipole components:[1, 27,29]

$$\Delta_s^w \varphi = g_s^w (\text{ion}) + g_s^w (\text{dip}) \qquad (4)$$

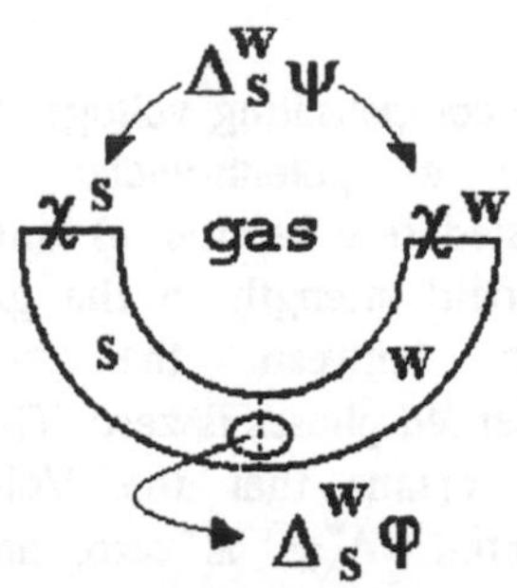

Figure 1. The electric potentials assumed to exist at liquid/liquid interfaces.

Usually $g_s^w(\text{ion}) \neq \Delta_s^w \psi$ and $g_s^w(\text{dip}) \neq \Delta_s^w \chi$. It appears, that under accessible experimental conditions there is little or no dependence of χ on ψ, i.e. the surface potential is independent of the free charge of phase.[1,30] However the dependence of the dipole component of the Galvani potential at the metal/solution interface, on the variation of charge (i.e. $g_s^M(\text{ion})$ potential) is often observed experimentally.[1, 27]

The surface potential of a liquid solvent s, χ^s, is defined as the difference of electrical potentials across the interface between this solvent and the gas phase, with the assumption that the outer potential of the solvent is zero.[1] The potential χ^s arises from a preferred orientation of the solvent dipoles in the free surface zone. At the solution surface the electric field responsible for the surface potential may arise from a preferred orientation of the solvent and solute dipoles, and from the ionic double layer.* This is discussed later, in section IV. For water, it is accepted that χ^w has a positive value; 0.13±0.02 V.[29] It implies that water molecules at the free surface have their hydrogen atoms oriented toward bulk liquid, thus facilitating the formation of hydrogen bonds.[31]

III. VOLTA POTENTIAL AND VOLTAIC CELLS

Volta potentials are measured by means of voltaic cells which are. systems composed of conducting, condensed phases in series, with a gas- or a vacuum (in the case of metals) gap situated between two liquid, phases. The gap contains gas like pure air or nitrogen, saturated with vapours of the liquid to be studied. Due to the presence of gas special methods for the investigation of voltaic cells are necessary (see section IV).

A single vertical bar (|) is used to represent a metal/metal or metal/solution phase boundary, while a dashed vertical bar (¦) represents junction between liquids. A double, dashed vertical bar (¦¦) represents a liquid junction, in which the diffusion potential has been assumed to be eliminated.

The basic principle of Volta potential measurements and investigations of voltaic cells, in comparison to galvanic cells, is presented for liquid/liquid

* The "surface potential" name is unfortunately also used often for the description the ionic double layer potential (i.e. the ionic part of the Galvani potential) at the interfaces of membranes, micro-emulsion droplets and micelles, measured usually by the acid-base indicator technique, e.g.[32-34]

interfaces in Fig. 2. This interface is created at the contact of aqueous and organic solutions (w and s, respectively) of electrolyte MX being in the partition equilibrium.[23, 35]

Galvanic Cell:

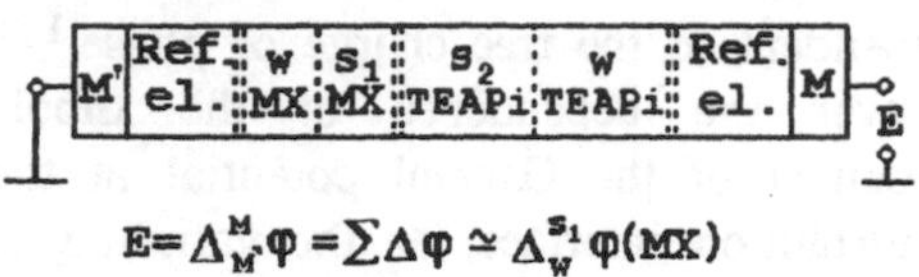

$$E=\Delta_{M'}^{M}\varphi=\sum\Delta\varphi\simeq\Delta_{w}^{s_1}\varphi(MX)$$

Voltaic Cell:

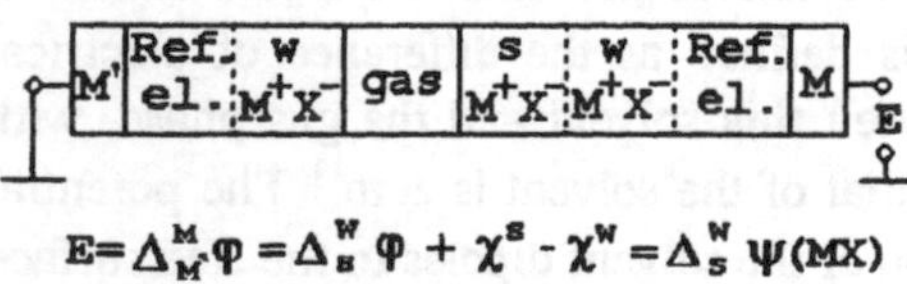

$$E=\Delta_{M'}^{M}\varphi=\Delta_{s}^{w}\varphi+\chi^{s}-\chi^{w}=\Delta_{s}^{w}\psi(MX)$$

Figure 2. Comparison of galvanic and voltaic cells with liquid/liquid interfaces

The compensating voltage, E, from a potentiometer is adjusted (see section 6) until the field strength in the gas space between the two condensed phases is zero. This state means that the Volta potential, $\Delta_{s}^{w}\psi$, is zero, and simultaneously that the compensating voltage equals the sum of all existing Galvani potentials (as it is also true for every galvanic cell) and the difference of surface potentials (instead of Galvani potential) between the conducting phases which contact the gas space. The application of two identical reference electrodes and the elimination of the liquid junction potentials by proper salt bridges, removes their contributions to the compensation potential. Using relation (3), after simple rearrangement we have

$$E=\Delta_{s}^{w}\psi(MX) \qquad (5)$$

Thus, the Volta potential may be operationally defined as the compensation voltage of the cell. Very often the terms "Volta potential" and "compensation voltage" are used interchangeably. It should be stressed that the compensation voltage of a voltaic cell is not always a direct measure of the Volta potential. That is, relation (5) is not general, but instead depends on the configuration of the cells. For this reason, an exact, thermodynamic relation to changes of the Gibbs energy is lacking, the term "compensation voltage" is also recommended instead of the "e.m.f.", which is commonly used for the reversible galvanic cells. The use of two-phase salt bridge containing tetraethylammonium picrate (TEAPi), in the galvanic cell shown in Fig. 2, is explained in section 5.

In the discussion of liquid voltaic cells it is necessary to distinguish two groups of immiscible liquid/liquid interfaces: water/polar organic solvent such as nitrobenzene, and water/non-polar organic solvent (water/oil or water/hydrocarbon systems). As schematically presented in Fig. 3 , the main difference is the presence of a dissociated electrolyte in the organic phase of the first group. As clearly shown by Davies and Rideal,[10] this controls the potential differences to be measured (Fig. 3). If the organic phase contains dissociated electrolyte an ionic double layer is created there, and Galvani potential changes measured. In the opposite case, the voltaic cell allows surface potential changes to be measured. This behaviour is fulfilled for systems at equilibrium, which contain non-polar oil phase. Between these extremes lie the intermediate cases of slightly polar solvents such as benzene saturated with water.[10] For these cases the results depend on time and the method of measurement.

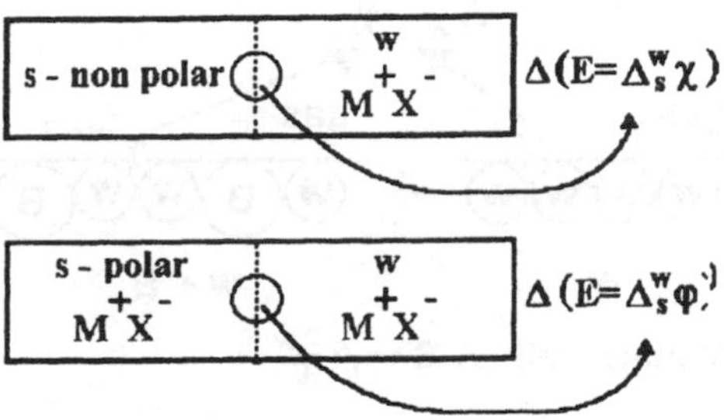

Figure 3. Potential changes measured at interfaces formed by non-polar solvent/water and polar solvent/water systems

IV. VOLTAIC CELLS WITH WATER/NONPOLAR LIQUID INTERFACES

Investigations of water/nonpolar liquid (w/o) systems can be considered as a special case of water/gas (for instance, w/a or water/air) interfaces. They are more difficult experimentally, but often simpler to be interpreted.[10-15] General discussion of the voltaic cells with the w/o type interfaces may be done on the basis of w/a type interfaces, for which investigations are more advanced.[10-17] The differences are relatively small, more quantitative than qualitative.

The adsorption of a dipolar organic compound, B, on a water surface can occur either by spreading B from the appropriate solution over water, (formation of a monolayer) or by expelling molecules of the compound from the bulk aqueous solution.[10-17] Monolayers are formed by relatively large, amphipathic molecules. These molecules have a hydrophobic moiety, which is most commonly a flexible hydrocarbon chain with ten or more carbon atoms, and a hydrophilic group. There is a large number of such compounds, including molecules of biological interest. The total number of adsorbed molecules per unit surface area, N_B, may be easily evaluated from the amount of B. The second method - adsorption from solution is commonly used for water soluble molecules. Surface tension measurements make it possible to calculate, from the Gibbs isotherm, the surface excess of such adsorbate.[10-17]

The nonpolar solvent/water interface has the advantage gas/water interfaces that interactions between adsorbed molecules due to dipole and Van der Waals's forces are negligible. Thus, at the oil/water interfaces behavior of adsorbates is near ideal, but quantitative interpretation may be uncertain, in particular for the higher chains which are dissolved in the oil phase to an unknown extent. The replacement of gas by the hydrocarbon phase may also modify the interactions between molecules in a spread film of long chain molecules.

Adsorption of dipolar substances at the w/a and w/o interfaces affects the surface potential of water (Fig. 4).

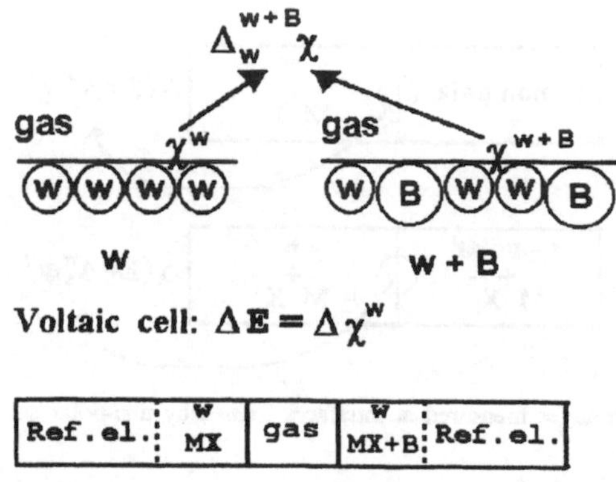

Figure 4. Influence of the adsorbed molecules **B** on the surface potential of water.

As seen in Fig. 4, the change in the compensation voltage due to adsorption is the surface potential difference, which is usually referred to as the surface potential and indicated by ΔV.[10-17]

$$\Delta E = \Delta\chi^{w} = \chi^{w} - \chi^{w+B} \qquad (6)$$

The oil phase (not presented in Fig. 4 - to simplify the illustration) is poured on the surface of the aqueous solution, hydrocarbon like heptane or decane forms a membrane few millimeters thick.[10] Because of the small difference in dielectric constant between the air and a hydrocarbon oil, adsorption at the oil/air interface should be small and is always neglected. The presence of the oil phase disturbs the water orientation at the interface [35] but, the change in χ^{w} is only a modification of the reference potential state.

Experimental investigation of the voltaic cell may be done directly as presented in Fig. 4 or by using two alternate measuring cells.[36,37] In the first case, the differential ionizing probe or the jet method can be used. In the second case, the ionizing electrode or the vibrating plate method are applied. These probes are two versions of the air electrode, which mediates measurement of voltaic cells, illustrated in Fig. 4. The air electrode, e.g. a vibrating plate, creates the two following cells:

$$\text{M} \,\Big|\, \text{Vib.pl.} \,\Big|\, \text{gas} \,\Big|\, \begin{matrix}\text{W}\\ \text{MX}\end{matrix} \,\vdots\vdots\, \text{Ref.el.} \,\Big|\, \text{M,E}_1 \qquad \text{(I)}$$

$$\text{M} \,\Big|\, \text{Vib.pl.} \,\Big|\, \text{gas} \,\Big|\, \begin{matrix}\text{W}\\ \text{MX+B}\end{matrix} \,\vdots\vdots\, \text{Ref.el.} \,\Big|\, \text{M,E}_2 \qquad \text{(II)}$$

and

$$\Delta E = E_2 - E_1 = \Delta\chi^w \qquad (7)$$

The presence of a supporting electrolyte MX in the aqueous phases assures stability of the measurements. However, MX must not adsorb at the surface to avoid an influence on $\Delta\chi^w$ potential.

The surface potential change $\Delta\chi^w$ is measured accurately, if the following conditions are fulfilled:[10,36,37]

1. Constant surface potential of the air electrode.
2. Constant surface potential of the aqueous phase or water/oil interface (dissolved electrolytes and possible contaminations from reference electrode should be negligible.
3. Constant reference electrode (usually a saturated calomel electrode) potential and constant diffusion potentials.

Before adding the surfactant, it is necessary to clean the surface of the aqueous solutions by sucking off the outer layer of water with a glass capillary, until a constant compensation voltage is obtained.

The surface potential change and the surface pressure are the most important quantities describing the surface state in the presence of an adsorbed substance. However, the significance in molecular terms of surface potential remains unclear. It is common in the literature to link $\Delta\chi^w$ with the properties of the neutral adsorbate by means of the Helmholtz equation [10-17]

$$\Delta\chi^w = N_B p_B^{\perp} / \varepsilon\varepsilon_0 \qquad (8)$$

where ε_0 and ε are the electric permittivity of vacuum and the relative permittivity of the interfacial region, respectively, and $p_B^{\perp}$ is the normal component of the molecular dipole moment of the substance B. Either from the known value N_B, or from the slope of the experimental relationship of $\Delta\chi^w$ vs. N_B , the quantity $\bar{p} = p_B^{\perp}/\varepsilon\varepsilon_0$ can be derived. This quantity may be treated as the *apparent* surface dipole moment of the adsorbate.

Little information is available on the local value of ε, which constitutes the main obstacle to an *a priori* calculation of $\Delta\chi^w$. An assumption is often made that $\varepsilon = 1$, because either the molecules are treated as isolated entities, or there is "lack of a better value".[10,38] It is known that $\bar{p}$ values derived from experimental $\Delta\chi^w$ data for insoluble monolayers, assuming $\varepsilon = 1$, are substantially different from the dipole moment for the same molecule in bulk solution.[10] This difference may be due to an inappropriate value of ε, reorientation of water molecules around the adsorbate, lateral interaction between adsorbed molecules in the monolayer.

Davies and Rideal proposed that the $\bar{p}$ term consists of three components[10]

$$\bar{p} = p_1^{\perp} + p_2^{\perp} + p_3^{\perp} \tag{9}$$

Later, Demchak and Fort[35] modified Eqn. (9) with the aim of including the effects above:

$$\bar{p} = (p_1^{\perp} / \varepsilon_1) + (p_2^{\perp} / \varepsilon_2) + (p_3^{\perp} / \varepsilon_3) \tag{10}$$

In Eqns. (9) and (10), $p_1^{\perp}$ is the contribution of the substrate water molecules, $p_2^{\perp}$ that of the adsorbate polar head, and $p_3^{\perp}$ that of the hydrophobic moiety of the adsorbed molecules, while ε_1, ε_2 and ε_3 are the effective local permittivities of the free surface of water, and of the regions in the vicinity of the polar head and of the hydrophobic group, respectively. The models have been used in a number of papers concerning adsorbed monolayers,[10-14] and water soluble short-chain substances.[39] Recently some improvements to the analysis, using Eqn. (10), has been proposed.[40] Vogel and Möbius presented a similar but simplified approach in which $\bar{p}$ is split into two components only.[41]

According to the macroscopic model, the adsorption potential shift is due to removing some solvent molecules, s, from the surface region to accommodate oriented molecules of adsorbate, **B.**[42] Using the assumptions listed in reference[14] the dependence for $\Delta\chi^s$ is in the form

$$\Delta\chi^s = \left[\frac{p_B}{\varepsilon_0 \varepsilon_{B(s)}} - \frac{np_s}{\varepsilon_0 \varepsilon_{s(B)}}\right] N_B + \left[\frac{np_s}{\varepsilon_0 \varepsilon_{s(B)}} - \frac{np_s}{\varepsilon_0 \varepsilon_s}\right] N_B^0 \tag{11}$$

where p_B, p_s and ε_B, ε_s are bulk dipole moment and relative dielectric constants for the solvent and substance, respectively, ε_0 is the permittivity of vacuum, and N_B is the surface amount of adsorbate. Parameter **n** is, in the limiting case, treated as the ratio of partial molar volumes.

For $N_B \to 0$, the second term in Eqn. (1) approaches 0, and we can obtain the slope of the relationship $\Delta\chi^s = f(N_B)$

$$\left(\frac{\partial \Delta\chi}{\partial N_B}\right)_{N_{B\to 0}} = \text{const}\left[\frac{p_B}{\varepsilon_B} - n\frac{p_s}{\varepsilon_s}\right] = \text{const}\ \bar{p} \tag{12}$$

The expression in brackets describes the physical sense of the apparent dipole moment $\bar{p}$. The model, up to now, has been used only to describe adsorption from solution, and have also been reviewed in ref. 43.

Eqns.(7) to (11) concern the case of neutral adsorbates, where there is no ionic double layer to contribute to the surface potential. In the case of ionic adsorbates, the measured potential $\Delta\chi^W$ consists of two terms. The first term is due to dipoles oriented at the interface, which may be described by the above formulas, and the second term presents the potential of the ionic double layer at the interface from the aqueous side[10,11]

$$\Delta\chi^w = \bar{p}/A_B + g^w(\text{ion}) \qquad (13)$$

The g^W(ion) is the electrical potential drop between the film of adsorbed long-chain ions and the bulk of aqueous solution. A_B is the reciprocal value of N_B, and expresses the surface area per ion.

The physical meaning of the g^W(ion) potential depends on the model of ionic double layer. The proposed models correspond to the Gouy - Chapman diffuse layer, with or without, allowance for the Stern modification and penetration of small counter ions above the plane of the ionic heads of the adsorbed large ions.[10-15] The experimental data obtained for the adsorption of dodecyl trimethylammonium bromide and sodium dodecyl sulphate strongly support the Haydon and Taylor model.[11,13,14,44] According to this model, there is a considerable space between the ionic heads and the surface boundary between, for instance, water and heptane. The presence of small inorganic ions in this space forms an additional diffuse layer which partly compensates the diffuse layer potential between the ionic heads and the bulk solution. Thus, Eqn. (12) may be considered as a linear combination of two linear functions, one of which [$\Delta\chi^W$ - g^W(ion)] crosses the zero point of the co-ordinates ($\Delta\chi^W$ and 1/A are equal to zero), and the other having an intercept on the potential axis. This, of course implies that the orientation of the apparent dipole moments of the long-chain ions is independent of **A**.

Studies of the adsorption of surface-active substances at the oil/water interface provide a convenient method for testing electrical double layer theory and for determining the state of water and ions in the neighbourhood of an interface. The change in the surface concentration of the large ions modifies the surface charge density. For instance, the surface ionic area of 1 nm^2 per ion corresponds to 16 microcoulombs per square centimetre.

Ion transfer processes are very important for extraction and ion selective electrodes,[7,10,18,20,21,23,45] and various redox and photochemical reactions occurring at the liquid/liquid interfaces have also been investigated.[24] They are good modelling systems for processes occurring in biological membranes. The reactions of electron transfer across the interfaces between immiscible liquids may be studied, if electron donors and acceptors are present in one or two of the phases in contact.

V. VOLTAIC CELLS WITH IMMISCIBLE ELECTROLYTE SOLUTION INTERFACE

For symmetrical electrolytes, a liquid/liquid interface at equilibrium is characterised by the standard Galvani potential, usually called the distribution potential. This very important quantity can be expressed in three equivalent forms: 1) using standard ionic potentials, 2) standard Gibbs energies of the ion transfer, 3) and employing limiting ionic partition coefficients [21-23, 25, 26]

$$\begin{aligned}\Delta_w^s\varphi^0(MX) &= \frac{1}{2}[\Delta_w^s\varphi^0(M^+) + \Delta_w^s\varphi^0(X^-)] \\ &= \frac{1}{2F}[\Delta_s^w G_{M^+}^0 - \Delta_s^w G_{X^-}^0] \\ &= \frac{RT}{2F}\ln\frac{B_w^{s,0}(M^+)}{B_w^{s,0}(X^-)} \end{aligned} \tag{14}$$

The water/nitrobenzene system, containing tetraethylammonium picrate (TEAPi) has been proposed as a convenient liquid junction bridge for liquid galvanic and voltaic cells.[23] The distribution potential of this system, and the diffusion potential at the interface between nitrobenzene and many organic solvents, are close to zero. It should be stressed that the application of salt bridges, which provide practically constant or negligible liquid junction potentials, constitutes a non-thermodynamic procedure which is necessary in many electrochemical experiments. In studies of interfaces between immiscible electrolyte solutions, only cells with salt bridges provide useful information.[23]

The interface separating two immiscible electrolyte solutions may also be made virtually ideally polarised by suitable choice of the electrolytes dissolved in the phases. For most of the water/nitrobenzene and water/1,2-dichloroethane systems, the presence of a strongly hydrophobic salt, such as. tetrabutylammonium tetraphenylborate in the organic phase, and a strongly hydrophilic lithium chloride in water constitute, within certain potential limits, a polarizable liquid/liquid interface. [7,20,23]

As noted in section 3 the compensation voltage does not always refer directly to the Volta potentials. The appropriate construction of voltaic cells, or more precisely - the proper mutual arrangement of phases, as well as application of reversible electrodes or salt bridges in the systems, allows measurement of not only the Volta potential but also the surface and the Galvani potentials. The measurements of $\Delta_s^w\chi$ and $\Delta_s^w\varphi$ potentials include also the state of zero charge potential and make also possible the estimation of the dipolar potentials $\Delta_s^w g(\text{dipole})$, Eqn. (4). This is schematically illustrated in Fig. 5. Of course, it should be remembered that these potential differences are only partially independent of one another, as they are obtained using the same nonthermodynamic assumptions on negligible diffusion potentials, and usually the same salt bridges eliminating these potentials.[23,37]

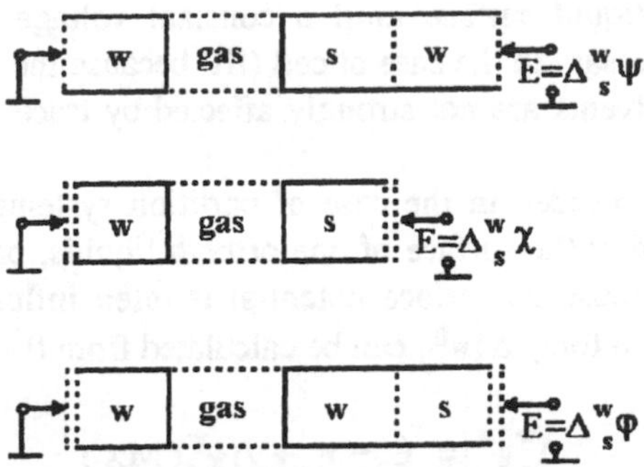

Figure 5. A possible configurations of the voltaic cells with liquid/liquid interfaces

The Volta potential at the water/non-aqueous solvent boundary, $\Delta_s^w\psi$, may be measured by the dynamic condenser method (section 6) as the difference in the compensation voltages of the following cells[23,37]

$$\mathrm{M} \,\Big|\, \mathrm{Vib.pl.} \,\Big|\, \mathrm{N_2} \,\Big|\, \overset{\mathrm{s}}{\mathrm{M^+ + X^-}} \,\vdots\, \overset{\mathrm{w}}{\mathrm{M^+ + X^-}} \,\Vert\, \mathrm{SCE} \,\Big|\, \mathrm{M.E_1} \qquad \mathrm{(III)}$$

$$\mathrm{M} \,\Big|\, \mathrm{Vib.pl.} \,\Big|\, \mathrm{N_2} \,\Big|\, \overset{\mathrm{w}}{\mathrm{M^+ + X^-}} \,\Vert\, \mathrm{SCE} \,\Big|\, \mathrm{M.E_2} \qquad \mathrm{(IV)}$$

where w and s denote the mutually saturated aqueous and organic phases, respectively, which contain salt MX; N_2 stands for the chemically inert gaseous phase, e.g. nitrogen or clean air; and SCE is the aqueous saturated calomel electrode. Measurements of these cells usually are done using glass vessels.[23,37] The contact at the miscible solutions, denoted ¦¦ is made from a glass sinter, gel or a fine capillary to avoid mixing.

The standard Volta potential, $\Delta_s^w\psi^0_{(MX)}$, in the partition systems, can be obtained from the difference in the compensation voltages $\mathbf{E_1}$ and $\mathbf{E_2}$, assuming the fulfilment of the following conditions[23,37]

1. Constant surface potential of the vibrating plate, e.g. the gold plate, protected with a layer of permaflon;
2. Constant surface potential of the water-saturated organic phase χ^s, i.e. its independence of the presence of electrolytes dissolved therein;
3. Constant surface potential of the nitrobenzene-saturated water phase χ^w, i.e. its independence of the presence of electrolyte therein;
4. Constant of the reference electrode (SCE) potential, and possible diffusion potential.

Conditions (1), (3), and (4) are typical for all investigations of voltaic cells, see section 4.

The surface of the aqueous solution should be purified by vacuum aspiration of the liquid surface until a constant voltage is attained. This operation is unnecessary in the case of cell (III) because the surface potentials of non-aqueous solvents are not strongly affected by trace impurities on the surface.

A correction is needed in the case of partition systems containing ions which are adsorbed at the surface of one or both liquids, particularly for the aqueous phase, because its surface potential is often influenced by organic ions.[23,37,46,47] Therefore, $\Delta_s^w \psi^0$, can be calculated from the equation

$$\Delta_s^w \psi^0 = E_1 - E_2 + \Delta \chi^w (MX) \qquad (15)$$

The $\Delta_s^w \varphi$ or $\Delta_s^w \psi$ data can be used for the estimation of ion solvation energies in water saturated solvents.[49]

The liquid/liquid partition systems discussed above are very similar to various membrane interfaces and may serve as a model for them. A good example is the distribution of a dissociated salt between an aqueous solution and a permeable organic polymer.[50]

The value of $\Delta \chi^w(MX)$ for any MX salt can be found as the difference between the compensation voltage of a type (IV) cell containing an aqueous phase of the particular partition system and the compensation voltage of the same cell with an electrolyte (e.g. NaCl or Na_2SO_4), which at the low concentrations does not change the surface potential of water saturated with the organic solvent.

The type (IV) cell can also be used to measure surface potential changes $\Delta \chi^w(MX)$ as a function of the amount of organic solvent added. For higher organic solvent concentrations (usually above 10%), one must use a voltaic cell containing the partition system water/nitrobenzene with TEAPi, instead of the usual aqueous KCl bridge. It is interesting to note that the ions like tetrabutylammonium cation and tetraphenylborate anion, which are commonly used in the investigations of immiscible electrolyte solutions, are very surface active and the correction for their influence on surface potential is substantial.[23,37,46,47]

The reliability of the experimental $\Delta_s^w \psi^0(MX)$ values was checked for systems containing nitrobenzene, nitromethane and 1,2 dichloroethane as organic solvent, by comparing of the differences in these values for various pairs of salts with the differences in the Galvani (i.e. distribution) potentials, $\Delta_s^w \psi^0$, for the same pairs. The following relationship should hold [23,37,46,47]

$$\Delta_{M_2X_2}^{M_1X_1} \Delta_s^w \psi^0 = \Delta_{M_2X_2}^{M_1X_1} \Delta_s^w \varphi^0 \qquad (16)$$

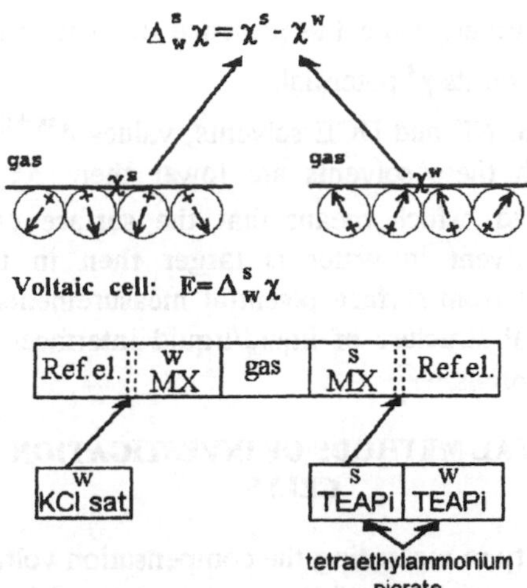

Figure 6. Differences between surface potentials of water and organic solvent

The difference between the surface potentials of an organic solvent and water may be measured by means of a voltaic cell, see Figs. 5 and 6.[5,23,37,48] If both liquid junction potentials are eliminated and supporting electrolytes MX are not adsorbed at the free surfaces of solvents the compensating voltage is

$$E = \Delta_s^w \chi \tag{17}$$

The liquid junction potential from the organic side may be practically negligible, due to the use of nitrobenzene/water partition system containing tetraethylammonium picrate.

The voltaic cells presented in the Fig. 6, have been studied by the dynamic condenser method (section 6), in the form of the following two cells with ($E = E_6 - E_5$).

Vib.pl. | air | $\overset{S}{MX}$ ⁞ Ref.el. | M.E_5 (V)

Vib.pl. | air | $\overset{W}{MX}$ ⁞ Ref.el. | M.E_6 (VI)

This approach allowed determination of the differences of the surface potentials between mutually saturated water and organic solvents such as nitrobenzene (NB),[23,37,46] nitroethane (NE),[47] 1,2-dichloroethane (DCE)[47] and isobutyl methyl ketone (IBMK).[5]

The data, which are in agreement with those calculated according to relation (3), show a very strong influence of the added organic solvent on the surface potential of water, while the presence of water in the nonaqueous phase has little effect on its χ^s potential.

In the case of NB, NE and DCE solvents, values $\Delta^{w+sw}\chi$ for the water phase saturated with these solvents are lower then $\Delta^w_s\chi$. For IBMK a maximum is observed, which means that the surface orientation of the molecules of the solvent in water is larger then in the pure IBMK. Information resulting from surface potential measurements may be used to analyse the interfacial structure of liquid/liquid interfaces and their dipole and zero-charge potentials.[23,28]

VI. EXPERIMENTAL METHODS OF INVESTIGATION OF VOLTAIC CELLS

The main difficulty in measuring the compensation voltage of the voltaic cells is a very large resistance of the systems caused by the presence of dielectric gas phase. There are two possible solutions to this problem: to reduce resistance, or to measure the work of charge transfer across the dielectric. The first possibility is accomplished by the ionizing method, and the second by the condenser and jet methods.

The ionizing electrode method, also called the radioactive or ionizing probe, requires a radioactive source to ionize the gas gap and a high impedance electrometric device.[10,15] Usually, as the mediating air electrode, gold foil coated with an alpha emitter, such as ^{241}Am, is used. The air gap between the air electrode and liquid surface is ionized so that a small current can flow. This allows direct compensation and measurement of the voltage of the system.[51,52] The simultaneous use of two ionizing probes, placed above the test and reference surfaces, makes possible the direct differential measurement of $\Delta\chi^w$.[52,53]

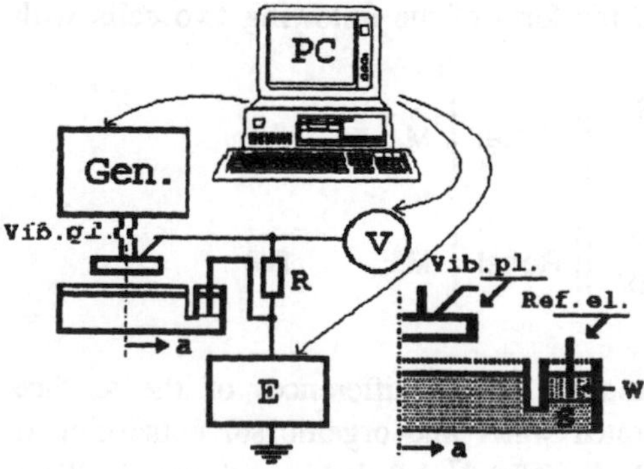

Figure 7. A block schematic diagram of the dynamic condenser method for voltaic measurements.

In the dynamic condenser, (vibrating plate or the vibrating condenser method, also called Kelvin, Zisman or Kelvin-Zisman probe) the capacity of a condenser created by the surface and the plate is continuously modulated by periodic vibration of the plate. The ac-output is then amplified, and fed back to the condenser to obtain null-balance operation.[36,54-57] Fig. 7 shows a liquid/liquid interface example.

In contrast to the ionizing method, the dynamic condenser method is based on well understood theory, and fulfils the condition of thermodynamic equilibrium. Its precision is limited by noise, stray capacitances, and variation of the surface potential of the air electrode surface. The precision of the dynamic condenser method is limited only by the nature of the surfaces of the electrode and investigated system. Adsorption - resistant air metal electrodes, often gold-plated and protected with a permaflon layer are commonly used to minimize drift of the surface potential of the vibrating electrodes and thereby secure stability and reproducibility of results.

Uncontaminated surfaces of aqueous solutions can be difficult to produce and maintain. Even minute traces of adsorbable organic impurities strongly influence the surface potential of water. Cleaning of the aqueous surface by aspirating the surface layer is usually necessary, but for the organic solutions is unnecessary.[36]

It is now possible to construct a computer set-up (Fig. 7) which combines good reproducibility, and a low time constant with theoretical sensitivity of ±0.05 mV for ca. 0.5 mm air gap distance, in which changes of E equal to ±0.5 mV are detectable. This construction is easier for solid than for liquid surfaces.

Recently scanning Kelvin probes and microprobes have been developed for high resolution surface analysis, which permit investigate the lateral distribution of the work functions of the surfaces of various phases to be investigated.[58-63] Up to now, they were used to determine corrosion potential profiles of metals and semiconductors under very thin films of electrolytic solution,[59] and for surface potential mapping of charged ionomer-polymer blends.[60-63]

The static capacitor method is in principle the true original Kelvin technique. In this method the tendency for charge to flow from the capacitor through the external circuit connecting the capacitator plates is detected, and then a backing-off potential is rapidly applied until the charge ceases .[64-66]

A theoretical approach that compares the ionizing probe to dynamic and static condenser methods has been described.[66] The dynamic condenser method gives probably the most realiable results. However, the ionising probe appears to be experimentally simpler for investigation of liquid surfaces, due to the delicate mechanical and signal measuring problems intrinsic to condenser methods. It has been shown that the two techniques give similar results.[30]

The principle of the jet method, which also utilizes a condenser, was originated by Kenrick, then improved by Randles,[3] and again later by Mc Tique et al.[67] may be summarised as follows. A jet of one liquid is directed down the axis of a tube, the inner surface of which is covered by a stream of the second liquid. If the reference electrodes are the same and the outer potentials at the two liquids are different, then a Volta electric field exists in the gap between them. The droplets carry away the charge on the jet, so that there must be continuos flow of charge into the jet. If this is connected to a high impedance electrometric system, and liquid surrounding the jet is connected to a potentiometer, a condition is established in which the outer potential of the jet equals that of surrounding liquid. The continuous renewing of the surface, which is the principal virtue of the jet method, renders the method particularly suitable to the solutions that do not contain spread monolayers. Experimental systems with the test solution flowing vertically have also been used.[68]

VII. FINAL REMARKS

As stated in the Introduction, the purpose of this chapter was to review the voltaic cell method of investigating liquid/liquid interfaces and treatment of the results. Previous research in the area of voltaic cells has considerably broadened our understanding of the properties of solid and liquid surfaces. This is and remains an important experimental approach for studying phenomena at the electrified surfaces and interfaces. The difficulty with the method, common to most electrochemical methods, is lack of sufficient molecular specificity. For practical purposes, the present state of voltaic cell investigations is a reasonable compromise between theoretical rigor and experimental accessibility. Nevertheless, more detailed and sophisticated analysis of the method and results, as well as new applications, are required. Complementary information provided by techniques more sensitive to surface orientation, such as surface light scattering[69] and other optical and spectroscopic methods, is expected.

Voltaic approaches to liquid/liquid interfaces are not common, despite the fact that such interfaces are good models of membrane systems. However, voltaic cells may soon enjoy a renaissance. More precise results are achievable and voltaic cells are applicable in a wide range of disciplines, from theoretical electrochemistry and surface physical chemistry to analytical applications and interpretation of phenomena occurring at the surface of biological membranes.

Acknowledgements - Financial support from the Polish Committee on Scientific Research (Grant No. 3 T09A 009 08) is gratefully acknowledged.

REFERENCES

1. **Parsons, R.**, Equilibrium properties of electrified interfaces, in *Modern Aspects of Electrochemistry*, Bockris, J. O'M. and Conway, B. M., Eds., Buttervorths, London, 1954, Vol. 1, chap.3.
2. **Hansen, W. N. and Kolb, D. M.**, The work function of emersed electrodes, *J. Electroanal. Chem.*, 100, 493, 1979.
3. **Randles, J. E. B.**, The real hydration energies of ions, *Trans. Faraday Soc.*, 52, 1573, 1956.
4. **Case, B. and Parsons, R.**, The real free energies of solvation of ions in some non-aqueous and mixed solvents, *Trans. Faraday Soc.*, 63, 1224, 1967.
5. **Koczorowski, Z. and Zagorska, I.**, The real and chemical energies of ion transfer from water to some organic solvents, *J. Electroanal. Chem.*, 193, 113, 1985.
6. **Zagorska, I. and Koczorowski, Z.**, Volta potential at metal-solid salt interface and real potentials of ions in solid electrolytes, *J. Electroanal. Chem.*, 101, 317, 1979.
7. **Koryta, J.**, Electrochemical polarization phenomena at the interface of two immiscible electrolyte solutions, *Electrochim. Acta*, 24, 293, 1979.
8. **Minc, S. and Koczorowski, Z.**, Measurements of the interphase potential differences water-polar oil by the dynamic condenser method, *Roczniki Chem.*, 34, 349, 1960.
9. **Minc, S. and Koczorowski, Z.**, Investigation of polar oil-water electrochemical interphase properties - I. Application of the dynamic condenser method for nitrobenzene-water distribution potential difference measurements, *Electrochim. Acta*, 8, 575, 1963.
10. **Davies, J. T. and Rideal, E. K.**, *Interfacial Phenomena*, Academic Press, N.York, 1963, chaps. 2, 4, 5 and 6.
11. **Haydon, D. A.**, The electrical double layer and electrokinetic phenomena, in *Recent Progress in Surface Science*, Danielli, J. F., Pankhurst, K. G. A. and Riddiferd, A. C., Eds., Academic Press., New York, 1964, chap. 3.
12. **Gaines, G. L.**, *Insoluble Monolayers at Liquid-Gas Interfaces*, Interscience, New York, 1966, chaps. 4 and 5.
13. **Llopis, J.**, Surface potential at liquid interfaces, in *Modern Aspects of Electrochemistry* No.6, Bockris, O'M. and Conway, B. E., Eds., Plenum Press, New.York, 1971, 71.
14. **Aveyard, R. and Haydon, D. A.**, *An Introduction to the Principles of Surface Chemistry*, Cambridge Univ.Press, London, 1973, chaps. 2 and 3.
15. **Adamson, A. W.**, *Physical Chemistry of Surfaces*, Wiley-Interscience, New York, 1982, chaps. 4 and 5.
16. **Chattoray, D. K. and Birdi, K. S.**, *Adsorption and Gibbs Surface Excess*, Plenum Press, New York, 1984, chaps. 5 and 6.
17. **Birdi, K. S.**, *Lipid and Biopolymer Monolayer at Liquid Interfaces*, Plenum Press, New York-London, 1988, chaps. 4 and 5.
18. **Popov, A. N.**, Counterions and adsorption of ion-exchange extractans at the water/oil interface, *The Interface Structure and Electrochemical Processes at the Boundary Between Two Immiscible Liquids*, Kazarinov, V. E., Ed., Springer Verlag, Berlin-Heidelberg, 1987, 143.
19. **Shchipunov, Ju. A. and Kolpakov, A. F.**, Phospholipids at the oil/water interface: Adsorption and interfacial phenomena in an electric field, *Adv. Colloid Interface Sci.*, 35, 31, 1991.
20. **Koryta, J.**, Electrochemistry of liquid membranes; Interfacial aspects, *Electrochim. Acta*, 32, 419, 1987.
21. **Boguslavsky, L. I. and Yaguzhinski, L. S.**, Bioelectrochemical phenomena and interface, in *Electrosynthesis and Bioelectrochemistry*, Frumkin, A. N., Ed., Nauka, Moscow, 1975, p. 305.
22. **Markin, V. S. and Volkov, A. G.**, Interfacial potentials at the interface between two immiscible electrolyte solutions. Some problems in definitions and interpretation, *J. Colloid Interface Sci.*, 131, 382, 1989.
23. **Koczorowski, Z.**, Galvani and Volta potentials at the interface separating immiscible electrolyte solutions in *The Interface Structure and Electrochemical Processes at the Boundary Between Two Immiscible Liquids*, Kazarinov, V. E., Ed., Springer Verlag, Berlin-Heidelberg, 1987, p. 77.
24. **Boguslavsky, L. I. and Volkov, A. G.**, Redox and photochemical reactions at the interface between immiscible liquids, *The Interface Structure and Electrochemical Processes at the*

Boundary Between Two Immiscible Liquids, Kazarinov, V. E., Ed., Springer Verlag, Berlin-Heidelberg, 1987, 179.

25. **Markin, V. S. and Volkov, A. G.**, Potentials at the interface between two immiscible electrolyte solutions, *Adv. Colloid Interface Sci.*, 31, 111, 1990.
26. **Senda, M., Kakiuchi, T. and Osakai, T.**, Electrochemistry at the interface between two immiscible electrolyte solutions, *Electrochim. Acta*, 36, 253, 1991.
27. **Trasati, S. and Parsons, R.**, Interphases in systems of conducting phases, *Pure & Appl. Chem.*, 58, 437, 1986.
28. **Koczorowski, Z.**, On the surface and zero charge potentials at the water-nitrobenzene interfaces, *J. Electroanal. Chem.*, 190, 257, 1985.
29. **Trasati, S.**, Relative and absolute electrochemical quantities. Components of the potential difference across the electrode/solution interface, *J. Chem. Soc. Faraday Trans. I,* 70, 1752, 1974.
30. **Pethica, B. A., Standish, M. M., Mingins, J., Smart, C., Iles, D. H., Feinstein, M. E., Hossain, S. A. and Pethica, J. B.**, The significance of Volta and compensation states and the measurement of surface potentials of monolayers, in *Advances in Chemistry*, No.144, *Monolayers*, Goddard, Ed., New York, 1975, p.123.
31. **Goodisman, J.**, *Electrochemistry: Theoretical Foundations*, Wiley-Interscience Publ., New York, 1987, 132.
32. **Hobson, R. A., Grieser, F. and Healy, T. W.**, Surface potential measurements in mixed micelle systems, *J. Phys. Chem.*, 98, 274, 1994.
33. **Cerbôn, J. and Calderôn, V.**, Changes of the compositional asymmetry of phospholipids associated to the increment in the membrane surface potential, *Biochim. Biophys. Acta*, 1067, 139, 1991.
34. **Murray, B. S., Drummond, G. J., Grieser, F. and White, L. R.**, Determination of electrostatic surface potentials of oil-in-water microemulsion droplets using a lipoidal acid-base spectroscopic probe, *J. Phys. Chem.*, 94, 6804, 1990.
35. **Khentov, V. Ya.**, Structure of the surface layer of an electrolyte solution at a hydrocarbon boundary, *Kolloid Zh.,* 60, 584, 1978.
36. **Minc, S., Zagórska, I. and Koczorowski, Z.**, Differences of surface potentials of electrolyte solutions in methyl alcohol and methyl cyanide determined by condenser and jet methods, *Roczniki Chem.*, 41, 1983, 1967.
37. **Koczorowski, Z. and Zagórska, I.**, Investigations on Volta potentials in water-nitrobenzene systems and on surface potentials of these solvents, *J. Electroanal. Chem.*, 159, 183, 1983.
38. **Demchak, R. J. and Fort Jr., T.**, Surface dipole moments of close packed un-ionized monolayers at the air-water interface, *J. Colloid Interface Sci.,* 46, 191, 1974.
39. **Dynarowicz, P. and Paluch, M.**, Electrical properties of some adsorbed films at the water-air interface, *J. Colloid Interface Sci.,* 107, 75, 1985.
40. **Oliveira Jr.,O. N., Riul, A. and Leal Fereira, G. F.**, Surface potentials of mixed Langmuir films: A model consistent with a domain-structured monolayer, *Thin Solid Films*, 242, 239, 1994.
41. **Vogel, V. and Mobius, D.**, Local surface potentials and electric dipole moments of lipid monolayers: contributions of the water/lipid and the lipid/air interfaces, *J. Colloid Interface Sci.,* 126, 408, 1988.
42. **Koczorowski, Z., Kurowski, S. and Trasatti, S.**, A macroscopic approach to the adsorption potential shift at the air/solution interface, *J. Electroanal. Chem.*, 329, 25, 1992.
43. **Dynarowicz, P.**, Recent developments in the modelling of the monolayers structure at the water/air interface, *Advances in Colloid and Interface Science*, 45, 215, 1993.
44. **Minc, S. and Koczorowski, Z.**, Surface potentials of ionized monolayers, *Roczniki Chem.*, 39, 469, 1965.
45. **Shchipunov, Yu. A.**, Hydrophobic and electrostatic interactions in adsorption of surface-active substances: Tetraalkylammonium salts, *Adv. Colloid Interface Sci.*, 28, 135, 1988.
46. **Zagorska, I. and Koczorowski, Z.**, Experimental study of Volta potentials in water/nitrobenzene systems with anion adsorption, *J. Electroanal. Chem.*, 204, 273, 1986.
47. **Zagorska, I., Koczorowski, Z. and Paleska, I.**, Volta potentials in water/1,2-dichloroethane and water/ nitroethane systems, *J. Electroanal. Chem.*, 282, 51, 1990.
48. **Koczorowski, Z., Zagorska, I. and Kalinska, A.**, Differences between surface potentials of water and some organic solvents, *Electrochim. Acta.*, 34, 1857, 1989.

49. **Koczorowski, Z. and Minc, S.,** Investigation of polar oil-water electrochemical interphase properties - II. Solvation energies of 1:1 electrolytes in water saturated nitrobenzene, *Electrochim. Acta*, 8, 645, 1963.
50. **Doblhofer, K.,** Thin polymer films on electrodes: A physicochemical approach, in *The Electrochemistry of Novel Materials*, Lipkowski, J. and Ross, P. N., Eds., VCH Publishers, Inc., New York 1994, 141.
51. **Dragèeviè, D. and Milunoviè, M.,** An apparatus for surface potential measurements of films at the liquid/air interface and its application, *Kem. Ind.*, 36, 429, 1987.
52. **Hühnerfuss, H.,** Hydrophobic and hydrophilic hydration effects determined by surface potential measurements, *J. Colloid Interface Sci.*, 128, 237, 1989.
53. **Plaisance, M. and Ter-Minassian-Saraga, L.,** A differential method of measurement the surface potential, *C. R. Acad. Sc. Paris* (in French), 270, 1269, 1970.
54. **Yamins, H. G. and Zisman, W. A.,** Measurements of surface potentials of monomolecular films, *J. Chem. Phys.*, 1, 656, 1933.
55. **Surplice, N. A. and D'Arcy, R. J.,** A critique of the Kelvin method of measuring work functions, *J. Phys. E: Sci. Instrum.* 3, 477, 1970.
56. **Engelhardt, H. A., Feulner, P., Pfnür, H. and Menzel, D.,** An accurate and versatile vibrating capacitor for surface and adsorption studies, *J. Phys. E: Sci. Instrum.*, 10, 1133, 1977.
57. **Harris, L. B. and Fiason, J.,** Vibrating capacitor measurement of surface charge, *J. Phys. E: Sci. Instrum.*, 17, 788, 1984.
58. **Palau, J. M. and Bonnet, J.,** Design and performance of a Kelvin probe for the study of topographic work functions, *J. Phys. E: Sci. Instrum.*, 21, 674, 1988.
59. **Yee, S., Orani, R. A. and Stratmann, M.,** Application of a Kelvin microprobe to the corrosion of metals in humid atmospheres, *J. Electrochem. Soc.*, 138, 55, 1991.
60. **Liess, H. D., Mäckel, R., Baumagärtner, H. and Ren, J.,** Scanning Kelvin probe as a high resolution surface analysis device, *Sensors and Actuators* B, 13-14, 739, 1993.
61. **Huang, S.M., Atanasoski, R.T. and Oriani, R.A.,** Detection of effects of low electric fields with the Kelvin probe, *J. Electrochim. Soc.*, 140, 1065, 1993.
62. **Fujihira, M. and Hirosuke, K.,** Scanning surface potentials microscope for characterization of Langmuir-Blodgett films, *Thin. Solid Films*, 242, 163, 1994.
63. **Nguyen, M. T., Kanazawa, K. K., Brock, P. and Diaz, A. F.,** Surface potential map of charged ionomer-polymer blends studied with a scanning Kelvin probe, *Langmuir*, 10, 597, 1994.
64. **Delchar, T., Eberhagen, A. and Tomkins, F. C.,** A static capacitor method for the measurement of the surface potential of gases on evaporated metal films, *J. Sci. Instrum.*, 40, 105, 1963.
65. **Jacobs, J. C., Buuron, A. J. M., Renders, P. J. M. and Snik, A. F. M.,** Surface potential measurements of insoluble monolayers using the static-capacitor method, *J. Colloid Interface Sci.*, 84, 270, 1981.
66. **Venselaar, J. L. M., Kruger, A. J., Verbakel, L. M. H. and Poulis, J. A.,** The static capacitor method of measuring the effective dipole moment of surfactant molecules, *J. Colloid Interface Sci.*, 70, 149, 1979.
67. **Farrel, J. R. and Mc Tigue, P.,** Precise compensating potential difference measurements with voltaic cell. The surface potential of water, *J. Electroanal. Chem.*, 139, 37, 1982.
68. **Doblhofer, K. and Cappadonia, M.,** Calibration of the Kelvin vibrator for measurements of electric work functions in a humid atmosphere, *J. Electroanal. Chem.*, 243, 337, 1988.
69. **Sauer, B. B., Chen, Y., Zografi, G. and Yu, H.,** Surface light scattering studies of dipalmitoyphoshadylcholine monolayers at the air/water interfaces, *Langmuir*, 4, 111, 1988.

Chapter 3

ION SOLVATION

Yizhak Marcus

I. INTRODUCTION

The behavior of ions in solution depends strongly on the extent and energetics of their solvation. The more strongly an ion is solvated, the less reactive it tends to be. If offered the choice between two phases containing different solvents, it tends to partition into the solvent in which it is more strongly solvated. If the ion is located in a mixed solvent, it may undergo selective solvation, so that the composition of its solvation shell differs from that of the bulk solvent. Phenomena dependent on the size of (solvated) ions (e.g., diffusion) will also depend on the extent of solvation (the number of solvent molecules surrounding an ion and bound to it) and the size of the solvent. In order to understand the behavior of the ions it is necessary to have information on the properties of the ions and of the solvents as well as on their mutual interactions.

The interactions between ions at long range are electrostatic in nature (attraction for ions of opposite sign, repulsion if of the same sign), therefore depend on the relative permittivity of the solvent. At very short range they are repulsive (between the electron shells of the ions that are considered non-compressible and non-penetrable). However, at intermediate ranges (of the order of ionic and solvent diameters) the interactions - ion pairing - can be both electrostatic and solvent-structure-mediated. The following deliberations pertain to such dilute solutions of the ions where no ion-ion interactions take place, and the individual ion interacts only with its surrounding solvent. This is the nature of the solvation process[1], the transfer of the ion from the ideal gas, where there are no interactions whatsoever, to the infinitely dilute solution in the solvent, where the ion interacts only with the solvent and affects solvent-solvent interactions in its immediate environment.

II. THE RELEVANT PROPERTIES OF IONS

The solvation (hydration) of an ion depends on its properties as well as on those of the solvent. An ion is characterized in the present context by the sign and the magnitude (in proton charge units) of its charge, by its size and shape, by its polarizability and ability to accommodate electron pairs in its outermost orbitals, by its ability to undergo hydrogen bonding, by its hydrophobicity, and by its effects on the structure of water. These quantities can all be given numerical values, and they are employed in the expressions that describe models of the solvated ion and of the solvation process. The

0-8493-7694-7/96/$0.00+$.50

temperature and pressure dependencies of these ionic quantities pertinent to solvation are generally ignored.

Ions can be classified as cations and as anions, and in many cases the expressions applying to these categories differ. However, zwitterions, such as glycine, require a category for themselves. A further classification into monoatomic and small polyatomic ions on the one hand and large, hydrophobic polyatomic ions on the other is useful, since the models applicable to these categories may differ. Some ions, such as acetate and methylammonium, are borderline, since they include hydrophobic and hydrophilic parts.

Monoatomic ions can be assigned radii, assumed to be independent of the medium in which the ion is immersed, be it a crystal, a glass or other amorphous phase, a liquid, or vacuum. It has been shown[2] that the crystal ionic radii r_c listed by Shannon and Prewitt[3], based on the Pauling model with an appropriate coordination number (4, 6 or 8, but mainly 6), are consistent with experimental interatomic distances ion - water oxygen atom in aqueous solutions with a constant "radius" of the water molecule. Symmetric tetrahedral and octahedral polyatomic ions can also be assigned radii pertaining to the circumscribing spheres, based on van-der-Waals diameters of the atoms or radicals attached to the central atom with an allowance for the size of the latter. For ions of lower symmetry the assignment of "size parameters" is difficult. Thermochemical radii[4], based on the effect of ionic size on the lattice energy of crystals involving the ions have been assigned. Such size parameters, also called "radii", are uncertain to some degree. A representative list of ionic radii, r, is presented in Table 1. The shape of an ion, as seen above, is more difficult to quantify. On the one hand there are the spherical (monoatomic) or near-spherical (symmetric tetrahedral or octahedral) ions, and on the other there are the low-symmetry ions (or ionic groups) such as thiocyanate and nitrate or those that are of great physiological importance, such as carboxylate and alkylammonium as well as hydrogen carbonate, dihydrogen phosphate, etc.[5] In the latter the hydrogen atoms are often ignored and for the former an ellipsoid of rotation enclosing the ion is taken to represent its shape. The geometric mean of the three axes of this ellipsoid is sometimes used in lieu of the "radius" of such an ion.

The polarizability of an ion is, again, a property that is assumed to be independent of the medium in which the ion is immersed. The polarizability à is closely related to the molar refractivity R: $\alpha = (3/4\pi N_A)R$, which, in turn is obtained from the refractive index n of solutions or crystals containing the ion: $R = V(n^2-1)/(n^2+1)$, where V is the molar volume. The dependence of R (or α) on the wavelength at which n is measured is generally ignored, but practically the sodium D-line is generally employed, and R_D is therefore used. The assignment of R or α to individual ions requires an arbitrary assignment of a value to one ion for the values of all the others to be obtained from additivity relationships. The value $R_D/(\text{cm}^3\text{mol}^{-1}) = 0.65$ for the sodium ion is used[6]. A representative list of ionic polarizabilites is shown in Table 1.

Table 1. The properties of representative ions

Cation	r^a	α^b	σ^c	$\alpha_{KT}{}^d$	$G_{HB}{}^e$	Anion	r^a	α^b	σ^c	$\beta_{KT}{}^d$	$G_{HB}{}^e$
H^+	f	-0.04	0.00			F^-	1.33	0.88	-0.66	2.95	+0.08
Li^+	69	0.03	-1.02	2.07	0.28	Cl^-	181	3.42	-0.09	1.00	-0.61
Na^+	102	0.26	-0.60	0.83	-0.03	Br^-	196	4.85	0.17	0.67	-0.80
K^+	138	1.07	-0.58	0.85	-0.52	I^-	220	7.51	0.50	0.30	-1.09
Rb^+	149	1.63	-0.53	0.49	-0.56	OH^-	133	1.84	0.00		0.28
Cs^+	170	2.73	-0.54	0.47	-0.69	SH^-	207	5.07	0.65		-0.54
$NH_4{}^+$	148	1.20	-0.60	1.00	-0.18	CN^-	191	3.13	0.41	1.37	-0.61
Ag^+	115	2.02	0.70	1.61	-0.02	$N_3{}^-$	195	4.44	0.66	0.80	-0.61
Tl^+	150	4.56	0.20	0.96	-0.52	SCN^-	213	6.74	0.85	0.33	-0.82
Me_4N^+	280	9.08	0.81		-0.47	$NO_2{}^-$	192	3.45	0.15		-0.52
Et_4N^+	337	17.7			-0.10	$NO_3{}^-$	179	4.53	0.03	0.09	-0.68
Pr_4N^+	379	24.0			0.56	$ClO_3{}^-$	200	4.80	0.03		-0.65
Bu_4N^+	413	31.5			1.04	$BrO_3{}^-$	191	6.03			-0.49
Ph_4P^+	424	45.0				$IO_3{}^-$	181	7.47			-0.02
Ph_4As^+	426	45.7	7.3		0.14	$ClO_4{}^-$	250	5.06	-0.30	0.08	-1.01
Mg^{2+}	72	-0.28	-0.41		0.78	$ReO_4{}^-$	267		-0.40		-0.98
Ca^{2+}	100	0.63	-0.66		0.34	$BF_4{}^-$	232	2.78	-0.30		-0.90
Sr^{2+}	113	1.05	-0.64		0.29	$MeCO_2{}^-$	190	5.50	-0.22	1.49	0.12
Ba^{2+}	136	2.05	-0.66	5.15	0.01	$BPh_4{}^-$	421	43.15	6.9		0.21
Mn^{2+}	83	0.87	-0.15		0.57	$HCO_2{}^-$	185	4.32			0.00
Fc^{2+}	78	0.83	-0.16		1.10	$HSO_4{}^-$	230	0.83			-0.38
Co^{2+}	75	0.81	-0.11		0.86	$H_2PO_4{}^-$	238	5.80			-0.10
Ni^{2+}	69	0.6	-0.11		0.90	S^{2-}	184	10.31	1.09		-0.65
Cu^{2+}	73	0.52	0.38	5.03	0.70	$CO_3{}^{2-}$	178	4.54	-0.50		0.28
Zn^{2+}	75	0.55	0.35	3.67	0.71	$SO_3{}^{2-}$	200	5.11	0.70		0.28
Cd^{2+}	95	1.28	0.58	2.19	0.59	$SO_4{}^{2-}$	240	5.47	-0.38		-0.21
Hg^{2+}	102	2.43	1.27	2.13	0.35	$CrO_4{}^{2-}$	255	4.80			-0.34
Pb^{2+}	118	4.72	0.41	4.63	0.03	$Cr_2O_7{}^{2-}$	320	17.12			-1.54
Al^{3+}	53	-0.47	-0.31		0.17	$SiF_6{}^{2-}$	259	4.36			-0.76
Cr^{3+}	62	1.23	-0.10		0.17	$PdCl_6{}^{2-}$	385				-1.35
Fe^{3+}	65	1.27	0.33		0.65	$PtCl_6{}^{2-}$	395	20.7			-1.05
Ga^{3+}	62	0.20	0.29		0.55	$PO_4{}^{3-}$	238	5.99	-0.78		0.93
In^{3+}	79	0.69	0.48			$AsO_4{}^{3-}$	248				0.63
Tl^{3+}	89	0.87	1.07		0.34	$Fe(CN)_6{}^{3-}$	380	21.13			-1.61
Y^{3+}	90	0.95	-0.69		0.77	$Fe(CN)_6{}^{4-}$	343	22.56			-1.02
La^{3+}	105	1.09	-0.75		0.78	$P_2O_7{}^{4-}$	300	9.20			-0.30
Cd^{3+}	94	1.90	-066		0.67						
Lu^{3+}	86		-0.64		0.86						
Th^{4+}	100	2.22	-0.57		0.83						

Notes for Table 1.
[a] Radius in pm, from refs. [3,26]. [b] Polarizability in 10^{-30} m^3 from ref. [6] and an unpublished compilation by the author. [c] The softness parameter, numerical, from ref.[7]. The Kamlet-Taft hydrogen bond acidity (α) or basicity ([b]), numerical, from ref.[8]. [e] The effect on water structure, numerical, from ref. [10]. [f] The radius of the hydronium ion, H_3O^+ is 112 pm for fitting thermodynamic quantities of hydration. [26]

Transition metal ions are able to accommodate electron pairs of donor atoms of solvents in their outer orbitals to form coordinative bonds. This ability, measured by the HOMO-LUMO energy gap, affect the energetics of the solvation of such ions. A related but more general property of ions, not confined to transition metal ions, is their softness. This was quantified as the softness parameter σ, the normalized difference between the ionization potential (for atoms forming cations) or electron affinity (for atoms or radicals forming anions) and the corresponding enthalpies of hydration[7]. A representative list of ionic softness parameters is shown in Table 1. Values are lacking, however, for most polyatomic ions and multivalent anions. It was shown that there exists some correlation between the σ and α of ions for which both values are known, and this may help fill approximately empty data slots.

The ability to undergo hydrogen bonding has been deduced from the Gibbs free energy of transfer of ions from water into nonaqueous solvents, in comparison with such values for nonelectrolyte solutes, to which Kamlet-Taft α_{KT} and β_{KT} values have been assigned from measurements with solvatochromic indicators[8]. Anions are hydrogen bond acceptors or Lewis bases, therefore have β_{KT} values whereas cations are Lewis acids (although not able to donate hydrogen bonds) and have α_{KT} values, but they are available only for a relatively short list of ions, shown in Table 1. The hydrophobicity of nonelectrolyte solutes is measurable by their partition constant P between 1-octanol and water, but this includes a strong component of ability to donate and accept hydrogen bonds. Furthermore, P values (actually, $\log_{10}P$ is employed) are not known for most ions (i.e., the small inorganic ones that are highly hydrophilic) but is pertinent mainly for large ions involving alkyl chains or aryl rings. For these, more or less independent of the counterions, $\Delta\log P = \log P_{ion} - \log P_{neutral}$ is between -3 and -4 for carboxylate and alkyl- (or aryl-) ammonium ions[9]. For the neutral compounds $\log P$ values have been tabulated and can be estimated from group contributions[9].

The effects of ions on the structure of water, i.e., their structure-making and -breaking abilities have been shown to be obtainable from their standard molar Gibbs free energies of transfer from water into (the slightly more structured) heavy water. The measure adopted is the ratio, G_{HB}, of $\Delta_{tr}G^0$ (ion, $H_2O \rightarrow D_2O$) to the difference in hydrogen bonding strength of light and heavy water, -929 J mol^{-1}. Since these quantities are known for only a few ions, but are linearly correlated with the viscosity B-coefficients of the ions, the latter are a good substitutes for this quantity[10]. Representative values of G_{HB} are shown in Table 1.

III. THE RELEVANT PROPERTIES OF SOLVENTS

The relevant properties of the solvents are available in published collections[11,12] and need not be repeated here. They include the following: the molar volume V, the isothermal compressibility k_T, the heat capacity at constant pressure c_p, the solubility parameter δ (or its square, the cohesion energy density), the polarizability α, the dielectric constant ε, the dipole moment μ, the Kirkwood dipole angular correlation parameter g (or some other measure of the solvent structuredness[13]), the Kamlet-Taft solvatochromic parameters for hydrogen bond donation ability α_{KT} and acceptance ability β_{KT}, and the polarity/ polarizability parameter π^* (or some other parameter, such as the Dimroth-Reichardt $E_T(30)$, that is linear with this property), and their softness μ_S[14]. Not all these quantities are independent of each other and caution must be taken to employ only mutually orthogonal properties in statistical analysis of solvent dependencies of ion solvation data.

Among the many solvents that are used in chemistry, only those from a rather limited list have had the solvation properties of ions in them investigated at all extensively. In the present context this means the transfer energetics from a reference solvent (mainly water) into the target solvent for both cations and anions. In the reference solvent the solvation should have been studied in all its aspects, and this restricts the choice practically to water, i.e., the hydration of the ions. The list of solvents includes water, the lower alkanols [methanol (MeOH), ethanol (EtOH), 1-propanol (PrOH)], ethylene glycol (EG), acetone (Me_2CO), propylene carbonate (PC), liquid ammonia, formamide (FA), N-methylformamide (NMF), N,N-dimethylformamide (DMF), N,N-dimethylacetamide (DMA), N-methylpyrrolidinone (NMPy), acetonitrile (MeCN), benzonitrile (PhCN), nitromethane ($MeNO_2$), nitrobenzene ($PhNO_2$), pyridine (Py), dimethylsulfoxide (DMSO), sulfolane (TMS), N,N-dimethylthioformamide (DMThF), hexamethylphosphoric triamide (HMPT), dichloromethane, chloroform, and 1,2-dichloroethane (DClE). Homologous and other derivatives of these solvents have been studied for a limited number of ions, mainly cations.

IV. QUANTITIES DESCRIBING IONIC HYDRATION

The following standard molar thermodynamic quantities pertaining to the hydration of ions have been studied for a large number of ions: the Gibbs free energy, the enthalpy, the entropy, and the heat capacity. The standard partial molar volume of the ions has also been studied for many ions. Less extensive studies include the isobaric thermal expansibility and the isothermal compressibility. Other quantities pertinent to the hydration of many ions are the transport properties: limiting equivalent conductivities and the *B*-coefficients of viscosity, whereas self-diffusion coefficients are less extensively known. For relatively few ions is the molar decrement of the relative permittivity of the water known, whereas the molar refraction is considered to be a property of the ion itself, independent of its solvation (see above). The standard molar thermodynamic quantities of hydration pertain to the standard states of 0.1 MPa pressure in the gas phase and 1 mol dm^{-3} in the aqueous solution. If no other temperature is mentioned, then 298.15 K should be understood in the following.

In practically all these cases (excepting conductivity and diffusivity) are the quantities for individual ions obtained from measured quantities for electrolytes split into the ionic contribution according to the additivity principle and based on an extra-thermodynamic assumption (or an equivalent one for non-thermodynamic quantities). The principle of additivity asserts that at a given temperature and pressure and at infinite dilution (i.e., for the standard thermodynamic quantities) the measured quantity is additive in the stoichiometrically weighted invariant properties of the ions because ion-ion interactions are absent. At final concentrations (that may be as low as 0.01 mol dm^{-1} or even lower) such interactions cause the measured quantities to be concentration dependent. Therefore extrapolation to infinite dilution is required, and a rule permitting accurate extrapolation is necessary. At the low concentration range involved the Debye-Huckel expressions are valid, and extrapolation with respect of the square root of the concentration is generally employed. However, the measured quantities generally become less accurate as the concentration of the electrolyte is allowed to diminish, and the payoff between accurate data and sufficiently low concentrations for short extrapolation is not easy to optimize.

A. THERMODYNAMICS OF ION HYDRATION

Conventional values of the thermodynamic quantities of hydration, based on the convention that the relevant thermodynamic quantities for the hydrogen ion are zero (at all temperatures) have been reported[15]. They need to be converted to so-called absolute values, by means of the extra-thermodynamic assumption, in order to represent as nearly as possible the hydration properties of the individual ions. The main problem with the obtaining of individual ionic thermodynamic quantities of hydration is the choice and validity of the extra-thermodynamic assumption. Conway[16] examined the various assumptions that had been proposed and recommended those that are the least objectionable. It must be stressed, however, that being assumptions, they cannot be put to rigorous tests and their choice is based mainly on the "reasonableness" of the resulting individual ionic values.

A method that appears to be optimal could be based on a reference electrolyte with singly charged cation and anion that are identical in all respects except the sign of the charge. The ions of such an electrolyte should have minimal interactions with the aqueous solvent, both electrostatic (the ions should therefore be large) and non-electrostatic, such as due to dispersion forces and interference with solvent structure (the ions should therefore be small and not polarizable). If such a reference electrolyte existed, it would have relatively small thermodynamic quantities of hydration that could be divided evenly between the cation and the anion to obtain the value for the individual ion. The additivity principle is then applicable to electrolytes involving the reference ion and a counter-ion to yield the value for the latter, hence for any ion. Unfortunately, such a reference electrolyte does not exist (the ionic size requirements mentioned above are contradicting) but approximations have been suggested. Tetrabutylammonium tetrabutylborate would fulfill several of the criteria (but not that of minimal interference with the water structure) but its anion is not very stable in aqueous solutions. Tetraphenylphosphonium tetraphenylborate (TPTB) has been employed for the present purpose (the tetraphenylarsonium salt (TATB) is a second choice), with recognizable drawbacks when the resulting ionic values are large compared with those of ordinary ions[17].

B. METHODS OF INVESTIGATION

The standard molar enthalpy of hydration of an electrolyte is obtained from measurements of its heat of solution in water and a theoretical calculation of its lattice enthalpy[17]. Data are available for those salts where such a calculation has been or can be carried out. The method suggested by Halliwell and Nyburg[18] can then serve for the splitting of the data to the ionic contributions. This method involves the extrapolation to zero of the difference between the conventional enthalpies of hydration of cations and anions having the same radius against the reciprocal of the cube of the sum of this radius and the diameter of a water molecule, to yield twice the absolute value of $\Delta_{hyd}H^\infty(H^+)$. A wider consideration of assumptions, including the small enthalpies of hydration of the tetraphenyl ions of TPTB mentioned above, has led to the value $\Delta_{hyd}H^\infty(H^+)$. = -1094±7 kJ mol^{-1}.[19]

The standard molar entropy of hydration of an ion is obtained from the third-law entropy of the gaseous ion, obtained from structural and spectroscopic data[20] and the standard partial molar entropy of the aqueous ion. Conventional values of the latter have been tabulated[15], based on the temperature coefficient of the standard potentials of electrodes involving the ions. Conversion to their absolute values has been based on the results from thermocells, where identical electrodes are immersed in half-cells of the same composition but at different temperatures[21]. The value accepted for $\bar{S}^\infty(H^+,aq)$ is -22.2±1.4 J K^{-1} mol^{-1}.[16] The standard molar entropy of hydration is then obtained with the theoretical value of $S^\circ(H^+,g)$ = 108.8 J K^{-1} mol^{-1} as $\Delta_{hyd}S^\infty(H^+)$ = -131±1 J K^{-1}mol^{-1}.

The standard molar Gibbs free energies of hydration of ions must conform to the relationship: $\Delta_{hyd}G^\infty = \Delta_{hyd}H^\infty - T\Delta_{hyd}S^\infty$. Hence, having selected the absolute enthalpy and entropy of hydration of the hydrogen ion, the Gibbs free energy of hydration: $\Delta_{hyd}G^\infty(H^+)$ = -1056±7 kJ mol^{-1} follows. A check on these choices can be made, if $\Delta_{hyd}G^\infty$ can be estimated independently. This can be done by means of the Volta potentials, across a nitrogen gap, between a flowing mercury jet in the center of a vertical tube and an aqueous electrolyte solution along its walls. The resulting value $\Delta_{hyd}G^\infty(H^+)$ = -1088±20 kJ mol^{-1}, not in complete agreement with the previous choices. Sorption of water vapor on the mercury may have changed its work function and been responsible for the discrepancy[16].

The standard partial molar heat capacities of electrolytes are determined by either measuring the specific heat of their dilute aqueous solutions or by measuring the temperature coefficient of their heats of solution in water at low concentrations. For the former method the apparent molar heat capacity is calculated and extrapolated to infinite dilution. For the latter determination the molar heat capacity of the pure salt is also necessary. Both methods require very sensitive instrumentation and the accuracy of the results is not as high as desirable. A wide range of $\bar{C}_p^{\infty}(H^+,aq)$ has been suggested, -71 to 142 J K^{-1} mol^{-1},[16] the most negative of which being based on the TPTB assumption. The ions of this electrolyte have the same intrinsic heat capacities (within 2 J K^{-1} mol^{-1}) and their interaction with the water should be similar, due to their hydrophobic nature and low electrostatic effects. With the theoretical value of $C_p(H^+,g) = 21$ J K^{-1} mol^{-1}, the value of $\Delta_{hyd}C_p(H^+) = -92\pm30$ J K^{-1} mol^{-1} is adopted here as valid.

The standard partial molar volumes of electrolytes are obtained from measurements of the densities of their dilute solutions via extrapolation of the apparent molar volumes to infinite dilution. The splitting into the individual ionic values can be based on the extrapolation of data for a series of salts of similar ions of varying radius with a common counter-ion to zero radius, yielding the partial molar volume of the counter-ion. This method was implemented, e.g., for the tetraalkylammonium bromides[16] yielding $\bar{V}^{\infty}(H^+,aq) = -5.5\pm0.5$ cm^3 mol^{-1}. This value is consistent with the vibration potential method of Zana and Yeager (accurate to within ±2 cm^3 mol^{-1})[24] and also with the TPTB assumption, taking into account the small difference in the actual sizes of its ions. Since all the ions have the same molar volume in the ideal gas phase ($RT/p = 24790$ cm^3 mol^{-1}), and since this is much larger than their partial molar volumes in solution, there is no point in dealing with $\Delta_{hyd}V^{\infty}$.

C. OTHER PROPERTIES RELEVANT TO HYDRATION

The limiting equivalent conductivities λ^{∞} of ions can be obtained from the equivalent conductivities of dilute solutions of the electrolytes and the corresponding transference numbers, extrapolated to infinite dilution. This is one of the very few measures of properties of individual ions that can be obtained directly from experiment without the necessity for an assumption. The additivity of the stoichiometrically weighted ionic equivalent conductivities (Kohlrausch's law) and the expressions for extrapolation to infinite dilution (Onsager's limiting law) are well established. The accuracy of the λ^{∞} values in water[25] is ±0.02 cm^2 ohm^{-1} mol^{-1} at ambient temperatures.

The viscosity B-coefficients are obtained from measurements of the viscosity η of dilute aqueous solutions of electrolytes as the limiting slope of the dependence of $[(\eta/\eta^{\circ})-1]/c^{1/2}$ on $c^{1/2}$, where η° is the viscosity of the solvent water and c is the concentration in mol dm^{-3}. Alternatively, the intercept of this dependence, the *A*-coefficient, can be calculated from the limiting equivalent conductivity of the electrolyte, so that *B* results from $[[(\eta/\eta^{\circ}) -1 - A\ c^{1/2}]/c$. It is then necessary to split the *B*-coefficient into the ionic contributions, but no valid theory is known specifying how to do it. If the cubes of the reciprocals of the mobilities (or the Stokes radii) of the ions are assumed to represent the effective volumes of the hydrated ions in the solution, then analogy with non-electrolyte behavior suggests that the *B*-coefficient should be split evenly for an electrolyte with equal limiting equivalent conductivities of its cation and anion. Aqueous rubidium bromide fills this requirement best at ambient temperatures. The accuracy with which ionic *B*-coefficients in aqueous solutions are known is ±0.001 dm^3 mol^{-1}.[10]

The final quantity to be discussed is the "hydration number". This cannot be measured experimentally but can be derived from experimental data when defined operationally. Hydration numbers may mean the average number of water molecules in immediate contact with the ions or the average number of water molecules that are affected by the field of the ion. In the latter case, they may be located in a "first hydration shell" or a second and even further ones. Water molecules are strongly coordinated to transition metal ions and are then restricted to locations in the coordination polyhedron. With other cations and all anions, the number of water molecules in contact with the ion is governed primarily by their packing ability (i.e., mutual repulsions of inpenetrable electron shells). Secondarily this number is governed by their mutual hydrogen bonding, affected somewhat by hydrogen bonding to the ion on the one hand and to water molecules beyond the first hydration shell, oriented by the ionic field, on the other.

The incompressible volume per ion of an electrolyte solution, less the intrinsic volume of the ion, divided by the volume of an electrostricted water molecule, has served as the basis for one operational definition and experimental measure of the hydration number. It is assumed that neither the ion itself nor the electrostricted water molecules in its hydration shell are further compressible by moderate external pressure. The incompressible volume is obtained from extrapolation to infinite dilution of $(1000/c)(1-\kappa/\kappa^{\circ})$, where the compressibility is $\kappa = -(\partial \ln V/\partial p)_T$ for the solution and k° is the corresponding quantity for water. Splitting of the resulting hydration number n of the electrolyte into the ionic contributions requires the assumption of additivity and assignment of a value to one ion. Some ion (e.g., thiocyanate) is deemed to be unhydrated and a value of $n= 0$ is assigned to it. A model (see below) has shown that hydration numbers can be calculated simply from $n = |z|\,[360/(r/\text{pm})]$.[26]

D. THE DATA

Table 2 shows the data for a selection of the more common ions; data for many other ions are available in the publications cited. It should be noted that the data shown for the Gibbs free energy, enthalpy, entropy, and heat capacity of hydration include corrections pertaining to the definition of the hydration process of an ion as proceeding from a fixed position in the ideal gas to a fixed position in water, relative to a process that includes translation in both phases. The thermodynamics of the process involving fixed positions pertains directly to the total interactions of the ion with the water, i.e., the hydration proper. The correction is +7.93 kJ mol^{-1} for $\Delta_{hyd}G^o$, +2.29 kJ mol^{-1} for $\Delta_{hyd}H^o$, -18.9 J K^{-1} mol^{-1} for $\Delta_{hyd}S^o$, and +7.0 J K^{-1} mol^{-1} for $\Delta_{hyd}C_p{}^o$.[26] The data shown for the Gibbs free energy and the enthalpy are rounded to the nearest 5 kJ mol^{-1}. Except for very few cases, the thermodynamic quantities of hydration are negative, due to the immobilization of the water molecules in the first hydration shell by electrostatic (in the case of transition metal ions, coordinative) bonding to the charged ions.

The limiting partial molar volumes of the ions are negative when the elctrostriction of the water molecules caused by the charge is larger than the intrinsic volume of the ion. The molar conductivity of monoatomic ions and some of the polyatomic ones is generally in the range $50z$ to $70z$ cm^2 Ω^{-1} mol^{-1} but it decreases with increasing size of the (hydrated) ion (i.e., with $r + \Delta r$). Negative B-coefficients are characteristic of water-structure- breaking ions (i.e., those with negative G_{HB}, cf. Table 1). The hydration numbers n pertain to total hydration, i.e., including electrostricted water molecules beyond the first hydration shell. These numbers are, on the average, $(0.6\pm0.4)z^2$ units larger for the cations and $(1.3\pm1.0)z^2$ units smaller for the anions than the numbers obtained from compressibility.

E. INTERPRETATION

The quantities describing the hydration of the ions have been interpreted in terms of a simple empirical model[26]. The model prescribes for all ions, irrespective of the sign and the magnitude of their charge and their size and shape a hydration shell of width: $\Delta r = [(d/2)^3 n + r^3]^{1/3} - r$, where $d = 276$ pm is the diameter of a water molecule, and $n = |z|\,[360/(r/\text{pm})]$, as specified above. Inside this shell the electrostricted water has empirically specified relative permittivity and its temperature and pressure derivatives that yield valid hydration Gibbs free energies and enthalpies and partial molar volumes of ions of charges $-3 \leq z \leq 4$. The entropies and heat capacities of hydration resulting from the model have an extra contribution from the effect of the ions on the structure of the water beyond the hydration shell, which is, in turn, consistent with the viscosity B-coefficients[10]. The ionic conductivities, in their turn, are consistent with the values of $r + \Delta r$ calculated with no regard to the sign of the charge: the former have a maximum where the latter have a minimum, and the conductivities of the cations and anions fall on the same curve, when plotted against r[27]. It is concluded that the model is capable of remarkably well predicting the various quantities of hydration of ions considered here.

Table 2a. Quantities describing the hydration of caions

Ion	$\Delta_{hyd}G^{oa}$	$\Delta_{hyd}H^{ob}$	$\Delta_{hyd}S^{oc}$	$\Delta_{hyd}C^{od}$	$\overline{V}^{\infty e}$	$\lambda^{\infty f}$	B^{g}	n^{h}
H_3O^+			-163	-85	-5.5	349.8	0.068	2.7
Li^+	-475	-530	-161	-23	-6.4	38.7	0.146	5.2
Na^+	-365	-415	-130	-42	-6.7	50.1	0.085	3.5
K^+	-295	-330	-93	-72	3.5	73.5	-0.009	2.6
Rb^+	-275	-305	-84	-94	8.6	77.8	-0.033	2.4
Cs^+	-250	-280	-78	-108	15.8	77.3	-0.047	2.1
NH_4^+	-285	-325	-131	-29	12.4	73.6	-0.008	2.4
Ag^+	-430	-480	-136	-59	-6.2	61.9	0.090	3.1
Tl^+	-300	-335	-91	-103	5.4	74.7	-0.036	2.4
Me_4N^+	-160	-215	-163	74	84.1	44.9	0.123	1.3
Et_4N^+	0	-205	-241	259	143.6	32.7	0.385	1.1
Pr_4N^+				576	208.9	23.4	0.916	0.9
Bu_4N^+		-225		900	270.2	19.5	1.275	0.9
Ph_4P^+		-45		779	285.8	20.2	1.073	0.8
Ph_4As^+	50	-45	-321	803	295.2	19.7	1.073	0.8
Mg^{2+}	-1830	-1945	-350	-172	-32.2	106.1	0.385	10.0
Ca^{2+}	-1505	-1600	-271	-183	-28.9	119.0	0.298	7.2
Sr^{2+}	-1380	-1470	-261	-191	-29.2	118.9	0.272	6.4
Ba^{2+}	-1250	-1330	-224	-202	-23.55	127.3	0.229	5.3
Mn^{2+}	-1760	-1870	-311	-168	-28.7	100.0	0.390	8.7
Fe^{2+}	-1840	-1970	-381	-202	-30.2	107.0	0.420	9.2
Co^{2+}	-1915	-2035	-356	-183	-35.0	110.0	0.376	9.6
Ni^{2+}	-1980	-2115	-370	-198	-35.0	98.0	0.375	10.4
Cu^{2+}	-2010	-2120	-339	-176	-36.0	107.2	0.368	9.9
Zn^{2+}	-1955	-2070	-337	-178	-32.6	105.6	0.361	9.6
Cd^{2+}	-1755	-1830	-3-4	-164	-31.0	108.0	0.360	7.6
Hg^{2+}	-1760	-1850	-194	-147	-30.3	127.2		7.1
Pb^{2+}	-1425	-1570	-228	-209	-26.5	139.0	0.233	6.1
Al^{3+}	-4525	-4715	-557	-363	-58.7	183.0	0.670	20.4
Cr^{3+}	-4010	-4670	-533	-208	-53.2	201.0	0.743	17.4
Fe^{3+}	-4265	-4460	-576	-218	-53.0	204.0	0.696	16.6
Ga^{3+}	-4515	-4305	-579	-214	-61.4			17.4
In^{3+}	-3980	-4125	-405	-231	-58.7	186.3		13.7
Tl^{3+}	-3970	-4125	-453	-249	-55.8			12.3
Y^{3+}	-3450	-3590	-502	-234	-57.3	186.0		14.4
La^{3+}	-3145	-3310	-474	-353	-55.6	209.1	0.582	10.3
Gd^{3+}	-3375	-3545	-481	-345	-56.4	201.9	0.646	11.5
Lu^{3+}	-3515	-3695	-523	-353	-61.5		0.681	12.6
Th^{4+}	-5815	-6055	-707	-441	-75.5	276.0	0.860	15.3

Notes for Table 2a and 2b.

[a] Standard molar Gibbs free energy of hydration,[26] in kJ mol^{-1}. [b] Standard molar enthalpy of hydration, [26] in kJ mol^{-1}. [c] Standard molar entropy of hydration,[26] in J K^{-1} mol^{-1}. [d] Standard molar heat capacity at constant pressure of hydration, [26] in J K^{-1} mol^{-1}. [e] Standard partial molar volume, [26] in cm^3 mol^{-1}. Limiting molar conductivity,[25] in cm^2 Ohm^{-1} mol^{-1}. [g] The *B*-coefficient of viscosity, [10] in dm^3 mol^{-1}. The hydration number, $n = 360 \cdot |z| /(r/\text{pm})$.[26]

Table 2b. Quantities describing the hydration of anions

Ion	$\Delta_{hyd}G^{oa}$	$\Delta_{hyd}H^{ob}$	$\Delta_{hyd}S^{oc}$	$\Delta_{hyd}C^{od}$	$\overline{V^{\infty}}^{e}$	$\lambda^{\infty f}$	B^{g}	n^{h}
F^-	-465	-510	-156	-59	4.3	55.4	0.127	2.7
Cl^-	-340	-365	-94	-70	23.3	76.4	-0.005	2.0
Br^-	-315	-335	-78	-74	30.2	78.1	-0.033	1.9
I^-	-275	-290	-55	-74	41.7	76.4	-0.073	1.6
OH^-	-430	-520	-180	-91	-0.2	198.3	0.120	2.7
SH^-	-295	-340	-117	-45	26.2	65.0	0.025	1.7
CN^-	-295	-345	-99		29.7	82.0	-0.024	1.9
N_3^-	-295	-300	-101		30.5	69.0	-0.018	1.9
SCN^-	-280	-310	-85	6	41.2	66.0	-0.025	1.7
NO_2^-	-330	-410	-110	-47	31.7	71.8	-0.024	1.9
NO_3^-	-300	-310	-95	-39	34.5	71.5	-0.045	2.0
ClO_3^-	-280	-295	-99	-38	42.2	64.6	-0.024	1.8
BrO_3^-	-330	-375	-114	-74	40.8	55.7	0.007	1.9
IO_3^-	-400	-450	-167	-59	30.8	40.5	0.138	2.0
ClO_4^-	-205	-245	-76	-9	49.6	67.4	-0.060	1.4
ReO_4^-	-330	-360	-90	-3	53.7	54.9	-0.055	1.3
BF_4^-	-190	-225	-85	-13	49.7		-0.093	1.6
$MeCO_2^-$	-365	-425	-189	43	46.2	40.9	0.236	1.9
BPh_4^-	50	-45	-327	781	283.1	19.9	1.115	0.9
HCO_2^-	-335	-380	-156	-26	28.9	44.5	0.130	2.0
HSO_4^-	-330		-148		37.1	50.0	0.127	1.6
$H_2PO_4^-$	-465	-520	-290	-19	34.6	33.0	0.340	1.5
S^{2-}	-1315	-1345	-141		2.8			3.9
CO_3^{2-}	-1315	-1395	-264	-196	6.7	138.6	0.278	4.0
SO_3^{2-}	-1295	-1375	-268	-222	16.6	159.8	0.282	3.6
SO_4^{2-}	-1080	-1035	-219	-193	25.0	160.0	0.206	3.0
CrO_4^{2-}	-950	-1010	-206	-177	30.7	166.0	0.169	2.8
$Cr_2O_7^{2-}$			-92	-77	84.4			2.3
SiF_6^{2-}	-930	-980	-162	-161	50.5		0.374	2.8
$PdCl_6^{2-}$	-695	-730	-115					1.8
$PtCl_6^{2-}$	-685	-740	-182		161.0			1.8
PO_4^{3-}	-2765	-2875	-440	-341	-14.1		0.590	4.5
AsO_4^{3-}			-404		0.9		0.520	4.4
$Fe(CN)_6^{3-}$			-165	-443	137.3	302.7	0.123	2.8
$Fe(CN)_6^{4-}$			-305	-249	96.0	442.0	0.371	4.2
$P_2O_7^{4-}$			-391		24.6	384.0		4.8

V. TRANSFER OF IONS INTO NON-AQUEOUS SOLVENTS

When an ion leaves its aqueous environment in order to be solvated by some non-aqueous solvent it is necessary to invest the required thermodynamic quantities of hydration (i.e., as if the transfer goes via the gas phase) with the corresponding quantities of solvation being then returned, once the ion is at equilibrium with the new environment. In fact, most of the investment is returned, and the thermodynamic quantities of transfer are (for the smaller ions) only ca. 1 to 10% of those for hydration, and can be both positive and negative. In many cases they can be measured (for electrolytes, not for individual ions) much more accurately than the thermodynamic quantities for solvation of ions from the gas phase in the non-aqueous solvents themselves. Such transfer quantities are, in principle, measurable for transfers from any one solvent (used as a reference solvent) into another, and methanol, acetonitrile, and N,N-dimethylformamide have been employed in this capacity of reference solvents. Since, however, the thermodynamic quantities of hydration of the ions are known as accurately as any data for solvation that have been measured directly or better, and are available for many more ions (cf. Table 2 and the references cited there), water is the reference solvent almost universally preferred nowadays.

The problem of the splitting of the thermodynamic quantities of transfer measured for electrolytes into the contributions of the individual ions is as serious as in the case of hydration. The extrathermodynamic assumption employed in recent years is generally that of a reference electrolyte, the quantities for which can be split evenly between the cation and the anion. In the case of electrochemical determinations, a rivaling assumption involves the half-cell potential of a reference redox couple that is insensitive to the solvent. The reference electrolyte employed most often is tetraphenylarsonium tetraphenylborate (TATB) with the corresponding tetraphenylphosphonium salt (TPTB) being a second choice. The small difference in size of the cation and anion and the small effect of the difference in the quadrupole moment[28] are generally ignored, amounting to $< \pm 2$ kJ mol^{-1} for the Gibbs free energy and enthalpy of transfer. In the case of the volume change on transfer, the size effect is taken into account (the reference cation is larger than the anion by 2 cm^3 mol^{-1}), due to the large intrinsic volumes of the reference ions[29]. For the heat capacity of transfer, the difference in the intrinsic (gas phase) heat capacities of the reference ions (3J K^{-1}mol^{-1}) is negligible compared with the uncertainties of the values for the electrolytes and can be ignored[30].

A. METHODS OF INVESTIGATION

The key quantity among the thermodynamic quantities of transfer of ions is the standard molar Gibbs free energy of transfer, $\Delta_{tr}G^o$, since its sign determines which of the two solvents the ion prefers. If the solute electrolyte is sparingly soluble in both the reference solvent, w, and the solvent into which it is being transferred, the target solvent, s, then the determination of its solubility in the two solvents is a preferred method of determination. This is because with sparingly soluble solutes the concentrations are sufficiently low for the Debye-Huckel expression to be applicable for the correction to infinite dilution (the reference state). Another proviso is that the solute does not form solvates, so that it is the same substance that is at equilibrium with the two saturated solutions. Then $\Delta_{tr}G^o = RT\ln(K_{sS}/K_{sW})$, where K_s is the solubility product. The reference electrolyte assumption (TATB) for the splitting of the $\Delta_{tr}G^o$ value for the electrolyte into the ionic contributions is well suited to this method. The very low aqueous solubility of TATB is given by $\log_{10}K_{sW} = -17.51\pm0.21$ at 25°C,[28] but its solubility in the target solvents, being higher but still sparing, is more readily determinable, e.g., in the propanediols[31]. A great advantage of the solubility method is that it is applicable for both cations and anions, so that the additivity of the ionic $\Delta_{tr}G^{o}$ values can be tested.

A related method involves the partition of the solute between the target solvent and the reference solvent, applicable when these two solvents are essentially mutually insoluble. Then concentrations below saturation are used, so that the method is applicable also to well soluble electrolytes. On the other hand, this transfer does not pertain to strictly neat solvents, and the differences between "dry" and "wet" solvents can be appreciable, as is the case with transfer from water into 1,2-dichloroethane[32].

Electrochemical methods are popular, and can be carried out with very good precision on dilute solutions of electrolytes, permitting ready extrapolation to infinite dilution. The difference of the standard electromotive forces of cells involving electrodes reversible with respect to the cation and anion, measured in the reference and the target solvent, then gives $\Delta_{tr}G^{o}$ directly. An alternative, if an electrode reversible to only one of the ions is available, is to employ a liquid junction between two half cells with the reversible electrodes and the two solvents. It is then necessary to devise the liquid junction and its composition in such a manner, which the assumption of a negligible liquid junction potential is acceptable. A liquid junction employing tetraethylammonium picrate in acetonitrile between acetonitrile as the reference solvent and another aprotic solvent as the target one was shown to lead to acceptable (i.e., compatible with the TATB assumption) results[33].

A further electrochemical method involves polarographic or voltammetric measurements of half-wave potentials, taken to represent the equilibrium standard potential with respect to a redox couple, the potential of which is assumed to be independent of the solvent. Earlier, the ferrocene/ferricinium couple was assumed to have this property, but this approach was criticized on the grounds that the ferricinium ion is too open and small for electrostatic effects on its solvation by different solvents to be negligible. This couple was later replaced by the bis(biphenyl)chromium (I)/(0) couple (BBCr)[34], and a large amount of work with this BBCr assumption has since been reported. A drawback of this assumption is that the electrochemical method involved relates to the transfer of cations only, and is not being tested by the presence of different anions. Otherwise it is difficult to prefer the BBCr or the TATB assumption: in many cases the differences between the resulting $\Delta_{tr}G^{o}$ are small but in others they are appreciable.

The standard molar enthalpy of transfer of an electrolyte, $\Delta_{tr}H^{o}$, is obtained from the difference in the calorimetrically measured standard heats of solution of the electrolyte in the reference and target solvents, again for solutes that do not form solvates in either solvent. Here the TATB assumption can be applied directly[35], whereas the BBCr assumption is not applicable. A less accurate method involves the temperature coefficient of

Table 3. The Gibbs free energies of ions transfer from water into selected non-aqueous solvents*.

Ion	MeOH	Me_2CO	PC	FA	DMF	MeCN	$MeNO_2$	$PhNO_2$	Py	DMSO	DMThF	HMPT	DCl
H^+	10		50	-10	-18	44	95	33	-28	-19	39	40	56
Li^+	4	10	24	-10	-10	25	48	38	18	-15	55		56
Na^+	8	10	15	-8	-10	15	32	36	16	-13	39	-17	52
K^+	10	4	5	-4	-10	8	15	21	14	-13	27	-16	46
Rb^+	10	4	-1	-5	-10	6	11	19	13	-10	16	-10	37
Cs^+	9	4	-7	-6	-11	6	6	18	11	-13	14	-7	
Ag^+	7	9	19	-15	-21	-31	21	30	-57	-35	-102	-44	5
Tl^+	4	3	11	-1	-12	8	18	17	-1	-21	-24	-26	26
Me_4N^+	6	3	-11	3	-5	3	-5	4		-2			16
Et_4N^+	1	-3	-13		-8	-7	-10	-5		-9			5
Pr_4N^+	-10		-22	-10	-17	-13	-20	-16					-9
Bu_4N^+	-21		-31		-29	-32		-31					-18
Ph_4As^+	-24	-32	-36	-24	-39	-33	-33	-36	-38	-37	-36	-39	-33
Ba^{2+}	17	20	46		-21	57			38	-27	71	-59	
Cu^{2+}	29	49	73	-4	-18	68	142	115	-50	-43		-52	
Zn^{2+}	27	83	81		-30	69	123	140	-2	-45	-85	-86	
Cd^{2+}	33	61	70	-28	-34	42	1011	93	-31	-58	-91	-36	
Hg^{2+}	48	2	80		-44	28	61	44	-79	-48	-168	-86	
Pb^{2+}	4	78	47	-12	-34	64	78	71	7	-52	-23	-38	
F^-	16	84	56	25	85	71		70		73			65
Cl^-	13	57	40	14	48	42	38	35	34	40	22	58	52
Br^-	11	42	30	11	36	31	29	29	21	27	15	46	38
I^-	7	25	14	7	20	17	19	18	19	10	15	30	25
CN^-	9	48	36	13	40	35	31	38		35	9		41
N_3^-	9	43	27	11	36	37	28		71	26		49	
SCN^-	6		7	7	18	14	15	16	20	10		20	19
NO_3^-	13	22				21		24					32
ClO_4^-	6	6	-3	-12	4	2	5	10	16	-1		-7	17
$MeCO_2^-$	16			20	66	61	56			50			
Pi^-	-6			-7		-3		-5	-5		-13		-3
BPh_4^-	-24	-32	-36	-24	-39	-33	-33	-38	-38	-37	-36	-39	-33
SO_4^{2-}	31	105			78	88		141	141	113			

*. In kJ mol^{-1}, on the mol dm-3 scale, using TATB assumption.

the solubilities in the two solvents. On the other hand, the standard molar entropy of transfer, $\Delta_{tr}S^o$, is obtained directly from the temperature coefficient of the polarographic or voltammetric half-wave potentials in thermocells. The assumption here is that the thermal diffusion potential with tetrabutylammonium perchlorate as a background electrolyte is negligible[36]. The enthalpy of transfer is then obtained from $\Delta_{tr}H^o = \Delta_{tr}G^o + T\Delta_{tr}G^o$ (with $\Delta_{tr}G^o$ involving the BBCr assumption), whereas with the TATB assumption it is the entropy that is obtained indirectly: $\Delta_{tr}S^o = (\Delta_{tr}H^o - \Delta_{tr}G^o)/T$.

The standard partial molar heat capacity and volume of electrolytes have been measured in non-aqueous solvents by the same methods employed in aqueous ones. The TATB (or preferably the TPTB) assumption has to be applied, since no viable alternative has been shown to be available. It is then assumed that the differences between the values of the reference cation and anion are altogether negligible with respect to the experimental errors (heat capacities) or are taken into account but assumed to be independent of the solvent (volumes). Because of the large intrinsic contributions of the internal modes (heat capacities) and volumes of the reference ions to the partial molar values in the solutions, these assumptions appear to be acceptable.

The *B*-coefficients of viscosity of electrolytes in non-aqueous solvents are measured in the same manner as in water, but the difference between the values in different solvents is not referred to as a quantity of transfer. Still the *B*-coefficients do provide information on the solvation properties of the electrolytes. The splitting into contributions from individual ions, however, cannot employ the mobilities of the alkali and halide ions (rubidium bromide or potassium chloride) as in aqueous solutions, since these differ considerably in non-aqueous solutions. The use of an electrolyte made up of large hydrophobic ions, such as TPTB, has been suggested for this purpose.

B. THE DATA

The standard molar Gibbs free energies of transfer of ions from water into several non-aqueous target solvents are listed in Table 3. The entries, $\Delta_{tr}G^o$ /(kJ mol^{-1}), pertain to 25°C and the mol dm^{-3} scale and are based on the TATB assumption unless otherwise noted. The enthalpies of transfer are shown in Table 4, and the entropies can be calculated from $\Delta_{tr}S^o = (\Delta_{tr}H^o - \Delta_{tr}G^o)/T$ and the entries in Tables 3 and 4. Note, however, that the list of solvents is not identical (no extensive $\Delta_{tr}H^o$ data for acetone, nitromethane and hexamethyl phosphoric triamide are available) and also the list of ions is somewhat shorter. Heat capacities and volumes of transfer are known for much fewer ions, and the values are shown in Tables 5 and 6.

Limiting ionic conductivities λ^∞ at 25°C in non-aqueous solvents are shown in Table 7, based mainly data by Krumgalz[37]. Ionic *B*-coefficients at 25°C in non-aqueous solvents are shown in Table 8, based on data by Jenkins and Marcus[38].

C. INTERPRETATION

The Gibbs free energies and enthalpies of transfer of ions from water to non-aqueous solvents have been interpreted in terms of the compensation of the large electrostatic effect in the solvation shell of the ion and more subtle effects of interaction of the ions with the reference and target solvents[39]. Abraham and Liszi[40] have pointed out that due to dielectric saturation, the relative permittivity and its temperature coefficient may be the same in this shell irrespective of the solvent. If this is indeed so, then on transfer of the ion from water to the target solvent there would be no change in the dominant electrostatic term arising from the change of solvent in the solvation shell. The electrostatic effect beyond this shell, i.e., beyond $r+\Delta r$ can be described by the Born equation as $[N_{Av}e^2/8\pi\varepsilon_o(r+\Delta r)](1/\varepsilon_W-1/\varepsilon_s)$, which is relatively small. The thickness of the first solvation shell, Δr, however, need not be the same in different solvents. This difference can be expressed in terms of the different molar volumes of water and the target solvent. A further effect depends on the consideration of the ions as Lewis acids (cations) and bases (anions) interacting with the water and solvents that also have Lewis acid and/or base properties[39].

Table 4. The enthalpies of transfer of ions from water into selected non-aqueoue solvents.*

Ion	MeOH	PC	$HCONH_2$	DMF	MeCN	Py	Me_2SO	DMThF
Li^+	-22	3	-6	-32	-8	-56	-27	22
Na^+	-21	-10	-17	-33	-13	-30	-29	-35
K^+	-19	-23	-18	-39	-23	-43	-35	-25
Rb^+	-17	-25	-18	-38	-25	-42	-35	-25
Cs^+	-14	-28	-18	-37	-26	-50	-33	-42
Ag^+	-21	-11	-23	-39	-53	-106	-53	-141
Tl^+	-54	-47	-38	-53	-49	-86		-65
Me_4N^+	0	-18	-2	-13	-15		-16	
Et_4N^+	7	0	6	3	-2	-4	4	-11
Pr_4N^+	15	11	16	13	9		16	
Bu_4N^+	20	21	26	20	18	8	26	4
Ph_4As^+	-1	-13	-1	-17	-11	-23	-11	0
Ba^{2+}	-61		-40	-86	-9	-26	-80	
Cu^{2+}	-33				12	-145	-57	
Zn^{2+}	-47		-24	-63	20	-86	-62	-54
Cd^{2+}	-42		-28	-63	8	-115	-71	-92
Hg^{2+}	-24				10	-160	-83	
Pb^{2+}	-16			-80	-5	-75	-85	-85
F^-	5		20	59			30	
Cl^-	8	26	4	18	19	28	20	1
Br^-	5	15	-2	1	8	11	5	12
I^-	-1	-2	-7	-15	-8	-7	-12	-1
N_3^-	1	17		-1	9		-3	
SCN^-	-3		-11	-10		-5		-1
NO_3^-	15				13	0	5	14
ClO_4^-	-3	-17	-20	-23	-17	-19	-18	-11
Pi^-	-1				-13	-11	-12	-31
BPh_4^-	-1	-13	-1	-17	-11	-23	-11	

*. In $kJ\ mol^{-1}$, using TATB assumption.

Table 5. Standard partial molar ionic heat capacities at constant pressure, C_p^{∞}/J K^{-1} mol^{-1}, in selected non-aqueoue solvents at 25°C.

Ion	MeOH	EtOH	PrOH	PC	NMF	DMF	MeCN	$MeNO_2$	Me_2SO
Li^+	-20	3	-89	27	-6	-14	52	200	-46
Na^+	42	91	13	57	47	32	81	134	-26
K^+	56	129		38	51	35	31	30	
Rb^+				36		34			-35
Cs^+	43	122		36	49	29	33	1	
Me_4N^+	138			159					
Et_4N^+	300	291	280	267		257	266		
Pr_4N^+	432	418	396	383		385			
Bu_4N^+	557	589	577	496		517	513		
Pe_4N^+	670	821	753	610			626		
Ph_4P^+	555	594	539	496	572	480	490	475	515
Ph_4As^+	596			512			501		
F^-	-131	-194						71	60
Cl^-	-102	-185	-247	44	10	108	55	61	58
Br^-	-76	-170	-211	44	27	84	38	107	95
I^-	-56	-93	-123	41	37	58	29	64	114
ClO_4^-	53			103		68	76		107
BPh_4^-	555	594	539	498	572	480	490	475	515

Table 6. Standard partial molar ionic volumes, V^{∞}/cm^{-3}mol-1, in selected non-aqueoue solvents at 25°C.

Ion	MeOH	EtOH	EG	PC	NMF	DMF	MeCN	$MeNO_2$	Me_2SO
Li^+	-18.5	-18.7	-8.7	-8.6	-8.2	-9.9	-16.2	-17.6	-5.3
Na^+	-18.2	-9.1	-3.6	-4.5	-3.5	-1.5	-16.0	-12.6	2.9
K^+	-7.4	-0.7	6.2	2.5	4.8	6.0	-5.0	-8.3	11.2
Rb^+	-3.0	5.2	11.8	6.8	8.6	10.1	-1.7	-3.4	17.2
Cs^+	3.4	13.1	20.0	13.4	14.6	16.6	5.0	2.0	22.6
NH_4^+	3.3	8.6			10.2	11.5	4.5		
Me_4N^+	66.9	76.1	78.9	80.9					83.0
Et_4N^+	125.9	138.0	137.7	142.2	139.3	140.9	134.8		140.0
Pr_4N^+	196.8	206.9	206.2	211.4	210.2	212.5	206.2		211.0
Bu_4N^+	263.6	274.5	275.3	280.2	279.3	282.1	274.5	284.9	282.0
Pe_4N^+	337.5	341.2		349.7			343.9		344.0
Ph_4P^+	263.1	263.3	285.3	287.9	286.5	284.0	274.4		289.3
Ph_4As^+	269.0		290.9	290.4		291.9	283.1		294.3
F^-	-0.9	-13.8	5.2	-5.2	6.0	-15.1	-26.4	13.0	-1.3
Cl^-	13.9	13.4	24.5	17.6	25.9	7.4	1.2	13.8	11.4
Br^-	22.0	15.4	31.0	23.8	31.2	9.7	6.8	21.2	16.7
I^-	29.2	26.3	40.4	36.4	40.9	23.6	20.6	34.1	31.1
SCN^-				41.9	46.0		24.7		
NO_3^-	29.5	24.4			36.8	18.7			25.5
ClO_4^-	39.5			46.0	46.3		32.1		42.8
BPh_4^-	251.1	251.3	283.9	285.9	284.5	282.0	272.4	282.9	287.3

Table 7. Limiting ionic conductivities, λ^{∞}/cm W^{-1} mol^{-1}, in selected non-aqueoue solvents at 25°C.

Ion	MeOH	EtOH	PC	$HCONH_2$	NMF	DMF	MeCN	$MeNO_2$	Py	Me_2SO
H^+	146.1	62.7		10.41		35.0		64.5		15.5
Li^+	39.6	17.1	7.14	8.32	10.1	26.1	68.8	53.9	25.9	11.77
Na^+	45.2	20.3	9.13	9.88	16.01	30.0	76.8	56.8	26.6	13.94
K^+	52.4	23.5	11.08	12.39	16.49	31.6	83.7	58.1	31.8	14.69
Rb^+	56,2	24.9	11.73	12.82	17.94	33.2	85.8			14.96
Cs^+	61.5	26.3	12.16	13.38	18.52	35.4	87.4			16.19
Ag^+	50.1	20.6	11.96			35.7	96.0	50.8	34.4	16.08
Tl^+			13.06	15.60		39.5	91.1	58.8		
NH_4^+	57.6	22.1		14.94	24.59	39.4	97.1	62.8	46.6	
Me_4N^+	68.7	29.6		12.84		39.9	94.5	56.1		17.93
Et_4N^+	61.1	28.7		10.44		36.6	85.0	48.8		16.39
Pr_4N^+	46.1	22.5		7.86		30.0	70.4	40.1		
Bu_4N^+	39.1	19.4	9.38	6.54		26.9	61.7	34.9	22.7	10.93
Cl^-	52.4	21.9	18.77	17.46	25.61	53.8	100.4	62.5	51.4	23.41
Br^-	56.5	24.5	19.41	17.51	28.16	53.4	100.7	62.8	51.2	23.76
I^-	62.6	27.0	18.82	16.90	28.39	51.1	102.6	63.6	49.0	23.59
SCN^-	61.9	27.5	22.21	17.51	28.65	59.2	113.3	72.1		28.93
NO_3^-	61.0	24.8	20.92	17.66		57.1	106.2	66.7	52.5	26.84
ClO_4^-	70.8	30.5	18.94	16.63	27.37	51.6	102.8	65.8	47.5	24.39
Pi^-	46.9	25.4	13.12		19.75	37.0	77.3	45.4	33.6	17.08
Bu_4B^-	38.9	19.7	9.39			26.4	61.4	35.0		11.88
BPh_4^-	36.5					24.4	57.3	32.8	20.5	12.6

Table 8. Ionic *B*-coefficients of viscosity, *B*/mol dm^{-1}, in selected non-aqueoue solvents at 25°C.

Ion	MeOH	PC	FA	NMF	DMF	HMPT	MeCN	Me_2SO	TMS	CH_2Cl_2
Li^+	0.34	0.79	0.31	0.07		1.13	0.43	0.61	0.57	
Na^+	0.31	0.61	0.42	0.09	0.72	1.17	0.45	0.53	0.80	
K^+	0.27		0.20	0.11	0.57	0.89	0.39	0.54	0.61	
Rb^+			0.17			0.88		0.52	0.54	
Cs^+	0.07		0.15	0.15		0.87		0.49	0.41	
Me_4N^+	0.02			-0.07				0.41		
Et_4N^+	0.14	0.26		0.04	0.55		0.33	0.48		0.40
Pr_4N^+	0.24	0.40		0.23	0.74		0.39	0.56		0.50
Bu_4N^+	0.38	0.59	0.51	0.37	0.84	0.99	0.50	0.61	0.29	0.69
Pe_4N^+	0.528	0.74		0.51	0.89	1.26	0.67	0.63		
Ph_4P^+						1.90	0.81			0.75*
Cl^-	0.048	0.25	0.17	0.52		0.74		0.26	0.49	0.33
Br^-	0.046	0.46	0.13	0.47		0.73	0.34	0.30	0.56	0.29
I^-	0.42	0.29	0.10	0.45	0.51	0.60	0.32	0.27	0.54	0.23
ClO_4^-		0.26			0.18	0.73			0.43	0.13
BPh_4^-		0.72			1.02	1.84	0.79		1.45	0.75

* For Ph_4As^+ rather than Ph_4P^+

The enthalpies of transfer of small cations are all negative because of the Born term and the larger electron pair donation ability of most of the solvents studied than that of water. For anions the enthalpy of transfer is negative but small, due to their larger inherent sizes, whereas for the hydrophobic ions it may become positive for the larger ones. The entropy of transfer is generally negative, since the water released from the hydration shell returns to highly structured, low-entropy, water, whereas the solvent that replaces it comes from a relatively unstructured (less structured) solvent. The combination of a negative enthalpy and a negative entropy of transfer may then lead to an either positive or negative Gibbs free energy.

The heat capacity change on transfer is a complicated function of the properties of the ions and of the solvents. For the monoatomic ions it is positive, except for transfer of Li^+ into some solvents and of the halide anions into protic solvents. It is negative for the transfer of the hydrophobic ions into all solvents. It generally becomes more positive or less negative as the size of the monoatomic ions increases and more negative as the size of the hydrophobic ions increases. The volume change of transfer depends on the compressibility of the solvent but also on other factors. It is a complicatedfunction of the properties of the ions and solvents, such as the strength of the hydrogen bonding of the solvent in the case of the transfer of anions. The ionic conductivities depend strongly on the viscosities of the solvents, but the product $\lambda^\infty \eta$ for a given ion is nearly constant (Walden's rule), reflecting the nearly invariant size of the solvated ion, i.e., $r + \Delta r$ (Stokes' law)[37]. The change of the ionic viscosity *B*-coefficients with the nature of the solvent is linear with the molar volume of the solvent for a given ion[41].

VI. PREFERENTIAL ION SOLVATION IN MIXED SOLVENTS

In a (binary) mixture of solvents ions generally are surrounded by an environment which differs in composition from that of the bulk solvent. This is due to preferential solvation of the ions by the components of the mixture, in a manner that is predictable from the solvation properties of the ions in the neat solvents and the mutual interactions of the solvents. Two theoretical approaches have been proposed to permit such predictions: the quasilattice quasi-chemical (QLQC) model and the inverse Kirkwood-Buff integral (IKBI) method. In the former[43], the binary solvent containing an ion at infinite dilution is supposed to have all particles occupying sites in a quasilattice, characterized by a lattice parameter (coordination number) Z, which may be composition-dependent. The pairwise interaction of a particle i with any of its neighbors j, e_{ij} is assumed to be independent of the natures of its other neighbors. The quasi-chemical formulation of the number of ii, jj, and ij pairs as a function of the energies e_{ii} , e_{jj} , and e_{ij} is also assumed[42]. If one of the components of the mixture is taken to be the reference solvent, then the Gibbs free energy of transfer into the mixture $\Delta_{tr}G^\circ$ can be related to that into the other (target) solvent ($\Delta_{tr}G^o$ at x=1), the composition of the solvent mixture, x, the excess Gibbs free energy of mixing of the two solvents at the equimolar composition $G^E(x=0.5)$, and the lattice parameter, Z. These quantities also determine the preferential solvation, i.e., the excess (deficiency) of the target solvent in the solvation shell of the ion over (below) the bulk composition[43].

The IKBI method deals with the correlation volume around the ion, in which the solvent composition differs from that of the bulk, not necessarily the first solvation shell. This volume is calculated iteratively from the dimensions (molar volumes) of the solvent molecules and the composition in this volume. This, in turn, is obtained from the first derivative of the Gibbs free energy of transfer from the reference to the target solvent, $d\Delta_{tr}G^o/dx$ and the second derivative of the excess Gibbs free energy of mixing of the two solvents, d^2G^E/dx^2. The Kirkwood-Buff integrals are then calculated from these data and the partial molar volumes of the solvents in the mixture at each composition x, to yield again the preferential solvation as defined above. These methods have been applied to several systems, e.g., aqueous MeOH, DMSO, and MeCO, and mixtures of the latter two and of each of them with DMF[43,44], with fair agreement between the approaches. It is clear that if $\Delta_{tr}G^o$ is positive then the reference solvent is preferred near the ion, if it is negative then the target solvent is the preferred one. This preference is modified, however, by the mutual interaction of the two solvents (expressed by G^E) in a quantitative but not a qualitative manner.

Other methods have also been applied to this problem, but their description and detailed data are outside the scope of this review.

VII. REFERENCES

1. **Ben-Naim, A. and Marcus, Y.**, Solvation thermodynamics of nonionic solutes, *J. Chem. Phys.* 81, 2016, 1984.
2. **Marcus Y.**, Ionic radii in aqueous solutions, *Chem. Rev.*, 88, 1475, 1988.
3. **Shannon, R. D. and Prewitt, C. T.**, Effective ionic radii in oxides and fluorides, *Acta Crystallogr.*, 25, 925, 1969.
4. **Jenkins, H. B. D. and Thakur, K. P.**, Reappraisal of thermochemical radii for complex ions, *J. Chem. Educ.*, 56, 576, 1979.
5. **Marcus, Y. and Loewenschuss, A.**, Standard entropies of hydration of ions, *Annu. Rep. C* 1984, 81, 1985.
6. **Heydweiller, A.**, Optische untersuchungen an wasserigen elektrolytlosungen, *Phys. Z.*, 26, 526, 1925.
7. **Marcus, Y.**, On enthalpies of hydration, ionization potentials, and the softness of ions, *Thermochim. Acta*, 104, 389, 1986.
8. **Marcus, Y.**, Linear solvation energy relationships. Correlation and prediction of the distribution of organic solutes between water and immiscible organic solvents, *J. Phys. Chem.*, 95, 8886, 1991.
9. **Leo, A., Hansch, C. and Elkins, D.**, Partition coefficients and their uses, *Chem. Rev.*, 71, 525, 1971.
10. **Marcus, Y.**, Viscosity B-coefficients, structural entropies and heat capacities, and the effects of ions on the structure of water, *J Solution Chem*, 23, 831, 1994.

11. **Marcus, Y.**, The properties of organic liquids that are relevant to their use as solvating solvents, *Chem. Soc. Rev.*, 22, 409, 1993.
12. **Riddick, J. A., Bunger, W. B. and Sakano, T. K.**, *Organic Solvents*, 4th Ed. New York: Wiley, 1986.
13. **Marcus, Y.**, The structuredness of solvents, *J. Solution Chem.*, 21, 1217, 1992.
14. **Marcus, Y.**, Linear solvation energy relationships. A scale describing the 'softness' of solvents, *J. Phys. Chem.*, 91, 4442, 1987.
15. **Wagman, D. D., Evans, W. H., Parker, V. B., Schumm, R. H., Halow, I., Bailey, S. M., Churney, K. L. and Nutall, R. L.**, The NBS tables of chemical thermodynamic properties, *J. Phys. Chem. Ref. Data*, 11, supp. 2, 1, 1982.
16. **Conway, B. E.**, The evaluation and use of properties of individual ions in solution, *J. Solution Chem.*, 7, 721, 1978.
17. **Marcus, Y.**, The thermodynamics of ion solvation. Part 4. Application of the TATB extrathermodynamic assumption to the hydration of ions and the properties of hydrated ions, *J. Chem. Soc., Faraday Trans.* 1, 83, 2985, 1987.
18. **Halliwell, H. F. and Nyburg, S. C.**, Enthalpy of hydration of the proton, *Trans. Faraday Soc.*, 59, 1126, 1963.
19. **Marcus, Y.**,The thermodynamics of solvation of ions. Part 2. The enthalpy of hydration at 298.15 K, *J Chem Soc, Faraday Trans 1*, 83, 339, 1987.
20. **Loewenschuss, A. and Marcus, Y.**, The entropies of gaseous polyatomic ions, *Chem. Rev.*, 84, 89, 1984.
21. **Eastman, M.**, Electromotive force of electrolytic thermocouples and thermocells and the entropy of transfer of ions, *J. Am. Chem. Soc.*, 50, 292, 1928.
22. **Trasatti, S.**,The absolute electrode potential: an explanatory note, *Pure Appl. Chem.*, 58, 955, 1986.
23. **Abraham, M. H. and Marcus, Y.**, The thermodynamics of solvation of ions. Part 1. The heat capacities of hydration at 298.15 K, *J. Chem. Soc., Faraday Trans. 1*, 82, 3255, 1986.
24. **Zana, R. and Yeager, E.**, Determination of ionic partial molal volumes from ionic vibration potentials, *J. Phys. Chem.*, 70, 954, 1966.
25. **Robinson, R. A. and Stokes, R. H.**, *Electrolyte Solutions*, 2nd Ed., London: Butterworths, 1959.
26. **Marcus, Y.**, A simple empirical model describing the thermodynamics of hydration of ions of widely varying charges, sizes, and shapes, *Biophys. Chem.*, 51, 111, 1994.
27. **Marcus, Y.**, Thermodynamics of solvation of ions. Part 5. Gibbs free energies of hydration at 298.15 K, *J. Chem. Soc., Faraday Trans.*, 87, 2995, 1991.
28. **Kim, J.-I.**, Preferential solvation of single ions. A critical study of the Ph_4AsPh_4B assumption for single ion thermodynamics in amphiprotic and dipolar-aprotic solvents, *J. Phys. Chem.*, 82, 191, 1978.
29. **Marcus, Y., Hefter, G. and Pang, T.-S.**, Ionic partial molar volumes in non-aqueous solvents, *J. Chem. Soc., Faraday Trans.*, 90, 1899, 1994.
30. **Marcus, Y. and Hefter, G.** ,Ionic partial molar heat capacities in non-aqueous solvents, *J Chem Soc, Faraday Trans*, to be submitted, 1995.
31. **Marcus, Y. and Migron, Y.**, Solubility of asymmetric quaternary and non-quaternary ammonium salts in water and non-aqueous solvents at 298.15 K and their transfer Gibbs free energies between them, *J. Chem. Soc., Faraday Trans.* 89, 2437-2439, 1993.
32. **Shao, Y., Stewart, A. A. and Girault, H. H.**, Determination of the half-wave potential of the species limiting the potential window. Measurements of the transfer Gibbs energies at the water/1,2-dichloroethane interface, *J. Chem. Soc., Faraday Trans.*, 87, 2593, 1991.
33. **Alexander, R., Parker, A. J., Sharpe, J. H. and Waghorne, W. E.**, Solvation of ions. XVI. Solvent activity coefficients of single ions. A recommended extrathermodynamic assumption, *J. Am. Chem. Soc.*, 94, 1148, 1972.
34. **Gritzner, G.**, Gibbs free energies of transfer (ΔG) for alkali metals and Tl , *Inorg. Chim. Acta*, 24, 5, 1977.
35. **Krishnan, C. V. and Friedman, H. L.**, Solvation enthalpies of various ions in water, propylene carbonate, and dimethyl sulfoxide, *J. Phys. Chem.*, 73, 3934, 1969.
36. **Gritzner, G. and Lewandowsky, A.**, Temperature coefficients of half-wave potentials and entropies of transfer of cations in aprotic solvents, *J. Chem. Soc., Faraday Trans.*, 87, 2599, 1991.

37. **Krumgalz, B. S.**, Separation of limiting equivalent conductances into ionic contributions in non-aqueous solutions by indirect methods, *J. Chem. Soc., Faraday Trans.*, 79, 571, 1983.
38. **Jenkins, H. B. D. and Marcus, Y.**, The viscosity B-coefficients of ions in solution, *Chem. Rev.*, 95, accepted, 1995.
39. **Marcus, Y., Kamlet, M.J. and Taft, R.W.**, Linear solvation energy relationships. Standard molar Gibbs free energies and enthalpies of transfer of ions from water into nonaqueous solvents, *J. Phys. Chem.*, 92, 3613, 1988.
40. **Abraham, M. H. and Liszi, J.**, Calculations on ionic solvation. Part 2. Entropies of solvation of gaseous ions using a one-layer continuum model, *J. Chem. Soc., Faraday Trans. 1*, 74, 2858, 1978.
41. **Feakins, D., Freemantle, D. J. and Lawrence, K.G.**, Transition state treatment of relative viscosities of electrolytic solutions, *J. Chem. Soc., Faraday Trans. 1*, 70, 795, 1974.
42. **Guggenheim, E.A.**, *Mixtures*, Clarendon press: Oxford, 1952
43. **Marcus Y.**, Preferential solvation of ions in mixed solvents. Part 4. Comparison of the Kirkwood-Buff and quasi-lattice quasi-chemical approaches, *J. Chem. Soc., Faraday Trans. 1*, 85, 3019, 1989.
44. **Labban, A. S. K. and Marcus, Y.**, The solubility and solvation of salts in mixed nonaqueous solvents. 1. Potassium halides in mixed approtic solvents, *J. Solution Chem.*, 20, 221, 1991.

Chapter 4

ADSORPTION ISOTHERMS AND THE STRUCTURE OF OIL/WATER INTERFACES

Vladislav S. Markin and Alexander G. Volkov

I. INTRODUCTION

The most common method for monolayer formation and deposition is adsorption. Traditional models for calculation of adsorption isotherms are based on the assumption that surface active compounds at the interface can substitute for adsorbed molecules of one solvent but can not penetrate the second phase [1-7]. Although this model is useful for metal/water interfaces, recent interest has focused on the surface chemistry of amphiphilic compounds which can penetrate both phases and replace adsorbed molecules of both solvents, for example water and oil [8-16]. For this reason, we present here a theoretical analysis of the generalized Frumkin adsorption isotherm for amphiphilic compounds.

It is quite difficult in general to define the standard Gibbs free energy of the adsorption equilibrium, ΔG^0_{ads}, for any substance adsorbing at the interface between two immiscible liquids. For a neutral substance i at the metal/solution interface, ΔG^0_{ads}, is usually defined as the Gibbs free energy change for the adsorption process when all species are in their standard states. It can be calculated as a difference between the standard chemical potentials in the adsorbed state and in the bulk solution minus the difference between the chemical potentials of the solvent in the adsorbed state and in the bulk solution:

$$\Delta G^0_{ads} = (\mu_i^{0,s} - \mu_i^0) - n(\mu_w^{0,s} - \mu_w^0) \tag{1}$$

where n is the number of solvent molecules which are displaced by one adsorbate molecule. For an amphiphilic substance that is adsorbed at the interface between two immiscible solvents, ΔG^0_{ads} can be estimated from the value of $\Delta\mu^0$, both in water (w) and in the oil (o). Let these solvents have the distribution coefficient P_i of the solute between two phases. Then

$$\Delta^w_{ads} G^0_{ads} = \mu_i^{0,s} - \mu_i^{0,w} - n_1 \Delta\mu_w^0 - n_2 \Delta\mu_o^0 \tag{2}$$

$$\Delta^{w'}_{ads} G^0_{ads} = \mu_i^{0,s} - \mu_i^{0,o} - n_1 \Delta\mu_w^0 - n_2 \Delta\mu_o^0 \tag{3}$$

0-8493-7694-7/96/$0.00+$.50

and

$$\Delta_o^w G_{ads}^0 = \mu_i^{0,o} - \mu_i^{0,w} = RT \ln P_i \tag{4}$$

Different definitions of Gibbs free energy of adsorption in the literature lead to different quantities and difference in interpretation of adsorption behavior of amphiphilic molecules.

We consider here the general case of adsorption equilibrium thermodynamics at the interface between two immiscible liquids..

II. SURFACE SOLUTION MODEL

The interface between two immiscible liquids may be considered to be a surface solution of surfactant in a special kind of solvent. In order to calculate the entropy of such a solution we will adopt a simplified lattice model and use lattice statistics, a widely used method for describing surface solutions.[1-3, 8] The transition from three-dimensional (3-d) to two dimensional (2-d) geometry, may cause errors in statistical formulas, if some peculiarities of 2-d solutions are overlooked.

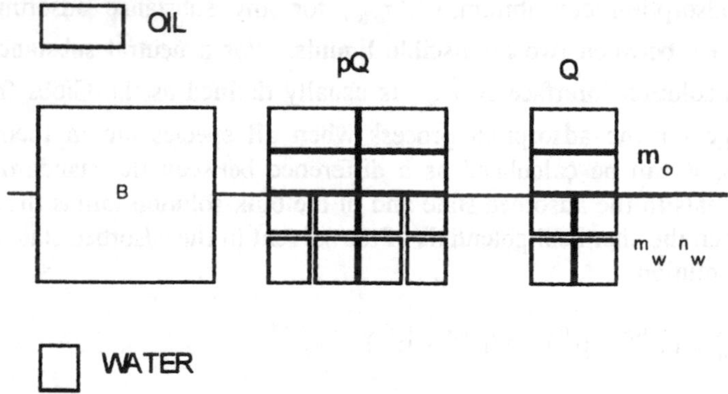

Figure 1. Structure of oil/water interface with adsorbed monolayer of amphiphilic surfactant B.

The main difficulty is as follows. When dealing with a monolayer of surfactant, one can consider this monolayer as a 2-d system. The solvent molecules do not form a monolayer, but rather a multilayer. Therefore transition from 3d- to 2d-geometry should be specified. Consider the molecules of both solvents which are substituted by a surfactant (Fig. 1). Suppose that these molecules can be assembled into columns consisting of m_o molecules of oil and m_w molecules of water. Suppose that one column of oil molecules matches the n_w molecules of water. This match of 1 oil column and n_w water columns will be considered in what follows as a quasi-molecule of solvent Q. These quasi-molecules constitute a "monolayer" of solvent. They consist of m_O oil molecules and $n_W m_W$ water molecules.

Designate the molecules of surfactant in the bulk as A, and in the monolayer as B. At the interface aggregation of surfactant molecules can take place, B <=> rA, such as dimerization of porphyrin molecules[11] or pheophytin [9] at the octane/water interface. Let the surfactant B replace *p* quasi-molecules at the interface. Therefore one can write

$$pQ + rA = B + pm_O(\text{oil}) + pn_W m_W(\text{water}) \tag{5}$$

The chemical potentials for (5) are

$$p\mu^s_Q + r\mu^b_A = \mu^s_B + pm_o\mu^b_o + pn_w m_w \mu^b_w \tag{6}$$

Taking the 2-d solution as ideal, we have

$$\mu^s_Q = \mu^{0,s}_Q + RT\ln X^s_Q \tag{7}$$

$$\mu^s_B = \mu^{0,s}_B + RT\ln X^s_B \tag{8}$$

In the bulk phase we have

$$\mu^b_A = \mu^{0,b}_A + RT\ln X^b_A \tag{9}$$

$$\mu^b_o = \mu^{0,b}_o + RT\ln X^b_o \tag{10}$$

$$\mu^b_w = \mu^{0,b}_w + RT\ln X^b_w \tag{11}$$

In all these equations X designates the mole ratio of corresponding substances. Substituting these equations into (6), one obtains:

$$p\mu^{0,s}_Q + r\mu^{0,b}_A - \mu^{0,s}_B - pm_o\mu^{0,b}_o - pn_w m_w\mu^{0,b}_w + RT\ln\frac{(X^b_A)^r}{(X^b_o)^{pm_o}(X^b_w)^{pn_w m_w}} = RT\ln\frac{X^s_b}{(X^s_Q)^p} \tag{12}$$

Using the standard Gibbs free energy of adsorption

$$\Delta^s_b G^0 = \mu^{0,s}_B - r\mu^{0,b}_A + pm_o\mu^{0.b}_o + pn_w m_w\mu^{0,b}_w - p\mu^{0,s}_Q \tag{13}$$

one obtains the adsorption isotherm:

$$\frac{X^s_B}{(X^s_Q)^p} = \frac{(X^b_A)^r}{(X^b_o)^{pm_o}(X^b_w)^{pn_w m_w}}\exp\left(-\frac{\Delta^s_b G^0}{RT}\right) \tag{14}$$

The problem of choosing standard states of particles in the bulk solution and at the interface in these processes was analyzed by Mohilner *et al.* [2].

We considered the 2-d solution of surfactant B in the solvent of quasi-particles Q, in which the mole ratios were defined as

$$X_B^s = \frac{N_B^s}{N_B^s + N_Q^s}; X_Q^s = \frac{N_Q^s}{N_B^s + N_Q^s} \tag{15}$$

Some authors prefer another set of definitions when real particles in the interface are considered. The equation for this state with real particles A, O, W becomes:

$$X_A^s = \frac{N_A^s}{N_A^s + N_O^s + N_w^s}, \tag{16}$$

$$X_Q^s = \frac{N_Q^s}{N_A^s + N_O^s + N_w^s}, \tag{17}$$

$$X_w^s = \frac{N_w^s}{N_A^s + N_O^s + N_w^s}, \tag{18}$$

and we can obtain

$$X_B^s = \frac{m_o X_A^s}{m_o X_A^s + X_o^s}; X_Q^s = \frac{X_o^s}{m_o X_A^s + X_o^s}. \tag{19}$$

The adsorption isotherm can then be presented in the form

$$\frac{m_o X_A^s}{(X_Q^s)^p}(m_o X_A^s + X_o^s)^{p-1} = \frac{(X_A^b)^r}{(X_o^b)^{pm_o}(X_w^b)^{pn_w m_w}} \exp\left(-\frac{\Delta_b^s G^0}{RT}\right) \tag{20}$$

In the past the adsorption isotherm was presented in terms of the fraction θ of the surface actually covered by the adsorbed surfactant. The detailed description of the transition to these terms for the case of organic adsorption at mercury-aqueous solution interface was presented by Mohilner *et al.*[2] The main idea of this approach can be used in our case.

If we introduce η as the ratio of areas occupied in the interface by the molecules of surfactant and oil, the mole fractions in surface solution can be presented as follows:

$$X_B^s = \frac{\Theta}{\Theta + \eta(1-\Theta)};\, X_o^s = \frac{\eta(1-\Theta)}{\Theta + \eta(1-\Theta)} \quad (21)$$

The adsorption isotherm takes the form:

$$\frac{\Theta}{\eta^p(1-\Theta)^p}[\Theta + \eta(1-\Theta)]^{p-1} = \frac{(X_A^b)^r}{(X_o^b)^{pm_o}(X_w^b)^{pn_w m_w}} \exp(-\frac{\Delta_b^s G^0}{RT}) \quad (22)$$

In this isotherm the mole fractions X_A^b, X_o^b, X_w^b of the components in the bulk solution are presented. In the general case they must be substituted with activities:

$$\frac{\Theta}{\eta^p(1-\Theta)^p}[\Theta + \eta(1-\Theta)]^{p-1} = \frac{(a_A^b)^r}{(a_o^b)^{pm_o}(a_w^b)^{pn_w m_w}} \exp(-\frac{\Delta_b^s G^0}{RT}) \quad (23)$$

If the molecules B can interact as pairs in the adsorbed layer and the energy of each new particle is proportional to its concentration, then their chemical potential, μ_B^s, instead of equation (8), should be presented as

$$\mu_B^s = \mu_B^{s,0} + RT \ln X - 2aRTX \quad (24)$$

where a is so called attraction constant [6,7]. Then after some algebra we obtain, instead of Eq. (22), the isotherm:

$$\frac{\Theta[\eta - (\eta - 1)\Theta]^{p-1}}{\eta^p(1-\Theta)^p} \exp(-2a\Theta) = \frac{(X_A^b)^r}{(X_0^b)^{pm_o}(X_w^b)^{pn_w m_w}} \exp(-\frac{\Delta_b^s G^0}{RT}) \quad (25)$$

Recall that η was introduced as the ratio of areas occupied in the interface by the molecule of surfactant to the same of oil and p was introduced as the number of columns of oil which could be supplanted with one molecule of surfactant (Fig. 1). Therefore p is a relative size of the surfactant molecule in the interfacial layer. It is reasonable to suppose that

$$\eta = p \quad (26)$$

If the concentration of surfactant in the solution is not high and the mutual solubility of oil and water is low, then we can use the approximation $X_o^b = X_w^b = 1$, so that the general equation (25) simplifies to

$$\frac{\Theta[p-(p-1)\Theta]^{p-1}}{p^p(1-\Theta)^p}\exp(-2a\Theta)=(X_A^b)^r\exp(-\frac{\Delta_b^s G^0}{RT}) \tag{27}$$

This is the final expression for the isotherm that we will call the amphiphilic isotherm. We may now compare it with the classical isotherms.

If $p = 1$ and r =1, the Frumkin isotherm is recovered:

$$\frac{\Theta}{(1-\Theta)}\exp(-2a\Theta)=(X_A^b)\exp(-\frac{\Delta_b^s G^0}{RT}) \tag{28}$$

Therefore, the amphiphilic isotherm (Eq. 24) could be considered as a generalization of the Frumkin isotherm, taking into account the replacement of some solvent molecules with larger molecules of surfactant. Of course, the amphiphilic isotherm includes all the features of the Frumkin isotherm and displays some additional ones. To elucidate them, it will be convenient to change the variable X_A^b to the relative concentration $y = X_A^b / X_A^b(\Theta = 0.5)$, where $X_A^b(0.5)$ is the concentration corresponding to the surface coverage $\theta = 0.5$:

$$y=\frac{\Theta[p-(p-1)\Theta]^{p-1}}{(p+1)^{p-1}(1-\Theta)^p}\exp(a-2a\Theta) \tag{29}$$

This equation gives the coverage fraction θ as a function of relative concentration y, while a and p are the parameters of this isotherm, the first being the attraction constant and the second - the size of surfactant. These parameters play a very important role because their impact on the shape of amphiphilic isotherm is very strong.

III. ANALYSIS OF THE GENERALIZED FRUMKIN ISOTHERM

As it is well known, the attraction constant in the Frumkin isotherm (Eq. 28) or in the amphiphilic isotherm (Eq. 29) with $p = 1$ determines the expanded-condensed transition in the adsorbed layer.[1] A family of amphiphilic isotherms (Eq. 29 with $p = 1$) with different parameters a is presented in Fig. 2. Because variables y and θ were specially chosen, all the curves cross all the points with coordinates (1, 0.5), which is also an inflection point for those curves that have one. The first curve with $a = 0$ represents the well-known Langmuir isotherm. With increasing a, the curves tend to become S-shaped, which is a manifestation of the condensation in the adsorbed layer. The expanded-condensed transition occurs for the first time when $a = 2$. This case is presented by the third curve in the Fig. 2A, which goes vertical at the crossing point. With increase of a, the curves display more pronounced S-shaped form. Therefore, increasing the attraction constant *a* makes the adsorbed layer more condensed.

Now let us change the size of surfactant *p*. In Fig. 2B, Fig. 2C and Fig. 2D the same family of isotherms is presented for *p* equal to 3, 8 and 40. The isotherms still cross at the same point, but increasing *p* suppresses the tendency of isotherms to be S-shaped. In Fig. 2B, with $p = 3$, only the fourth curve with $a = 2.84$ displays the beginning of phase transition. In Fig. 2C, with $p = 8$, it occurs only at the fifth curve with $a = 3.168$. In Fig. 2D, with $p = 40$, it happens only at the last isotherm with $a = 3.333$.

Therefore, increasing the surfactant size *p* prevents condensation of the interfacial layer. The reason is that the larger surfactant molecules must

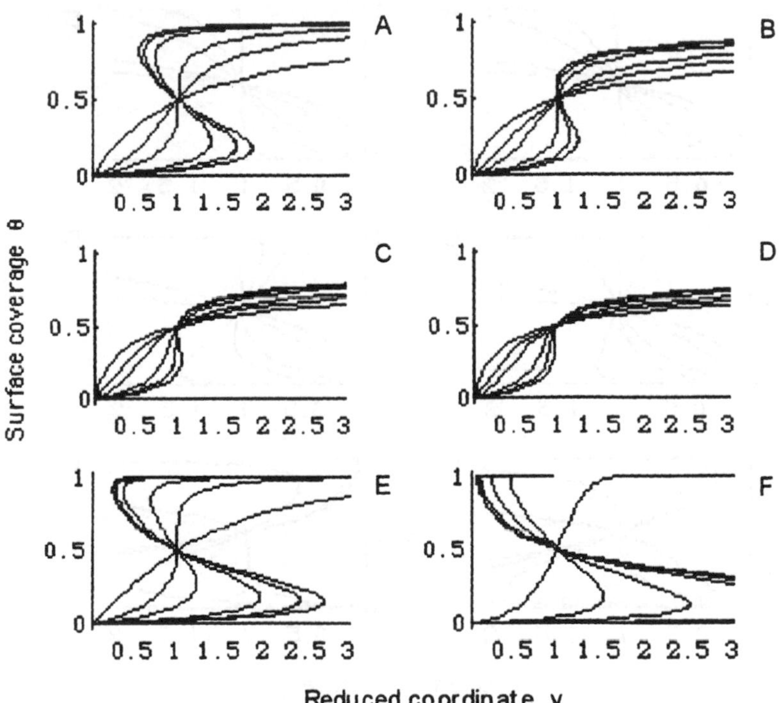

Figure 2. Theoretical dependencies of the extent of the surface coverage θ in reduced coordinates $y = c/c_{\theta = 0.5}$.

supplant more solvent molecules from the interfacial layer, which is unfavorable because the entropy of interface should decrease in this process. This becomes especially clear at higher concentrations. One can see in these figures that with increasing *p* the upper part of the bunched curves is depressed, while the lower part deforms much less. Therefore the larger surfactant molecule is less able to saturate the layer at high concentration in comparison to the smaller molecules.

We began the consideration of the surfactant size effect with $p = 1$, when surfactant is equal in size to the solvent molecule, and increased surfactant size. We will now consider the effect of decreasing of surfactant size. Fig. 2E presents the same family of isotherms with $p = 0.5$ and Fig. 2F with $p = 0.1$. One can see that smaller p values enhanced the tendency of curves to become S-shaped. In Fig. 2E the phase transition began at the second curve with $a = 1.299$ and in Fig. 2F even the Langmuir isotherm with $a = 0$ displays a concave portion of the curve.

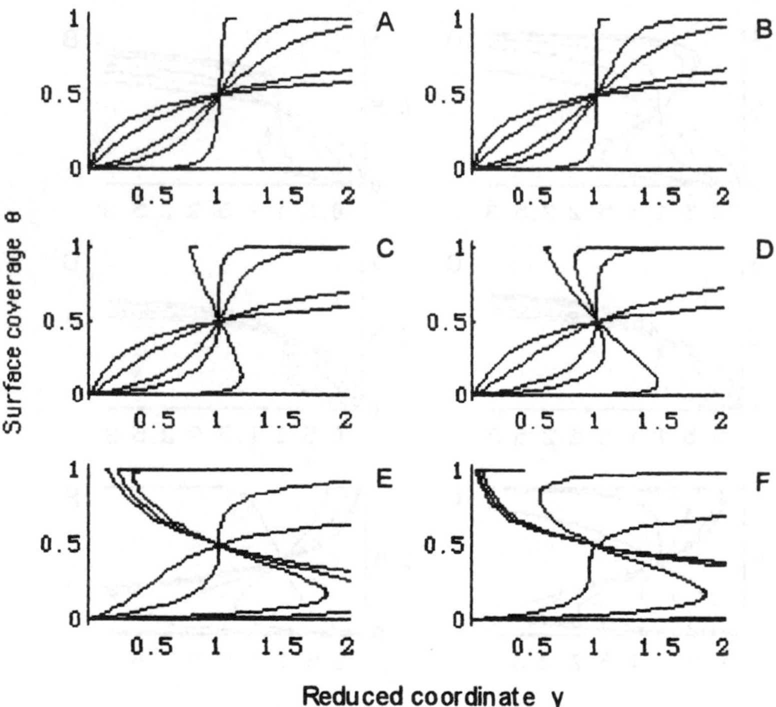

Figure 3. Theoretical dependencies of the extent of surface coverage θ in reduced coordinates $y = c/c_{\theta = 0.5}$.

We can also consider isotherms with parameter p correspondingly equal to 40, 1, 0.2, 0.1 and 0.01. Fig. 3A presents the family of isotherms for zero attraction constant ($a = 0$): there are no S-shaped curves and therefore no phase transitions to the condensed state. If we insert a very small attraction constant $a = 0.0336$, curve 5 in Fig. 3B displays the beginning of phase transition due to the very low value of parameter $p = 0.01$. Fig. 3C corresponds to $a = 0.321$. Here the isotherm with $p = 0.1$ displays the beginning of phase transition. The shift of the incipient phase transition can be followed in Fig. 3D, Fig. 3E and Fig. 3F with attraction constants corresponding to 0.609, 2.000 and 3.333.

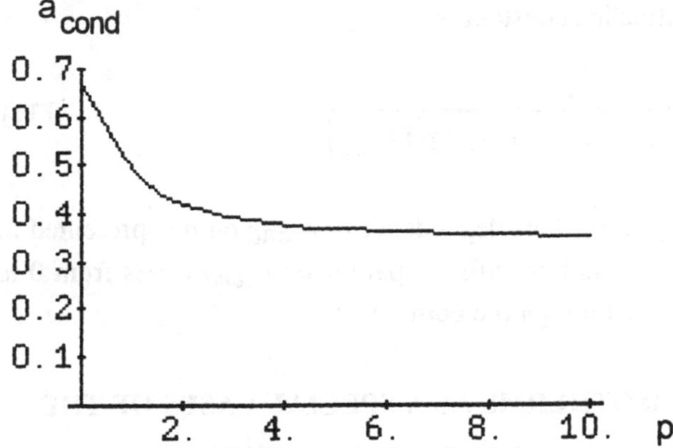

Figure 4. The dependence of the extent of the surface coverage θ_{cond} on relative size of the surfactant molecule in the interfacial layer.

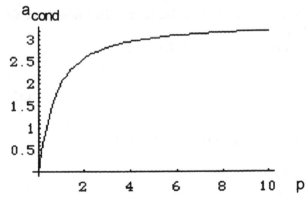

Figure 5. The dependence of attraction constant a_{cond}, corresponding to the beginning of condensation on relative size of the surfactant molecule in the interfacial layer.

In the Frumkin isotherm (28) the inflection point coincides with the crossing point of all the curves (1, 0.5). This is not necessarily the case in the generalized Frumkin amphiphilic isotherm. Analysis shows that the coverage θ_{cond}, at which the condensation can begin, does not depend on attraction constant a but is a function of p as given by the equation below:

$$\Theta_{cond} = \frac{2p - 1 - \sqrt{p^2 - p + 1}}{3(p-1)} \tag{30}$$

When p varies from 0 to ∞ the value of θ_{cond} changes from 2/3 to 1/3 as presented in Fig. 4. And when $p = 1$, critical covering becomes $\theta_{cond} = 0.5$.

In the Frumkin isotherm condensation begins when $a = a_{cond} = 2$. With the amphiphilic isotherm, condensation depends on the size of surfactant p and begins when the attraction constant is

$$a_{cond} = \frac{1}{2\theta_{cond}(1-\theta_{cond})[1-(1-1/p)\theta_{cond}]} \tag{31}$$

with θ_{cond} given by Eq. (30). This dependence of a_{cond} on p is presented in Fig. 5. When p changes from 0 to infinity, parameter a_{cond} varies from 0 to 27/8, and the curve passes through the point (1,2).

IV. CLASSICAL ISOTHERMS AS A SPECIAL CASES OF THE GENERALIZED ADSORPTION ISOTHERM

It is straightforward to derive classical isotherms of adsorption from the amphiphilic isotherm (Eq. 27).

1. The Henry isotherm, when a = 0, r = 1, p = 1, $\Theta \ll 1$:

$$\Theta = X_a^b \exp\left(-\frac{\Delta_b^s G^o}{RT}\right) \tag{32}$$

2. The Freundlich isotherm [5], when a = 0, p = 1, $\Theta \ll 1$:

$$\Theta = (X_a^b)^r \exp\left(-\frac{\Delta_b^s G^o}{RT}\right) \tag{33}$$

3. The Langmuir isotherm [4], when a = 0, r = 1, p = 1:

$$\frac{\Theta}{1-\Theta} = X_a^b \exp\left(-\frac{\Delta_b^s G^o}{RT}\right) \tag{34}$$

4. The Frumkin isotherm [6,7], when r = 1, p = 1:

$$\frac{\Theta}{1-\Theta}\exp(-2a\Theta) = X_a^b \exp(-\frac{\Delta_b^s G^o}{RT}) \qquad (35)$$

V. ADSORPTION ISOTHERM AND THE STRUCTURE OF INTERPHASE

Chlorophyll *a* and pheophytin *a* are well-known surfactant molecules that contain a hydrophobic chain (phytol) and a hydrophilic head group (Fig. 6). The amphiphilic isotherm yields adsorption parameters for amphiphilic compounds shown in Table 1. The value of p less than 1.0 indicates that adsorbed molecules of *n*-octane are parallel to the interface between octane

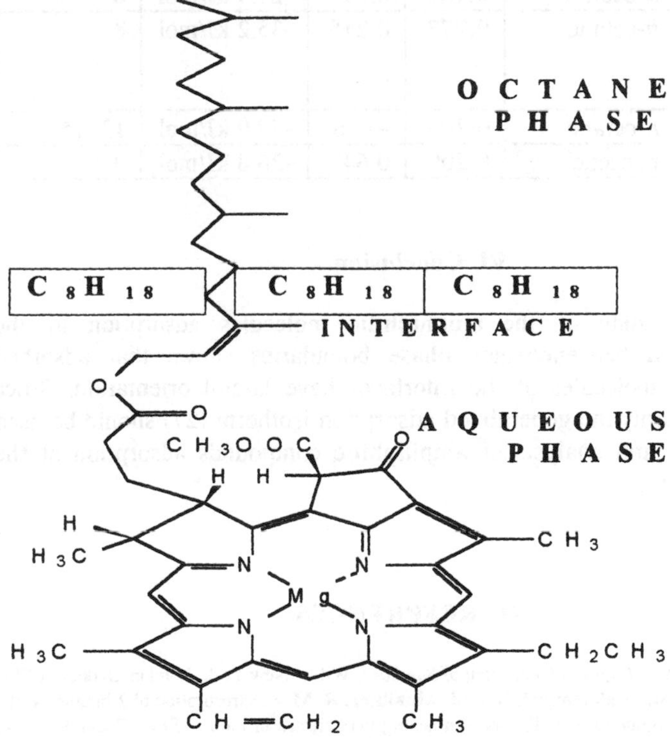

Figure 6. Structure of the octane/water interface in the presence of chlorophyll *a*, an amphiphilic compound, which can substitute 1/6 of the lateral oriented adsorbed molecule of octane C_8H_{18}.

and water (Fig. 6) Substitution of one adsorbed octane molecule requires about 4-5 adsorbed chlorophyll or pheophytin molecules. This result and our previous study of adsorption of amphiphilic compounds such as chlorophyll *a* [8] and pheophytin [9, 13, 15] are supported by molecular dynamic studies in the systems decane/water [17], nonane/water [18] and hexane/water [19]. The structure of both water and octane at the interface is different from the bulk. Adsorbed at the interface octane molecules (C_8H_{16}) have a lateral orientation at the interface, as it shown in Figure 6.

Table 1.
Adsorption parameters p, a, and Gibbs free energy of adsorption of amphiphilic molecules at the oil/water interface.

Amphiphilic compound	Nonaqueous solvent	p	a	ΔG°	Reference
chlorophyll *a*	*n*-octane	0.180	0.59	-27.4 kJ/mol	8
hydrated oligomer of chlorophyll *a*	*n*-octane	0.273	0.215	-35.2 kJ/mol	8
pheophytin *a*	*n*-octane	0.209	-0.36	-29.9 kJ/mol	13, 15
pheophytin *a*	benzene	0.200	0.643	-26.8 kJ/mol	9

VI. Conclusion.

Experimental study of the amphiphilic molecules adsorption at the octane/water and benzene/water phase boundaries shows that adsorbed organic solvent molecules at the interfaces have lateral orientation. Since parameter $p<1$, only the generalized adsorption isotherm (27) should be used for calculation and analysis of amphiphilic compounds adsorption at the oil/water interface.

VII. REFERENCES

1. **Adamson, A. W.,** *Physical Chemistry of Surfaces*, Wiley, New York, London, Sydney, 1976.
2. **Mohilner, D. M., Nakadonari, H. and Mohilner, R. M.** Electrosorption of 2-butanol at the mercury-solution interface. 2. Theory of noncongruent electrosorption. *J. Phys. Chem.* 81 , 224, 1977.
3. **Guggenheim, E.** A., *Thermodynamics*, 3rd edn., North-Holland, Amsterdam, 1957.
4. **Langmuir, L.,** The adsorption of gases on plane surfaces of glass, mica and platinum. *J. Amer. Chem. Soc.* 40, 1369, 1918.
5. **Freundlich, H.**, *Colloid and Capillary Chemistry*, Methuen, London, 1926
6. **Frumkin, A.** N., *Electrocapillary Phenomena and Electrode Potentials*, Odessa, 1919.

7. **Damaskin, B. B., Petrii, O. A. and Batrakov, V. V.,** *Adsorption of organic compounds on electrodes*, Plenum Press, New York, London, 1971.
8. **Markin, V. S., Gugeshashvili, M. I., Volkov, A. G., Munger, G. and Leblanc, R. M.,** The standard Gibbs free energy of adsorption equilibrium and isotherms of adsorption of amphiphilic molecules and clusters at the oil/water and gas/water interfaces. Adsorption of dry and hydrated chlorophyll, *J. Colloid Interface Sci.*, 154, 264, 1992.
9. **Volkov, A. G., Markin, V. S., Leblanc, R. M., Gugeshashvili, M. I., Zelent, B. and Munger, G.,** Monolayers of pheophytin *a* at the oil/water, gas/water and SnO_2/water interfaces: adsorption and photoelectrochemistry. The general isotherm of adsorption of amphiphilic molecules. *J. Solution Chemistry*, 23, 223, 1994.
10. **Clarke, R. J.,** An adsorption isotherm for the interaction of membrane-permeable hydrophobic ions with lipid vesicles. *Biophys. Chem.*, 42, 63, 1992.
11. **Volkov, A. G., Bibikova, M. A., Mironov, A. F. and Boguslavsky, L. I.,** Adsorption and catalytic properties of iron coproporphyrin II complex at the octane/water interface *Bioelectrochem. Bioenerg.*, 10, 477, 1983.
12. **Volkov, A. G., Gugeshashvili, M. I., Kandelaki, M. D., Markin, V. S., Zelent, B., Munger ,G. and Leblanc, R. M.,** Artificial photosynthesis at octane/water interface in the presence of hydrated chlorophyll a oligomer thin film *Proc. Soc. Photo-Opt. Instrum. Eng.*, 1436, 68, 1991.
13. **Markin, V. S., Gugeshashvili, M. I., Volkov, A. G., Munger, G. and Leblanc, R. M.,** Isotherm of adsorption of amphiphilic molecules and clusters at the oil/water and gas/water interfaces. *J. Electrochem. Soc.* 139, 455, 1992.
14. **Higgins, D. A. and Corn, R. M.,** Second harmonic generation studies of adsorption at a liquid-liquid electrochemical interface. *J. Phys. Chem.* 97, 489, 1993
15. **Markin, V. S., Gugeshashvili, M. I., Volkov, A. G., Munger, G. and Leblanc, R. M.,** Isotherm of adsorption of amphiphilic molecules and clusters at the oil/water and gas/water interfaces. Adsorption of pheophytin *Extended Abstracts, Fall Meeting, Toronto, Canada, October 1992,* The Electrochemical Society, Inc., Vol. 92-2, p. 978, 1992.
16. **Markin, V. S. and Volkov, A. G,** Electrocapillary phenomena at interface between two immiscible liquids, *Progress Surf. Sci.* 30, 233 (1989).
17. **Vanbuuren, A. R, Marrink, S. J. and Berendsen, H. J. C.,** A molecular dynamics study of the decane/water interface, *J. Phys. Chem.*, 1993, 97, 9206
18. **Michael, D. and Benjamin I.,** Solute orientational dynamics and surface roughness of water/hydrocarbon interfaces, *J. Phys. Chem.*, 1995, 99, 1530.
19. **Carpenter, I. L. and Hehre, W. J.,** A molecular dynamics study of the hexane/water interface, *J. Phys. Chem.*, 1990, 94, 531.

Chapter 5

THE ELECTRICAL DOUBLE LAYER AT LIQUID-LIQUID INTERFACES

Aaron Watts and T. J. VanderNoot

I. INTRODUCTION

There have been many reviews of liquid-liquid interfaces in the electrochemical literature. The most recent review of the electrical double layer at a range of interfaces is that by Parsons [1]. In view of the extensive treatment by previous authors, this review will not consider the thermodynamics of liquid-liquid interfaces. Furthermore, we will not consider adsorption of surfactants at liquid-liquid interfaces, since this is considered in another chapter.

Traditional electrochemical experiments have contributed much to our understanding of the electrical double layer at liquid-liquid interfaces. Unfortunately, many times the information has been ambiguous at best. This review will focus upon the structure of the liquid-liquid interface, but it will draw upon information from outside the traditional electrochemical literature. This will lead to a more realistic picture of the interfacial region in liquid-liquid systems. Some of our conclusions may disagree with conventional views.

A. MODEL OF GOUY, CHAPMAN, AND STERN

The original models of Gouy [2] and Chapman [3] (GC) were derived for the metal-electrolyte interface. In their model, which applied only for dilute solutions, ions were considered as point charges and the solvent was simply a dielectric continuum. With these assumptions, the Poisson-Boltzmann equation was solved to yield a relationship between potential and surface charge density. The modification by Stern [4] introduced an inner layer which consisted of oriented solvent dipoles or specifically adsorbed ions. This meant ions could only approach the metal surface to within their hydrated radius without being specifically adsorbed or partially desolvated.

However, the liquid-liquid interface is radically different from the metal-electrolyte interface. In the metal-solution case, the metal can be considered to have an effectively infinite relative permittivity, unlike the second solution phase in the liquid-liquid case. Thus, the liquid-liquid interface will be composed of two *interacting* double layers. The idea of a distance of closest approach or inner layer is also not applicable to a liquid-liquid interface where ion penetration or transfer can occur. Liquid-liquid electrochemistry has suffered from the analogies with the metal-solution interface.

B. MODEL OF VERWEY AND NIESSEN

The model proposed by Verwey and Niessen (VN) [5] was essentially an adaptation of the Gouy-Chapman model, with the interface considered as a

0-8493-7694-7/96/$0.00+$.50

mathematical plane. The two diffuse double layers were considered to be independent of one another. Only the condition of potential continuity was satisfied at the interface. The properties of each diffuse layer were calculated from the Gouy-Chapman model.

The principal result of the VN model was that the potential which appeared across each phase was proportional to the product of the concentration and the relative permittivity. This meant that the major portion of the potential would appear across the organic phase, which typically has a lower concentration and lower relative permittivity. However, the unequal potential drop did not imply that the thicknesses or charges of the two diffuse double layers were significantly different.

The limitations of the Gouy-Chapman model apply equally to the VN model. The concept of the interface as a plane was also unphysical.

C. MODIFIED VERWEY-NIESSEN MODEL

The VN model was modified by Gavach et al. [6], who suggested the presence of an ion-free inner layer of oriented solvent molecules. Samec et al. [7] extended this model by including ion penetration and image forces. The numerous attempts to determine the potential drop across the inner layer generally gave negligible values.

D. MIXED SOLVENT LAYER MODEL

Girault and Schiffrin [8] presented an alternative model which contradicted the idea of an inner layer of oriented solvent molecules. They suggested that the interfacial region was not molecularly sharp, but consisted of a mixed solvent region where there was a gradual change in the solvent properties.

II. MODELS OF ELECTROLYTES AND DOUBLE LAYERS

A. MODIFIED POISSON-BOLTZMANN (MPB) MODEL

The modified or nonlinear Poisson-Boltzmann model is an attempt to incorporate ion-ion correlations and finite ion size by retaining higher order terms in the Poisson-Boltzmann equation. Unfortunately, this increases the complexity of the equations which can only be solved numerically. Alternative approaches used integral equations such as the Hypernetted Chain (HNC) method. However, the solvent is still treated as a dielectric continuum and, as such, it will not accurately reflect solvent induced fluctuations nor discreteness effects. Solvent orientation and polarizability are also ignored. Discrete ions in a dielectric continuum solvent is known as a *restricted primitive model*. Valleau et al. [9] have reviewed and compared the various theoretical treatments based on the primitive model of electrolytes. They pointed out that despite the refinements, the MPB model was still essentially similar to the Debye-Huckel model.

Bhuiyan et al. [10] solved the MPB model for 1:1 and 2:2 electrolytes near a hard wall of unit permittivity and compared this to results from Monte Carlo simulations. When the wall was uncharged, this would approximate a gas or organic phase, both of which have lower relative permittivities than water. The results showed a surface deficit of ions repelled by image forces and ion-ion correlation effects. The ion exclusion zone was approximately 1 nm thick. The disagreement with the Monte Carlo simulations increased as the concentration increased. Both image forces and the degree of ionic screening increased as the ion charge increased.

Outhwaite et al. [11] numerically solved the MPB equation near a planar wall of uniform charge. These authors considered small separations between ions (exclusion volumes) but neglected image forces. They found damped oscillations in both the mean electrostatic potential, ψ, and ion distribution function, which were in contrast to the Modified Gouy-Chapman model. The magnitude of the oscillations and the degree of stratification of charge near the wall increased with concentration. Increasing charge on the wall also enhanced ordering.

Miklavic and Attard [12] solved the MPB equation for a restricted primitive electrolyte between uniformly charged hard walls of variable separation. However, the surface charge was uniform rather than discrete. They found that ion-ion correlations influenced the ability to screen the surface charge. This shows that ion-ion correlations will need to be a factor in any model of the diffuse layer.

Cui et al. [13,14] have recently applied the MPB4 model to the water-nitrobenzene and water-1,2 dichloroethane (DCE) interfaces. This work was prompted by their observation of the poor agreement between experimental data and the values calculated from the GC/MVN models. The MPB4 model included the effects of ion size and image forces, but they also included a term to represent the inner-layer potential distribution, which they attributed to ionic penetration and ion-ion correlations across the interface. They found that the potential drop in the diffuse layers increased with increasing surface charge density, and the rate of change was greater at lower concentration. In both cases, the potential drop was greater across the organic phase than the aqueous phase. The extent of the organic diffuse layer seemed inversely proportional to the relative permittivity of the organic phase [14]. The interfacial capacitance increased with concentration and the agreement with experimental data was much better than the GC/MVN models. For both cases, the inner layer potential drop was independent of concentration. The inner layer potential was smaller in nitrobenzene than in 1,2 DCE, which suggested that the importance of the inner layer depended inversely upon the relative permittivity of the organic phase. Thus, the inner layer made a more significant contribution to the interfacial properties for 1,2 DCE than for nitrobenzene.

Although the Modified Poisson-Boltzmann model is unrealistic in terms of its treatment of the solvent, the results clearly indicate charge stratification or layering near a charged surface. This charge layering is reminiscent of ionic ordering in crystal lattices. If the surface is uncharged with a low relative permittivity, then ions will be excluded from the interface by image forces.

B. QUASI-LATTICE MODELS

The crystal-like ordering of ions in electrolyte solutions is suggested by the charge layering which is observed in the MPB models. It is also implied from X-ray and neutron scattering from aqueous solutions [15, 16].

Enderby and Neilson [15] reviewed the structure of molten salts and strong aqueous electrolytes. They considered X-ray and neutron scattering data as well as Monte Carlo simulations of restricted primitive models (solvent continuum). In the simulations, ion-ion interactions were accurately represented, but ion-solvent interactions would require discrete solvent molecules. The Monte Carlo simulations showed oscillations in the ion-ion radial distribution functions, indicating that the ions were correlated.

The disadvantage of both X-ray and neutron scattering from aqueous solutions is that every atom will scatter, so the analysis of the scattering data is a very complex problem, since all pairwise correlations must be considered. X-ray scattering is sensitive to heavier atoms whereas neutron scattering is sensitive to lighter atoms. The major result was that ions in concentrated solutions were ordered. However, the ion-water contribution to the total scattering was 30% (X-ray) and 10% (neutron) and, as such, it is difficult to unambiguously distinguish ion-ion and ion-water terms. This was compounded at lower concentrations. Enderby and Neilson concluded that primitive models were not good enough.

Murphy [16] proposed a bimorphic quasi-lattice model. He assumed body centered cubic or face centered cubic structures. Soft (long range) repulsive forces were invoked theoretically as the principal factor stabilizing the ionic lattice. There were oscillations in the charge cloud density at all concentrations and the layer separation decreased as concentration increased. However, he suggested a 3 dimensional (3D) to planar (2D) second order phase transition occurred with decreasing concentration. Thermal agitation would continually disrupt equilibrium lattice positions, so that, on average, the lattice would reform with random orientations leading to radial symmetry. His model was capable of fitting experimental ionic activity coefficients.

An interesting model of 1:1 electrolyte solutions was developed by Bennetto and Spitzer [17]. The ion with its solvation shell was replaced by a polarizable dielectric sphere with a net charge, but a non-uniform surface charge density. The solvated ions were then fixed on lattice sites of specified geometry (dipole, fcc, tetrahedral). The remainder of the solvent was a dielectric continuum which filled the space between the lattice sites. The linearized PB equation was then solved for this system. The authors considered the difference between a structured or asymmetric ion cloud with a spherical ion cloud. As the concentration increased, the electric field of the central test ion was screened more effectively, with a consequent reduction in the solvation strength. Mean ionic activity coefficients decreased with increasing structure or asymmetry in the ionic cloud. Deviations from the predictions of the Debye-Huckel model were more significant when the solution was structured. The degree of structure will decrease with decreasing concentration and increasing ion separation. Thermal fluctuations of the solvent will disrupt the structures, which will reform continuously. This work showed the importance of solvation in promoting lattice-like structures in solution.

Horsak and Slama [18] modelled electrolyte solutions as two interpenetrating sub-lattices (cationic and anionic). Sites on a body centered cubic or face centered cubic lattice could be occupied by cations, anions, or solvent molecules depending upon the respective mole fraction. The lattice energy was calculated using only nearest neighbour interactions. Obviously, the lattice type defined the coordination. The long range ion-ion interactions gave rise to a constant similar to the Madelung constant in solid ionic crystals. Horsak and Slama found that the mean ionic activity depended upon the cube root of concentration. They also argued that the exponents of 1/2 in the Debye-Huckel model or 1/3 in their work, were indistinguishable based upon available data. Therefore, the Debye-Huckel model is not certain at low concentrations. Their lattice model gave good agreement with measured solvent activities. Horsak [19] then extended the above model to a system composed of a salt (LiCl) and two miscible solvents (methanol and water).

Zhang et al. [20] carried out Monte Carlo simulations of the Solvent Primitive Model. The ions (1:1 electrolyte) were charged hard spheres and the solvent was also a hard sphere but without a dipole moment. The solution was confined between two hard walls, one with a uniform surface charge density and the other neutral. The simulation used 30 ions and 130 solvent molecules. They found that there were fluctuations in the ion density out to 3.5 ion diameters from the charged wall. The presence of discrete solvent molecules at the walls strongly induced a structure of four to five layers of ions near each wall. The solvent played an essential role in the diffuse layer structure. The density oscillations in the solvent were modulated by the presence of the ions. Surface potentials were lower than those calculated by the Gouy-Chapman model or results for restricted primitive models.

Torrie and Valleau [21] carried out Grand Canonical Monte Carlo simulations of 1:1 restricted primitive electrolytes near a hard wall with a uniform surface charge density. They further assumed the wall had the same relative permittivity as the solvent. They found that at low surface charge densities the MGC model gave reasonable predictions of the charge density profiles, but the potential profile was less accurate when compared to the MC results. The errors of the MGC model increased with increasing concentration and/or surface charge density. The major effects were that the MGC model overestimated the potential drop and the thickness of the diffuse layer. However, the discrepancies were attributed to the neglect of ion-ion correlations in the MGC model and not finite ion size effects. Neglect of ion-ion correlations has the effect of overestimating the electrolytic screening. Both MPB and HNC models gave better, but not ideal, agreement with the MC results. Again, the discrepancies occurred at higher concentrations and surface charge densities, where packing of counterions near the wall will be more important. The MC results also gave indications of charge stratification in the solution, which arose from packing problems and repulsion near the charged wall. The counterion density could reach values as high as 50% of a close packed layer. It is possible that if Torrie and Valleau had considered image forces in their simulations, the effect of charge stratification might have been more pronounced.

In concluding this section it is obvious that the use of the Modified Gouy-Chapman or Modified Verwey-Niessen models in the calculation of surface charge densities and interfacial potential drops is incorrect. Similarly, the use of the Debye-Huckel model to calculate mean ionic activity coefficients is also to be avoided, since it is based upon the same assumptions and mathematical theory as the MGC and MVN models. At moderate to high concentrations, we could expect significant charge stratification in the electrolytes on both sides of the liquid-liquid interface with intra- and inter-phase ion-ion correlations.

III. SIMULATIONS OF SOLVENTS AND INTERFACES

A. MOLECULAR DYNAMICS SIMULATIONS

The aim of molecular dynamics (MD) simulations is to calculate time resolved molecular trajectories of the molecules in a system. This involves pairwise calculation of the energies of interaction between all the atoms in each molecule and the solution of the Newtonian laws of motion. Normally, only a limited number of molecules can be simulated and interactions beyond a certain "cutoff" distance are ignored. This cutoff distance may introduce artifacts into the simulation since long range effects have been artificially truncated. Periodic boundary conditions are also usually employed for the boundaries of the volume. A further limitation of current MD simulations is that the polarizabilities of the molecules are not considered, which could lead to inconsistent results [22]. There are two types of molecular dynamics simulations which are of relevance to liquid-liquid interfaces. The first type is the simulation of a solvent confined between walls. In this case, the hard walls can be considered as analogous to a second incompressible fluid. The second type is the simulation of two immiscible solvents.

1. Solvent Between Walls

There have been several MD simulations of solvents confined between hard walls. In all cases a small number of molecules has been used. For example, the simulations have used 150 [22], 113 [23], or 216 [24,25] molecules. It must be appreciated that such small numbers of molecules will lead to large statistical uncertainties [22] in the results.

The type of wall and the type of interaction between the wall and the solvent have been quite varied. Typically, the separations between the walls have been quite small (20 to 30 Å). Uncharged non-polar walls, which are analogous to a solid hydrocarbon, have been used in two cases. In one case a 6-12 Lennard-Jones interaction potential was used [24] and in the second a 3-9 Lennard-Jones potential [25]. In the latter paper, the authors argued that the 3-9 potential was the correct form for a molecule interacting with an infinite wall. A purely repulsive wall with an exponential interaction potential has been used [22]. This was equivalent to an elastic wall and the authors found that the results did not depend upon the hardness of the wall. A wall with 6-12 Lennard-Jones interaction plus electrostatic interactions [23] has also been studied. In this work, the surface charges were discrete and were intended to mimic the charges in either minerals or the head groups of a lecithin monolayer.

Regardless of the exact nature of the wall and the interaction potential, a common result was the observation of oscillation in the solvent density near the wall. In one case only was it noted that the amplitude of the density oscillation decreased as the simulation time increased [24], which suggested to these authors that the oscillations might be an artifact caused by insufficient equilibration. However, it must be pointed out that Monte Carlo simulations of water near walls have also shown density oscillations and these simulations determine energetically favorable configurations rather than time-resolved molecular trajectories. Furthermore, the density oscillations might depend upon the water-wall interaction potential. Purely hydrophobic walls produced density oscillations [25] even with uncharged Lennard-Jones spheres. The simulations with water gave damped oscillations whose amplitude was of the order of 10% and which extended 10 Å into the bulk [25]. The simulations with the exponential repulsive interaction also showed density oscillations which extended approximately 10 Å from the wall [22]. Softening of the wall-water repulsion had no significant effect on the density profiles [22]. This latter result suggests that "softer" organic liquids might still induce density fluctuations in water. In the simulations of charged walls, density oscillations or layering of water molecules extending 5-6 layers into the bulk (≈ 9 Å) was observed [23]. An important result was that the major force was the electrostatic interaction with the wall. The higher density of water near the wall was due to orientation by the discrete surface charges [23]. A similar effect might operate at the liquid-liquid interface when electrolytes were present in both phases.

Concomitant with the density oscillations discussed above, dipolar solvent molecules such as water exhibited a preferential orientation near the wall. The preference was for the dipole to orient parallel to the wall [22, 24]. The orientational preference was broad spanning a range of dipole orientations with respect to the wall from 60° to 120° [25]. The dipole avoided an orientation perpendicular to the wall [25]. The preferential orientation extended approximately 6 to 10 Å into the bulk [24, 25]. Basically, the water near the wall showed greater order in a plane parallel to wall than would be expected from a simple termination of the bulk phase [22]. This orientational structure has been attributed to an attempt to optimize hydrogen bonding interactions of the water molecules near the wall [25]. The structure was similar to ice I [25]. In none of the reported work was an attempt made to calculate the surface potential which should exist as a result of the preferential dipolar orientation.

Near a hydrophobic wall the number of nearest neighbors, n_{NN}, dropped to 50% of the bulk value, but the number of hydrogen bonds, n_{HH}, only dropped to 75% of the bulk value [25]. Thus, there was a relative enhancement of hydrogen bonding near the walls which was consistent with the observed reorientation [25]. However, the situation was different when the wall possessed discrete electrostatic charges. There was a decrease of hydrogen bonding near the electrostatic surface [23], although the data indicated an increase in the ratio of n_{HB}/n_{NN}. The decreased level of hydrogen bonding was believed to be caused by the stronger orientation in the electric fields near the discrete surface charges [23]. It is not surprising that solvent orientation by surface charges is greater than that by hydrogen bonding, since this occurs in the solvation of ions.

The structure induced in the water near the walls was observed to have other effects as well. Near the walls, the reorientational relaxation time was twice as long as in the bulk [22]. The diffusion coefficients perpendicular to the wall, D_{perp}, and parallel to the wall, D_{para}, were also affected. In one case D_{perp} was half the value of D_{para} which remained close to bulk values [22]. In a second case, D_{para} was greater near the wall than in bulk solution, but D_{perp} was approximately the same as bulk [24]. It was suggested that the 25% fewer hydrogen bonds allowed faster lateral diffusion [24]. In either case, the perpendicular diffusion coefficient was observed to be less than the corresponding parallel value.

The results discussed above have several implications for liquid-liquid interfaces. If the liquid hydrocarbon is considered analogous to a wall, then we might expect to see ordering in the water near the interface. This would consist of oscillations in the density, preferential orientation and differences in nearest neighbor and hydrogen bonding interactions. Of particular interest, is the fact that the parallel and perpendicular diffusion coefficients should show a spatial variation near the liquid-liquid interface. It must be noted that the observed effects may be smaller when the wall is a liquid hydrocarbon.

2. Liquid-Liquid Interfaces

A limited number of molecular dynamics simulations have been made of the liquid-liquid interface. The same general conditions and limitations apply to these simulations as for the MD simulations of water near hard walls. It has been pointed out that a more accurate simulation should include polarizabilities of the solvents [26].

As in the case of the MD simulations of solvents near hard walls (section III.A.1) the number of molecules in the MD simulations of liquid-liquid interfaces has been limited (cf. Table 1).

In many of the MD simulations, density oscillations could be observed extending into the bulk phase. This might be a similar effect to that observed with the hard wall simulations or it might be an artifact of the sampling statistics. In general, the bulk phases possessed bulk properties [26-29]. It was observed in one simulation that the interfacial density decreased as the intermolecular repulsion between the two solvents increased [30].

The interfacial thickness will be comprised of three contributions: molecular discreteness; the intrinsic compositional profile; and thermally induced surface fluctuations. The contributions from molecular discreteness and the intrinsic compositional profile, which arises even with mean field or continuum models, are difficult to quantitatively assess. The sharpness of the interface changed dramatically as the Lennard-Jones energy parameter decreased, leaving only electrostatic interactions [26]. The surface tension also increased as the Lennard-Jones energy parameter decreased [26]. From the density profiles, the average thickness of the interfacial region was approximately 10 Å [26,27,29].

TABLE 1
Numbers of Molecules in Molecular Dynamics Simulations

Non-polar Solvent	Polar Solvent	Reference
50 decane	389 water	26
108 1,2 DCE	343 water	27,28
187 hexane	1200 water	29
864 L-J spheres	864 L-J spheres	30
256 non-polar diatomics	256 polar diatomics	31
256 non-polar diatomics	256 polar diatomics + 1:1 electrolyte	32

In the simulations of liquid-liquid interfaces, the finite thickness of the interfacial region was not attributed to mixed solvation. The interfacial thickness has been interpreted as being sharp at the molecular level with the finite thickness due to capillary waves [26-29]. This interpretation of local surface deformations as being caused by capillary waves was originally due to Linse [33]. His analysis was based upon the sub-division of the simulation box into smaller domains and the determination of the maximum and minimum positions of one molecule of each phase. Unfortunately, due to the very small numbers of molecules in each sub-divided box as well as using the extremal positions of molecules, this approach would suffer from very poor sampling statistics. In our opinion, the conclusion that the interfacial roughness is due to capillary waves can not be trusted based upon the current sizes of simulation. It has been indicated that the use of periodic boundary conditions will suppress long wavelength fluctuations [34] and it will not be possible to see capillary waves whose length is greater than the simulation box size [33]. In view of these facts, it seems that the finite interfacial thickness in the simulations is essentially the intrinsic thickness predicted by the mean field theory of Fisk and Widom [35]. The interface will be only slightly thickened by capillary waves.

The MD simulations show that interfacial preferential orientation exists. Radial distribution functions showed increased structure (correlation) in the water and organic solvents at the interface relative to the bulk [27,29]. For water molecules at the interface, there were fewer nearest neighbors [27,29]. The number of hydrogen bonds was also lower at the interface [26, 27] but the hydrogen bonds seemed to be stronger [27]. Thus, water molecules reoriented at the interface to maximize the hydrogen bond interactions in the surface layer [26, 29]. Decane seemed to prefer a lateral orientation at the interface [26] but hexane did not exhibit any orientational preference [29].

As well as maximizing the hydrogen bonding interactions, the water dipoles also showed a preferential orientation parallel to the interface [27, 32] and this preferential orientation extended several molecular layers into the aqueous phase [27]. Nevertheless, near an ion in the aqueous or organic phase, the water molecules would be expected to orient with respect to the charge [32]. The reason for the preferential dipolar orientation might be the minimization of the electrostatic interaction with the non-polar organic solvent. This would mean that there would be a negligible surface potential associated with oriented solvent molecules at the interface. None of the simulations included any calculation of the surface potential arising at the interface.

Similar to the results which were observed for MD simulations near hard walls, the interfacial diffusion coefficients were anisotropic. In one case, D_{perp} was the same as the bulk diffusion coefficient, but D_{para} was higher than the value in the bulk [30]. In another case, D_{perp} was less than the bulk value, but D_{para} was approximately the same as bulk [27]. D_{perp} was believed to be lower due to orientational and positional constraints at the interface [27]. In either case, D_{perp} appears to be lower than D_{para}.

Due to the small size of the simulations, mutual solubility of the two solvents will not be observed. For 1% (mole/mole) water in 1,2 DCE, we would expect only 1 or 2 water molecules at most in the organic phase. Furthermore, the simulation would need to run long enough to allow these isolated molecules to diffuse into the bulk organic phase. In one simulation of water and hexane, a small number of hexane molecules were completely surrounded by water molecules, but there were no isolated water molecules in hexane [29]. This was inconsistent with the known mutual solubilities of hexane and water [29].

Although the simulations indicated interfacial ordering and preferential orientation, this degree of ordering at the interface would not contribute significantly to an interfacial barrier to ion transfer [27]. The interfacial roughness would also lead to an overestimation of the image forces at the interface in electrostatic models which assumed a flat interface [27].

All of the above MD simulations have not simulated polarizable solvents. The effect this would have on the interfacial properties are unknown. The effects of electric fields and/or electrolytes upon the interfacial properties are also unknown.

B. MONTE CARLO SIMULATIONS

Monte Carlo (MC) simulations consider molecular configurations and equilibrium properties rather than time evolution of molecular positions. As with the MD simulations, the simulation boxes have been small with periodic boundary conditions. Typically, one molecule is perturbed at a time and the new energy of the molecular ensemble is calculated. One MC simulation [36] which has been frequently quoted as demonstrating that the interface was molecularly sharp was an extremely simplified 2D lattice model. The large scale positional interchanges between pairs of molecules were unrealistic and neglected nearest neighbor interactions. Furthermore, the 2D square lattice would tend to enforce a smooth interface.

1. Solvent Between Walls

The only reported MC simulations of a solvent between hard walls used a small number of molecules (40, 80, and 150) [37]. As pointed out by the authors, this would lead to large statistical uncertainties [37]. The walls were infinitely repulsive and were 20 Å apart. Density oscillations near walls extending several molecular diameters into the bulk were observed. The extent depended upon the water-wall interaction potential. At the wall, water showed a preferential orientation with the hydrogen towards the wall. Surprisingly, the number of hydrogen bonds increased near the wall.

2. Liquid-liquid Interfaces

Monte Carlo simulations of liquid-liquid interfaces have used small numbers of molecules, 648 [33] or 307 [38]. The one other MC simulation used a 30x30 2D square lattice filled with two solvents [36]. This simulation, although interesting, was quite crude. In particular, the square lattice would enforce interfacial smoothness.

Linse simulated the benzene-water interface [33]. He found that there was a 10 Å thick region where the density varied smoothly from one solvent to the other. Linse argued that capillary waves contribute significantly to interfacial thicknesses [33]. He concluded that the molecularly sharp interface was broadened by capillary waves [33]. However, he did state that the concepts of a gradual compositional change and capillary waves were meaningless ideas for such small interfacial areas [33]. In reality, capillary waves will be more pronounced at a liquid-liquid interface because differences in density and surface tension will be smaller than at gas-liquid or solid-liquid interfaces [33]. Gao and Jorgensen [38] found that interfacial roughness and molecular interpenetration were difficult to separate for a hexanol-water interface [38]. The interfacial zone was 6 to 8 Å, although the overlap was confined to the α carbon [38].

In the data of both Linse [33] and Gao and Jorgensen [38] density oscillations could be observed which extended into the bulk aqueous phases. Linse [33] assumed these oscillations were not due to the presence of the organic phase, but were a statistical artifact. Gao and Jorgensen [38] noted that the density oscillations extended into the bulk with 3 Å wavelength, similar to simulations of solvents near a hard wall. If an organic solvent can give an effect similar to that of a hard wall, then it might be expected that the density oscillations would be damped with a smaller amplitude than those near a hard wall.

As with the MD simulations, it was found that the number of hydrogen bonds decreased near the interface, but the strength was greater which led to clustering[33].

Linse [33] noted the formation of interfacial trimers of water. In the simulation of the water-hexanol interface, hydrogen bonding between the water and hexanol molecules extended over 7 Å and two water molecules were involved in hydrogen bonding with each hexanol [38].

The dipole of water was preferentially oriented parallel to the interface [33, 38]. The hexanol was also more ordered at the interface than in bulk [38]. The surface potential of the interfacial region was not calculated, although we would expect it to be negligible due to the orientation of the dipoles parallel to the interface.

The Monte Carlo simulations did not reveal any mutual solubility of the two phases. Whether this is an effect of the intermolecular potentials used or insufficient sampling of configurations is impossible to assess.

3. Diffuse Layers at Liquid-liquid Interfaces

Torrie and Valleau [39] carried out MC simulations of restricted primitive electrolytes on both sides of a liquid-liquid interface. The interface was an impenetrable barrier with no net charge. This corresponded to an ideally polarizable interface without any adsorption. They pointed out that when the relative permittivities of the two phases are not equal there will be surface polarization at the interface due to image forces. The simulation results showed that the ions in the aqueous phase experienced repulsive image forces at the interface while the ions in the organic phase experienced attractive image forces at the interface. Thus, image forces will be important in liquid-liquid systems and will tend to thin the organic diffuse layer and thicken the aqueous diffuse layer. In a simple sense, ions are attracted to a polar solvent.

Torrie and Valleau [39] also found that ion-ion correlations between the two diffuse layers were significant! This inter-phase correlation led to thinner diffuse layers than if each diffuse layer saw a uniform surface charge density at the interface. This effect would be more pronounced for solvents with lower relative permittivities. The inter-layer correlations also increased with concentration. However, repulsive effects will also become more important at higher concentrations and will tend to thicken the diffuse layers. These two effects will be competitive.

As a result of these simulations, Torrie and Valleau [39] criticized both the MGC and MVN models. The MGC model will predict inaccurate values for the diffuse layer thickness, surface charge density, and potential when the solvent has a low relative permittivity. Consequently, the MVN model will also be incorrect because one solvent has a low relative permittivity. The MVN and MGC models give uncorrelated mean field behavior and neglect ion-ion correlations. In particular, the two models ignore inter- and intra-layer ion-ion correlations. However, the diffuse layers cannot be considered to be independent.

IV. EXPERIMENTAL METHODS

A. SURFACE TENSION AND ELECTROCAPILLARITY

The measurement of surface tension of the liquid-liquid interface is an important quantity for several reasons. Most importantly, the thermodynamic theory is well developed and relates surface tension to both the surface charge density and the interfacial capacitance. Changes in the surface tension also conveniently indicate adsorption of both charged and uncharged species at the interface.

The surface tension of liquid-liquid interfaces has been measured by numerous methods, some of which will be discussed. Reid et al. used the maximum bubble pressure method [40].

1. Drop Weight and Drop Time

Drop weight or drop time methods have been used successfully [41–44]. The drop weight and drop time methods rely upon the assumption of a spherical drop geometry. These methods are also not suited to situations where there is slow adsorption.

Kakiuchi and Senda[41,42] studied LiCl in water and tetra-butylammonium tetraphenylborate (TBATPB) in nitrobenzene. They considered the possible contributions of base electrolyte transfer (TBA^+ and TPB^-) at the limits of the potential window [42]. Based upon surface tension and interfacial capacitance data, they concluded that the interface was virtually ideally polarizable [42]. However, careful inspection of the data does reveal discrepancies at the ends of the potential window, suggesting that ion transfer was becoming more significant. Kakiuchi and Senda also found that the surface tension increased with increasing concentration of the base electrolytes and there were corresponding shifts in the pzc [41]. The agreement with the Gouy-Chapman model was poor, which led them to assume an ion free inner layer with ion exclusion [41].

Blank and Feig [43] studied the adsorption of amino acids and cetyl-trimethylammonium bromide at the water-nitrobenzene interface using drop weights. In their discussion they distinguished between interfacial accumulation due to adsorption (large interfacial barrier to ion transfer) or concentration changes due to transference (small interfacial barrier to ion transfer).

2. Wilhelmy Plate

The other principal method which has been used to measure surface tensions of liquid-liquid interfaces is the Wilhelmy plate [43–45]. An interesting modification which avoids some of the traditional problems involves the determination of the curvature of the cylindrical meniscus by laser reflection [45].

3. Drop Profiles

The determination of surface tension from drop profiles was developed by Girault and Schiffrin [46,63]. Their method was much more promising because it did not rely upon any assumptions about drop geometry and, in principle, it could be used in real-time to monitor the dynamic changes in surface tension. The drop profile method avoided the limitations of the static Du Nouy ring and Wilhelmy plate which rely upon perfect wetting and zero contact angle [46]. The analysis of the drop profile involved the video capture of the drop image and subsequent digitization [46]. The method gave precise results although the data analysis seemed somewhat cumbersome and inefficient.

Girault and Schiffrin [63] used the drop profile method to study the interface between an organic phase (heptane, nitrobenzene, or 1,2 DCE) and aqueous electrolytes (LiCl, NaCl, KCl, Mg_2SO_4). They noticed a surface excess of water which they interpreted as exclusion of ions from the interface. The surface excess of water decreased as the polarity of the organic solvent increased. This was interpreted as an indication of interfacial mixing. A more plausible explanation of the ion exclusion is repulsion of the aqueous ions from the uncharged and non-polar organic interface by image forces.

Kakiuchi et al. [47] used the drop profile method to study the adsorption of dilauroylphosphatidylcholine at the water-nitrobenzene interface. They determined that the monolayer was in a liquid-expanded state [47].

The presence of capillary waves at the liquid-liquid interface will tend to disrupt any monolayer structures formed at the interface, so we believe that the liquid-expanded state will be the most commonly observed state of adsorbed monolayer surfactants, unless the intermolecular interaction forces are very strong.

4. Thermal Ripplons and Capillary Waves

The mean field theory of Fisk and Widom [35] predicts an intrinsic thickness for a liquid-liquid interface, but it was unclear as to its exact source. The surface tension would depend upon the density profile across the interface with sharper density profiles corresponding to higher surface tensions. The thickness of the interfacial region would increase as the difference in densities between the two solvents decreased.

The liquid-liquid interface is elastic and flexible. Thermal fluctuations in both solvents would give rise to a large range of surface vibrations of varying wavelength. Gravity and surface tension act as the restoring forces [48, 49] and viscosity is the damping force [48, 50]. The amplitude of these thermal ripplons or capillary waves increases as the interfacial surface tension decreases. When the surface tension becomes very small (or zero) the two solvents will mix. Thus, a decrease in surface tension corresponds to an increase in interfacial roughness

B. ELECTROCHEMICAL TRANSIENT TECHNIQUES

1. Pulse Methods

Although pulse methods have been used in the study of the double layer at liquid-liquid interfaces, they are not to be recommended. One problem is the large uncompensated solution resistance which hinders fast rise-times [51]. A second problem is the occurrence of mechanical instabilities with changes in potential due to variation in the surface tension [51]. In the case of galvanostatic pulses, both the interfacial capacitance and surface tension vary quite strongly with potential. When the potential variation is quite small, then the interface may still be considered to be at equilibrium. If the current pulse is not sufficiently small, then the variation in potential will be quite large and only values, which are an average over the range of potentials, will be determined. This latter criticism applies to the use of galvanostatic pulses to determine interfacial capacitance at the water-nitrobenzene interface [52]. With the current magnitudes used, variation in potential was approximately 200 mV. The potentiostat also employed a "smoothing capacitor" between the organic phase counter and reference electrodes. The effects this would have upon the measurements is uncertain.

2. Impedance Methods

Impedance methods have been used very often in studies of both the interfacial double layer properties and ion transfer kinetics. Unfortunately, four electrode potentiostats and cells are prone to serious instrumental artifacts. Most of the published impedance data are not reliable.

Silva and Moura [53] were the first to openly question the reliability of liquid-liquid impedance data. They commented upon the large semi-circles in the complex plane impedance plots, which some took to represent slow transfer kinetics. They also noted that the angles of the low frequency imaginary impedance were potential dependent, being nearly perpendicular in the middle of the potential window but 45° at the ends. Silva and Moura attributed the artifacts to capacitive coupling between the two reference electrodes.

Wiles et al. [54] tested a variety of four electrode liquid-liquid cell designs. They determined that the instrumental artifacts which were observed in impedance measurements had a relatively simple cause. The high resistances of both the bulk organic phase and the organic phase in the Luggin capillary of the organic reference arm coupled with stray and input capacitances in the four electrode potentiostat. This was clearly proven by the use of passive electrical circuits with high resistances which gave the same effects observed in liquid-liquid measurements. Unfortunately, there is little which can be done to improve the conductivity of the organic phase. Furthermore, the exact nature and extent of any artifacts will depend upon the combination of electrochemical cell and potentiostat employed.

In view of the severity of the artifacts caused by coupling of the organic solution resistance with the stray and input capacitance of the potentiostat, VanderNoot et al. [55] reported an improved design of four electrode potentiostat. They showed how the capacitive contribution could be conveniently assessed. They also indicated how apparent inductive behavior could arise due to frequency response limitations in the current follower sub-circuits.

Kakiuchi and Senda [56] discussed impedance at liquid-liquid interfaces. They pointed out that one must account for the parallel transfer of base electrolyte which will contribute to the measured impedance even in the middle of the potential window. As a result one cannot use the simple relationship to extract C_{DL} from Z" or Y".

Even in the absence of instrumental artifacts, the complex plane impedance plots are rather featureless curves. VanderNoot and Schiffrin [57] showed how complex non-linear least squares regression could be used to analyse impedance data from liquid-liquid systems. The method allowed discrimination between the base electrolyte transfer and interfacial capacitance. One possible difficulty with impedance data from liquid-liquid systems was that the time constants for both the diffusional and ion transfer processes were comparable, which complicated the extraction of ion transfer rate constants.

Since the series of papers dealing with the instrumental artifacts in impedance measurements, there have been two important and trustworthy papers. Yufei et al. [58] studied interfacial ion pairing (specific adsorption) at the liquid-liquid interface. They used a two electrode cell and potentiostat to avoid impedance artifacts. The data was also analyzed using non-linear regression of data to extract C_{DL} in the presence of parallel ion transfer. The pzc was observed to vary with both the cation and its concentration. They interpreted the results in terms of interfacial ion pair formation. In analysing their data, they used the Gouy-Chapman model, but the data disagreed with the calculated GC results which they took to indicate specific adsorption. They attempted to calculate ion association constants using Bjerrum theory and they only considered the organic half of interface. However, the calculated ion association constants were too high compared to the measurements.

In a related study, Pereira et al. [59] investigated the differential capacitance of the water-1,2 DCE interface using a four 4 electrode cell and potentiostat. They indicated the importance of accounting for the parallel transfer of base electrolyte ions, but it was unclear from the paper whether they had in fact done so. However, they did study the effects of ions in both the aqueous and organic phases. In the case of aqueous cations, the interfacial capacitance, C_{DL}, increased as the ionic radius decreased. There was no obvious correlation for aqueous anions. Organic cations were found to specifically adsorbed as evidenced by a shift of the pzc. C_{DL} increased with either increasing concentration in both phases or decreasing ionic radius. The interfacial capacitance was determined by ion pairing at the ends of the potential window. Pereira et al. [59] noted that the results were inconsistent with two GC diffuse layers, even if image forces were included. They also commented upon the fact that the relationship between C_{DL} and the Gibbs energy of transfer and ionic radii suggested interfacial ion pairing, just as Yufei et al. [58].

The same instrumental artifacts which plague impedance measurements will also apply to ac voltammetric measurements.

C. SPECTROELECTROCHEMISTRY

1. Laser Scattering

Laser scattering from liquid surfaces is well suited to in-situ measurements in electrochemical cells. Optical light scattering investigates surface properties on the μm to mm length scale [60]. Essentially the laser light is scattered from the capillary waves which are present at liquid surfaces. Since it is a scattering experiment, the major experimental problems are mechanical vibration [48] and dust and particulates. The observed wavelengths of the capillary waves will depend upon the wavelength of the laser. Below a critical wavelength, λ_c, the decay of the thermally induced fluctuation is over-damped and non-oscillatory, whereas above

λ_c the decay is under-damped and oscillatory [49, 50]. The critical wavelengths for a variety of liquids lie in range 50 nm to 1 μm [49].

The determination of the interfacial surface tension from laser scattering off the liquid-liquid interface has only been reported twice. Katyl and Ingard [49] studied the surface tension of the methanol-hexane interface as a function of temperature. Near the critical temperature where the two phases became miscible, there was a linear decrease in the surface tension. In a similar experiment, McClure and Pegg [48] studied the interface between nitroethane and 3-methyl-pentane.

2. Ellipsometry

Ellipsometry measures changes in the polarization of light reflected from an interface [61]. It provides information the interfacial or optical thickness[62, 63] and refractive indices of phases [63]. Only a few papers have reported the use of ellipsometry with liquid-liquid interfaces.

Schmidt [62] used ellipsometry to study the interfaces formed between: CS_2 and methanol; methanol and cyclohexane/deuterated cyclohexane; and nitrobenzene and n-decane. The transition region between two fluid phases will be the sum of bulk correlation lengths plus capillary waves. The ellipticities were 20 to 30% higher than those predicted from theoretical mean field values. When a contribution from capillary waves was included the theoretically calculated ellipticity was too large. No further analysis was made.

Bonn and Wegdam [64] studied the interface between cyclohexane and methanol. They argued that the ellipticity was a measure of the optical thickness of the interface which was the sum of the intrinsic thickness (mean field theory) and capillary waves. Unfortunately, the transition from short wavelength bulk-like fluctuations to long wavelength capillary wave-like fluctuations will not be clear. The short wavelength fluctuations give rise to the intrinsic profile (molecular length scales) and the long wavelength capillary waves are associated with the macroscopic interface.

Electroreflectance measurements, which are related to ellipsometry, have not been made at liquid-liquid interfaces.

3. Non-linear Optical Spectroscopy

Second Harmonic (SHG) and Sum Frequency (SFG) Generation are two relatively new non-linear optical spectroscopic techniques. Both are based upon non-linear optical processes which are only allowed in a non-centrosymmetric environment. Molecules in a bulk phase exist in a symmetric environment and will not give rise to non-linear optical effects. Molecules at an interface or surface exist in an anisotropic environment and non-linear optical processes are allowed. Thus, both SHG and SFG are surface selective, even in the presence of overlying bulk phases. The response will be characteristic of the interface and any adsorbed molecules. There is some uncertainty concerning the thickness of the interfacial region which is anisotropic. The probable answer will be any portion of the interfacial region which is non-bulk. The attraction of these two techniques, apart from their surface specificity, is that they can be adapted to in-situ electrochemical measurements.

Sum frequency generation measurements from liquid-liquid interfaces have not been reported in the literature. There are three examples of second harmonic generation from liquid-liquid interfaces.

The first reported application of SHG measurements to liquid-liquid interfaces was reported by Bell et al [65]. They investigated the adsorption of p-nitrophenol at both the air-water and heptane-water interfaces. They indicated that the laser intensity must be low enough to avoid local surface heating or photodecomposition. The uv absorption of p-nitrophenol showed maximum absorption near 310 nm, so there was resonant enhancement with the 600 nm laser. The order parameters suggested a rather broad distribution of orientations of the p-nitrophenol with an average tilt of 40° to 50° to the interface.

Conboy et al. [66] reported SHG from the alkane-water interface in a total internal reflection (TIR) mode. Their results showed molecular ordering at the interface. Alkane chains with an even number of carbon atoms were more ordered at the interface than alkanes with an odd number of carbon atoms. This correlated well with heats of fusion. From their results, they were unable to determine the orientation at the interface.

Higgins and Corn [67] have reported SHG measurements from a liquid-liquid interface under electrochemical control. They investigated the adsorption of 2-(n-octadecylamino)-naphthalene-6-sulfonate (ONS) at the 1,2 DCE-water interface. They used a simplified four electrode cell and four electrode potentiostat. Surface tension measurements were made while the interface was under potentiostatic control using a Wilhelmy plate. The hysteresis in the surface tension with potential was due to ion transfer. When ONS was added, the pzc shifted positively and the surface tension decreased with increasing positive potential, which indicated that the ONS was adsorbing from the organic phase. From the interface in the presence of only base electrolytes there was no observable SHG signal. However, there was a measurable SHG signal from the anionic form of ONS and the increase in the SHG response correlated well with the decrease in the surface tension. The SHG response was only sensitive to the anionic form of ONS at the interface but not the zwitterionic form. Conversely, surface tension measurements were sensitive to both forms of ONS. Thus, by a combination of SHG and surface tension measurements it was possible to determine the surface concentrations of the two species at the interface.

4. Raman Spectroscopy

Takenaka and coworkers have used successfully total-internal-reflection resonance Raman spectroscopy to study the adsorption of surfactants at the water-CCl_4 interface [68-70]. In their earliest work, they investigated the co-adsorption of the cetyltrimethylammonium cation (CTA^+) and the methyl orange anion [68]. Surface tension measurements showed the formation of a 1:1 interfacial monolayer due to combined Coulombic and van der Waal's forces. Resonance Raman spectroscopy was able to detect the signal from the methyl orange in the interfacial monolayer. There was no signal observed from methyl orange in the bulk or from the interface when only methyl orange was present in the solution. From parallel and perpendicular polarization measurements, the methyl orange molecule was oriented at the interface with the long axis 50-60° with respect to the surface normal.

Nakanaga and Takenaka [69] then investigated the adsorption of the surface active anionic azo dye Suminol Milling Brilliant Red BS (BRBS). Surface tension measurements showed the formation of a condensed monolayer at the interface. The Raman measurements showed a transition from liquid-expanded to condensed as the concentration increased. Polarization measurements gave a tilt angle of approximately 86°. However, the orientation seemed to change with surface concentration, suggesting that the molecule was orienting vertically as the surface pressure increased. The addition of 0.01 M NaCl or $BaCl_2$ to the aqueous phase effectively "salted out" the BRBS, leading to condensed monolayers at lower bulk concentrations [70]. The orientation angles of the molecule were 55-65° with NaCl and 80-86° with $BaCl_2$, indicating that the electrolytes affected both the amount and orientation of BRBS at the interface [70]. The work by Takenaka and coworkers show that resonance Raman spectroscopy is a useful tool to study adsorption at the liquid-liquid interface. There have been no reports of resonance Raman measurements made upon liquid-liquid interfaces which were under potential control.

5. Fluorescence Emission

There has been one reported use of fluorescence emission to study the adsorption of acridine orange at the liquid-liquid interface [71]. Wirth and Burbage[71] investigated the interface between water and n-hexadecane, isopropylcyclohexane, *cis*-decalin, and *trans*-decalin. They found that there was a small range of orientation angles yet the out-of-plane reorientation was strongly hindered. Calculations of the amplitude of the interfacial capillary waves gave values of 4.5 Å, but this roughness would have given a much larger range of orientation angles. They interpreted this in terms of the acridine orange molecule (16 Å) being smaller than the average wavelength of the capillary waves. Thus the acridine orange was a local probe of the surface roughness. They also indicated that the surface roughness will depend upon the molecular (granularity) of the solvents. The in-plane reorientation was less hindered than the out-of-plane reorientation, but it showed no correlation with the bulk viscosity. They suggested that the molecular granularity of the interface might be the cause.

This work shows that fluorescence emission is a useful tool to study adsorption at the liquid-liquid interface. There have been no reports of its use at liquid-liquid interfaces which were under potential control.

6. X-ray Reflectivity

X-ray reflectivity measurements can provide information concerning liquid interfaces similar to that which can be obtained from laser scattering. X-rays study surface properties on length scales from 100 Å to 1 μm. X-ray scattering has not been applied to the study of liquid-liquid interfaces, although there is no reason why it could not be used. It has been used successfully to investigate the vapor-liquid interface. The thickness of the vapor-water interface was dominated by interfacial roughness due to thermally excited capillary waves [60, 63]. The capillary wavelengths lay in the range $400 < \lambda < 80000$ Å [60]. The macroscopic capillary wave model gave a good representation of the long wavelength portion of surface excitations, but it was uncertain whether the capillary wave model could be extended to shorter wavelengths.

The vapor-alkane (C_{20} to C_{36}) interface has also be studied [72]. The capillary wavelengths for the vapor-C_{20} interface at 40°C lay in the range $7<\lambda<6 \times 10^8$ Å.

Both water and alkanes had capillary wavelengths of 10 Å or greater at the vapor-liquid interface. It is reasonable to assume that the wavelengths of the capillary waves at the liquid-liquid interface will be comparable in magnitude. The amplitudes of the capillary waves at the liquid-liquid interface can be expected to be larger than at the vapor-liquid interface because the differences in density and surface tension are smaller.

7. Neutron Reflectivity

Neutron scattering from liquid interfaces has been reviewed by Penfold and Thomas [73]. Neutron scattering and absorption varies with the isotope and it is high for H where the extinction length is 1 mm. Thus, at grazing incidence the long path-length through either the water or organic solvent will result in large losses. The neutron absorption is lower for D, but the cost of deuterated solvents and the need for a neutron source means that neutron scattering is of limited practical use in electrochemical studies of liquid-liquid interfaces.

Lee et al. [74, 63] studied the interface between deuterated octane-deuterated water in the absence and presence of a surfactant. The spatial resolution of their experiments was several Å. The data acquisition time was typically 3 hours. To minimize neutron absorption in the grazing incidence measurements, the upper oil phase was made ultrathin and the solvents were deuterated. The surfactant was not deuterated. The scattering was dominated by capillary waves and the average surface roughness was a superposition of a range of sinusoidal deformations. With the adsorption of the surfactant, the surface tension decreased with a concomitant increase in the interfacial roughness. As the temperature increased the roughness also increased, but the oscillations became smoother.

V. CONCLUSIONS

A. STRUCTURE OF THE INTERFACIAL REGION

After consideration of the evidence presented in the previous sections, we are now in a position to outline a more realistic model of the liquid-liquid interface.

With regard to the pure solvents, there will probably be an interfacial mixed solvent region of approximately 1 nm where the density profiles of the two solvents vary continuously. There will not be any sudden transition or discontinuity. The solvents on either side of the interface may be ordered with density oscillations extending several nm from the interface. The solvent molecules will tend to adopt preferential orientations at the interface but these preferred orientations may be modified by electrostatic interactions with ions or surfactants.

In terms of the electrolytic double layers, there will be two interacting quasi-lattice diffuse layers in either solvent whose dimensions will be of the order of 3 nm (at 0.01 M). Within the diffuse region, the ions will tend to be structured or stratified. At lower concentrations the ionic structuring will be less pronounced.

Both the solvent and ionic structures will be seriously disrupted by capillary waves whose total amplitude may reach tens or hundreds of nm. The range of capillary wavelengths may span tens of nanometers to the μm range. In some sense, the liquid-liquid interface might be considered to be fractal. The amplitude of the capillary waves will increase with: decreasing surface tension; decreasing differences between the surface tensions and/or densities of the two solvents; and increasing temperature.

Concentration gradients associated with any transferring ions will exist on the μm length scale. Within the interfacial region, the parallel and perpendicular diffusion coefficients will vary.

There is no convenient analytic theory at present, but the lack of an improved theory is no excuse to continue using the MGC or MVN models which are clearly inadequate!

B. IMPLICATIONS OF INTERFACIAL STRUCTURE

The interfacial situation outlined in the previous section is probably too complex to model in a simple analytic way. Computer simulations may allow empirical relationships to be developed, which can then be used in experimental situations.

There will be no well defined inner and outer Helmholtz planes. Rather, there will be a region of space where there is continuous variation in solvent and ionic properties. The existence of ion free solvent layers at the interface is highly unlikely and there will probably be differing degrees of ion penetration of the interface. As the concentration increases, the screening length will decrease, but the diffuse layer will become more structured due to quasi-lattice effects. Image forces will be only important for distances less than the screening length. But the concept of image forces will be difficult to apply since there is no sharp boundary between phases.

The presence of capillary waves will modify both the solvent and ionic interfacial structures. The capillary waves will also vary with potential, since the interfacial surface tension varies with potential. The capillary waves will be larger near the ends of the potential window.

C. VALIDITY OF CONVENTIONAL MODELS

The Debye-Huckel model has very limited applicability at concentrations typically used in liquid-liquid experiments and this is especially true for the organic phase. The use of the Debye-Huckel model to calculate mean ionic activity coefficients is dubious and will introduce bias into any calculations using these quantities.

The Gouy-Chapman, Verwey-Niessen, and modified Verwey-Niessen models are equally incorrect at concentrations typically used in liquid-liquid experiments. The use of these models is not justified and will give incorrect results. The use of the Gouy-Chapman model to calculate surface charge densities and potentials of the diffuse layers is not valid. Any calculation of an inner potential difference based upon the Gouy-Chapman model is meaningless.

The experimental data in the literature is generally satisfactory barring instrumental artifacts in the impedance data. Any derived results or conclusions based upon the use of the Debye-Huckel, Gouy-Chapman, or Modified Verwey-Niessen models will be incorrect.

D. ADSORPTION

In considering the adsorption of species at the interface the exact interfacial positions will be ambiguous. Specific ionic adsorption via interfacial ion pairing is more likely to be ion association within an interfacial region of 1-2 nm, rather than ions aligning themselves on either side of a molecularly sharp interface. To speak of positions at the interface is ambiguous.

Due to the presence of capillary waves which will disrupt the interfacial structure, surfactants will be unable to form tightly packed monolayer structures. Rather we would expect to see liquid-expanded structures with a fair degree of solvent penetration. The formation of pores in adsorbed lecithin monolayers [75] might then be the result of capillary fluctuations, so that activation energies would reflect variations in solvent viscosity rather than lateral interactions amongst phospholipids.

E. KINETICS OF ION TRANSFER

If the view of the interfacial structure outlined above (section V.A) is correct, there will be no single barrier to ion transfer, especially in terms of potential. Rather there will be a gradation in properties across the interface. The Butler-Volmer theory which assumes an activated state will not be applicable. A diffusion-migration process would be a more accurate description.

The kinetic theory proposed by Kakiuchi et al. [76-78] based upon a Goldman-type current potential characteristic is more consistent with the structure of the interface. In their model, they considered a thin layer of solution which exhibited a greater friction (smaller diffusion coefficient) to ion motion. The Nernst-Planck equation for diffusion-migration was solved. A key feature of this model is that ion transfer is an activation-less process. It is possible to estimate the heterogeneous rate constant, k_0, from the ratio of the diffusion coefficient to the thickness of the layer. If we assume a value of 1×10^{-5} cm^2 s^{-1} for the diffusion coefficient and a total thickness of 10 nm for the interfacial region, then the estimated value of k_0 is 10 cm s^{-1}, which is not unreasonable. There is the possibility that k_0 might vary with concentration because the interfacial and diffuse layer structures will change with concentration.

F. KINETICS OF ELECTRON TRANSFER

With regard to interfacial electron transfer reactions, there will not be a well defined interfacial thickness over which the electron will tunnel. The concept of a distance of closest approach is ambiguous, since there will be no sharp molecular interface to separate the two reactants. Furthermore, the concepts of solvent reorganization, de-solvation, and re-solvation will also be unclear in the interfacial region. There is a distinct possibility that electron transfer reactions may involve the formation of an interfacial outer-sphere complex without the need of an interfacial electron tunnelling event.

VI. REFERENCES

1. **Parsons, R.**, Electrical double layer: recent experimental and theoretical developments, *Chem. Rev.* 90, 813, 1990.
2. **Gouy, G.**, Constitution of the electric charge at the surface of an electrolyte, *C. R. Acad. Sci.*, 149, 654, 1910.
3. **Chapman, D. L.**, A contribution to the theory of electrocapillarity, *Philos. Mag.*, 25, 475, 1913.
4. **Stern, O.**, Zur theorie der elektrolytischen doppelschicht, *Z. Elektrochem.*, 30, 508, 1924.
5. **Verwey, E. J. W. and Niessen, K. F.** , The electrical double layer at the interface of two liquids, *Philos. Mag.*, 28, 435, 1939.
6. **Gavach, C., Seta, P. and d'Epenoux, B.**, The double layer and ion adsorption at the interface between two non-miscible solutions Part I: interfacial tension measurements for the water-nitrobenzene tetraalkylammonium bromide systems, *J. Electroanal. Chem.*, 83, 225, 1977.
7. **Samec, Z., Marecek, V. and Homolka, D.**, The double layer at the interface between two immiscible electrolyte solutions Part II: structure of the water/nitrobenzene interface in the presence of 1:1 and 2:2 electrolytes, *J. Electroanal. Chem.*, 187, 31, 1985.
8. **Girault, H. H. and Schiffrin, D. J.**, Thermodynamic surface excess of water and ionic solvation at the interface between immiscible liquids, *J. Electroanal. Chem.*, 150, 43, 1983.
9. **Valleau, J. P., Cohen, L. K. and Card, D. N.**, Primitive model electrolytes II: the symmetrical electrolyte, *J. Chem. Phys.*, 72, 5942, 1980.
10. **Bhuiyan, L. B., Bratko, D. and Outhwaite, C. W.**, Electrolyte surface tension in the modified Poisson-Boltzmann approximation, *J. Phys. Chem.*, 95, 336, 1991.
11. **Outhwaite, C. W., Bhuiyan, L. B. and Levine, S.**, Theory of the electric double layer using a modified Poisson-Boltzmann equation, *J. Chem. Soc., Faraday Trans. 2*, 76, 1388, 1980.
12. **Miklavic, S. J. and Attard, P.**, A practical approach to solving the double-layer problems that includes effects of ion size and correlation, *J. Phys. Chem.*, 98, 4320, 1994.
13. **Cui, Q., Zhu, G. and Wang, E.**, The application of the MPB4 theory to the interface between two immiscible electrolyte solutions Part 1: the differential capacitance of the water/nitrobenzene interface, *J. Electroanal. Chem.*, 372, 15, 1994.
14. **Cui, Q., Zhu, G. and Wang, E.**, The application of the MPB4 theory to the interface between two immiscible electrolyte solutions Part 2: the differential capacitance of the water/1,2-dichloroethane interface, *J. Electroanal. Chem.*, 383, 7, 1995.
15. **Enderby, J. E. and Neilson, G. W.**, Structural properties of ionic liquids, *Adv. In Phys.*, 29, 323, 1980.
16. **Murphy, G. W.**, Bimorphic lattice theory of electrolyte solutions, *J. Chem. Soc., Faraday*

Trans. 2, 78, 881, 1982.

17. **Bennetto, H. P. and Spitzer, J. J.**, Theory of electrolytes, *J. Chem. Soc., Faraday Trans. 1*, 74, 2385, 1978.
18. **Horsák, I. and Sláma, I.**, A lattice model of electrolytes for the whole concentration range, *Collect. Czech. Chem. Commun.*, 52, 1672, 1987.
19. **Horsák, I.**, Extension of a lattice model of electrolytes to a ternary system of a salt and two solvents: the system CH_3OH-H_2O-LiCl, *Collect. Czech. Chem. Commun.*, 54, 1464, 1989.
20. **Zhang, L., Davis, H. T. and White, H. S.**, Simulations of solvent effects on confined electrolytes, *J. Chem. Phys.*, 98, 5793, 1993.
21. **Torrie, G. M. and Valleau, J. P.**, Electrical double layers I: Monte Carlo study of a uniformly charged surface, *J. Chem. Phys.*, 73, 5807, 1980.
22. **Marchesi, M.**, Molecular dynamics simulation of liquid water between two walls, *Chem. Phys. Lett.*, 97, 224, 1983.
23. **Kjellander, R. and Marcelja, S.**, Perturbation of hydrogen bonding in water near polar surfaces, *Chem. Phys. Lett.*, 120, 393, 1985.
24. **Sonnenschein, R. and Heinzinger, K.**, A molecular dynamics study of water between Lennard-Jones walls, *Chem. Phys. Lett.*, 102, 550, 1983.
25. **Lee, C. Y., McCammon, J. A. and Rossky, P. J.**, The structure of liquid water at an extended hydrophobic surface, *J. Chem. Phys.*, 80, 4448, 1984.
26. **Van Buuren, A. R., Marrink, S-J. and Berendsen, H. J. C.**, A molecular dynamics study of the decane/water interface, *J. Phys. Chem.*, 97, 9206, 1993.
27. **Benjamin, I.**, Theoretical study of the water/1,2-dichloroethane interface: structure, dynamics and conformational equilibria at the liquid-liquid interface, *J. Chem. Phys.*, 97, 1432, 1992.
28. **Benjamin, I.**, Mechanism and dynamics of ion transfer across a liquid-liquid interface, *Science*, 261, 1558, 1993.
29. **Carpenter, I. L. and Hehre, W. J.**, Molecular dynamics study of the hexane/water interface, *J. Phys. Chem.*, 94, 531, 1990.
30. **Meyer, M. , Mareschal, M. and Hayoun, M.**, Computer modelling of a liquid-liquid interface, *J. Chem. Phys.*, 89, 1067, 1988.
31. **Benjamin, I.**, Dynamics of ion transfer across a liquid/liquid interface: a comparison between molecular dynamics and a diffusion model, *J. Chem. Phys.*, 96, 577, 1992.
32. **Benjamin, I.**, Solvent dynamics following charge transfer at the liquid/liquid interface, *Chem. Phys.*, 180, 287, 1994.
33. **Linse, P.**, Monte Carlo simulation of liquid-liquid benzene-water interface, *J. Chem. Phys.*, 86, 4177, 1987.
34. **Allen, M. P. and Tildesley, D. J.**, *Computer Simulation Of Liquids*, Clarendon Press, Oxford, 1987, p25.
35. **Fisk, S. and Widom, B.**, Structure and free energy of the interface between fluid phases in equilibrium near the critical point, *J. Chem. Phys.*, 50, 3219, 1969.
36. **Yurtsever, E. and Karaaslan, H.**, Monte Carlo simulation of model three-component liquid systems, *Ber. Bunsenges. Phys. Chem.*, 91, 600, 1987.
37. **Jönsson, B.**, Monte Carlo simulations of liquid water between two rigid walls, *Chem. Phys. Lett.*, 82, 520, 1981.
38. **Gao, J. and Jorgensen, W. L.**, Theoretical examination of hexanol-water interfaces, *J. Phys. Chem.*, 92, 5813, 1988.
39. **Torrie, G. M. and Valleau, J. P.**, Double layer structure at the interface between two immiscible electrolyte solutions, *J. Electroanal. Chem.*, 206, 69, 1986.
40. **Reid, J. D., Vanýsek, P. and Buck, R. P.**, Potential dependence of capacitance at a polarizable (blocked) liquid/liquid interface, *J. Electroanal Chem.*, 161, 1, 1984.
41. **Kakiuchi, T. and Senda, M.**, Structure of the electrical double layer at the interface between nitrobenzene solution of tetrabutylammonium tetraphenylborate and aqueous solution of lithium chloride, *Bull. Chem. Soc. Jpn.*, 56, 1753, 1983.
42. **Kakiuchi, T. and Senda, M.**, Polarizability and electrocapillary measurements of the nitrobenzene-water interface, *Bull. Chem. Soc. Jpn.*, 56, 1322, 1983
43. **Blank, M. and Feig, S.**, Electric fields across water-nitrobenzene interfaces, *Science*, 141, 1173, 1963.
44. **Joos, P. and Vanden Bogaert, R.**, Alternating electric current across a nitrobenzene-water

interface I: adsorption kinetics, *J. Colloid Interface Science*, 56, 206, 1976.

45. **Ishida, K., Kinoshita, S. and Mori, Y. H.**, Surface tensiometer utilizing laser-beam reflection at cylindrical liquid menisci, *Rev. Sci. Instrum.*, 64, 1324, 1993.
46. **Girault, H. H., Schiffrin, D. J. and Smith, B. D. V.**, Drop image processing for surface and interfacial tension measurements, *J. Electroanal. Chem.*, 137, 207, 1982.
47. **Kakiuchi, T. Nakanishi, M. and Senda, M.**, The electrocapillary curves of the phosphatidylcholine monolayer at the polarized oil-water interface II: double layer structure of dilauroylphosphatidylcholine monolayer at the nitrobenzene-water interface, *Bull. Chem. Soc. Jpn.*, 62, 403, 1989.
48. **McLure, I. A. and Pegg, I. L.**, Laser light-scattering spectroscopy on thermally excited capillary waves at liquid/liquid interfaces in binary liquid mixtures near critical end-points, *J. Mol. Struct.*, 80, 393, 1982.
49. **Katyl, R. H. and Ingard, U.**, Light scattering from thermal fluctuations of a liquid surface, in *In Honour Of Philip M. Morse*, Feshbach, H. and Ingard , K.U., Eds., The MIT Press, Cambridge, Massachusetts, 1969, p. 70.
50. **Katyl, R. H. and Ingard, U.**, Scattering of light by thermal ripplons, *Phys. Rev. Lett.*, 20, 248, 1968.
51. **Wandlowski, T., Marecek, V., Holub, K. and Samec, Z.**, Ion transfer across liquid-liquid phase boundaries: electrochemical kinetics by faradaic impedance, *J. Phys. Chem.*, 93, 8204, 1989.
52. **Marecek, V. and Samec, Z.**, Evaluation of ohmic potential drop and capacity of interface between two immiscible electrolyte solutions by the galvanostatic pulse method, *J. Electroanal. Chem.*, 149, 185, 1983.
53. **Silva, F. and Moura, C.**, On the measurement of the impedance of ITIES: the nitrobenzene-water and 1,2-dichloroethane-water interfaces, *J. Electroanal. Chem.*, 177, 317, 1984.
54. **Wiles, M. C., Schiffrin, D. J., VanderNoot, T. J. and Silva, A. F.**, Experimental artifacts associated with impedance measurements at liquid/liquid interfaces, *J. Electroanal. Chem.*, 278, 151, 1990.
55. **VanderNoot, T. J., Schiffrin, D. J. and Whiteside, R. S.**, Design and evaluation of a 4-electrode potentiostat/voltage clamp suitable for ac impedance measurements at the interface of immiscible electrolytes, *J. Electroanal. Chem.*, 278, 137, 1990.
56. **Kakiuchi, T. and Senda, M.**, Polarizability and nonpolarizability of oil-water interfaces with relevance to ac impedance measurements, *Collect. Czech. Chem. Commun.*, 56, 112, 1991.
57. **VanderNoot, T. J., and Schiffrin, D. J.**, Non-linear regression of impedance data for ion transfer across liquid/liquid interfaces, *Electrchim. Acta*, 35, 1359, 1990.
58. **Yufei, C., Cunnane, V. J., Schiffrin, D. J., Mutomäki, L. and Kontturi, K.**, Interfacial capacitance and ionic association at electrified liquid/liquid interfaces, *J. Chem. Soc., Farady Trans.*, 87, 107, 1991.
59. **Pereira, C. M., Martins, A., Rocha, M., Silva, C. J. and Silva, F.**, Differential capacitance of liquid/liquid interfaces: effect of electrolytes present in each phase, *J. Chem. Soc. Faraday Trans.*, 90, 143, 1994.
60. **Schwartz, D. K., Schlossman, M. L., Kawamoto, E. H., Kellogg, G. J., Pershan, P. S. and Ocko, B. M.**, Thermal diffuse X-ray scattering studies of the water vapor interface, *Phys. Rev. A.*, 41, 5687, 1990.
61. **Bosch, S.**, Double layer ellipsometry: an efficient numerical method for data analysis, *Surf. Sci.*, 289, 411, 1993.
62. **Schmidt, A.**, Structure of a fluid interface near the critical point, *Phys. Rev. A*, 38, 567, 1988.
63. **Lee, L. T., Langevin, D., Mann, E. K. and Farnoux, B.**, Neutron reflectivity at liquid interfaces, *Physica B*, 198, 83, 1994.
64. **Bonn, D. and Wegdam, G. H.**, Capillary waves and ellipsometry experiments, *J. Phys. I. France*, 2, 1755, 1992.
65. **Bell, A. J., Frey, J. G. and VanderNoot, T. J.**, Second harmonic generation by *p*-nitrophenol at water/air and water/heptane interfaces, *J. Chem. Soc., Faraday Trans.*, 88, 2027, 1992.
66. **Conboy, J. C., Daschbach, J. L. and Richmond, G. L.**, Studies of alkane/water interfaces by total internal reflection second harmonic generation, *J. Phys. Chem.*, 98, 9688, 1994.
67. **Higgins, D. A. and Corn, R. M.**, Second harmonic generation studies of adsorption at a

liquid-liquid electrochemical interface, *J. Phys. Chem.*, 97, 489, 1993.

68. **Takenaka, T. and Nakanaga, T.**, Resonance Raman spectra of monolayers adsorbed at the interface between carbon tetrachloride and an aqueous solution of a surfactant and a dye, *J. Phys. Chem.*, 80, 475, 1976.
69. **Nakanaga, T. and Takenaka, T.**, Resonance Raman spectra of monolayers of a surface-active dye adsorbed at the oil-water interface, *J. Phys. Chem.*, 81, 645, 1977.
70. **Takenaka, T.**, Effect of electrolyte on the molecular orientation in monolayers adsorbed at the liquid-liquid interface: studies by resonance Raman spectra, *Chem. Phys. Lett.*, 55, 515, 1978.
71. **Wirth, M. J. and Burbage, J.D.**, Reorientation of acridine orange at liquid alkane/water interfaces, *J. Phys. Chem.*, 96, 9022, 1992.
72. **Ocko, B. M., Wu, X. Z., Sirota, E. B., Sinha, S. K. and Deutsch, M.**, X-ray reflectivity study of thermal capillary waves on liquid surfaces, *Phys. Rev. Lett.*, 72, 242, 1994.
73. **Penfold, J. and Thomas, R. K.**, The application of the specular reflection of neutrons to the study of surfaces and interfaces, *J. Phys. A. Condens. Matter*, 2, 1369, 1990.
74. **Lee, L.T. , Langevin, D. and Farnoux, B.**, Neutron reflectivity of an oil-water interface, *Phys. Rev. Lett.*, 67, 2678, 1991.
75. **Cunnane, V. J., Schiffrin, D. J., Fleischmann, M., Geblewicz, G. and Williams, D.**, The kinetics of ionic transfer across adsorbed phospholipid layers, *J. Electroanal. Chem.*, 243, 455, 1988.
76. **Kakiuchi, T.**, Dc and ac responses of ion transfer across an oil-water interface with a Goldman-type current-potential characteristic, *J. Electroanal. Chem.*, 344, 1, 1993.
77. **Kakiuchi, T.,, Noguchi, J. and Senda, M.**, Double-layer effect on the transfer of some monovalent ions across the polarized oil-water interface, *J. Electroanal. Chem.*, 336, 137, 1992.
78. **Kakiuchi, T.**, Current-potential characteristics of ion transfer across the interface between two immiscible electrolyte solutions based on the Nernst-Planck equation, *J. Electroanal. Chem.*, 322, 55, 1992.

Chapter 6

SECOND HARMONIC GENERATION AT LIQUID/LIQUID INTERFACES

Pierre F. Brevet and Hubert H. Girault

I. INTRODUCTION

Optical Second Harmonic Generation (SHG) has proven its versatility in the past being used in fields as diverse as surface physics and electrochemistry, dealing with solids and liquids.[1-4] From a fundamental point of view, SHG is forbidden in the bulk of any centrosymmetric media and therefore is inherently a surface phenomenon for such media. This also means that only a very thin layer of material contributes to the nonlinear process, a fact that explains why signal levels are usually weak.

Current interest is the application of this technique to a field of growing interest, namely liquid/liquid electrochemistry.[5] Liquid/liquid interfaces offer to the biologist a simple experimental system to model an interface. Many parameters can be externally controlled, the dielectric constant, the applied potential, for example, and yet many features at the interface have never been investigated at the molecular level. For instance, the structure and the dynamics at the interface are modified as compared to the bulk phase, by the asymmetry of the surface forces. Many phenomena are highly likely to be influenced by this asymmetry, in particular charge transfer across the interface. Both the structure of the interface, through solvation effects, frictional forces or intermolecular forces and the dynamics of the solvent relaxation will ease or hinder the transfer, as will other parameters, the nature of the phases, the adsorbates and the external conditions, namely the temperature or the applied potential.

An optical nonlinear technique, like Surface SHG or Surface infra-red Sum Frequency Generation (SFG), is surface specific, in the range of a few nanometers on both sides of the interface, non destructive and can probe very short time scales. Although the literature is very scarce on this topic, we intend to show in this review what SHG can offer to the field of liquid/liquid electrochemistry. Section II is a brief overview of the historical background. First observation of SHG dates back to the beginning of the sixties and since then it has been applied to many surface studies. Because of the scarcity of experimental results and the extensive underlying theory, we have decided to give an extended theoretical part in Section III. We have endeavored to present the theory in a simple way, using the phenomenological model of the nonlinear polarization sheet. It will suit the needs of this review and highlight

0-8493-7694-7/96/$0.00+$.50

most of the important features. Only important results are presented as equations and therefore the reader should find the basic formalism to analyze SHG experimental results. Section IV is devoted to the main experimental geometries used by the different groups involved in the field so far, with particular emphasis on the Total Internal Reflection geometry which offers a good means of overcoming weak SH intensities. Then in the following sections we will present the experimental results. In Section V, we deal with the problem of the structure of the neat liquid/liquid interfaces. Indeed, the problem of contributions from higher order terms in the nonlinear polarization is sometimes unavoidable but we will show how useful information can also be extracted from these contributions. In Section VI we present the investigation of adsorbates at the liquid/liquid interfaces. Most of the experimental results published so far fall into this category. In Section VII we address one of the key questions of interfacial studies. It is well known that surfaces present disymmetries, in particular for the forces on both sides of the interface, and that these latters affect chemical equilibria at surfaces. Using the example of the air/water interface, we show how this problem can be tackled. We adopt the same procedure in Section VIII for the study of the dynamics of relaxation at the interface. The air/water interface has already been investigated by SHG and yielded confirmation of differences between bulk and interfacial relaxation. Although the air/water interface is dramatically different than the liquid/liquid interface, we believe that the methodology is still suited for the latter. Finally in Section IX we present briefly another technique, closely related to SHG, namely infra-red Sum Frequency Generation, a technique which cannot be omitted in such a review. Based on the same nonlinear phenomena as SHG, this technique can yield much more selective information.

II. HISTORICAL OVERVIEW

Optical Second Harmonic Generation was first observed by P.A. Franken *et al* in 1961 in a quartz crystal.[6] The quartz crystal is a noncentrosymmetric medium but shortly after, in 1962, R.W. Terhune *et al* observed SHG from the centrosymmetric crystal of calcite.[7] In the following years, many experiments involved a wide range of other media, from metals[8] to liquids[9] in 1969. Theoretical developments were derived by N. Bloembergen and coworkers in a series of papers. The first paper published in 1962 presented the solution of the nonlinear Maxwell equations in homogeneous nonlinear media, as well as the solution for the harmonic wave generated from a thin slab of nonlinear material.[10] In 1968, a model was finally derived for second harmonic generation at the boundary of two centrosymmetric media.[11] However, the model developed was based on the assumption that the leading order for the SH response arose mainly from the bulk of the media through the quadrupolar terms in the nonlinear polarisation. This was consistent with the experimental data available at that time which didn't show any large surface sensitivity. But in 1969, F. Brown and F. Matsuoka observed that they could get a much stronger signal from freshly evaporated silver films under vacuum conditions than silver films in ambient air. They explained their observation by introducing an additional dipole electric term in the nonlinear polarization. Further work provided confirmation of the surface sensitivity of SHG by using adsorbate layers on metal surfaces.[1,12,13]

Since SHG is an optical technique, buried interfaces like metal/solution interfaces are accessible and this property has been widely used in electrochemistry to study electrode surfaces during potential sweeps. Many processes occur immediately at the interface and SHG has thus proven to be a very versatile tool to probe in-situ surface reactions. Adsorption and desorption can be detected while the interfacial potential is swept.[14] Sensitivity down to a fraction of a monolayer has been observed and simple ions, like halides or alkali/earth metals cations, as well as aromatic molecules like pyridine have been extensively studied.[15,16] Surface reconstruction can also be followed since surface symmetries can be determined by sample rotation around the surface normal.[17,18] This work has helped in the development of a theoretical framework for the SH response from the metal surfaces in vacuum or in solution. J. Rudnick and E.A. Stern first emphasized the consequences of the broken symmetry at the interface.[19] Later a hydrodynamic model allowed for a more realistic description of the surface under excitation[20] and recent developments using the jellium model have introduced the effects of the interaction of the electronic tail at the metal surface with the solution.[21,22] The problem of adsorbate layers are now being investigated and first models reported.[21]

The possibility of examining the molecular properties of an adsorbate layer has been recognized for some time and the advantage of resonant SHG on surface species selectivity acknowledged.[23,24] It was realized that not only the molecular hyperpolarizabilities could be inferred but also the molecular orientational parameters. This has led to a large amount of work on Langmuir-Blodgett films on substrates[25] or even just simple monolayers of dye molecules on quartz substrates.[26] This was accompanied by a renewed interest in simulation, in particular for the introduction of phenomenological models taking into account the properties of linear media in which the SH active monolayer could be embedded. The problem of the optical dielectric constant for the monolayer itself was raised, an acute problem in the case of resonant experiments.[27]

More recently, SHG has been used to look at air/liquid surfaces.[28] It has brought a wealth of information on the structure of neat surfaces as well as those with adsorbates. With the availability of laser sources of short light pulses, the dynamics of processes occurring at the interface have been investigated.[29,30] The recent advances in SHG at the air/liquid interface have demonstrated the potential of the technique in the field of liquid/liquid electrochemistry. So far, the literature on this topic has been rather scarce but there is no doubt that this technique will continue to develop. Now more sophisticated techniques, like infra-red Sum Frequency Generation, can be as surface sensitive as SHG, but are also much more selective on the species probed. With the time resolution only determined by the light pulse duration, such nonlinear techniques should prove to be the ideal tool to investigate both the structure and the dynamics of the liquid/liquid interfaces for which many questions have still to be addressed at the molecular level.

III. THEORY

A. MICROSCOPIC ORIGIN OF NONLINEAR PHENOMENA

Nonlinear optical phenomena arise from the nonlinear nature of the forces binding electrons to nuclei. If we look at a simple system made up of a nucleus and one electron (see Figure 1), we can describe the attractive force F between the two particles with a harmonic oscillator force law:

$$F = k(x)\,x \tag{1}$$

where x is the displacement and $k(x)$ the strength of the force. Since at large distances from the nucleus the electron is likely to feel nonlinear forces due to its environment or the attractive force itself, we have introduced a possible dependence of the force constant on the distance. Only at small x values does equation (1) describe a linear force law of a harmonic oscillator. For larger x distances, linearization starts to break down and one must introduce higher order terms.

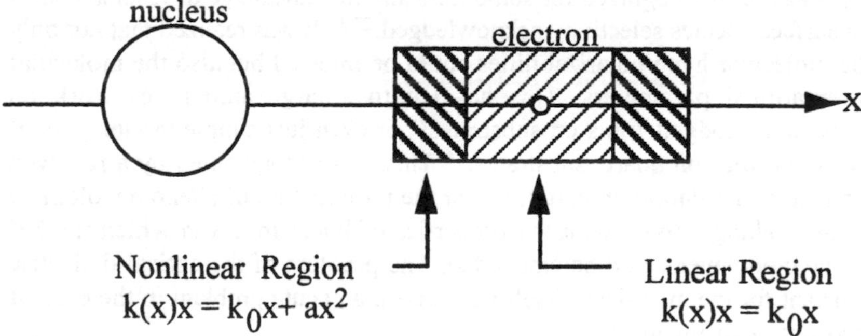

Figure 1: Microscopic model for the origin of the nonlinear response in atomic or molecular systems.

Up to the second term, we obtain for the equation of motion:

$$\frac{d^2x}{dt^2} + 2\gamma\frac{dx}{dt} + \omega_0^2 x + ax^2 = -\frac{e}{m}E(t) \tag{2}$$

for the system undergoing excitation by an external electromagnetic field $E(t)$. ω_0 is the characteristic frequency of the oscillator and γ a damping coefficient. This form has been reduced to a one-dimensional equation on the Ox axis, and e and m are the electronic charge and the electron mass respectively. The a coefficient gives the strength of the non linearity effect. This equation can be solved using perturbation theory (analogous to the Rayleigh-Schrödinger resolution), by introducing a parameter λ, ranging from 0 to infinity, representing the strength of the perturbation. The solution can then be written as:

$$x = \sum_i \lambda^i x^{(i)} \tag{3}$$

and we get for the first order of the displacement x:

$$x^{(1)} = -\frac{e}{m}\frac{E(t)}{\left[\omega_0^2 - \omega^2 - 2i\omega\gamma\right]} \tag{4}$$

The linear polarization of the medium, taken as the superposition of non interacting systems identical to this one, can be written as:

$$p^{(1)} = -Nex^{(1)} = -\frac{Ne^2}{m}\frac{E(t)}{\left[\omega_0^2 - \omega^2 - 2i\omega\gamma\right]} \tag{5}$$

where N is the number of systems per unit volume. Note that this equation can be further analyzed to extract an expression for the dielectric constant ε. For the second order of the displacement, in noncentrosymmetric media, we get:

$$x^{(2)} = -\frac{ae^2}{m^2}\frac{\left[E(t)\right]^2}{\left[\omega_0^2 - 4\omega^2 - 4i\omega\gamma\right]\left[\omega_0^2 - \omega^2 - 2i\omega\gamma\right]^2} \tag{6}$$

and therefore the nonlinear polarization can be written:

$$p^{(2)} = -Nex^{(2)} = -\frac{Nae^3}{m^2} \frac{\left[E(t)\right]^2}{\left[\omega_0^2 - 4\omega^2 - 4i\omega\gamma\right]\left[\omega_0^2 - \omega^2 - 2i\omega\gamma\right]^2} \tag{7}$$

We clearly see a dependence on the square of the external field and resonances at both the harmonic and the fundamental frequencies. We will see later the quantum mechanical equivalent of this expression.

This model is rather simple, since it involves only one frequency in the molecular system, but the basic features have been taken into account. Note that in a centrosymmetric system, a would be null and therefore we would have to carry over the development of equation (3) to the next order.

B. FIRST MODELS OF THE NONLINEAR SLAB.

The first model applied to Surface Second Harmonic Generation was derived in the early sixties by N. Bloembergen et al.[10] Dedicated to the generation of nonlinear electromagnetic waves at the boundary of dielectric media, it included a section devoted to the generation of nonlinear waves within a slab of nonlinear material, lying between two adjacent linear media. In such a description, an electromagnetic plane wave at the fundamental frequency is incident onto the slab from the linear medium 1. It is then refracted into the slab where it induces both a linear polarization and a nonlinear polarization. This latter nonlinear polarization acts as the source of the harmonic wave at twice the fundamental frequency. From the nonlinear Maxwell equations, one can write a nonlinear wave equation whose general solution consists of two harmonic homogeneous plane waves, propagating in opposite directions, and one inhomogeneous plane wave. The matching of both the electric and the magnetic fields at the two boundaries of the slab and the two linear media yields a reflected wave in medium 1 and a transmitted wave in medium 2. The calculations led to rather simple formulae in the particular case of a very thin slab whose thickness was much smaller than the wavelength of the fundamental wave. Interesting properties of the harmonic response from the slab were deduced. For example, it was shown that the S-polarized reflected and transmitted SH waves were of identical amplitude whereas that equality was spoiled in the case of the P-polarized waves. These derivations also led to the conclusion that multiple reflections within the slab had to be taken into account in order to yield the correct SHG intensities. Indeed, the reflected wave amplitude can vary from zero to twice the value deduced from a calculation for a semi-infinite medium. Some time later, T. F. Heinz presented in detail the boundary conditions in the particular case of a slab of vanishing thickness. In this work, the slab was described as a sheet of nonlinear induced polarization.[31] This approach, although rigorous, is difficult to use in practice when one wants to derive equations relative to a specific experimental geometry. A much more attractive presentation was therefore presented[32,33]. It consists in a phenomenological presentation of the system where the slab is still described as a nonlinear polarization sheet but the electromagnetic wave amplitudes are obtained by extensive use of the Fresnel coefficients, including multiple reflections at the boundaries between the slab and the two linear media. However, phase differences due to different light paths are ignored, although they have been included in other works.[34] Such a model has inherent drawbacks but all the features presented here can be described with this formalism. The main advantage of such a description is its ability to be quite simply modified according to the experimental geometry.

C. THE MODEL OF THE POLARIZATION SHEET

One can describe this model with a sheet of nonlinear polarization having an infinitely thin thickness and lying between two linear dielectric media (see Figure 2). The model, as originally derived, was mainly proposed for systems of monolayers on a substrate. In our particular case of interest, we can slightly modify the model to embed the nonlinear sheet into a linear medium having its own optical properties. This can be of great advantage if resonant SSHG is dealt with, in particular to introduce the physical properties of a mixed solvent layer. This also leaves some flexibility in the description of the liquid/liquid interface, allowing for a space region where the optical dielectric constant varies from one bulk value to the other. This region could, in principle, be correlated to the mixed solvent layer.[35] However for a simpler description, the slab dielectric constant will be taken as independent of the space coordinates.

The nonlinear polarization sheet is described through the following relations:[36]

$$\boldsymbol{P}_s^{(2)}(\boldsymbol{r},t) = \boldsymbol{P}_s^{(2)}(2\omega)\exp\left[-i\left(2\omega t-\kappa\cdot\boldsymbol{R}\right)\right]\delta(z-0) \quad + \quad c.c. \tag{8}$$

where the space coordinate vector $\boldsymbol{R}$ lies in the (Ox, Oy) plane and $\delta(z-0)$ is the Dirac delta function. κ is the component of the fundamental field wave vector in the same plane and in particular:

$$\kappa = \frac{\sqrt{\varepsilon(\omega)}}{c}\omega\sin\theta(\omega) \tag{9}$$

and for simplicity, κ can be taken along the Ox axis. $\boldsymbol{P}_s^{(2)}(2\omega)$ is then given by:

$$\boldsymbol{P}_s^{(2)}(2\omega) = \chi_s^{(2)}:\boldsymbol{E}(z=0,\omega)\boldsymbol{E}(z=0,\omega) \tag{10}$$

and the electric fields are taken within the slab. $\chi_s^{(2)}$ is the macroscopic dipole electric susceptibility tensor of the interface. The amplitudes of these fields are actually the sum of the transmitted incident fundamental wave and the many reflected waves within the slab. If we reduce the problem to the first reflection, we get the sum of the transmitted fundamental wave and the wave reflected at the boundary between the slab and the second linear media after transmission from medium 1 to the slab.

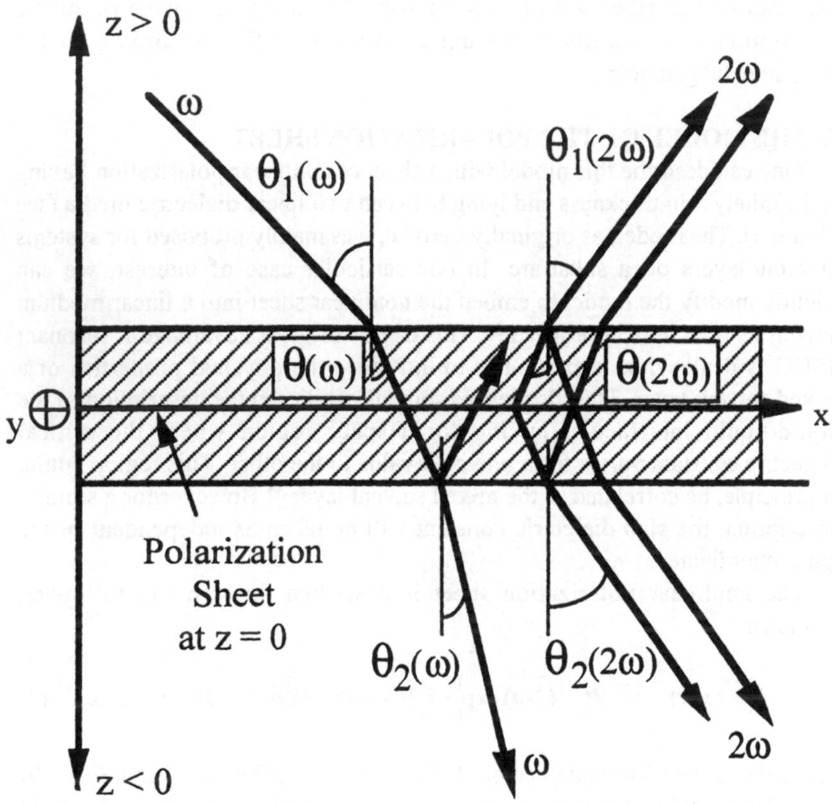

Figure 2: Schematic model for Surface SHG. The nonlinear polarization sheet lying at z=0 is embedded in a linear medium of optical dielectric constants $\varepsilon(\omega)$ and $\varepsilon(2\omega)$. Lower and upper linear media are described with their respective linear dielectric constants $\varepsilon_1(\omega)$, $\varepsilon_1(2\omega)$ and $\varepsilon_2(\omega)$, $\varepsilon_2(2\omega)$ respectively. Multiple reflections on both the fundamental and the harmonic waves are shown.

According to the resolution of the nonlinear Maxwell equations, the induced nonlinear polarization is thus the source of two waves at twice the frequency of the fundamental wave: one propagating downwards towards medium 2 as a transmitted wave and one propagating upwards towards medium 1 as a reflected wave. Their general form also involves multiple reflections within the slab. Expressions for the transmitted and the reflected SH waves can then be formally described by:

$$I(2\omega)=\frac{32\pi^3\omega^2}{c^3}\frac{\sqrt{\varepsilon_i(2\omega)}}{\left[\varepsilon(2\omega)-\varepsilon_i(2\omega)\sin^2\theta_i(2\omega)\right]}$$
$$\left|e_i(2\omega)\cdot\chi_s^{(2)}:e(\omega)e(\omega)\right|^2 I^2(\omega) \qquad (11)$$

where $I(\omega)$ is the power density of the fundamental wave and $I(2\omega)$ the power density of the SH signal. Vectors $e(\omega)$ and $e(2\omega)$ both embed angular dependencies as well as Fresnel factors. This expression is valid for both reflection and transmission if one uses the correct form of equation (11): *i=1* for reflection and *i=2* for transmission. This expression slightly differs from the form derived by previous authors[37] because SH generation was assumed within the slab. In the particular case of the reflection geometry and with generation in medium 1 with an assumed optical dielectric constant $\varepsilon_1(2\omega)$ equal to unity at the harmonic frequency, one returns to the expressions previously quoted in the literature. From this expression, we can see that the SH intensity depends on the square of the input intensity, and that liquid/liquid experiments require the inclusion of the second factor unless work is carried out at a given interface. We need now to introduce the symmetry properties of the interface in order to develop equation (11) for practical use.

The susceptibility tensor $\chi_s^{(2)}$ is a third rank tensor and thus possesses 27 components. But since it is a macroscopic quantity, it should exhibit the macroscopic symmetry properties of the system under investigation. In the case of liquid/liquid interfaces, which are isotropic interfaces, we can also assume the surface plane to be a mirror plane. The symmetry class we should look at is therefore the mm2 crystal class with degeneracy of the x and y axes.[38] In this case, there are only four independent non vanishing elements of the susceptibility tensor, namely $\chi_{s,XZX}^{(2)},\chi_{s,XXZ}^{(2)},\chi_{s,ZXX}^{(2)}$ and $\chi_{s,ZZZ}^{(2)}$. Following the geometry described in Figure 2, the Oz axis corresponds to the surface normal and we have chosen the Ox axis anywhere in the plane of the surface. For this symmetry class, the Ox and Oy axes are interchangeable. For SHG, the two last indices can be freely rotated, and therefore only three elements are necessary: $\chi_{s,XXZ}^{(2)},\chi_{s,ZXX}^{(2)}$ and $\chi_{s,ZZZ}^{(2)}$. We also have to emphasize that the three tensor components can be complex quantities This is due to the occurrence of resonances, which depend on the wavelength of the pump beam. Equation (11) can now be fully developed. It yields, in the case where the pump intensity in measured in medium 1:

$$I(2\omega)=\frac{32\pi^3\omega^2}{c^3}\frac{\sqrt{\varepsilon_i(2\omega)}}{\varepsilon_1(\omega)\left[\varepsilon(2\omega)-\varepsilon_i(2\omega)\sin^2\theta_i(2\omega)\right]}\Big|a_1\chi^{(2)}_{s,XXZ}\sin 2\gamma\sin\Gamma$$
$$+(a_2\chi^{(2)}_{s,XXZ}+a_3\chi^{(2)}_{s,ZXX}+a_4\chi^{(2)}_{s,ZZZ})\cos^2\gamma\cos\Gamma$$
$$+a_5\chi^{(2)}_{s,ZXX}\sin^2\gamma\cos\Gamma\Big|^2 I^2(\omega) \tag{12}$$

with $i=1$ for reflection and $i=2$ for transmission in the factor for the optical dielectric constants. We have introduced the two polarization angles, namely γ for the input fundamental field and Γ for the output SH field. The a_i, $i=1..5$ coefficients depend on the geometry[33]. With the geometry described in Figure 2, we get in reflection mode:

$$\begin{aligned}
a_1 &= e_y(\omega)e_z(\omega)e_y(2\omega)\\
a_2 &= -2e_z(\omega)e_x(\omega)e_x(2\omega)\\
a_3 &= e_x(\omega)e_x(\omega)e_z(2\omega)\\
a_4 &= e_z(\omega)e_z(\omega)e_z(2\omega)\\
a_5 &= e_y(\omega)e_y(\omega)e_z(2\omega)
\end{aligned} \tag{13}$$

with the fundamental vector:

$$\begin{aligned}
e_x(\omega) &= (r^p_{m2}-1)t^p_{1m}\cos\theta(\omega)\\
e_y(\omega) &= (1+r^s_{m2})t^s_{1m}\\
e_z(\omega) &= (1+r^p_{m2})t^p_{1m}\sin\theta(\omega)
\end{aligned} \tag{14}$$

and the harmonic one:

$$\begin{aligned}
e_x(2\omega) &= (R^p_{m2}-1)T^p_{ml}\cos\theta(2\omega)\\
e_y(2\omega) &= (1+R^s_{m2})T^s_{ml}\\
e_z(2\omega) &= (1+R^p_{m2})T^p_{ml}\sin\theta(2\omega)
\end{aligned} \tag{15}$$

For completeness, the Fresnel factors are:[39]

$$r^s_{ij}=\frac{w_i-w_j}{w_i+w_j}$$

$$r^p_{ij}=\frac{w_i\varepsilon_j-w_j\varepsilon_i}{w_i\varepsilon_j+w_j\varepsilon_i}$$

$$t_{ij}^{s} = \frac{2w_i}{w_i + w_j}$$
$$t_{ij}^{p} = \frac{2w_i\sqrt{\varepsilon_i\varepsilon_j}}{w_i\varepsilon_j + w_j\varepsilon_i} \tag{16}$$

with

$$w_i = \sqrt{\varepsilon_i}\cos\theta_i \tag{17}$$

Fresnel factors taken in capital letters mean that they must be calculated at the harmonic frequency. For the transmission mode, the a_i, $i = 1..5$ retain the expression given by equation (13). The fundamental vectors describing the incoming fields are unchanged upon changing the geometry for the SH signal detection. Therefore, only the harmonic vectors change and we can now write:

$$e_x(2\omega) = (1 - R_{m1}^{p})T_{m2}^{p}\cos\theta(2\omega)$$
$$e_y(2\omega) = (1 + R_{m1}^{s})T_{m2}^{s}$$
$$e_z(2\omega) = (1 + R_{m1}^{p})T_{m2}^{p}\sin\theta(2\omega) \tag{18}$$

Equations (12) can be further simplified if one takes the two limiting cases of the S-output polarization (Γ=90°) and P-output polarization (Γ=0°). In the case of the S-polarized output, the SH response behaves like a sine square function of the input polarization angle γ, peaked at $\pi/4$. The P-polarized output behaves like the sum of a sine square and a cosine square function, the actual shape of the curve depending on the coefficients and therefore on the susceptibility components as well as the angle of incidence and the linear optical constants of the different media. In principle, only three points are necessary to extract experimental values for the susceptibility components $\chi_{s,XXZ}^{(2)}, \chi_{s,ZXX}^{(2)}$ and $\chi_{s,ZZZ}^{(2)}$. In practice, one fits experimental curves to equation (12). Nevertheless, there still subsists an absolute phase uncertainty which can be lifted if phase interferences experiments are performed.[40] In many systems, like phenol molecules adsorbed at the air/liquid interfaces, physical considerations can lead to the exclusion of some possibilities. In the case of the phenol molecules, the -OH group is likely to be anchored on the aqueous side thus defining the absolute phase.

D. NONLOCAL CONTRIBUTIONS FROM THE BULK

We have seen above that in centrosymmetric media, under the electric dipole approximation, the signal arises only from the interface where the symmetry is broken. This is a first order approximation because higher order terms involving field gradients can also be the source of a harmonic response.

In general, in any medium, the induced nonlinear polarization can be written as a multipole expansion:[41,42]

$$\boldsymbol{P}_{eff}^{(2)}(2\omega) = \boldsymbol{P}^{(2)}(2\omega) - \nabla \cdot \boldsymbol{Q}^{(2)}(2\omega) + \frac{c}{i\omega} \nabla \times \boldsymbol{M}^{(2)}(2\omega) + \ldots \tag{19}$$

where $\boldsymbol{Q}^{(2)}(2\omega)$ and $\boldsymbol{M}^{(2)}(2\omega)$ denote respectively the electric quadrupole polarization and the magnetization:

$$\begin{aligned} \boldsymbol{Q}^{(2)}(2\omega) &= \chi_Q^{(2)} : \boldsymbol{E}(\omega)\boldsymbol{E}(\omega) \\ \boldsymbol{M}^{(2)}(2\omega) &= \chi_M^{(2)} : \boldsymbol{E}(\omega)\boldsymbol{E}(\omega) \end{aligned} \tag{20}$$

The magnetic contributions can be neglected as far as SHG is concerned but studies on ferromagnetism have been reported.[43] $\boldsymbol{Q}^{(2)}(2\omega)$ is a second rank tensor and therefore the electric quadrupole susceptibility $\chi_Q^{(2)}$ is a fourth rank tensor. The nonlinear polarization of electric dipole origin consists into two terms:

$$\boldsymbol{P}^{(2)}(2\omega) = \chi_D^{(2)} : \boldsymbol{E}(\omega)\boldsymbol{E}(\omega) + \chi_P^{(2)} : \boldsymbol{E}(\omega)\nabla\boldsymbol{E}(\omega) \tag{21}$$

The first term is the usual induced electric dipole nonlinear polarization but the second term describes the harmonic response of dipole electric origin from possible field gradients. We have used two different susceptibility tensors, namely $\chi_D^{(2)}$ and $\chi_P^{(2)}$ to account for the influence of field gradients on the susceptibility tensors. In the bulk of liquid media, the first one of these terms vanishes due to the centrosymmetry property. The others terms of equations (19) involving field gradients also disappear because, in homogeneous media, no field gradients are expected. In this respect, the interface between two nonlinear centrosymmetric media is rather different from the bulk. In this thin region, the symmetry is broken and therefore electric dipole harmonic response is allowed. Concurrently, field gradients occur because of the mismatch of the optical dielectric constants. In principle the symmetry breaking and the mismatch of the dielectric constant should be the two sources of the nonlinear polarization. But we have to introduce a third contribution which arises from the gradient of the quadrupole electric susceptibility tensor.[42] This term originates from the divergence of the electric quadrupole polarization $Q^{(2)}(2\omega)$. The tensor $\chi_Q^{(2)}$ should be dependent upon a distribution function, itself function of relative position and orientation of molecules within the bulk. It should be written with a generic form $f(r_1,\alpha_1,r_2,\alpha_2)$, r_1,α_1 and r_2,α_2 being the position and the orientation of two correlated molecules. Leaving aside the contribution from the quadrupole electric hyperpolarizability of the molecules themselves, the tensor $\chi_Q^{(2)}$ should then give information on molecular correlation in the vicinity of the interface. We must emphasize here that it is the gradient of this tensor, as one moves from one bulk phase to the other across the interface, which gives rise to the effective nonlinear polarization. Therefore one has to think about disparities between the correlation functions of the two adjacent phases rather than the correlation functions themselves. The effective nonlinear polarization as described through equation (19) is now written at the interface:

$$\begin{aligned}P_{eff}^{(2)}(2\omega) = \chi_s^{(2)}:E(\omega)E(\omega) + \gamma_1\nabla\left[E(\omega)E(\omega)\right] + \gamma_2\nabla\left[E(\omega)E(\omega)\right] \\ -\nabla\left[\chi_Q^{(2)}\right]:E(\omega)E(\omega) \qquad (22)\end{aligned}$$

taking into account fundamental field gradients on both sides of the nonlinear polarization sheet. The γ_i, $i=1,2$ coefficients now include the two susceptibility tensors $\chi_Q^{(2)}$ and $\chi_P^{(2)}$. This form is not very helpful in the sense that only field gradients appear and not the fields within the sheet. Nevertheless, it has been shown that one can rewrite such a formulation by making use of a surface equivalent harmonic polarization with the fields taken in the sheet[31,36]. As a consequence, one can reduce equation (22) to an effective form similar to equation (10):

$$P_{eff}^{(2)}(2\omega) = \chi_{eff}^{(2)}:E(\omega)E(\omega) \qquad (23)$$

and the effective tensor components, under the same mm2 symmetry, are:

$$\begin{aligned}\chi_{eff,XXZ}^{(2)} &= \chi_{s,XXZ}^{(2)} + \chi_{Q1,1}^{(2)}\frac{\varepsilon(\omega)}{\varepsilon_1(\omega)} - \chi_{Q2,1}^{(2)}\frac{\varepsilon(\omega)}{\varepsilon_2(\omega)} \\ \chi_{eff,ZXX}^{(2)} &= \chi_{s,ZXX}^{(2)} + (\gamma_1 + \chi_{Q1,2}^{(2)})\frac{\varepsilon(2\omega)}{\varepsilon_1(2\omega)} - (\gamma_2 + \chi_{Q2,2}^{(2)})\frac{\varepsilon(2\omega)}{\varepsilon_2(2\omega)} \\ \chi_{eff,ZZZ}^{(2)} &= \chi_{s,ZZZ}^{(2)} + (\gamma_1 + \chi_{Q1,3}^{(2)})\frac{\varepsilon(2\omega)\varepsilon^2(\omega)}{\varepsilon_1(2\omega)\varepsilon_1^2(\omega)} \\ &\quad - (\gamma_2 + \chi_{Q2,3}^{(2)})\frac{\varepsilon(2\omega)\varepsilon^2(\omega)}{\varepsilon_2(2\omega)\varepsilon_2^2(\omega)} \qquad (24)\end{aligned}$$

where we have also used the symmetry properties of the quadrupole electric susceptibility tensor[38]:

$$\begin{aligned}\chi^{(2)}_{QI,1} &= \chi^{(2)}_{QI,ZXXZ}\\ \chi^{(2)}_{QI,2} &= \chi^{(2)}_{QI,ZZXX}\\ \chi^{(2)}_{QI,3} &= \chi^{(2)}_{QI,ZZZZ}\end{aligned} \tag{25}$$

The main feature in equation (24) is the different dependence of the three components on contributions from the bulk. The $\chi^{(2)}_{eff,ZXX}$ and the $\chi^{(2)}_{eff,ZZZ}$ components exhibit a dependence on both the quadrupolar electric tensor and the fundamental field gradients through the γ_i, $i=1,2$ coefficients embedding the susceptibility tensors $\chi^{(2)}_Q$ and $\chi^{(2)}_P$ whereas the $\chi^{(2)}_{eff,XXZ}$ component does not show any sensitivity towards the fundamental field gradients. This has been noted before, but within this complete development, it is also demonstrated that this last component possesses a nonlocal contribution from the bulk.

The main result from this theoretical formulation, is to show that there is a competition between surface and bulk for the origin of the harmonic response. It is obvious that the smaller the mismatch of the optical dielectric constant, the smaller the field gradients will be. Therefore contributions from the bulk should be much weaker at liquid/liquid interfaces than at air/liquid interfaces, assuming small disparities between the correlation functions.

E. FIELD-INDUCED SURFACE SH RESPONSE.

In liquid/liquid studies, one usually controls the potential between the two adjacent phases with a four electrode potentiostat. With such a system, one can modify the excess surface charge directly at the interface. In a more conventional electrochemical cell, at the metal/electrolyte interface, it has been shown that such an excess surface charge could lead to a specific harmonic response.[44] The same response is expected at the liquid/liquid interface, although the strength of this phenomena should be much weaker. In principle, a nonlinear polarization at twice the fundamental frequency is expected from the third harmonic generation process involving a combination between the fundamental optical fields and the static electric field arising from the applied potential:

$$\boldsymbol{P}^{(2)}_s(2\omega) = \chi^{(3)}_s : \boldsymbol{E}(\omega)\boldsymbol{E}(\omega)\boldsymbol{E}_{dc} \tag{26}$$

If we now assume the interface to be an infinite surface plane, and using Gauss's theorem, we can simply introduce the surface charge σ. It yields:

$$P_s^{(2)}(2\omega) = \chi_s^{(3)} \frac{\sigma}{\varepsilon_0} : E(\omega)E(\omega)z \qquad (27)$$

This expression is only dependent on the optical fundamental fields within the polarization sheet and therefore we can readily add this new contribution to equation (24) for the effective susceptibility tensor. Since the tensor components are expected to behave linearly with the surface charge, we should expect a parabolic shape for the SH intensity as a function of the surface charge. Unfortunately this nonlinear response depends on the fourth rank tensor $\chi_s^{(3)}$ which is one or two orders of magnitude weaker than the third rank tensor, $\chi_s^{(2)}$. Unless this latter third rank tensor is very weak, the contribution from this field-induced SH response will be negligible and therefore difficult to detect.

F. MICROSCOPIC DESCRIPTION OF THE SURFACE SH RESPONSE.

So far we have dealt with macroscopic electromagnetic fields and macroscopic susceptibility tensors. This development is very useful to understand the origin of the nonlinear response but doesn't go far enough to give any insight into the physical nature of the system at the molecular level. This is unfortunate since all phenomena are in essence microscopic. We will now present a molecular level approach for second harmonic generation at liquid/liquid interfaces.

In the macroscopic theory of the nonlinear Maxwell equations, every microscopic quantity is averaged over a macroscopically small volume. But this latter value can still be considered large on the molecular scale. As a consequence, we have to note that the macroscopic electromagnetic fields are not the applied fields on molecules. The real applied fields are the local fields.[45] Nevertheless, in liquid media where optical dielectric constants are rather weak, local fields corrections are often unnecessary.

It is possible to correlate molecular hyperpolarizabilities to the dipole electric surface susceptibility tensor $\chi_s^{(2)}$. The nonlinear response from the surface molecules is not a collective effect as with the response of the free electron gas of the metal/electrolyte interface. On the contrary, it is the simple superposition of the response from all the molecules. Since the laboratory frame, where the electromagnetic fields are considered, is different from the molecular frame, where the interaction between the applied fields and the molecules is effective, we have to introduce a frame transformation tensor. To be complete, we can also use a distribution function of the molecules for the usual three Euler angles ϕ, θ and ψ (see Figure 3):[46,47]

$$\chi_s^{(2)} = N_s < f(\phi,\theta,\psi)T(\phi,\theta,\psi) > \beta \qquad (28)$$

where N_S is the number of molecules per unit surface and $T(\phi, \theta, \psi)$ the transformation tensor. N_S coefficient enter the formula as a scaling factor. This means that the SH response from the interface, if purely surface specific, can be a measure of the surface concentration.[48] In principle, this is only valid in the case where the adsorbed molecules do not undergo any orientational reorganization with increasing surface concentration. It is also obvious that the $\chi_s^{(2)}$ tensor closely follows the molecular β tensor. In particular, this latter tensor can have strong enhancements close to resonances. Perturbation theory in quantum mechanics is necessary to rigorously calculate this tensor for molecules in the gas phase.[49] Simpler calculations involving a two-levels system with the ground state and the first excited state of the molecule have been used. This model yields:[50]

$$\beta_{ijk}(\omega) = \frac{-e^3}{2h^2}\left[\frac{\Delta r_n^i r_{ng}^j r_{ng}^k}{\omega_{ng}^2 - \omega^2} + r_{ng}^i (r_{ng}^j \Delta r_n^k + r_{ng}^k \Delta r_n^j)\frac{\omega_{ng}^2 + 2\omega^2}{(\omega_{ng}^2 - 4\omega^2)(\omega_{ng}^2 - \omega^2)}\right] \quad (29)$$

where Δr_n^i is the difference in the permanent dipole moment between the excited state n and the ground state g. r_{ng}^j is the transition moment between the two states n and g, ω_{ng} the energy difference between these two states and e and h, the charge of the electron and Planck's constant respectively. This relation clearly shows that resonances can occur at both frequencies, fundamental or harmonic. This feature is of particular interest in the sense that the fundamental frequency can be far from any resonance, which is important to avoid any absorption in the bulk of a phase, and yet the harmonic frequency still at resonance with certain adsorbates to obtain resonance enhancements for the surface signal. In practice, with large probe molecules, electronic structures become more and more complicated and simple models break down. Therefore we have to go back to the complete calculation, or assume that the major contribution comes from one particular feature. This can be the case for aromatic molecules for which UV-Vis spectra exhibit strong resonances in the near UV range. These resonances usually correspond to a π–π^* transition and models, such as the one derived by Pople, Pariser and Parr (PPP), can be used to extract excited states energies and wavefunctions.[51,52] From equation (29), we can then calculate the hyperpolarizability tensor β. Note that any calculation using equation (29) directly would make the approximation of the independence of the molecular environment.[53] Most of the SHG active molecules used as adsorbed surface probes are based on the same model: a donor and an acceptor group linked with one or more aromatic rings. In such systems, the number of non zero independent components of the β tensor is highly reduced. In many systems, like phenol or p-nitrophenol, we are left with only three components, namely β_{xxz},β_{zxx} and β_{zzz}.

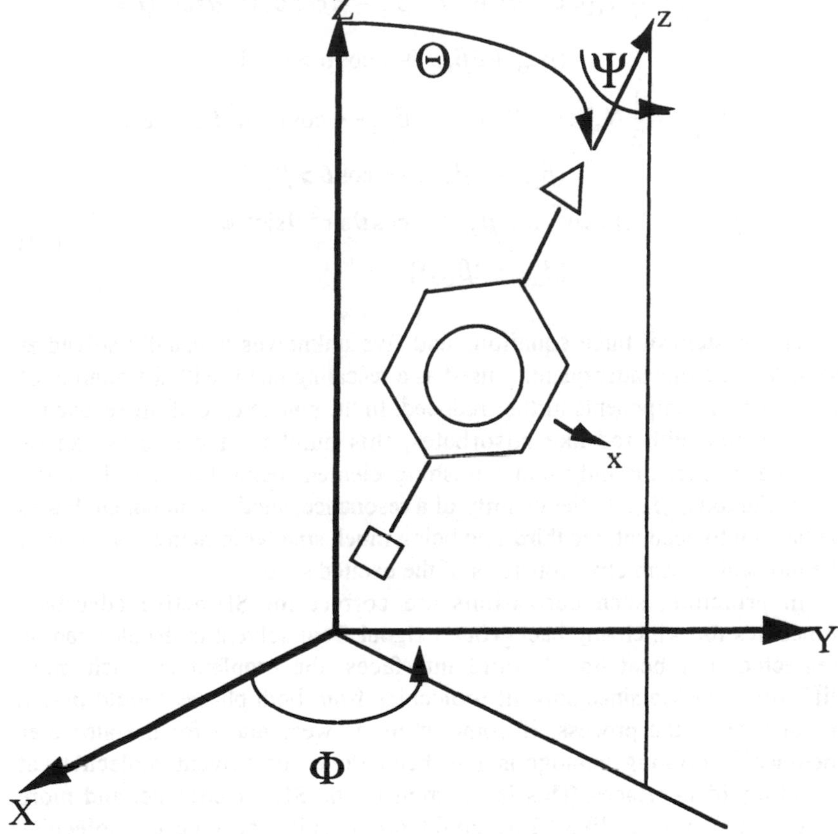

Figure 3: Euler angles (ϕ, θ, ψ) to relate the laboratory frame (X,Y,Z) with the molecular frame (x,y,z). In particular, the θ angle directly relates the molecular axis Oz to the laboratory surface normal OZ.

Therefore equation (28) can be simplified using some restrictions. The angle ϕ has been averaged in order to follow the assumption of surface isotropy and the two other angles, θ and ψ, are restricted to a defined domain. According to Figure 3, θ is the angle between the molecular axis and the surface normal, and ψ the angle of rotation around the molecular axis. In most studies on molecular orientation, the angle ψ is either averaged or assumed so that the aromatic ring lies perpendicular to the surface, although it could, in principle, provide a measurement of the position of the plane of the aromatic ring at the interface, for instance perpendicular or parallel to the surface plane. With such derivations, we obtain[31]:

$$\begin{aligned}
\chi^{(2)}_{s,XXZ} &= \frac{1}{2} N_s [< \cos\theta \sin^2\theta > \beta_{zzz} - < \cos\theta \sin^2\theta \sin^2\psi > \\
&\qquad (\beta_{zxx} + 2\beta_{xxz}) + < \cos\theta > \beta_{xxz}] \\
\chi^{(2)}_{s,ZXX} &= \frac{1}{2} N_s [< \cos\theta \sin^2\theta > \beta_{zzz} - < \cos\theta \sin^2\theta \sin^2\psi > \\
&\qquad (\beta_{zxx} + 2\beta_{xxz}) + < \cos\theta > \beta_{zxx}] \\
\chi^{(2)}_{s,ZZZ} &= N_s [< \cos^3\theta > \beta_{zzz} + < \cos\theta \sin^2\theta \sin^2\psi > \\
&\qquad (\beta_{zxx} + 2\beta_{xxz})]
\end{aligned} \tag{30}$$

This system of three equations and five unknowns is usually solved at fixed N_S and this latter quantity used as a rescaling factor with the number of the β tensor components further reduced. In the simple case of off-resonance experiments with rod-like adsorbates, this number of elements can be reduced to one, the only non vanishing element being the one along the molecular axis, β_{zzz}. In the vicinity of a resonance, another component has to be taken into account, the third one being much smaller in many cases due to the molecular symmetry properties of the excited state.

In principle, such derivations are correct for SH-active adsorbate molecules for which any background signal from solvent molecules can be neglected. For neat liquid/liquid interfaces, the problem is much more difficult to tackle since solvent molecules from both phases should play a major role in the process. If some attempts were made for the air/water interface[28], nothing analogous has been done for solvent molecules at liquid/liquid interfaces. This is inherent to the SHG technique, and more specific techniques, like SFG, could probe only one type of molecules yielding the desired information.[54] Finally we would like to stress here that the orientational angle is largely dependent on other system parameters. The most important of these parameters is the optical dielectric constant of the nonlinear polarization sheet. The necessity of external independent experiments to extract the optical dielectric constant of adsorbate species has already been mentioned in the past,[26] and often different values for the orientational angle are obtained, depending on the value used for the dielectric constant.[55] Such techniques do exist but are not very easy to put in practice. It consists of measuring the UV-Vis spectrum of the interfacial layer and reconstructing the spectrum of the complex optical dielectric constant as a function of wavelength through a Kramers-Kronig analysis.[56]

IV. EXPERIMENTAL APPARATUS

A schematic diagram of a typical SHG apparatus is given in Figure 4. Main features are a high peak power laser source, a working and a reference arm and a computer controlled detection system, usually a monochromator-photomultiplier system hooked to a boxcar integrator or a photon counter.

Since Surface SHG is not a very efficient process, signal levels are very weak. Indeed, the SSHG efficiency is in the order of 10^{-12}% and thus an incident power density of 10^8 W.cm^{-2} only yields an output SH response of a few tens of photons per pulse.[57] To counterbalance these low levels, we have to rely on high peak power lasers. Many experiments have been performed with nanosecond pulsed neodynium doped Yttrium Aluminum Garnet (Nd^{3+}-YAG) lasers because they are commonly available in laboratories. With a pulse length of less than 10 nanoseconds and an energy per pulse of more than 10 mJ, such laser sources allow peak powers in the range of 1 MW per pulse. This is large enough if we are interested in resonant enhanced surface SHG from adsorbed molecules but, as often noted, this is too weak a peak power to be able to get a detectable signal from neat liquid/liquid interfaces. We can increase the peak power by jumping into the picosecond time scale. Nd^{3+}-YAG lasers delivering 10 mJ per pulses of 25 picoseconds duration allow peak powers in the range of 0.4 GW per pulse. Even with these peak powers, we usually have to focus the pump laser beam from a diameter of more than a centimeter down to few millimeters. This is a careful operation since it can greatly increase both thermal effects on the sample and undesired SH response from the optics. Results achieved on molecular orientation in both the nanosecond and the picosecond timescale have given similar results, a strong argument to support minimal disordering due to surface energy deposition.[58]

Several geometrics have been used in SHG experiments at liquid/liquid interfaces, mainly differing in the incident angles employed. With normal glass cells, the interface is usually irradiated from the top of the cell. This implies smaller incident angles, and consequently smaller signal levels due to the nonlinear reflection coefficient which is only favored at wide angles. To fire through the cell walls, a quartz cell is required if the fundamental pump beam is already in the middle of the visible range, namely around 532 nm, since the SH response is in the UV. Such a setup necessitates careful light polarization measurements because of possible depolarization upon transmission. Normal incidence is thus preferable, a setup achievable with a cylindrical cell.[59] From linear optical theory, it is known that incidence from the medium with the highest optical index upon the medium of lowest index induces Total Internal Reflection (TIR).[39] In this configuration, no light propagation is allowed in the medium with the low index, and the only remaining electromagnetic wave decays exponentially with the distance away from the interface. The dramatic enhancements in reflected signal levels have been used recently to probe the structure of neat liquid/liquid interfaces.[59] Fresnel coefficients are complex quantities in this geometry but the expressions given in Section III, equations (12) to (18), are still valid.

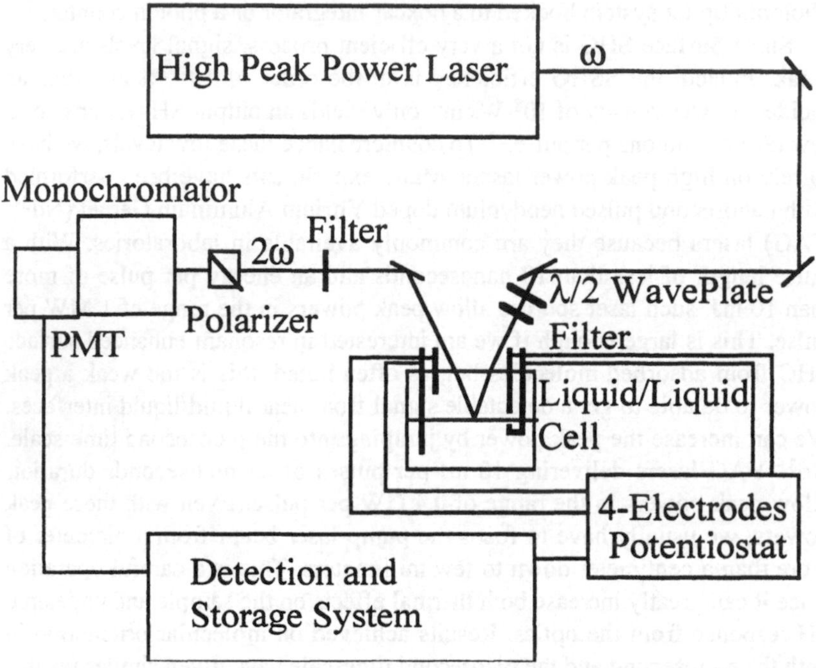

Figure 4: Typical schematic diagram for an SHG apparatus. A high peak power laser impinges onto the liquid/liquid interface in an electrochemical cell. The SH signal is then collected through a set of optical components and a monochromator and detected with a photomultiplier tube. The potential applied between the two liquid phases is controlled by a 4-electrodes potentiostat.

Very few experiments have been performed at polarized liquid/liquid interfaces, but these results are very promising. The setup has been described in detail elsewhere and consists mainly in a four-electrode potentiostat.[60]

Depending on signal levels, detection systems are chosen between an integrating technique, like boxcar averaging, or photon counting. This latter technique is generally used for very weak signals of a few photons per pulse. Usually the main experimental problem to overcome is the separation of the SH signal from the residual signal of the fundamental beam. Although linear reflection at liquid/liquid interfaces is not an efficient process, this signal is always much larger than the SH response. First experiments used a $CuSO_4$

cell on the detection path, but efficient separation can also be achieved with a set of filters or a spatial dispersing prism. Absolute calibration can also be performed by extracting a few percentage of the pump beam and doubling it with a quartz crystal.

V. SURFACE SH ORIGIN FROM NEAT LIQUID/LIQUID INTERFACES.

Surface SHG has been claimed to be a very surface sensitive technique, but, as presented in the theoretical part, non negligible contributions from the bulk can affect results. Therefore, in the case of liquid/liquid interfaces, it was important to experimentally distinguish between surface and bulk contributions. First experiments dealt with adsorbates. Such probe molecules were chosen as highly SHG-active and thus the resulting signals were essentially surface specific.

Therefore very recent work has been carried out on the neat liquid/liquid interfaces. The chosen solvents were those commonly used in liquid/liquid electrochemistry, namely water, 1,2-dichloroethane (DCE) or alkanes. The problem of competition between surface and bulk nonlinear response is even more acute in these systems, because DCE and alkanes are centrosymmetric molecules and as such, should not exhibit strong hyperpolarizabilities. So far two extensive studies have been performed using SHG experiments and one has been performed with an SFG experiment. Conclusions drawn from the latter are worth mentioning here. It is also interesting to compare the results with the closely related experiments on the air/liquid interfaces where the liquid phase is one of the three mentioned above.

In air/liquid experiments, the asymmetry between the two phases is highly pronounced. On one side sits the air with its optical dielectric constant equal to unity and which is independent of the pump wavelength. Such properties are not strictly true but are assumed valid. Experimental values for the $\chi^{(2)}_{eff}$ tensor elements extracted from experimental curves have been obtained for the three phases, water, DCE and hexane. Values for the air/water system are in close agreement for the different authors, yielding at 20°C:[28]

$$\begin{aligned} \chi^{(2)}_{eff,XXZ} / \chi^{(2)}_{eff,ZXX} &= 2.30 \\ \chi^{(2)}_{eff,XXZ} / \chi^{(2)}_{eff,ZZZ} &= 0.34 \end{aligned} \tag{31}$$

They clearly show that the elements $\chi^{(2)}_{eff,XXZ}$ and $\chi^{(2)}_{eff,ZXX}$ are unequal. Far from any resonance, we should observe the Kleinman rule[61] which states that these two elements are equal if the signal arises from the interfacial layer of water molecules. For the wavelengths of these experiments, performed in the visible region, water does not possess any absorption band. Therefore results should follow the Kleinman rule unless the SH response is not surface specific. Looking at the complete form for the effective $\chi^{(2)}_{eff}$ tensor elements, namely equation (24), we see that fundamental field discontinuities and molecular correlations can severely affect the results. This suggests a strong nonlocal contribution from the bulk. Further experiments involving the temperature dependence of the tensor components have been performed. A decrease of the components with increasing temperature was observed, a fact correlated with the decrease of the surface dipole electric response from the interfacial water molecules through disordering of the first water layers. Since the magnitude of the decrease was still relatively small compared to the overall magnitude of the components, the conclusions were that contributions from the bulk were dominant. We have to note here that SFG measurements performed on the same air/water system did not exhibit such bulk dominant behavior.[54] This could be explained by the experimental setup where the two fundamental beams are perpendicularly polarized. In this case, one of the main contributions from the bulk, the one involving the gradient of the scalar product of the two fundamental fields, then vanishes and the signal is once again surface specific. In the case of one-beam-SHG, this configuration is not allowed and thus the contribution from the bulk cannot be avoided. In the more particular arrangement of SHG with two noncollinear beams,[62] this contribution from the bulk should disappear if perpendicular polarization is used.

The neat liquid/liquid interfaces, water/alkanes and water/DCE systems, have undergone systematic investigations in two different geometries. One set of experiments has been performed in the TIR geometry, which compensates for low peak power.[59] The other set has been done with a much higher peak power, in the picosecond time domain.[36] Results show that the magnitude of the susceptibility tensors for the air/liquid systems are much larger than the magnitude of the tensors for the liquid/liquid systems. This is attributed to the disappearance of the contribution from the bulk arising from the electromagnetic fundamental field discontinuity. Indeed, the better matching of the two optical dielectric constants has been dramatically reduced, the ratio being of the order of one half for the air/liquid systems but closer to unity for the liquid/liquid systems. Note that it has been shown for a different system, that of liquids on fused silica, that a perfect matching strongly decreases the SH response from the interface but this latter response does not vanish altogether since the asymmetry of the interface still exists.[63] According to the Kleinman rule, the ratio of the two elements $\chi^{(2)}_{eff,XXZ}$ and $\chi^{(2)}_{eff,ZXX}$ for the liquid/liquid interface should be unity in the case of perfect matching of the optical dielectric constants. Consequently, departure from unity is a measure of the residual contribution from the bulk, arising from the molecular correlation in the vicinity of the interface. Water/DCE and water/odd-alkanes systems, namely heptane/water and nonane/water interfaces, exhibit ratios departing from unity. Consequently, these results suggest that these interfaces are less ordered than the water/even-alkanes ones, namely hexane/water, octane/water and decane/water interfaces.[36,59]

VI. MOLECULAR ORIENTATION AT LIQUID/LIQUID INTERFACES.

We have seen above in Section III the formalism through which molecular orientation parameters can be extracted from Surface SHG measurements. In the case of neat liquid/liquid interfaces, it is rather difficult to extract such quantities since both phases participate in the formation of the interface. At most, as presented recently, one can give a qualitative approach to give an idea on the weight of each phase to the overall nonlinear response. In the case of the water/alkanes interface, it has been argued that the main weight originated from the alkane molecules, since varying the length of the alkane chains induced non negligible variations on the ratios of the $\chi^{(2)}_{eff,XXZ}$ and $\chi^{(2)}_{eff,ZXX}$ susceptibility tensor components.[59] We have to mention though that absolute orientation has been achieved in the case of the neat air/water interface. This particular case is of course much simpler since only water molecules participate into the formation of the interface.

Studies at the liquid/liquid interfaces have mainly aimed at extracting orientational parameters of adsorbates. It was been noticed early that SSHG could be a sensitive technique to measure surface concentrations. The macroscopic susceptibility tensor $\chi^{(2)}_{s}$ is proportional to the surface concentration N_S, see equation (28), and consequently we can measure surface concentrations *in situ* with this optical technique. Indeed such measurements have been performed,[64] although this was achieved previously at other interfaces.[65] At the water/DCE interface, adsorption of the probe molecule 2-(n-octadecylamino)-naphtalene-6-sulfonate (ONS), a strong surfactant molecule, has been monitored as the interfacial potential was swept from 200 mV to 500 mV vs Ag/AgCl reference electrode, the oil phase being positive. The increase in the SHG signal was correlated with the decrease in the interfacial tension, itself attributed to the increase in the ONS surface concentration. In many cases, the relationship between the surface coverage θ and the applied potential $\phi_w - \phi_o$ can be described with a Frumkin isotherm:[66]

$$\ln\left(\frac{\theta}{1-\theta}\right) = \ln\left(\frac{a_{ONS}}{a_{org}}\right) - \frac{\Delta G^0}{RT} + \frac{bF}{RT}\left(\phi_w - \phi_o\right) - \frac{c\theta}{RT} \qquad (32)$$

where a_{ONS} and a_{org} are the activities of ONS in the organic phase and that of the organic phase itself respectively, ΔG^0 the Gibbs adsorption energy from the organic phase to the interface at zero potential difference, namely $\phi_w = \phi_o$, and b the fraction of the applied potential felt by ONS, c being the

Frumkin interaction parameter. Fits of experimental data to such expressions yielded both the Gibbs adsorption energy and the b parameter. The large value for b, $b = 0.67$ as compared to the value of 0.24 as calculated from the Gouy-Chapman theory for the case of ONS remaining at the outer Helmholtz plane of the organic phase, indicated a penetration of the ONS adsorbate into the water phase. Surface concentration monitoring has recently been applied in analytical chemistry at an aqueous solution/solvent polymeric membrane to study the formation of cation-ionophore complexes.[67] Surface SHG has proven in this case its advantage over other optical techniques, like Fourier Transform Infra Red Attenuated Total Reflection (FT-IR-ATR), because the effective depth probed by the nonlinear technique is much smaller, in the order of 10 nm or less as compared to 100 nm to 1 mm for more conventional linear techniques.

The first study on molecular orientation at the liquid/liquid interface was performed as early as 1988 for sodium 1-dodecylnaphtalene-4-sulfonate (SDNS) at the decane/water and water/carbon tetrachloride (CCl_4) interfaces.[5] Experiments were performed with a pumping wavelength of 532 nm and the SHG signal collected at 266 nm. The nonlinear hyperpolarizability tensor for this long chain molecule was shown to reduce to the component along the molecular axis Oz, namely β_{zzz}. This could be too simplistic a view, since many molecules possessing an aromatic ring present a resonance in this near UV-region. Nevertheless, the presence of the sulfonate group and the hydrocarbon chain aligned on opposite sides of the naphtalene chromophore suggests that such a simple rod-like model is rather realistic. The system (30) derived in section III is thus further reduced:

$$\chi^{(2)}_{s,XXZ} = \chi^{(2)}_{s,ZXX} = \frac{1}{2} N_s < \cos\theta \sin^2\theta > \beta_{zzz}$$
$$\chi^{(2)}_{s,ZZZ} = N_s < \cos^3\theta > \beta_{zzz} \tag{33}$$

and in particular, the ratio of the two components of the susceptibility tensor, $\chi^{(2)}_{s,ZXX}$ and $\chi^{(2)}_{s,ZZZ}$, yield a weighted average value for the orientation angle of the molecular axis Oz against the surface normal OZ. So far many authors have assumed a sharp angle distribution and thus have used a delta Dirac function. This is obviously an oversimplified description, but this allows a straightforward calculation of an averaged angle $< \theta >$ More complicated angular distribution functions have been proposed, like gaussian type functions, but the orientational angles corresponding to the peak of these distributions can be quite shifted from the value obtained with a sharp distribution.[47] This question is even more intriguing if we emphasize that the calculation of the $\chi^{(2)}_s$ tensor elements are subject to the uncertainty of the optical dielectric constant of the nonlinear slab in the proposed model. In this case, values can differ by 10° or more. It might be then sensible to leave some freedom of rotation in these systems of adsorbed molecules. Data obtained for SDNS at different interfaces showed that SDNS molecules can take flatter positions when the static dielectric constant of the organic phase is increased. This was explained by the screening effect of the static dielectric constant of the organic phase to the hydrocarbon tail-tail interactions. Nonetheless, other intermolecular forces, namely hydrophobicity or hydrophilicity, should also play an important role as demonstrated by other authors at the air/water interface.[66] It has also be noticed that adsorbed molecules tend to tilt to smaller angles at sharp interfaces whereas for more diffuse interfaces such constraints are relaxed. Interfacial thicknesses which increase in the case of diffuse interfaces can also be correlated with the interfacial tension decrease.[5]

More recent experiments on orientational measurements have been performed in resonant SHG mode. The same procedure can be successfully applied to get the orientational angle, although this time equations (23) must be used with two elements of the hyperpolarizability tensor. In such studies, either large surfactant molecules, like 4-octyloxybenzoic acid (OBA) or n-octyl-4-hydroxybenzoate (OHB), or much smaller ones like phenol derivatives, for instance p-nitrophenol, can be used.[55,68] Depending on the acceptor and donor groups present at either end of the aromatic ring, different hyperpolarizability tensor components will be enhanced at resonance. In this case, the orientational angle can be monitored as one changes the oil phase or one of the substituent groups. Recently, theoretical considerations on such intermolecular forces have been presented at the water/DCE interfaces using molecular dynamics calculations.[69,70]

VII. INTERFACIAL CHEMICAL EQUILIBRIUM.

We have seen how the structure of the neat liquid/liquid interfaces as well as adsorbed layers can be probed but we now have to wonder whether we could use this technique to address the question of interfacial chemical equilibrium. In the theoretical developments, we have emphasized the problem of the asymmetry of the intermolecular forces at the interface. In particular we have shown how information on the structural order at the interface can be accessed from the departure from the Kleinman rule. Previous studies on interfacial chemical equilibria have been performed on acid-base reactions at the air/water interface. It has been shown that the presence of the water vapor phase, reducing the polarity of the medium on the air side as compared to the water side, was a key factor in decreasing the stability of the charged species.

In the particular case of a dissociation equilibrium between an acid HA and its anionic form A^-:

$$HA + H_2O \Leftrightarrow A^- + H_3O^+ \tag{34}$$

we can write the interfacial pH as pH_S:

$$pH_s = pH_B + \frac{e\Psi_0}{2.3kT} \tag{35}$$

where pH_B is the bulk pH and Ψ_0 is the interfacial potential, and the interfacial equilibrium pK_a as pK_a^S:

$$pK_a^s = pH_s + \log\frac{[HA]}{[A^-]} \tag{36}$$

In the case where the acid form is the neutral p-nitrophenol molecule, studies of the bulk pH dependence of the neutral p-nitrophenol surface concentration have yielded a value of 7.9 for the bulk pH value at which the SH intensity decreases to half the maximum value obtained at low bulk pH. If this is compared to the bulk pH value, equal to 7.15, at which the concentration of the bulk acid form has decreased to half its value, we conclude that the presence of the vapor phase at the interface has shifted the equilibrium towards the side of the neutral molecules.[71] The Gibbs energy of adsorption can be split into two parts, a chemical and an electrostatic one:

$$\Delta G^0_{ads} = \Delta G^0_{chem} + \Delta G^0_{elec} \tag{37}$$

where the electrostatic part is given by:

$$\Delta G^0_{elec} = N_{Av} ez\Psi_0 \tag{38}$$

N_{Av} being Avogadro's number. A simple Gouy-Chapman model can be used to give an expression for the interfacial potential:[66]

$$\Psi_0 = \frac{2kT}{ze}\sinh^{-1}\left(\frac{1.36\text{x}10^{-14} N_s}{\sqrt{C_B}}\right) \tag{39}$$

where N_s is the surface concentration of charged molecules and C_B the bulk concentration. The electrostatic work to bring a charged molecule to an already charged interface is therefore positive and increases the Gibbs energy of adsorption for the anionic form. The net result is an increase in the ratio of neutral to charged molecules. At liquid/liquid interfaces, the asymmetry is likely to be much weaker although the organic phase, usually DCE, is a non polar organic phase and therefore we should still expect some shift in chemical equilibria. Experimental data are scarce but similar studies are under progress.[72]

As an important class of chemical reactions, electron transfer reactions are of particular importance in biological systems. Control over the rate of the reaction, difficult in the case of homogeneous transfers, can be achieved in heterogeneous transfers since acceptors and donors can be physically separated from each other. Photoinduced electron transfer reactions have been extensively studied as a special sub-class of electron transfers since these reactions allow external triggering through light illumination. The experiment consists of the simple two steps scheme:

$$\begin{aligned} &D + h\nu \rightarrow D^{*} && \text{(i)} \\ &D^{*} + A \rightarrow D^{+} + A^{-} && \text{(ii)} \end{aligned} \qquad (40)$$

The oxidizing agent is often based on the ion [tris(2,2'-bipyridinyl)Ruthenium(II)]$^{2+}$ ($[Ru(bpy)_3]^{2+}$). It can be easily photoexcited, its extinction coefficient being in the range of 10^4 M^{-1}cm^{-1} at 450 nm,[73] either from a laser or a simple Xenon lamp.[74] In a recent work, a surfactant molecule was synthesized with dedicated properties: hydrophobicity, ability to adsorb at the interface and optical SH activity dependent upon the oxidation state. This molecule, trans-1-ferrocenyl-2-[4-(trimethylammonio)phenyl]ethylene tetraphenylborate ($\mathbf{1}^{+}.BPh_4^{-}$) was subsequently oxidized at the interface by the $[Ru(bpy)_3]^{2+}$ complex dissolved in the water phase. No SH signal was detected when illumination of the water phase was turned off whereas an SH signal was recorded when the light was turned on. This was explained by first photoexcitation of the $[Ru(bpy)_3]^{2+}$ complex in the bulk of the water phase which then diffused to the interface where the electron transfer with the $\mathbf{1}^{+}$ surfactant subsequently occurred. This latter molecule being SH active in its oxidized $\mathbf{1}^{2+}$ state, a strong nonlinear response was observed.[75]

These studies have shown the ability for Surface SHG to monitor different types of chemical reactions: acid-base reactions or electron transfer. In the first place, it can bring a wealth of information on the interfacial equilibrium, which can be dramatically different from the bulk equilibrium due to the asymmetry of the surface forces, in particular the change of solvent polarity. In photoinduced electron transfer, where the inherent properties of the interface between two immiscible electrolytes are very useful to control the reaction, surface SHG provides surface sensitivity to allow the monitoring of interfacial changes.

VIII. DYNAMICS AT LIQUID/LIQUID INTERFACES.

We have seen so far how to investigate liquid/liquid interfaces, their structure and the local chemical equilibria. We believe that this technique is also able to address the problem of the dynamics at the interface. Indeed, the asymmetry of the intermolecular forces at the interface is usually large enough to shift the chemical equilibria in favor of the reactants or the products, as compared to the bulk equilibria. If this phenomenon is large enough, the dynamics of the relaxation motions is highly likely to be also affected.

To date, no time-resolved surface SHG experiments have been performed at the liquid/liquid interfaces, on the timescale of the light pulse durations available in laboratories, namely nano- or picoseconds. However several experiments have been performed at the air/quartz and liquid/quartz interfaces using Malachite green[29,76] and also at the air/water interface on rotational relaxation and energy transfers[30,77] and can illustrate the technique.

One of these classical experiments consist of looking at the photoisomerization of the dye molecule 3,3'-diethyloxadicarbocyanine iodide (DODCI) at the air/water interface.[77] A pump pulse excites the cis-DODCI molecule from the S_0 state to the S_1 state. The molecule then relaxes to the ground S_0 state of the cis-isomer or undergo a change to an intermediate twisted form. This latter intermediate form can then decay back to the cis- or the trans-isomer. A time-delayed probe pulse was used to generate an SH response from the DODCI molecules at the air/water interface, and a decrease of the signal was observed at short time delays followed by a recovery at longer times. The experiments were done with pulses of 15 ps duration. This allowed for the study of relaxation dynamics whose time scale is expected to fall in this range. The decrease of the SH signal was attributed to the depletion in the population of the cis-isomer S_0 ground state by the pump pulse. The recovery was then associated with the excited state relaxation. A characteristic time of 220 ps for the surface isomerization was deduced, as compared to the bulk value of 520 ps. The isomerization of the DODCI molecule is likely to be affected by the intermolecular forces between the dye molecules and the surrounding water molecules. In particular, during its isomerization, the DODCI molecule undergoes twisting around one of its bonds, a motion which is highly affected by molecular friction. A shorter relaxation time at the interface than in the bulk would therefore suggest a smaller friction at the interface.

Asymmetry forces, and molecular friction in particular, are defined by the two adjacent phases. In the example above, one of the two adjacent phases is air. This induces a marked difference between the two phases which is observed through dramatic differences in the relaxation rates. The question is still unanswered at the liquid/liquid interface were the discrepancies are expected to be much smaller due to the higher density of liquids. Nevertheless, such raw data could be valuable in the search for a molecular model of the transfer of species from one phase to the other. In these motions, solvation phenomena are key factors in the understanding of the process. A more definite insight could be achieved by use of femtosecond lasers to improve the time resolution. Such short laser light pulses have proven to be well suited to investigate solvent relaxation.

IX. SURFACE SUM-FREQUENCY GENERATION.

We cannot complete our survey without presenting another nonlinear technique, namely Surface Sum Frequency Generation (SSFG). If SSHG involves the same beam twice in the same process, or two beams at the same frequency in noncollinear SSHG experiments, SSFG involves two beams at two distinct frequencies.

If two beams at two distinct frequencies ω_1 and ω_2 impinge on the same spot at the surface of a nonlinear medium, they induce a nonlinear polarization which can be written under the general form:[38]

$$\boldsymbol{P}_s^{(2)}(\boldsymbol{r},t) = \chi_s^{(2)}(\boldsymbol{r},t){:}\boldsymbol{E}(\boldsymbol{r},t)\boldsymbol{E}(\boldsymbol{r},t) \quad (41)$$

If we take a simple monochromatic plane wave form for the fundamental fields, we write:

$$\boldsymbol{E}_i(r,t) = \boldsymbol{E}_i e^{-i\omega_i t} + c.c. \quad (42)$$

where c.c. stands for complex conjugate and $i=1$ for the first beam at frequency ω_1 and $i=2$ for the second beam at frequency ω_2. To simplify the notation, we have omitted the explicit space dependence. We can develop equation (41) to get the different frequency components for the nonlinear polarization. We get:

$$\begin{aligned} \boldsymbol{P}_s^{(2)}(r,t) = {} & \chi_s^{(2)}(0){:}\left[\boldsymbol{E}_1\boldsymbol{E}_1^* + \boldsymbol{E}_1^*\boldsymbol{E}_1 + \boldsymbol{E}_2\boldsymbol{E}_2^* + \boldsymbol{E}_2^*\boldsymbol{E}_2\right] \\ & + \chi_s^{(2)}(2\omega_1){:}\left[\boldsymbol{E}_1\boldsymbol{E}_1 e^{-i2\omega_1 t} + c.c\right] \\ & + \chi_s^{(2)}(2\omega_2){:}\left[\boldsymbol{E}_2\boldsymbol{E}_2 e^{-i2\omega_2 t} + c.c\right] \\ & + \chi_s^{(2)}(\omega_1+\omega_2){:}\left[\boldsymbol{E}_1\boldsymbol{E}_2 e^{-i(\omega_1+\omega_2)t} + \boldsymbol{E}_2\boldsymbol{E}_1 e^{-i(\omega_1+\omega_2)t} + c.c\right] \\ & + \chi_s^{(2)}(\omega_1-\omega_2){:}\left[\boldsymbol{E}_1\boldsymbol{E}_2^* e^{-i(\omega_1-\omega_2)t} + \boldsymbol{E}_2\boldsymbol{E}_1^* e^{-i(\omega_1-\omega_2)t} + c.c\right] \end{aligned} \quad (43)$$

The total electromagnetic field at any point $\boldsymbol{r}$ in the nonlinear medium is the superposition of the two fields $E_1(\boldsymbol{r},t)$ and $E_2(\boldsymbol{r},t)$ described through equation (42). Thus it yields five terms which correspond to five different nonlinear phenomena. The first term correspond to Optical Rectification (OR), that is the establishment of a static electric field at the interface. The second and the third terms are SHG processes for each fundamental incident beam whereas the two last terms are respectively Sum Frequency Generation (SFG) and Difference Frequency Generation (DFG). These latter two phenomena are very interesting in the sense that a simple generalization of the molecular hyperpolarizability tensors as given by equation (29) presented above, will show that the SH response from an adsorbate monolayer will undergo resonances at the three frequencies ω_1, ω_2 and $\omega_1+\omega_2$ or $\omega_1-\omega_2$ depending on the nonlinear process. The selection of the two fundamental frequencies is a matter of choice, but experimental contingencies have favored infra-red SFG where an infra-red photon and a visible photon are converted into another visible photon. This technique now offers surface selectivity since in this case the infra-red photon can probe a definite molecular bond within the surface molecules.[54,78]

SFG is a first order nonlinear phenomena and as such possesses the same surface sensitivity as SHG. Moreover, because it is inherently a two beam process, it is easy to chose two perpendicularly polarized beams so as to minimize nonlocal contributions from the bulk. Indeed recent results have exhibited this features and present a different picture of the neat air/water interface than the one obtained with SHG. This ability to probe a well defined bond should allow infra-red vibrational spectra of the liquid/liquid interface, thus assessing very precisely the origin of the nonlinear response.

X. CONCLUSION

From the overview we have presented here we have shown how an optical nonlinear technique like SHG or SFG can offer surface sensitivity and selectivity at liquid/liquid interfaces. Optical linear processes are often cumbersome to use because signals are always a combination of surface and bulk contributions and therefore deconvolution of the two contributions requires special experimental configurations, like Total Internal reflection (TIR) or Attenuated Total Reflectance ATR). In the case of nonlinear techniques, the surface sensitivity is inherent to the technique when one is concerned with centrosymmetric media. In this respect, the study of liquid/liquid interfaces is very promising. Added to the localized origin of the SH response, the timescale of the interaction process between light and matter is only limited by the duration of the light pulse. Therefore, timescale as short as 100 fs should be readily available, a timescale short enough to offer monitoring of the interfacial dynamics.

Many problems previously addressed at other types of interface, for example, charge transfer across the interface, both electron transfer or ion transfer, intramolecular energy transfers or solvent relaxation, can be revisited at the liquid/liquid interface. In-situ SHG experiments, combined with standard electrochemical techniques to control the interfacial potential, should prove to be successful as evidenced by the published articles which have appeared in these recent years.

XI. ACKNOWLEDGMENTS

The authors would like to thank A.A. Tamburello Luca, Ph. Hébert and G. Wellington for their collaboration during the writing of this manuscript and R.M. Corn for comments. This work is supported by the Swiss National Fund (under grant n° 21-36624.92), the European Community Human Capital and Mobility (under grant n° CHRx-CT92-0076) and the Office Fédéral de l'Education et des Sciences (under grant n° 93.0067).

REFERENCES

1. **Shen, Y. R.**, Surface second harmonic generation: a new technique for surface studies, *Annu. Rev. Phys. Chem.*, 40, 327, 1989.
2. **Richmond, G. L.**, Optical second harmonic generation as in situ probe of electrochemical interfaces in *Electroanalytical Chemistry*, Bard, A. J., Ed., Marcel Dekker Inc, New York, Vol 17, 1991.
3. **Corn, R.M. and Higgins, D. A.**, Optical second harmonic generation as a probe of surface chemistry, *Chem. Rev.*, 94, 107, 1994.
4. **Eisenthal, K. B.**, Equilibrium and dynamic processes at interfaces by second harmonic and sum frequency generation, *Annu. Rev. Phys. Chem.*, 43, 627, 1992.
5. **Grubb, S. G., Kim, M. W., Rasing, T. and Shen, Y. R.**, Orientation of molecular monolayers at the liquid-liquid interface as studied by optical second harmonic generation, *Langmuir*, 4, 452, 1988.
6. **Franken, P. A., Hill, A. E., Peters, C. W. and Weinreich, G.**, Generation of optical harmonics, *Phys. Rev. Lett.*, 7, 118, 1965.
7. **Terhune, R. W., Maker, P. D. and Savage, C. M.**, Optical harmonic generation in calcite, *Phys. Rev. Lett.*, 8, 404, 1962.
8. **Brown, F. and Matsuoka, F.**, Effect of adsorbed surface layers on second harmonic light from silver, *Phys. Rev.*, 185, 985, 1969.
9. **Wang, C. C.**, Second harmonic generation of light at the boundary of an isotropic medium, *Phys. Rev.*, 178, 1457, 1969.
10. **Bloembergen, N. and Pershan, P. S.**, Light waves at the boundary of nonlinear media, *Phys. Rev.*, 128, 606, 1962.

11. **Bloembergen, N., Chang, R. K., Jha, S. S. and Lee, C. H.**, Optical second harmonic generation in reflection from media with inversion symmetry, *Phys. Rev.*, 74, 813, 1968.
12. **Chen, J. M., Bower, J. R., Wang, C. S. and Lee, C. H.**, Optical second harmonic generation from submonolayer Na-covered Ge surfaces, *Opt. Commun.*, 9, 132, 1973.
13. **Song, K. J., Heskett, D., Dai, H. L., Liebsch, A. and Plummer, E. W.**, Dynamical screening at a metal surface probed by second harmonic generation, *Phys. Rev. Lett.*, 61, 1380, 1988.
14. **Heinz, T. F., Chen, C. K., Ricard, D., Shen, Y. R.**, Optical second harmonic generation from a monolayer of centrosymmetric molecules adsorbed on silver, *Chem. Phys. Lett.*, 83, 180, 1981.
15. **Heskett, D., Urbach, L. E., Song, K. J., Plummer, E. W. and Dai, H. L.**, Oxygen and Pyridine on Ag(110) studied by second harmonic generation: coexistence of two phases within monolayer pyridine coverage, *Surf. Science*, 197, 225, 1988.
16. **Stolberg, L., Richer, J., Lipkowski, J. and Irish, D. E.**, Adsorption of pyridine at the polycrystalline gold-solution interface, *J. Electroanal. Chem.*, 207, 213, 1986.
17. **Guidotti, D., Driscoll, T. A. and Gerritsen, H. J.**, Second harmonic generation on centrosymmetric semiconductor, *Solid State Commun.*, 46, 337, 1983.
18. **Heinz, T. F., Loy, M. M. T. and Thompson, W. A.**, Study of Si(111) surfaces by optical second harmonic generation: reconstruction and surface phase transformation, *Phys. Rev. Lett.*, 54, 63, 1985.
19. **Rudnick, J. and Stern, E. A.**, Second-harmonic radiation from metal surfaces, *Phys. Rev. B*, 4, 4174, 1971.
20. **Sipe, J. E., So, V. C. Y., Fukui, M. and Stegeman, G.**, Analysis of second-harmonic generation at metal surfaces, *Phys. Rev. B*, 21, 4389, 1980.
21. **Dzhavakhidze, P. G., Kornyshev, A. A., Liebsch, A. and Urbakh, M.**, Theory of second harmonic generation at the metal-electrolyte interface, *Phys. Rev. B*, 45, 9339, 1992.
22. **Schmickler, W. and Urbakh, M.**, Electronic distribution and second-harmonic generation at the metal-electrolyte interface, *Phys. Rev. B*, 47, 6644, 1993.
23. **Heinz, T. F., Tom, H. W. K. and Shen, Y. R.**, Determination of molecular orientation of monolayer adsorbates by optical second harmonic generation, *Phys. Rev. A*, 28, 1883, 1983.
24. **Heinz, T. F., Chen, C. K., Ricard, D. and Shen, Y. R.**, Spectroscopy of molecules monolayers by resonant second harmonic generation, *Phys. Rev. Lett.*, 48, 478, 1982.
25. **Rasing, T., Shen, Y. R., Kim, M. W. and Grubb, S. G.**, Observation of molecular reorientation at a two dimensional liquid phase transition, *Phys. Rev. Lett.*, 55, 2903, 1985.
26. **Guyot-Sionnest, P., Shen, Y. R. and Heinz, T. F.** Comments on "Determination of the nonlinear optical susceptibility c(2) of surface layers" by B. Dick et al., *Appl. Phys. B*, , 42, 237, 1987.
27. **Zhang, T. G., Zhang, C. H. and Wong, G. K.**, Determination of molecular orientation in molecular monolayers by second harmonic generation, *J. Opt. Soc. Am. B*, 7, 902, 1990.
28. **Goh, M. C., Hicks, J. M., Kemnitz, K., Pinto, G. R., Bhattacharyya, K., Eisenthal, K. B. and Heinz, T. F.**, Absolute orientation of water molecules at the neat water surface, *J. Phys. Chem.*, 92, 5074, 1988.
29. **Meech, S. R. and Yoshihara, K.**, Time-resolved surface second harmonic generation: a test of the method and its application to picosecond isomerization in adsorbates, *J. Phys. Chem.*, 94, 4913, 1990.

30. **Sitzman, E. V. and Eisenthal, K. B.**, Picosecond dynamics of a reaction at the air-water interface studied by surface second harmonic generation, *J. Phys. Chem.*, 92, 4579, 1988.
31. **Heinz, T. F.**, Second order nonlinear optical effects at surfaces and interfaces in *Modern Problems in Condensed Matter Science*, Agranovich, V. M. and Maradudin, A. A., Eds., North-Holland, Vol 29, Ch. 5, 1991.
32. **Sipe, J. E.**, New Green function formalism for surface optics, *J. Opt. Soc. Am. B*, 4, 481, 1987.
33. **Mizrahi, V. and Sipe, J. E.**, Phenomenological treatment of surface second harmonic generation, *J. Opt. Soc. Am. B*, 5, 660, 1988.
34. **Marlow, F., Werner, L. and Hill, W.**, Radiation fields in a surface layer model: application to optical SHG, *Surf. Science*, 249, 365, 1991.
35. **Girault, H. H. and Schiffrin, D. J.**, Thermodynamic surface excess of water and ionic solvation at the interface between immiscible liquids, *J. Electroanal. Chem.*, 150, 43, 1983.
36. **Tamburello Luca, A. A., Hébert, Ph., Brevet, P. F. and Girault H. H.**, Surface second harmonic generation at air/solvent and solvent/solvent interfaces, *J. Chem. Soc. Faraday Trans.*, in press.
37. **Shen, Y. R.**, *Principles of Nonlinear Optics*, Wiley, New York, 1984.
38. **Boyd, R. M.**, *Nonlinear Optics*, Academic Press, San Diego 1992.
39. **Born, M. and Wolf, E.**, *Principle of Optics*, Pergamon Press, Oxford 1980.
40. **Kemnitz, K., Bhattacharyya, K., Hicks, J. M., Pinto, G. R., Eisenthal, K. B. and Heinz T. F.**, The phase of the second harmonic light generated at an interface and its relation to absolute molecular orientation, *Chem. Phys. Lett.*, 131, 285, 1986.
41. **Pershan, P. S.**, Nonlinear optical properties of solids: energy considerations, *Phys. Rev.*, 130, 919, 1963.
42. **Guyot-Sionnest, P., Shen, Y. R.**, Bulk contribution in surface second harmonic generation, *Phys. Rev. B*, 38, 7985, 1988.
43. **Spierings, G., Koutsos, V., Wierenga, H. A., Prins, M. W. J., Abraham, D. and Rasing, T.**, Optical second harmonic generation study of interface magnetism, *Surf. Science*, 287, 747, 1993.
44. **Corn, R. M., Romagnoli, M., Levenson, M. D. and Philpott, M. R.**, The potential dependence of surface plasmon-enhanced second-harmonic generation at thin film silver electrodes, *Chem. Phys. Lett.*, 106, 30, 1984.
45. **Ye, P. and Shen, Y.R.**, Local field effect on linear and nonlinear optical properties of adsorbed molecules, *Phys. Rev. B*, 28, 4288, 1983.
46. **Goldstein, H.**, *Classical Mechanics*, Addison-Wesley, New York, 1950.
47. **Mazely, T. L. and Hetherington III, W. M.**, Second order susceptibility tensors of partially ordered molecules on surfaces, *J. Chem. Phys.*, 86, 3640, 1987.
48. **Rasing, T., Stehlin, T., Shen, Y. R., Kim, M. W. and Valint P.**, Adsorption kinetics of surfactant molecules at a air-liquid interface, *J. Chem. Phys.*, 89, 3386, 1988.
49. **Ward, J. F.**, Calculation of nonlinear optical susceptibilities using diagrammatic perturbation theory, *Rev. Mod. Phys.*, 37, 1, 1965.
50. **Oudar, J. A. and Zyss, J.**, Structural dependence of nonlinear optical properties of methyl (2,4-dinitrophenyl) aminopropanoate crystals, *Phys. Rev. A.*, 26, 2016, 1982.
51. **Pariser, P. and Parr, R. G.**, A semi-empirical theory of the electronic spectra and electronic structure of complex unsaturated molecules. I., *J. Chem. Phys.* , 21, 466, 1953.

52. **Pople, J. A.**, Electron interaction in usaturated hydrocarbons, *Trans. Faraday Soc.*, 49, 1375, 1953.
53. **Yu, J. and Zerner, M. C.**, Solvent effect on the first hyperpolarisabilities of conjugated organic molecules, *J. Chem. Phys.*, 100, 7487, 1994.
54. **Du, Q., Superfine, R., Freysz, E. and Shen Y. R.**, Vibrational spectroscopy of water at the vapor/water interface, *Phys. Rev. Lett.*, 70, 2313, 1993.
55. **Bell, A. J., Frey, J. G. and VanderNoot, T. J.**, Second harmonic generation by p-nitrophenol at water/air and water/heptane interface, *J. Chem. Soc. Faraday Trans.*, 88, 2027, 1992.
56. **Higgins, D. A., Byerly, S. K., Abrams, M. B. and Corn, R. M.**, Second harmonic generation studies of methylene blue orientation at silica surfaces, *J. Phys. Chem.*, 95, 6984, 1991.
57. **Shen, Y. R.**, Surface properties probed by second harmonic and sum frequency generation, *Nature*, 337, 519, 1989.
58. **Higgins, D. A., Abrams, M. B., Byerly, S. K. and Corn, R. M.**, Resonant second harmonic generation studies of *p*-nitrophenol adsorption at condensed phase interfaces, *Langmuir*, 8, 1994, 1992 and **Tamburello Luca, A. A., Hébert, Ph., Brevet, P. F. and Girault, H. H.**, unpublished results.
59. **Conboy, J. C., Daschbach, J. L. and Richmond, G. L.**, Studies of alkane/water interfaces by total internal reflection second harmonic generation, *J. Phys. Chem.*, 98, 9688, 1994.
60. **Samec, Z., Marecek, V. and Weber, J.**, Charge transfer between two immiscible electrolyte solutions. Part II. The investigation of Cs+ ion transfer across the nitrobenzene/water interface by cyclic voltammetry with iR drop compensation, *J. Electroanal. Chem.*, 100, 841, 1979.
61. **Kleinman, D. A.**, Nonlinear dielectric polarization in optical media, *Phys. Rev.*, 126, 1977, 1962.
62. **Muenchausen, R. E., Keller, R. A. and Nogar, N. S .**, Surface second harmonic and sum-frequency generation using a noncollinear excitation geometry, *J. Opt. Soc. Am. B*, 4, 237, 1987.
63. **Guyot-Sionnest, P. and Shen, Y. R.**, Local and nonlocal surface nonlinearities for surface optical second harmonic generation, *Phys. Rev B*, 35, 4420, 1987.
64. **Higgins, D. A. and, Corn R. M.**, Second harmonic generation studies of adsorption at a liquid-liquid electrochemical interface, *J. Phys. Chem.*, 97, 489, 1993.
65. **Hicks, J. M., Kemnitz, K., Eisenthal, K. B. and Heinz, T. F.**, Studies of liquid surfaces by second harmonic generation, *J. Phys. Chem.*, 90, 560, 1986.
66. **Tohda, K., Umezawa, Y., Yoshiyagawa, S., Hashimoto, S. and Kawasaki, M.**, Cation permselectivity at the phase boundary of ionophore-incorporated solvent polymeric membranes as studied by optical second harmonic generation, *Anal. Chem.*, 67, 570, 1995.
67. **Castro, A., Bhattacharyya, K. and Eisenthal, K. B.**, Energetics of adsorption of neutral and charged molecules at the air/water interface by second harmonic generation: hydrophobic and solvation effects, *J. Chem. Phys.*, 95, 1310, 1991.
68. **Higgins, D. A., Naujok, R. R. and Corn, R. M.**, Second harmonic generation measurments of molecular orientation and coadsorption at the interface between two immiscible electrolyte solutions, *Chem. Phys. Lett.*, 213, 485, 1993.
69. **Pohorille, A. and Benjamin, I.**, Molecular dynamics of phenol at the liquid-vapor interface of water, *J. Chem. Phys.*, 94, 5599, 1991.

70. **Pohorille, A. and Benjamin, I.**, Structure and energetics of model amphiphilic molecules at the water/liquid-vapor interface. A molecular dynamics study, *J. Phys. Chem.*, 97, 2664, 1993.
71. **Bhattacharyya, K., Sitzmann, E.V. and Eisenthal, K. B.**, Study of chemical reactions by surface second harmonic generation: *p*-nitrophenol at the air-water interface, *J. Chem. Phys.*, 87, 1442, 1987.
72. **Naujok, R. R., Higgins, D. A., Hanken, D. A. and Corn, R. M.**, Optical second harmonic generation measurements of molecular adsorption and orientation at the liquid-liquid electrochemical interface, *J. Chem. Soc. Faraday Trans.*, in press.
73. **Kavarnos, G. J.**, *Fundamentals of Photoinduced Electron Transfer*, VCH, New York, 1993.
74. **Brown, A. R., Yellowlees, L. J. and Girault, H. H.**, Photoinitiated electron-transfer reactions across the interface between two immiscible electrolyte solutions, *J. Chem Soc. Faraday Trans.*, 89, 207, 1993.
75. **Kott, K. L., Higgins, D. A., McMahon, R. J. and Corn, R. M.**, Observation of photoinduced electron transfer at liquid-liquid interface by optical second harmonic generation, *J. Am. Chem. Soc.*, 115, 5342, 1993.
76. **Meech, S. R. and Yoshihara, K.**, Picosecond dynamics at the solid-liquid interface: a total internal reflection time-resolved surface second harmonic generation study, *Chem. Phys. Lett.*, 174, 423, 1990.
77. **Sitzmann, E. V. and Eisenthal, K. B.**, Dynamics of intermolecular electronic energy transfer at an air/liquid interface, *J. Chem. Phys.*, 90, 2831, 1989.
78. **Du, Q., Freysz, E. and Shen, Y. R.**, Surface Vibrational spectroscopic studies of hydrogen bonding and hydrophobicity, *Science*, 264, 826, 1994.

Chapter 7

QUANTUM THEORY OF CHARGE TRANSFER

Yu. I. Kharkats and A. M. Kuznetsov

I. INTRODUCTION

The development of the quantum theory of charge transfer processes in polar media over last 10-15 years has led to a deeper understanding the details of the mechanisms of the elementary processes and facilitated the application of the theory to the description of new systems. The interface between two immiscible liquids, in particular, represents a system for which recent theoretical results are pertinent. This paper provides a brief discussion of the theory of charge transfer inherent to such complicated systems. A detailed and comprehensive description of earlier results related to charge transfer processes may be found in references [1-3].

II. PHYSICAL MECHANISM OF CHARGE TRANSFER AND THE ROLE OF POLAR MEDIUM.

General principles and approaches to charge transfer processes at the interface of two liquids are similar to those of bulk solutions. They involve the Born - Oppenheimer approximation, the Franck - Condon principle, and the Fermi rule for non-adiabatic processes and stochastic motion along the reaction coordinate for adiabatic reactions.

The Born - Oppenheimer approximation is used to separate electron or proton motion from faster and slower medium modes with which they interact. Usually polarization of liquids is divided into fast (electronic) polarization (P_f) and slow polarization (P_s) which includes other types of the motion in the liquid.

In a uniform medium the fast polarization is constant everywhere and can be excluded from dynamic considerations[3]. The systems under discussion differ in that the fast polarization may change in different liquids due to small variations of the refractive index. It influences therefore the profile of the potential energy for the electron $V_e(x)$. However the electron energies in the donor and acceptor species are usually not calculated but are extracted from the experimental data (optical or electrochemical). These energy levels correspond to an equilibrium configuration of surrounding molecules of the medium. Due to thermal fluctuations in the medium the positions of the electron energy levels vary, thus providing the transitional configuration P_s^* required by the Franck - Condon principle, at which matching of the levels occurs $\varepsilon_A(P_s^*)=\varepsilon_B(P_s^*)$.

0-8493-7694-7/96/$0.00+$.50

It is worth noting that although a liquid may be nonpolar, it does not follow that the electron energy level of an ion in this liquid does not fluctuate at all. Due to long-range Coulomb forces the electron interacts with the fluctuations of the polarization of the other liquid. Moreover it may also be affected by the motion of the counter-ions that tend to form ionic pairs in weakly polar solvents [4].

The transition probability per unit time W_R for non-adiabatic electron transfer between two species located at a distance R from each other may be calculated with the Fermi golden rule, which may be represented in the form

$$W_R = (\beta / i\hbar) V^2 \exp[\beta F_i(R^*)] \int_{c-i\infty}^{c+i\infty} d\theta \mathrm{Tr}\{\exp[-\beta(1-\theta)H_i^a]\exp[-\beta\theta H_f^a]\} \quad (1)$$

where V is the electron resonance integral, $\beta=1/k_BT$, F_i is the Gibbs free energy of the initial state, the trace is calculated over vibrational states, and adiabatic Hamiltonians of the initial and final states have the form

$$H_i^a = H_s - \int d^3r P(r) E_i^V(r) + \varepsilon_i$$
$$H_f^a = H_s - \int d^3r P(r) E_f^V(r) + \varepsilon_f \quad (2)$$

Here H_s is the Hamiltonian describing the state of the inertial polarization of both media P(r), ε_i and ε_f are the energies of the electron in the donor and in the acceptor with due account of its interaction with the fast polarization of the liquids, and $E_i^V(r)$ and $E_f^V(r)$ are the electric fields (in "vacuum") due to the initial and final charge distributions in the reacting species. The second (integral) terms in eq.(2) represent the interaction of the inertial polarization P (dynamic variable) with charged species.

Using the chronological operator T, eq.(1) may be transformed to the form[5]

$$W_R = (\beta / i\hbar) V^2 \int_{c-i\infty}^{c+i\infty} d\theta f_m(\theta) \quad (3)$$

where

$$f_m(\theta) = \exp[-\beta F(\theta)] \exp[-\beta\theta E_r - \beta\theta\Delta F(R^*)] \quad (4)$$

Here $\Delta F(R^*)$ is the free energy of the transition and E_r is the reorganization energy of the medium

$$E_r = -\left(\frac{1}{2}\right)\int d^3r d^3r' \sum_{\alpha,\beta} \Delta E^V_\alpha(r)\Delta E^V_\beta(r') D_{\alpha\beta}(r,r',\omega=0), \qquad \alpha,\beta = x, y, z \tag{5}$$

and $\Delta E^V(r) = E_f^V(r) - E_i^V(r)$.
The quantity $\exp[-\beta F(\theta)]$ in eq.(4) denotes the quantum statistical averaging over the initial states with the Hamiltonian H_i^a

$$\exp[-\beta F(\theta)] = \langle T_\tau \exp[\int_0^{\beta\theta} d\tau \int d^3r \delta P_i(r,\tau)\Delta E^V(r)]\rangle_i =$$

$$\exp(\beta F_i) Tr\{\exp(-\beta H_i^a) T_\tau \exp[\int_0^{\beta\theta} d\tau \int d^3r \delta P_i(r,\tau)\Delta E^V(r)]\} \tag{6}$$

where $\delta P_i(r,\tau) = P(r,\tau) - P_{0i}(r,\tau)$ is the operator in the Heisenberg representation describing the deviation of the inertial polarization from its initial equilibrium value $P_{0i}(r,\tau)$ where

$$P_{0i\alpha}(r) = -\sum_\beta D^R_{\alpha\beta}(r,r',\omega=0) E^V_{i\beta}(r') d^3r', \alpha,\beta = x, y, z \tag{7}$$

Here $D_{\alpha\beta}^R(r,r';\omega)$ is the Fourier component of the retarded temperature Green's function

$$D^R_{\alpha\beta}(r,r';t) = -i\theta(t)\langle[P_\alpha(r,t)P_\beta(r',0)]\rangle = D^R_{\beta\alpha}(r,r';-t) \tag{8}$$

For the effective Hamiltonians H_i^a and H_f^a of the type (2) the calculation of the average in eq.(6) leads to the expression involving only pair correlation function[5]

$$\exp[-\beta F(\theta)] = \exp\{-\frac{1}{2}\sum_{\alpha,\beta}\int d^3r d^3r' \Delta E^V_\alpha(r)\Delta E^V_\beta(r')\int_0^{\beta\theta} d\tau \int_0^{\beta\theta} d\tau' D_{\alpha\beta}(r,r';\tau,\tau')\} \tag{9}$$

where $D_{\alpha\beta}(x,x') = -\langle T_\tau \, \delta P_\alpha(x)\delta P_\beta(x')\rangle$ is the temperature causal Green's function for the operators of the polarization of the medium, and

$$\delta P_i(x) = \exp(\tau H_i^a)\delta P_i(r)\exp(-\tau H_i^a) \tag{10}$$

A similar expression may be obtained in the long-wave-length approximation without use of the explicit form of the Hamiltonians H_i^a and H_f^a [6]. Taking into account the relation between the causal and retarded Green's functions we obtain for $F(\theta)$[7]

$$\beta F(\theta) = \phi(\theta) - \beta\theta E_r \tag{11}$$

where

$$\phi(\theta) = -(1/\pi\hbar)\int d^3r d^3r' \sum_{\alpha,\beta} \Delta E^V_\alpha(r)\Delta E^V_\beta(r')*$$

$$* \int_{-\infty}^{\infty} \frac{d\omega}{\omega^2} \operatorname{Im} D^R_{\alpha\beta}(r,r';\omega) \sinh[\frac{\beta\hbar\omega(1-\theta)}{2}] \sinh(\frac{\beta\hbar\omega\theta}{2}) / \sinh(\frac{\beta\hbar\omega}{2}) \tag{12}$$

Usually the frequency spectrum of the polarization fluctuations almost entirely lies in the classical region $(\hbar\omega << k_B T)$. Neglecting the quantum "tail" we obtain

$$\phi(\theta) \approx \beta\theta(1-\theta)E_r \tag{13}$$

$$F(\theta) = -[\theta E_r - \theta(1-\theta)E_r] = -\theta^2 E_r \tag{14}$$

The calculation of the integral over θ in eq.(3) in this limit gives

$$W_R = [V^2 / \hbar(k_B T E_r / \pi)^{1/2}] \exp[-\beta|F(\theta^*)|] \tag{15}$$

where F(θ) is determined by eq.(14) and θ^* is equal to

$$\theta^* = \frac{1}{2} + \frac{\Delta F(R^*)}{2E_r} \tag{16}$$

Another aim of our discussion is to determine the physical meaning of the reorganization energy E_r defined by eq.(5). Eq.(6) shows that for the barrierless process ($\theta^*=1$) the quantity F(1) is equal to the change of the free energy of the system due to the polarization of the medium by the external field ΔE^V (the free energy related with the inertial polarization is meant throughout). Since the absolute value of F(1) is equal to E_r, this means that the reorganization energy represents the change of the free energy of the system due to the change of the polarization by the quantity $\Delta P(r)=P_{0f}(r)-P_{0i}(r)$. Using the relationship

$$\Delta P_\alpha(r) = -\sum_\beta D^R_{\alpha\beta}(r,r';\omega=0)\Delta E^V_\beta(r')d^3r' \tag{17}$$

we may write the reorganization energy in the form

$$E_r = \frac{1}{2}\int d^3r\Delta E^V(r)\Delta P(r) \tag{18}$$

At $\theta^* \neq 1$ in the classical limit eq.(4) may be written as follows

$$\exp[-\beta F(\theta)] = \langle T_t \exp\{\int_0^\beta dt \int d^3r\delta P_i(r,t)[\theta\Delta E^V(r)]\}\rangle \tag{19}$$

$F(\theta^*)$ therefore represents the change of the free energy of the medium due to its polarization by the field $\theta^*\Delta E^V = \theta^*[E_f^V(r) - E_i^V(r)]$. The absolute value of $F(\theta^*)$ is equal to the reorganization energy of the medium due to the change of the inertial polarization by the value

$$\Delta P_{\theta^*\alpha}(r) = \theta^*\Delta P_\alpha(r) = -\int \sum_\beta D^R_{\alpha\beta}(r,r';\omega=0)\theta^*\Delta E^V_\beta(r')d^3r' \tag{20}$$

corresponding to the transitional configuration[1,3,5]. Introducing the reorganization energy required to attain the transitional configuration

$$E_r(\theta^*) = \frac{1}{2}\int d^3r[\theta^*\Delta E^V(r)]\Delta P_{\theta^*}(r) =$$

$$-\frac{1}{2}\sum_{\alpha,\beta}\int d^3rd^3r' D^R_{\alpha\beta}(r,r';\omega=0)[\theta^*\Delta E^V_\alpha(r)][\theta^*\Delta E^V_\beta(r')] \tag{21}$$

Eq.(15) may be rewritten in the form

$$W_R = [|V|^2 / \hbar(k_BTE_r/\pi)^{1/2}]\exp[-E_r(\theta^*)/k_BT] \tag{22}$$

which shows the meaning of the activation factor as the free energy of attaining the transitional configuration.

The reorganization energy E_r determined by eq.(5) involves the "vacuum" electric field ΔE^V due to the difference of the charge distributions in the reaction products and reactants, and Green's function $D_{\alpha\beta}^R$. It is more convenient to express it through the dielectric properties of the liquids and electrostatic inductions due to the donor and acceptor in the initial and final states [8].

III. OUTER-SPHERE SOLVENT REORGANIZATION ENERGY.

In order to express the reorganization energy of the solvent through its dielectric properties let us consider the change of the polarization at slow and fast application of the external (vacuum) field $\Delta E^V(r)$ [8]. In the former case we have

$$\Delta P_t(r) = [\Delta D(r) - \Delta E(r)] / 4\pi \tag{23}$$

and for the latter

$$\Delta P_0(r) = [\Delta D_0(r) - \Delta E_0(r)] / 4\pi \tag{24}$$

where is ΔP_t and ΔP_0 denote the total and inertialess polarizations respectively, and ΔD, ΔE and ΔD_0, ΔE_0 the inductions and electric fields at slow and fast application of the field ΔE^V, which are related by eqs.(25) and (26)

$$\Delta E_\alpha(r) = \sum_\beta \int d^3r' \, \varepsilon^{-1}_{s\alpha\beta}(r,r') \Delta D_\beta(r') \tag{25}$$

$$\Delta E_{0\alpha}(r) = \sum_\beta \int d^3r' \, \varepsilon^{-1}_{0\alpha\beta}(r,r') \Delta D_{0\beta}(r') \tag{26}$$

where $\varepsilon_{s\alpha\beta}^{-1}(r,r')$ and $\varepsilon_{o\alpha\beta}^{-1}(r,r')$ are the inverse static and optical dielectric tensors of the inhomogeneous nonlocal medium.

It is important for further analysis to distinguish between the longitudinal and transverse fields. The Fourier components of the longitudinal field involve vectors that are parallel to **k**. The vector amplitude of the Fourier component for the transverse field is perpendicular to **k**. The vacuum electric field is longitudinal $\Delta E^V(r) = \Delta E^V_\parallel(r)$. The electric induction $\Delta D(r)$ in non-uniform media in general involves both components. Its longitudinal component is equal to the vacuum field ΔE^V. Therefore, we have for the longitudinal components of the electric field

$$\Delta \mathbf{E}_\parallel(\mathbf{r}) = \Delta \mathbf{E}^V(\mathbf{r}) - 4\pi \Delta \mathbf{P}_\parallel(\mathbf{r}) \tag{27}$$

The transverse component of $\Delta \mathbf{E}$ is zero, therefore we have

$$\Delta \mathbf{D}_\perp(\mathbf{r}) = 4\pi \Delta \mathbf{P}_\perp(\mathbf{r}) \tag{28}$$

In a non-uniform medium $\Delta P_{t\perp}$ and $\Delta P_{0\perp}$ are generally non-zero and not equal to each other, which accounts for the difference between ΔD, ΔD_0 and ΔE^V.

It may be seen that for two vector fields A(r) and B(r) eq.(29) holds

$$\int \vec{A}_{\parallel}(\vec{r})\vec{B}_{\perp}(\vec{r})\, d^3r = \int \vec{A}_{\parallel}(\vec{k})\vec{B}_{\perp}(-\vec{k})d^3k = 0 \tag{29}$$

Therefore we have

$$\int \Delta\vec{D}(\vec{r})\Delta\vec{E}^V(\vec{r})d^3r = \int d^3r[\Delta E^V]^2 \tag{30}$$

and

$$\int d^3r\Delta\vec{E}(\vec{r})\Delta\vec{E}^V(\vec{r}) = \int d^3r\Delta\vec{E}(\vec{r})\Delta\vec{D}(\vec{r}) \tag{31}$$

Introducing then eqs.(23) and (24) into eq.(18) and using eqs.(30) and (31) we obtain

$$E_r = \frac{1}{8\pi}\int d^3r[\Delta\vec{E}_0(\vec{r}) - \Delta\vec{E}(\vec{r})]\Delta\vec{E}^V(\vec{r}) = \frac{1}{8\pi}\int[\Delta\vec{E}_0\Delta\vec{D}_0(\vec{r}) -$$

$$\Delta\vec{E}(\vec{r})\Delta\vec{D}(\vec{r})]d^3r \tag{32}$$

or finally

$$E_r = \frac{1}{8\pi}\sum_{\alpha,\beta}\int d^3rd^3r'[\varepsilon^{-1}_{0\alpha\beta}(r,r')\Delta D_{0\alpha}(r)\Delta D_{0\beta}(r') - \varepsilon^{-1}_{s\alpha,\beta}(r,r')\Delta D_{\alpha}(r)\Delta D_{\beta}(r')] \tag{33}$$

This is the expression for the outer-sphere reorganization energy obtained earlier in[9,10].

The Gibbs free energy function describing the fluctuations of the inertial polarization is a quadratic form in P(r). However for a non-uniform medium it becomes very complicated even in the case where the dielectric functions of the two media have a piece-wise form[8].

In the case where the electrostatic induction is independent of the dielectric properties of the medium (e.g., in the uniform medium or at the interface between the dielectric and the metal) eq.(33) reduces to

$$E_r = \frac{1}{8\pi}\sum_{\alpha,\beta}[\int d^3rd^3r'\{\varepsilon^{-1}_{0\alpha\beta}(r,r') - \varepsilon^{-1}_{s\alpha\beta}(r,r')\}\Delta D_{\alpha}(r)\Delta D_{\beta}(r')] \tag{34}$$

IV. ELECTRON TRANSFER AT THE INTERFACE AND SPECIFIC FORMS OF THE SOLVENT REORGANIZATION ENERGY

General relationships for the probability (or rate constant) of the electron transfer at the interface are given in [11]. We shall dwell upon below on the case where the electron transfer occurs from one liquid to another. Then the reaction rate has the form

$$K = k_0 c_A^{I} c_B^{I} \exp\left\{-\frac{J_{is}^{II} - J_{is}^{I}}{k_B T} - \frac{V_i^{II}}{k_B T} - \frac{(E_r + \Delta F + J_{fs}^{II} - J_{is}^{II} + V_f^{II} - V_i^{II})^2}{4E_r k_B T}\right\} \tag{35}$$

where c_A^{I} and c_A^{I} are the bulk concentrations of the reactants in one of liquids (I), V_i^{II} and V_i^{II} are the works required for the reactants and reaction products, respectively, placed at infinite separation in different liquids, to approach at the reaction distance, and

$$J_{is}^{I} = \frac{z_1 e^2}{2a\varepsilon_1} + \frac{z_2 e^2}{2b\varepsilon_1};$$

$$J_{is}^{I} = \frac{z_1 e^2}{2a\varepsilon_1} + \frac{z_2 e^2}{2b\varepsilon_1} \tag{36}$$

The quantities J_{is}^{I} are obtained from eqs.(36) by substitutions $z_1 \to z_1 + n$ and $z_2 \to z_2 - n$ where n is the number of the electron transferred. ΔF is the reaction free energy, and a and b are the radii of the ions A and B.

The reorganization energy E_r calculated according to eq.(33) has the form[12]

$$\begin{aligned} E_r = {} & \frac{e^2}{2a}\left(\frac{1}{\varepsilon_{01}} - \frac{1}{\varepsilon_{s1}}\right) + \frac{e^2}{2b}\left(\frac{1}{\varepsilon_{02}} - \frac{1}{\varepsilon_{s2}}\right) - \\ & \frac{e^2}{4h_1}\left(\frac{\varepsilon_{02} - \varepsilon_{01}}{\varepsilon_{01}(\varepsilon_{02} + \varepsilon_{01})} - \frac{\varepsilon_{s2} - \varepsilon_{s1}}{\varepsilon_{s1}(\varepsilon_{s2} + \varepsilon_{s1})}\right) - \\ & \frac{e^2}{4h_2}\left(\frac{\varepsilon_{01} - \varepsilon_{02}}{\varepsilon_{02}(\varepsilon_{01} + \varepsilon_{02})} - \frac{\varepsilon_{s1} - \varepsilon_{s2}}{\varepsilon_{s2}(\varepsilon_{s1} + \varepsilon_{s2})}\right) - \\ & \frac{2e^2}{h}\left(\frac{1}{\varepsilon_{01} + \varepsilon_{02}} - \frac{1}{\varepsilon_{s1} + \varepsilon_{s2}}\right) \end{aligned} \tag{37}$$

where h_1 and h_2 are the distances between the first and second ions and the interface, and $h=h_1+h_2$. The subscripts 1 and 2 refer to the first and second liquids respectively, and 0 and s denote the optical and static dielectric constants. If the liquids are identical eq.(37) reduces to the usual expression for the reorganization energy in the uniform medium.

The work terms V_i^{II} and V_f^{II} are calculated according to eq.(38) [11]

$$V_i^{II} = \frac{1}{8\pi}\int d^3r E_i D_i - \frac{z_1 e^2}{2a\varepsilon_{s1}} - \frac{z_2 e^2}{2b\varepsilon_{s2}}$$
$$V_f^{II} = \frac{1}{8\pi}\int d^3r E_f D_f - \frac{(z_1+n)e^2}{2a\varepsilon_{s1}} - \frac{(z_2-n)e^2}{2b\varepsilon_{s2}} \qquad (38)$$

and have the form

$$V_i^{II} = \frac{2z_1 z_2 e^2}{(\varepsilon_{s1}+\varepsilon_{s2})(h_1+h_2)} + \frac{z_1^2 e^2(\varepsilon_{s1}-\varepsilon_{s2})}{4\varepsilon_{s1}(\varepsilon_{s1}+\varepsilon_{s2})h_1} + \frac{z_2^2 e^2(\varepsilon_{s2}-\varepsilon_{s1})}{4\varepsilon_{s2}(\varepsilon_{s1}+\varepsilon_{s2})h_2} \qquad (39)$$

$$V_f^{II} = \frac{2(z_1+n)(z_2-n)e^2}{(\varepsilon_{s1}+\varepsilon_{s2})(h_1+h_2)} + \frac{(z_1+n)^2 e^2(\varepsilon_{s1}-\varepsilon_{s2})}{4\varepsilon_{s1}(\varepsilon_{s1}+\varepsilon_{s2})h_1} + \frac{(z_2-n)^2 e^2(\varepsilon_{s2}-\varepsilon_{s1})}{4\varepsilon_{s2}(\varepsilon_{s1}+\varepsilon_{s2})h_2}$$

Eqs.(35)-(39) determine the rate of charge transfer between two liquids. It should be noted that the boundary between two liquids imposes some steric restrictions on the reaction which leads to a decrease of the reaction volume [12]. In the uniform medium the reaction volume for the spherically symmetric ions is formed by a spherical layer of a thickness ΔR and radius $R=a+b$. At the boundary of two immiscible liquids the solid angle embraced by the reaction layer is smaller than 4π and depends on the degree of penetration of the reactants in the other liquid.

V. ION TRANSFER ACROSS THE INTERFACE OF TWO PHASES.

The calculation of the rates of ion transfer through the interface between two liquids is a complicated problem and the treatment is different depending on the type of the process. The physical mechanism of the transfer of light ions (H^+, Li^+ etc.) between heavy molecular fragments is similar to that for the electron transfer. The behavior of these ions is quantum mechanical and the transitions occur between their various vibrational states. The equation for the transition probability is similar to that for the electron transfer reactions and may be found elsewhere [1,3,11]. The Franck- Condon factor involves here the squared overlap integral for the initial (m) and final (n) vibrational states of the transferable ion $\langle\chi_n^f|\chi_m^i\rangle^2$ and the free energy of the transition between these states involves the difference of vibrational energies E_n^f - E_m^i. The total transition probability is the sum of partial transition probabilities taking into account the occupation of the excited vibrational levels.

The transfer of heavier ions occurs presumably in a classical way. Due to "collisions" with the medium molecules their motion is of diffusional (stochastic) nature. A phenomenological stochastic approach is often used for the description of the ion motion in liquids. It uses Smoluchowski or Langevin equations for the motion in a potential V(x) under the action of random forces. The potential barrier is usually assumed to be one-dimensional and is not calculated. For quasi-steady state conditions Kramers' solution for the rate constant may be used[11]. Although this approach gives a rather general solution for the transition probability for a sufficiently high potential barrier of arbitrary shape, it provides no information about this potential barrier itself.

Therefore the microscopic calculations of molecular dynamics have been used recently, in which the classical Newton equations are solved for some number of interacting molecules (medium molecules interacting with the ion). The complexity of the problem for polar liquids is due to the fact that long-range electrostatic forces allow the ion to interact with a large number of medium molecules. Their microscopic description is impossible at present level of computational technique. One of the ways to take into account this part of the liquid is to consider it as a macroscopic dielectric medium characterized by the complex dielectric function $\varepsilon(\omega)$. The low-frequency limit of the latter is the static dielectric constant ε_s. This value was frequently used to take into account the screening of the interactions between molecules involved in the molecular dynamics (MD) calculations. However, the characteristic time scale for the molecular motion is of the same order of magnitude as the time characterizing the dispersion of the dielectric properties.

A consistent way of incorporating dielectric properties into MD calculations has been suggested[13]. It starts from the dynamic consideration of the whole system including the solute and some number of discrete medium molecules (which will be referred to below as "molecular complex"), and all the other medium described in terms of the polarization P(r,t).

A molecular complex and some quantity of the molecules of the medium characterized by a set of coordinates $x=\{x_1,x_2,\ldots,x_n,..\}$ are considered as a supermolecule immersed into a continuum medium. The dynamics of this supermolecule is of the major interest. It is considered on a microscopic level with the use of some interatomic or intermolecular potentials. It is assumed that the motion of the atoms of the supermolecule is classical and may be described by Newton equations.

The Hamiltonian of the system in general has the form

$$H = H_{sm}(x) + H_P(Q) + V(x,Q) \tag{40}$$

where $H_{sm}(x)$ is the Hamiltonian of the supermolecule, $H_P(Q)$ is the Hamiltonian describing the dynamics of the medium polarization characterized by a set of coordinates $Q=\{Q_1,Q_2,...Q_k,..\}$ and $V(x,Q)$ is the energy of the interaction of these two subsystems.

In what follows we will separate the polarization of the medium into two parts P_{class} and P_{quant}, which behavior is classical and a quantum respectively. A Born - Oppenheimer approximation is used below in order to separate the motions of the quantum polarization P_{quant} and supermolecule . Although the time steps used in MD calculations are small ($\sim 10^{-15}$ sec) and may be comparable with the characteristic times of the motion of quantum part of the polarization, the corresponding change of the configuration of the supermolecule is very small and does not change significantly the interaction field acting on the quantum polarization. Therefore we may expect that the Born - Oppenheimer approximation will be valid.

Thus assuming that the quantum part of the polarization follows adiabatically the dynamics of slower supermolecule and applying the Born - Oppenheimer approximation, we may exclude P_{quant} from the dynamic consideration. In this approximation its role reduces to an equilibrium solvation of any instant configuration of the supermolecule and an effective potential energy for the latter takes the form

$$U_{sm}=U_{sm}^{0}(x) + F_{solv}^{quant}(x) \tag{41}$$

where $U_{sm}^{0}(x)$ is the potential energy of the isolated supermolecule and the free energy of solvation by quantum part of the polarization F_{solv}^{quant} in the Born approximation has the form

$$F_{solv}^{quant}(x) = -(1-\frac{1}{\varepsilon_0})\frac{1}{8\pi}\int d^3rD^2(r;x_1,x_2,\ldots) \tag{42}$$

Here ε_0 is a high-frequency limit of the dielectric constant and $D(r;x_1,x_2,...)$ is the electrostatic induction created by the supermolecule at its given configuration $(x_1,x_2,...)$. Therefore after the separation of the terms corresponding to the quantum polarization the Hamiltonian H_P will involve only variables q_κ describing the classical part of the medium polarization P_{class}.

In what follows an effective Hamiltonian method (EHM) will be used for the description of the dynamics of the classical polarization and its interaction with the supermolecule[1,3]. In the EHM the polarization of the medium is represented as a set of the harmonic oscillators characterized by the "mass-weighted" coordinates q_κ and vibrational frequencies ω_κ. (Coordinates q_κ are related with usual coordinates r_κ as follows: $q_\kappa^2 = m_\kappa r_\kappa^2$). The potential energy of these oscillators has the form

$$U_{osc} = \frac{1}{2}\sum_{\kappa}\omega_{\kappa}^{2}q_{\kappa}^{2} - \sum_{\kappa}v_{\kappa}(x)q_{\kappa} \tag{43}$$

where the first term describes the potential energy of the free oscillators and the second describes their interaction with the supermolecule, $v_\kappa(x)$ being the coupling constants depending on the coordinates $x=\{x_1,x_2,...\}$ of the supermolecule.

Summation rules exist which relate the coupling constants and frequencies with observable quantities[1,3]. Thus the total Hamiltonian may be written as follows

$$H_{eff} = K_{sm} + U_{sm}(x) + K_{q_\kappa} + \frac{1}{2}\sum_{\kappa}\omega_{\kappa}^{2}q_{\kappa}^{2} - \sum_{\kappa}v_{\kappa}(x)q_{\kappa} \tag{44}$$

where K_{sm} and K_q are the kinetic energies of the supermolecule and classical polarization respectively.

It is known that for the system described by the Hamiltonian of eq.(44) closed equations of motion for the x-subsystem may be obtained. Our aim is to express them through the properties of the medium and supermolecule.

Classical equations of motion for each particle constituting the supermolecule and for the effective oscillators describing the classical part of the medium polarization are

$$m_1\partial^2 x_n / \partial t^2 + \partial U_{sm} / \partial x_n = \sum_{\kappa} q_\kappa \partial v_\kappa / \partial x_n + F_m \tag{45}$$

$$\partial^2 q_\kappa / \partial t^2 + \omega_\kappa^2 q_\kappa = v_\kappa(x(t)) \tag{46}$$

here F_m is a random force, and $x(t)=\{x_1(t),x_2(t),...,x_n(t),...\}$.

Eq. (46) for the effective oscillators may be solved exactly for arbitrary dependence of x on t

$$q_\kappa(t) = \left[q_\kappa(0)\cos\omega_\kappa t + \frac{1}{\omega_\kappa}\left(\frac{d}{dt}q_\kappa\right)_0 \sin\omega_\kappa t\right] + \frac{1}{\omega_\kappa}\int_0^t dt'\, v_\kappa(x(t'))\sin\omega_\kappa(t-t') \tag{47}$$

where $q_\kappa(0)$ and $(dq_\kappa/dt)_0$ are the values of the coordinates and velocities at $t=0$.

Inserting eq.(47) in eq.(45) we obtain closed equations for the supermolecule. After averaging over the initial values of the coordinates and velocities and introducing of the equilibrium values $q_{\kappa 0}(x(t))$ of the coordinates of the effective oscillators

$$q_{\kappa 0}(x(t)) = v_\kappa(x(t))/\omega_\kappa^2 \tag{48}$$

we obtain

$$\begin{aligned} & m_n\partial^2 x_n / \partial t^2 + \partial U_{sm} / \partial x_n = \\ & = 2\frac{\partial}{\partial x_n}\int_0^t dt' \sum_\kappa \omega_\kappa \sin\omega_\kappa(t-t')\left[\frac{1}{2}\omega_\kappa^2 q_{\kappa 0}(x(t)) q_{\kappa 0}(\bar{x}(t'))\right] + F_{rn} \end{aligned} \tag{49}$$

where only $q_{\kappa 0}(x(t))$ (but not $q_{\kappa 0}(\bar{x}(t'))$) is differentiated over x.

Eq.(49) may be further transformed using the summation rule[1,3]

$$\frac{1}{2}\sum_\kappa \omega_\kappa^2 q_{\kappa 0}\bar{q}_{\kappa 0} f(\omega_\kappa) = \frac{1}{8\pi}\int d^3r D(r)\bar{D}(r)\frac{2}{\pi}\int_0^{\omega_*} d\omega \frac{\operatorname{Im}\varepsilon(\omega)}{\omega|\varepsilon(\omega)|^2} f(\omega) \tag{50}$$

where $q_{\kappa 0}$ and $\bar{q}_{\kappa 0}$ are arbitrary sets of the normal coordinates values, D(r) and $\bar{D}(r)$ are corresponding electrostatic inductions due to charged particles in the medium, $\varepsilon(\omega)$ is the complex dielectric function of the medium, $f(\omega)$ is a function of ω, and ω_* is the frequency separating quantum and classical polarization regions.

Then we obtain

$$\begin{aligned} & m_1\partial^2 x_n / \partial t^2 + \partial U_{sm} / \partial x_n = 2\frac{\partial}{\partial x_n}\int_0^t dt' \frac{2}{\pi}\int_0^{\omega_*} d\omega \frac{\operatorname{Im}\varepsilon(\omega)}{\omega|\varepsilon(\omega)|^2}\omega\sin\omega(t-t') * \\ & * \frac{1}{8\pi}\int d^3r D(r; x(t)) D(r; \bar{x}(t')) + F_{rn} \end{aligned} \tag{51}$$

where D(r;x) is the electrostatic induction due to the supermolecule.

Eq.(51) shows that the role of the medium in general may not be reduced to the introduction of a dielectric constant into the interaction potentials of the particles of the supermolecule. The medium creates an effective potential that is nonlocal in time. A simple approximation is considered below when the dielectric function of the medium has a Debye form

$$\varepsilon(\omega) = \varepsilon_0 + \frac{\varepsilon_s - \varepsilon_0}{1 - i\omega\tau_D} \tag{52}$$

where ε_s is the static dielectric constant and τ_D is the Debye relaxation time. Then we may put $\omega_* \to \infty$ and

$$\frac{\operatorname{Im} \varepsilon}{|\varepsilon|^2} = \left(\frac{1}{\varepsilon_0} - \frac{1}{\varepsilon_s}\right) \frac{\omega\tau}{1+\omega^2\tau^2} \tag{53}$$

where

$$\tau = \frac{\varepsilon_0}{\varepsilon_s}\tau_D \quad (54)$$

is the longitudinal relaxation time.
Inserting eq.(53) into eq.(51) and calculating the integral over ω we obtain

$$m_1\partial^2 x_n / \partial t^2 + \partial U_{sm} / \partial x_n = 2\frac{\partial}{\partial x_n}\frac{1}{\tau}\int_0^t dt' \, e^{-(t-t')/\tau} *$$

$$* \left(\frac{1}{\varepsilon_0} - \frac{1}{\varepsilon_s}\right)\frac{1}{8\pi}\int d^3r D(r; x(t)) D(r; \overline{x}(t')) + F_{rn} \tag{55}$$

We see that only if the relaxation time tends to zero, e.g., the polarization reacts adiabatically to the change of the configuration of the supermolecule, we have

$$\frac{1}{\tau} e^{-(t-t')/\tau} \to \delta(t-t') \tag{6}$$

and eq.(55) takes the form

$$m_1\partial^2 x_n / \partial t^2 + \partial U_{sm} / \partial x_n + \partial F_{solv}^{class}(x(t)) / \partial x_n = F_{rn} \tag{57}$$

where

$$F_{solv}^{class}(x(t)) = -\left(\frac{1}{\varepsilon_0} - \frac{1}{\varepsilon_s}\right)\frac{1}{8\pi}\int d^3r D^2(r; x(t)) \tag{58}$$

is the free energy of solvation of the supermolecule by the classical polarization, which involves both the solvation free energies of the individual particles and their interaction via the classical polarization.

Together with the second term in the left-hand side of eq.(57) it gives the total effective potential energy for the supermolecule

$$U_{sm}^{eff} = U_{sm}^0 + F_{solv}^t \tag{59}$$

where

$$F^{t}_{solv} = -\frac{1}{8\pi}\left(1-\frac{1}{\varepsilon_s}\right)\int d^3rD^2(r;x(t)) \tag{60}$$

is the free energy of solvation of the supermolecule by total polarization. It involves the total solvation free energies of the individual particles of the supermolecule (the image forces) and their interactions via the total polarization. The latter being added to the potential energy U_{sm}^{0} leads to the appearance of the static dielectric constant in the Coulomb terms describing the interaction of the particles with each other.

However, in general eq.(55) involves memory effects that depend on the relaxation time τ. The dynamics described by eqs.(51) and (55) is more complicated than that obtained with the use of dielectric constants.

In some cases the imaginary part of $\varepsilon(\omega)$ in eq.(53) may be approximated as a sum of two terms

$$\frac{\mathrm{Im}\,\varepsilon}{|\varepsilon|^2} = \left(\frac{1}{\varepsilon_0}-\frac{1}{\varepsilon_{int}}\right)\frac{\omega\tau_1}{1+\omega^2\tau_1^2} + \left(\frac{1}{\varepsilon_{int}}-\frac{1}{\varepsilon_s}\right)\frac{\omega\tau_2}{1+\omega^2\tau_2^2} \tag{61}$$

where ε_{int} is an intermediate value of the dielectric constant separating two absorption bands with different relaxation times τ_1 and τ_2. If both absorption bands lie in classical region, eq.(55) takes the form

$$\begin{aligned} m_1\partial^2x_n/\partial t^2 + \partial U_{sm}/\partial x_n = {} & 2\frac{\partial}{\partial x_n}\frac{1}{\tau_1}\int_0^t dt'\, e^{-(t-t')/\tau_1} * \\ & * \left(\frac{1}{\varepsilon_0}-\frac{1}{\varepsilon_{int}}\right)\frac{1}{8\pi}\int d^3rD(r;x(t))D(r;\overline{x}(t')) + \\ & +2\frac{\partial}{\partial x_n}\frac{1}{\tau_2}\int_0^t dt'\, e^{-(t-t')/\tau_2} * \\ & * \left(\frac{1}{\varepsilon_{int}}-\frac{1}{\varepsilon_s}\right)\frac{1}{8\pi}\int d^3rD(r;x(t))D(r;\overline{x}(t')) + F_{rn} \end{aligned} \tag{62}$$

Thus if the relaxation time τ_1 is small, eq.(62) takes the form

$$\begin{aligned} & m_1\partial^2x_n/\partial t^2 + \partial U_{sm}/\partial x_n - \frac{\partial}{\partial x_n}\left(\frac{1}{\varepsilon_0}-\frac{1}{\varepsilon_{int}}\right)\frac{1}{8\pi}\int d^3rD^2(r;x(t)) = \\ & 2\frac{\partial}{\partial x_n}\frac{1}{\tau_2}\int_0^t dt'\, e^{-(t-t')/\tau_2}\left(\frac{1}{\varepsilon_{int}}-\frac{1}{\varepsilon_s}\right)\frac{1}{8\pi}\int d^3rD(r;x(t))D(r;\overline{x}(t')) + F_{rn} \end{aligned} \tag{63}$$

Thus the fast part of the medium polarization follows adiabatically the motion of the molecular complex adding the equilibrium solvation free energy to the potential energy of the supermolecule, whereas for small time intervals $\Delta t \ll \tau_2$ the term due to the slow polarization may be considered to be approximately constant, creating an external field for the supermolecule. However, when Δt becomes comparable with τ_2 the variation of this term must be taken into account.

The above discussion shows that by using the effective Hamiltonian method, closed equations describing the dynamics of a molecular complex in polar medium can be obtained. These equations may serve as a starting point for molecular dynamics simulations of various systems. They show that the mere introduction of a dielectric constant into the interaction potentials is insufficient for the description of the time evolution of the molecular complex. The reaction of the medium involves effects of memory and depends on the value of the relaxation time τ_2.

References

1. **Dogonadze, R. R. and Kuznetsov, A. M.**, Kinetics of chemical reactions in polar solvents, in *Itogi Nauki i Tekhniki, ser. Physical Chemistry. Kinetics*, Vol. 2, Bondar',V. V., Ed., VINITI, Moscow, 1973.
2. **Ulstrup, J.** *Charge Transfer in Condensed Media*, Springer-Verlag, Berlin-Heidelberg-New York, 1979.
3. **Kuznetsov, A. M.**, *Charge Transfer in Physics, Chemistry and Biology*, Gordon & Breach, Reading, 1995.
4. **Kuznetsov, A. M.**, A quantum mechanical theory of proton and electron transfer in weakly polar solvents, *J. Electroanal. Chem.*, 204, 97, 1986.
5. **Kuznetsov, A. M.**, The free energy of activation of nonadiabatic reactions of electron transfer and the parameters of the reorganization of the solvent, *Electrokhimiya*, 17, 84, 1981.
6. **Ovchinnikov, A. A. and Ovchinnikova, M. Ya.**, On the theory of elementary reactions of electron transfer in polar liquid, *Zhur. Eksp. Teor. Fiz.*, 56, 1278 1969.
7. **Dogonadze, R. R., Kuznetsov, A. M. and Marsagishvili, T. A.**, The present state of charge transfer in condensed phase, *Electrochim. Acta*, 25, 1 1980.
8. **Kuznetsov, A. M. and Medvedev, I. G.**, Activation free energy of the nonadiabatic process of electron transfer and the reorganization energy of the inhomogeneous nonlocal medium, J. Phys. Chem., in press.
9. **Marcus, R. A.**, Free energy of nonequilibrium polarization systems, *J. Phys. Chem.*, 98, 7170, 1994.
10. **Liu, Y.-P. and Newton, M. D.**, Reorganization energy for electron transfer at film-modified electrode surfaces: a dielectric continuum model, *J. Phys. Chem.*, 7162, 1994.
11. **Kuznetsov, A. M. and Kharkats, Yu. I.**, Problems of quantum theory of charge transfer reactions at the interface between two immiscible liquids, in ***The interface structure and electrochemical processes at the boundary between two immiscible liquids***, Kazarinov, V. E., Ed., Springer-Verlag, Berlin-Heidelberg-New York-London-Paris-Tokyo, 1987, p. 11.
12. **Marcus, R. A.**, Reorganization free energy for electron transfers at liquid-liquid and dielectric semiconductor-liquid interfaces, *J. Phys. Chem.*, 94, 1049, 1990.
13. **Kuznetsov, A. M. and Krishtalik, L. I.**, Equations of motion for charged particles in polar liquids, in press.

Chapter 8

KINETICS OF CHARGE TRANSFER

Zdeněk Samec

I. INTRODUCTION

The primary purpose of this review is to summarize the results of various studies of the kinetics of charge transfer across an interface between two immiscible electrolyte solutions (ITIES). Attention has focused mainly on simple ion transfer processes,

$$X^z_i\,(w) \rightleftharpoons X^z_i(o) \tag{1}$$

where X^z_i is an ion with the charge number z_i, and w or o denote the aqueous or the organic solvent phase, respectively and, to a lesser extent, on the simple electron transfer between a redox couple O1/R1 in water and a redox couple O2/R2 in oil, i.e.

$$O1(w) + R2(o) \rightleftharpoons R1(w) + O2(o) \tag{2}$$

When the bulk concentrations of all the reactants in eq. (1) or (2) differ from zero, contact equilibrium potential difference will be established, which is given by the Nernst-type equation for ion transfer [1],

$$\Delta_o^w\varphi = \Delta_o^w\varphi_i^0 + (RT/z_iF)\ln(a_i^o/a_i^w) \tag{3}$$

where R is the gas constant, T is the absolute temperature, F is the Faraday constant, z_i is the ion charge number and a_i^o or a_i^w are the ion activities in o or w, respectively. The standard ion transfer potential $\Delta_o^w\varphi_i^0$ is determined by the standard Gibbs energy of transfer of the ion i from the aqueous to the organic solvent phase, $\Delta^O_W G^0_i$,

$$\Delta_o^w\varphi_i^0 = -(1/z_i F)\,\Delta^O_W G^0_i \tag{4}$$

$\Delta_o^w\varphi_i^0$ and $\Delta^O_W G^0_i$ are not experimentally accessible quantities or, more precisely, they can be measured relative to the standard ion transfer potential and the standard Gibbs energy of transfer of a reference ion, respectively. Their absolute values are then inferred on the basis of a non-thermodynamic hypothesis[2,3]. An equation analogous to eq. (3) holds for the electron transfer[4], i.e.

$$\Delta_o^w\varphi = E_2^{o,0} - E_1^{w,0} + \Delta_o^w\varphi_{H+}^0 + (RT/nF)\ln(a_{O2}^o a_{R1}^w / a_{R2}^o a_{O1}^w) \tag{5}$$

where $E_1^{o,0}$ and $E_2^{w,0}$ are the standard redox potentials of O1/R1 in w and O2/R2

0-8493-7694-7/96/$0.00+$.50

in o related to the standard H^+/H_2 reference electrode in the respective phases, $\Delta_o^w\varphi_{H+}^0$ is the standard proton transfer potential, cf. eq. (4) and n is the number of electrons transferred in reaction (2).

Section II deals with the ion transfer kinetics. The apparent kinetic parameters are defined first and the results of their measurements are summarized. Then, the corrections of the apparent kinetic parameters for the effect of the electrical double layer are discussed and the theory of the elementary ion transfer step is outlined. Electron transfer kinetics will be dealt with in Section III in a similar manner.

II. ION TRANSFER

A. APPARENT KINETIC PARAMETERS

1. Definitions

Heterogeneous reaction (1) is currently supposed to follow the first-order rate law

$$J = k_f c^w - k_b c^o \quad (6)$$

where J is the interfacial ion flux, c^w or c^o are the ion concentrations on its aqueous or organic solvent side, and k_f or k_b are the heterogeneous rate constants (e.g., in cm s^{-1}) for the forward or the backward ion transfer, respectively. By taking into account the principle of microscopic balancing, the forward and the backward rate constants can be related to each other by[4],

$$k_f / k_b = \exp(-\Delta^o_w \bar{G}^0_i / RT) = \exp[zF(E - E^0)/RT] \quad (7)$$

where $\Delta^o_w\bar{G}^0_i = \Delta^o_w G^0_i - zF\Delta^w_o\varphi = -zF(\Delta^w_o\varphi - \Delta^w_o\varphi^0_i)$ is the standard electrochemical Gibbs energy change for the ion transfer (1). Eq. (7) holds irrespectively of the actual dependence of the rate constant on the potential E. For the sake of comparison, two apparent kinetic parameters are usually introduced. First one is the standard rate constant k^s_0 at the equilibrium potential $E = E^0$,

$$k^s_0 = k_f(E{=}E^0) = k_b(E{=}E^0) \quad (8)$$

Second parameter is the apparent charge transfer coefficient α_f (sometimes denoted as α_{app}), which characterizes the potential dependence of the forward rate constant,

$$\alpha_f = (RT/zF)(\partial \ln k_f / \partial E) \quad (9)$$

Its value at $E{=}E^0$ will be denoted as α_{f0}.

2. Experimental results

Kinetic studies of ion transfer have been aimed mainly to clarify the effect of the electrical potential difference. Besides, because the rate of both bulk and interfacial ion transport should depend on the properties of the medium, effects of the temperature, viscosity and dielectric permittivity were also examined. Kinetic data for series of homologous ions provided some insight into the ion transfer dynamics in terms of the ion mobility and solvation. Finally, phase behavior and ion permeability of monolayers of amphiphilic molecules formed at polarized liquid/liquid interfaces were investigated as suitable models of ion transfer across biological boundaries. Most of the experimental work was done using the water/nitrobenzene system, while kinetic studies of the water/1,2-dichloroethane interface are few.

Experimental approaches to the ion transfer kinetics are based on the classical galvanostatic[5] or potentiostatic[6] techniques, such as chronopotentiometry[7,8], chronocoulometry[9], cyclic voltammetry[6], convolution potential sweep voltammetry[10], phase selective a.c. voltammetry[11] or equilibrium impedance measurements[12]. These techniques were applied mostly to liquid/liquid interfaces with a macroscopic area (typically around 0.1 cm^2). Later on, microelectrode methodology has been introduced[13,14] and further developed[15-17]. Experimental difficulties in obtaining reliable kinetic parameters at macroscopic interfaces can arise from high solution resistance (typically of order 10^2 - 10^3 Ω) compared to the kinetic resistance (typically less than 10 Ω), as well as from the non-homogeneous polarization due to the curved interface and/or an improper electrode configuration, or from the electro-mechanical phenomena induced by the potential-dependent surface tension[12,18]. Artifacts in the a.c. impedance measurements of the liquid/liquid interfaces, which can originate from an improper design of the electrolytic cell were discussed[19]. It was concluded that the main origin of the observed high frequency dispersion is the high value of the resistance of the potential probe for the organic phase. An ideally flat liquid/liquid interface has been recognized as an essential requirement, together with the symmetric configuration of electrodes[18,20,21] and low-impedance potential probes[19]. A first attempt to construct such a cell[20] suffers from the improper use of Pt wires as reference electrodes, which probably prevented the authors from obtaining meaningful kinetic data. More advanced approaches to the cell design have relied on a two-[18] or four-electrode[21] galvanic cell. In either case, it is necessary to measure precisely the solution resistance, which is either subtracted numerically under the zero d.c. conditions, or instrumentally under the non-zero d.c. conditions from the total impedance, by using positive feedback[6]. Kinetic information can be then inferred from the impedance data, by using a nonlinear regression technique[22]. A convenient software for performing the nonlinear least square fitting of impedance data is available[23,24].

The first kinetic measurements were made without the proper ohmic drop compensation or subtraction and/or without the ideal polarization of the liquid/liquid interface being considered[8,25-27], and rather low values of the standard rate constant k^s_0 were obtained (10^{-3} - 10^{-4} cm s^{-1}). In more advanced kinetic measurements, the ohmic drop was either numerically subtracted[7], or compensated[6,9-11,28,29] with the help of the positive feedback. The feedback adjustment was based either on the assumption that the separation of the current peaks measured by the slow potential sweep voltammetry should reach the value of (59/z) mV [6,9,10,28], or on the value of the solution resistance obtained by an a.c. bridge technique[11,29]. However, the former adjustment is not very sensitive, whereas the estimated accuracy of 10 Ω [11] in the latter case may not be sufficient, because the kinetic resistances are of a comparable magnitude. Hence, the values of the standard rate constant (10^{-2} - 5×10^{-1} cm s^{-1}) reported in these studies can be also underestimated, though probably to a lesser degree. Later on, the phase angle measurements by a.c. polarography were shown to provide a very sensitive test for the correct adjustment of the positive feedback[18]. Kinetic analysis based on this technique[18,30-32], or on the equilibrium impedance measurements[12,33,34] yielded k^s_0 around 0.1 cm s^{-1}. Owing to a very good agreement between kinetic data inferred for the same ion transfer reactions[12,18,33,34], these results could serve as suitable basis for theoretical considerations until other techniques yield more reliable data. In this respect, fluctuation analysis[15] or ion transfer fluorometry[35,36] appear to be promising. Although the most recent kinetic studies at microITIES[37] point to a much faster ion transfer kinetics with $k^s_0 > 1$ cm s^{-1}, the preliminary results of a fluctuation analysis in a similar system[38] confirm that the order of magnitude of the standard rate constant is 0.1 cm s^{-1}.

For univalent ions, the plots of the logarithm of the apparent rate constant k_f against the potential difference (Tafel plots) have reciprocal slopes of about 118 mV per decade[6,9,11,18,29-31,34,39]. Tafel plots derived from d.c. or a.c. voltammetric measurements in a sufficiently broad potential range are usually curved[31,39]. One of the characteristic features of ion transfer kinetics is the minor effect of the ion structure or size (diameter). Table 1 summarizes the apparent kinetic parameters for several homologous series of univalent ions. Typically, the apparent standard rate constant k_0^s is of the order of 0.1 cm s^{-1} and the apparent charge transfer coefficient at the standard potential difference $\alpha_{0f} = 0.5 \pm 0.1$. While the ion transport rate in the bulk of the solution reflects clearly a change in the ion size, no straightforward effect on the interfacial ion transport is seen. If the ion transfer across the interface were essentially similar to the ion transport in the bulk of the solution[9], a linear relationship would be observed between k_0^s and the ion mobility. However, k_0^s can both decrease and increase with the ion mobility[18]. A conclusion was drawn that the hydrodynamic friction due to the solvent-ion interactions dynamics and the viscous momentum transport exerted on the transferring ion by the solvent layers at the interface play a significant role in the ion transfer dynamics[18].

Effect of temperature on ion transfer across the water/ nitrobenzene interface was studied for a series of six quaternary ammonium and phosphonium cations and two anions using cyclic voltammetry and equilibrium impedance measurements[33]. Standard entropies ($\Delta^O_W S^0_i$) and enthalpies ($\Delta^O_W H^0_i$) of ion transfer have been evaluated from the experimentally accessible reversible half-wave potential ($E_{1/2}^{rev}$) and standard Gibbs energy of transfer ($\Delta^O_W G^0_i$),

$$- z F (dE_{1/2}^{rev} / dT) = \Delta^O_W S^0_i - \Delta^O_W S^0_{ref} \quad (10)$$

$$\Delta^{O}_{W}G^{0}_{i} = \Delta^{O}_{W}H^{0}_{i} - T\,\Delta^{O}_{W}S^{0}_{i} \tag{11}$$

Table 1

Standard potential differences $\Delta^{w}_{o}\varphi^{0}$ and apparent kinetic parameters k_0^{a} and α_{fo} for the transfer of cations and anions across the water/nitrobenzene interface[a]

Ion	$\Delta^{w}_{o}\varphi^{0}$ (V)	$10 \times k_0^{a}$ ($cm\ s^{-1}$)	α_{fo}	ref.
Me_3NH^+	0.092	0.86	0.44	18
choline	0.079	0.83	0.47	18
Me_4N^+	0.030	0.90	0.50	18
		1.36	0.58	34
		1.20	-	33
$EtMe_3N^+$	0.003	0.78	0.50	18
$Et_2Me_2N^+$	- 0.022	0.83	0.43	18
Me_3PrN^+	-0.027	0.91	0.54	18
Et_3MeN^+	-0.042	1.12	0.52	18
Me_3BuN^+	-0.063	1.03	0.54	18
Et_4N^+	-0.067	1.5	0.55	18
		0.9	0.64	34
		1.1	-	33
Et_3PrN^+	-0.093	0.88	0.50	18
$EtPr_3N^+$	-0.143	0.80	0.42	18
Pr_4N^+	-0.170	0.47	0.44	18
		1.36	0.60	34
Me_4P^+	0.009	1.48	0.55	34
Me_3EtP^+	-0.020	1.26	0.51	34
		1.14	-	33
Me_3PrP^+	-0.050	1.26	0.58	34
		1.05	-	33
Me_3BuP^+	-0.084	0.89	0.57	34
Me_2V^{2+}	-0.015	0.48	0.50	34
Et_2V^{2+}	-0.043	0.53	0.49	34
Pr_2V^{2+}	-0.058	0.68	0.55	34
Pi^-	0.039	0.83	0.56	12
		0.37	0.45	29
PF_6^-	-0.007	1.63	0.50	31
ClO_4^-	-0.083	0.9	0.57	34
	-0.110	1.08	0.53	31
BF_4^-	-0.153	1.73	0.44	31
SCN^-	-0.189	0.91	0.45	31

[a] Experimental conditions : temperature 293[12,33,34] or 298 K[18,29,31], base electrolyte concentrations in both phases 0.05 [12,33,34] or 0.1[18,29,31] mol dm^{-3}.

The structure-breaking properties of small ions and enhancement of water structure in the presence of large cations are manifested in both entropic and enthalpic contributions, which both increase with the ion size, cf. Table 2. Ion diffusion coefficients at various temperatures were evaluated from voltammetric data. The temperature dependence of the rate constant k_{ft} corrected for the effect of the double layer, and of the ion diffusion coefficient provided the apparent activation energies of the ion transfer $E_{tr}^{a} = -R\,\partial \ln k_{ft}/\partial(1/T)$, and of diffusion $E_d^{a} = -R\,\partial \ln D/\partial(1/T)$, respectively (Table 2), which will be discussed in the next chapter.

Table 2
Thermodynamic functions and apparent activation energies for various ion transfer reactions at the water/nitrobenzene interface at 293 K (adapted from ref. 33)

Ion	$\Delta^o_w G^0_i$ kJ/mol	$\Delta^o_w H^0_i$ kJ/mol	$\Delta^o_w S^0_i$ J/mol K	E_w^* kJ/mol	E_d^* kJ/mol	$\Delta\bar{G}^*_i$ kJ/mol
Me_4N^+	2.9	-5.3	-27.4	19.3	18.8	4.7
Et_4N^+	-6.4	-3.9	-3.9	19.8	16.8	5.4
Bu_4N^+	-26.5	0.6	-	-	-	-
Me_4P^+	0.9	-11.6	-41.8	-	-	
Me_3EtP^+	-1.9	-7.8	-19.6	13.6	16.9	1.5
Me_3PrP^+	-4.8	-6.4	-5.2	20.1	19.5	4.4
Me_3BuP^+	-8.1	-3.0	17.0	-	-	-
Pi^-	-4.1	-4.6	-1.6	19.2	19.0	3.2
ClO_4^-	7.9	-12.6	-68.8	-	-	-

Other remarkable effects of the medium are related to the viscosity and dielectric constant. In particular, the transfer of acetylcholine across the water/1,2-dichloroethane interface has been studied as a function of the viscosity of the aqueous phase varied by adding sucrose (0 - 48 wt%)[9]. Both ion diffusion coefficient and apparent standard rate constant k_0^s were found to be inversely proportional to the viscosity and their temperature provided almost equal apparent activation energies (enthalpies) of about 21 kJ mol^{-1}. Plots of log k_0^s or the log D against the change in the standard Gibbs energy of ion transfer $\delta\Delta^O_W G^0_i$ due to the presence of sucrose were found to have similar slopes. Analogously, the transfer of acetylcholine from water to nitrobenzene was studied as a function of composition of the organic solvent, which was varied by adding nonpolar tetrachloromethane[28]. With increasing concentration of CCl_4 (0 - 86 wt%) both dielectric constant and viscosity of the organic phase decrease, which has an effect on the apparent standard rate constant k_0^s, ion diffusion coefficient in the organic phase D^o and the standard Gibbs energy of ion transfer $\Delta^O_W G^0_i$. It has been shown[40] that either effect appears to be a direct consequence of the stochastic theory[41,42]. Apparently, the correlation of the apparent standard rate constant with the standard potential difference (or standard Gibbs energy change) may not have a straightforward physical meaning when the solution viscosity varies. In particular, the parameter to be tested is not k_0^s, but the product of the rate constant and the viscosity, $k_0^s\,\eta$[40].

Ion transfer across phospholipid monolayers at liquid/liquid interfaces has been studied with the aim to elucidate mechanism and kinetics of ion transport across bilayer lipid membranes (BLM). The main advantage of using these systems is in the possibility of controlling the interfacial potential difference, which in the case of the BLM has to be inferred indirectly[43]. In the pioneering study[44], the facilitated Na^+ ion transfer across the water/ nitrobenzene interface in the presence of dibenzo-18-crown-6 has been found to be inhibited by adsorbed egg lecithin molecules at temperatures below 5 °C. Since the change in the ion transfer rate has been thought to be due to the phase transition of the phospholipid which normally occurs at a higher temperature, a conclusion was made that the transition is influenced by the adjacent nitrobenzene phase. Analogously, the Et_4N^+ ion transfer across the water/1,2-dichloroethane interface is inhibited in the presence of egg lecithin[45]. A simple model has been proposed[43], in which the rate-determining step is the formation of a pore in the phospolipid layer with the critical radius equal at least to the radius of the transferrable ion. These studies have indicated the importance of the phase behavior of the monolayer, as well as its chemical and structural characterization[46-48]. With this aim, monolayer characteristics and the ion permeability of saturated monolayers of six L-α-phosphatidyl-cholines: dilauroyl- (DLPC), dimiristoyl- (DMPC), dipalmitoyl- (DPPC), distearoyl- (DSPC), diarachidoyl- (DAPC), and dibehenoyl-phosphatidylcholine (DBPC), have been studied by measuring the a.c. impedance at the polarized water/nitrobezene interface[47]. The DLPC and DMPC monolayers are in a liquid-expanded state between 5 and 30 °C, whereas the DSPC, DAPC and DBPC are in a liquid-condensed state in the same temperature range. The DPPC monolayer exhibits a temperature-induced phase transition at 13 °C. The monolayers in the liquid-condensed state reduce the rate of transfer of both Me_4N^+ and Et_4N^+. This result indicates that a phosphatidylcholine monolayer exerts a hydrodynamic friction on transferring ions. In contrast, monolayers in the liquid-expanded state accelerate the transfer of both ions, for which an explanation was seen in the change of ion distribution or the solvent structure-related friction[47]. The role of these two factors has been studied in detail by using the same method for the transfer of a cation (Et_4N^+) and an anion (ClO_4^-) across a dilauroyl-phosphatidylethanolamine (DLPE) monolayer[46]. The advantage in using DLPE is that it forms a denser monolayer that phosphatidylcholines, and that the presence of an amino group in the hydrophilic head of DLPE makes it possible to change the surface charge density by changing the pH in the aqueous phase. The ion permeability was found to depend on packing density of the monolayer, surface charge density, and charge and size of transferring ions. When the condensed monolayer was present, a decreased ion transfer rate was detectable for Et_4N^+, but not for ClO_4^-, which has a smaller radius[46]. The negatively charged DLPE monolayer accelerates the transfer of the former ion and reduces appreciably the transfer of the latter ion. The effect is reversed in the case of a positively charged DLPE monolayer. The authors concluded that the ion permeability is primarily determined by the hydrodynamic friction and the double layer effect arising from the sign and density of the surface charge of adsorbed phospholipid molecules.

Simple ion transfer, eq. (1), is often coupled to a chemical reaction, such as the ion association or the formation of a complex at the ITIES, e.g.,

$$X^z\,(w) + Y^s\,(o) \rightleftharpoons XY^{z+s}(o) \tag{12}$$

where Y^s is a counter ion or a ligand with the charge number s. Only a few kinetic data for such a type the charge transfer reaction have been reported, which concern mainly the transfer of alkali[37,49-51] or alkaline earth[52] metal cations facilitated by polyether macrocyclic or acyclic ligands. These data are rather controversial, as the reported values of the apparent standard rate constant differ as much as 0.001 cm s^{-1} [50] and 3 cm s^{-1} [37] for the same reaction.

B. TRUE KINETIC PARAMETERS

1. Static and dynamic effects of the electrical double layer

Due to the existence of the electrical double layer, the concentration of an ion near the interface varies, which should influence the ion transfer rate. The static effect of an electrical double layer is accounted for by assuming an equilibrium ion distribution up to a point located close to the interface, from which the ion becomes driven by the local potential gradient to cross the interface. The assumption of a three-step (four-position) mechanism has been introduced by Gavach et al[53], but the idea can be traced back to a review by Buck[54]. Following this assumption, eq. (1) can be expanded into

$$X^z(w) \rightleftharpoons X^z(a) \rightleftharpoons X^z(b) \rightleftharpoons X^z(o) \qquad (13)$$

where the positions a and b are located in the interfacial region. Gavach et al.[53] suggested that the positions a and b are those of the outer Helmholtz planes x_2^W and x_2^O in the two phases in contact, and that the ion transfer from a to b is the rate determining step. This suggestion was adopted by several authors[4,55,56], while others[57] left the exact locations of a and b open to further discussion. Unless we refer to the latter model, we will assume that $a = x_2^W$ and $b = x_2^O$.

The apparent rate constant k_f was expressed[57] by an equation, which is equivalent to the classical Frumkin correction,

$$k_f = k_{ft}\,(c^a/c^W) = k_{ft} \exp\,[-(\Delta^a_W G^0_i + z F\,\Delta^a_W\varphi)/RT] \qquad (14)$$

where k_{ft} is the rate constant for the rate-determining step (i.e., the true or corrected rate constant), c^a is the concentration of the transferred ion at the location a, $\Delta^a_W G^0_i$ is the standard Gibbs energy for the ion transfer from the bulk aqueous phase to the position a, and $\Delta^a_W\varphi$ is the corresponding difference in the electrostatic potential. This approach is consistent with the idea of the mixed solvent layer introduced earlier[57a], which would imply a partial resolvation of the ion prior to the rate-determining step, and would give substance to the Gibbs energy term in eq. (14). However, molecular dynamics studies[58,59] point to a molecularly sharp boundary of two immiscible liquids. Consequently, the solvation structure of the ion near the boundary is probably the same as in the bulk of the solution, and the term $\Delta^a_W G^0_i$ should equal to zero.

The temperature dependence of the rate constant k_{ft} in eq. (14) was supposed[4] to have the form of the Arrhenius equation,

$$k_{ft} = Z \exp\,(-\Delta^{*}_{a}\bar{G}^0_i\,/RT) \qquad (15)$$

where the standard activation Gibbs energy $\Delta^{*}_{a}\bar{G}^{0}_{i}$ is proportional to the standard electrochemical Gibbs energy change $\Delta^{b}_{a}\bar{G}^{0}_{i}$ between locations a and b, i.e.,

$$\Delta^{*}_{a}\bar{G}^{0}_{i} = \Delta\bar{G}^{*}_{i} + \alpha\ \Delta^{b}_{a}\bar{G}^{0}_{i} \tag{16}$$

Effect of the electrical double layer on the elementary ion transfer step from a to b is then recovered upon expressing the Gibbs energy change $\Delta^{b}_{a}\bar{G}^{0}_{i}$ as the sum of the standard Gibbs energy of transfer $\Delta^{o}_{w}G^{0}_{i}$ from w to o and the electrostatic energy change between a and b,

$$\Delta^{b}_{a}\bar{G}^{0}_{i} = \Delta^{o}_{w}G^{0}_{i} - zF\Delta^{a}_{b}\varphi \tag{17}$$

where $\Delta^{a}_{b}\varphi$ is a part of the interfacial potential difference $\Delta^{w}_{o}\varphi$,

$$\Delta^{w}_{o}\varphi = \Delta^{a}_{b}\varphi + \Delta^{b}_{o}\varphi - \Delta^{a}_{w}\varphi \tag{18}$$

By using eqs. (15), (16) and (17), the following equation was derived[4] for k_f,

$$k_f = k^s \exp\left[\alpha zF(\Delta^{w}_{o}\varphi - \Delta^{w}_{o}\varphi^{0}_{i})/RT\right] \tag{19}$$

where

$$k^s = k_0\ \exp\{-zF[(1-\alpha)\Delta^{a}_{W}\varphi + \alpha\Delta^{b}_{O}\varphi]/RT\} \tag{20}$$

and

$$k_0 = k^{0}_{0}\exp(-\Delta\bar{G}^{*}_{i}/RT) \tag{21}$$

Note that the parameters k^s and α are not identical to the apparent rate constant k^{s}_{0} and the apparent charge transfer coefficient α_f defined by eq. (8) and (9), respectively. Since k^s can depend on the potential E indirectly through the exponential term with the potential differences across the space charge regions in eq. (20), $k^{s}_{0} = k^{s}(E{=}E^{0})$. The relationship between α_f and α can be derived from eqs. (19) and (20),

$$\alpha_f = \alpha(\partial\Delta^{a}_{b}\varphi/\partial E) + (\partial\alpha/\partial E)(\Delta^{a}_{b}\varphi - \Delta^{W}_{O}\varphi^{0}_{i}) - (\partial\Delta^{a}_{W}\varphi/\partial E) \tag{22}$$

When the potential difference across the inner layer $\Delta^{a}_{b}\varphi = \Delta^{W2}_{O2}\varphi$ is negligible, and the parameter α is a constant, the apparent charge transfer coefficient α is controlled only by the potential difference across the space charge region, $\alpha_f \approx -\partial(\varphi_2^{w} - \varphi^{w})/\partial E$, cf. eq. (22). According to the Gouy-Chapman theory, this potential difference can be expressed as a function of $\Delta^{W}_{O}\varphi$ [55]

$$\varphi_2^{W} - \varphi^{W} \approx -(1/2)(\Delta^{W}_{O}\varphi - \Delta^{W2}_{O2}\varphi) \mp (RT/z_b F)\ln(\epsilon^{O}c^{O}/\epsilon^{W}c^{W})^{1/2} \tag{23}$$

where ϵ^{O} or ϵ^{W} are the dielectric permittivities of the organic solvent and water, and c^O or c^W the concentrations of a z_b:z_b supporting electrolyte in the organic or the aqueous phase, respectively and, hence, $\alpha_f \approx 1/2$. In such a case, the experimentally observed Butler-Volmer behavior would not be of any relation to the properties of the energy barrier, but rather to the double layer structure. However, more recent studies[60] of the electrical double layer have indicated that the potential difference across the inner layer represents an appreciable part of the interfacial potential difference $\Delta^W{}_O\varphi$. Besides, the parameter α can depend on the potential E[31,39].

In addition to the static effect, the dynamic (Levich) effect of the electrical double layer has been treated theoretically[61]. By assuming the steady-state ion transport, the Nernst-Planck equation was integrated in the diffuse layer to yield the rate equation analogous to eq. (6). However, the expressions for the forward and backward rate constant, k_f and k_b, comprise a factor depending on the ion mobilities in the aqueous and the organic solvent phase, and on the sign and magnitude of the potential difference across the diffuse layer. Eq. (20) appears to be a limiting case of this more general approach.

2. Experimental results

In order to account for the effect of the electrical double layer on the apparent charge transfer coefficient, the Frumkin-type correction was applied to kinetic data in the earliest kinetic analyses[10,53]. As a result, the corrected rate constant k_{ft} was found to be practically independent of the potential E[7,10,62], which would correspond to the almost constant value of the inner-layer potential difference $\Delta^{W2}{}_{O2}\varphi$. However, more accurate measurements of the picrate ion transfer[12,29] revealed a systematic change in both the corrected rate constant k_{ft} and $\Delta^{W2}{}_{O2}\varphi$ and their significant correlation. The effect was reexamined for the Cs^+ ion transfer with a similar result[39].

On the other hand, the influence of the base electrolyte concentration on the ion transfer rate cast some doubts on the validity of the classical Frumkin correction[32]. Based on eq. (20), the apparent standard rate constant k_0^s should vary with the base electrolyte concentration in a way that is opposite for cations and anions, as well as opposite for ions of the same sign but with the standard potential difference on the positive and negative side relative to the p.z.c.[32]. At the same time, the apparent charge transfer coefficient α_{f0} should decrease with increasing base electrolyte concentration. In contrast, experimental rate constants for various ions show a tendency to increase slightly, while α_{f0} does not vary at all[32]. However, the predicted plots were calculated on assuming that the parameter α is a constant independent of the potential difference[32]. When this condition is relaxed, so that the charge transfer coefficient α can decrease with the inner-layer potential difference[31,39], the terms comprising the potential differences across the space charge regions in eq. (20) can compensate for each other. These mutual compensations can be seen, e.g. in the Cs^+ ion transfer kinetics, for which both apparent kinetic parameters are practically independent of the base electrolyte concentration, yet the corrected Tafel plots coincide[39].

The existence of the relationship described by eq. (16) can be anticipated for any kinetic process, which proceeds from an initial to a final state through a single transition state[63]. A more general form of eq. (16) is the Brønsted relationship[62],

$$\Delta^{*}_{a}\bar{G}^{0}_{i} = \Delta\bar{G}^{*}_{i} + \beta_0\, \Delta^{b}_{a}\bar{G}^{0}_{i} + (1/2)(\partial\beta/\partial\Delta^{b}_{a}\bar{G}^{0}_{i})_0\, (\Delta^{b}_{a}\bar{G}^{0}_{i})^2 + .. \tag{24}$$

where $\beta = \partial\Delta^{*}_{a}\bar{G}^{0}_{i}/\partial\Delta^{b}_{a}\bar{G}^{0}_{i}$ is the microscopic Brønsted coefficient. Obviously, the Brønsted coefficient β differs in value from the parameter α, except for the case that the former coefficient is independent of the Gibbs energy change $\Delta^{b}_{a}\bar{G}^{0}_{i}$. It has been concluded[7,62], that the physical significance of the parameters α_f and α is rather obscure, and that the analysis of the molecular mechanism of the rate-determining step should rely rather on the Brønsted coefficient β, which characterizes the symmetry of the energy barrier[63,64]. Indeed, when the Frumkin-type correction is applied to apparent kinetic data, the logarithm of the corrected rate constant k_{ft} exhibits a significant correlation with $\Delta^{b}_{a}\bar{G}^{0}_{i}$ for ions which differ in size, structure and sign of charge, with the slope corresponding to $\beta \approx 0.5$[7,33,34,62].

C. THEORETICAL CONSIDERATIONS

Theory of the elementary ion transfer step across an ITIES has been based on the multi barrier or stochastic models, which refer to the activation of a diffusion path mechanism, respectively. The existence of a multidimensional energy barrier, which the ion must overcome in crossing the ITIES, has been generally anticipated. However, the origin, shape, height and the location of this barrier have been a matter of continuing discussion. A reference has been made either[4] to Marcus's nonequilibrium thermodynamic[65] or Levich's quantum-mechanica[66]l theories of charge transfer in polar media, or[57] to Eyring's transition state theory of multistep ion transfer in liquids[67]. The former two theories rely explicitly on the role of various subsystems (ions, intramolecular degrees of freedom, solvent molecules), but their application to a specific ion transfer step would require exact definition of the reaction system and detailed knowledge of the wave functions of the subsystems[68]. On the other hand, Eyring's theory of transport processes is easier to extend to interfacial ion transfer. This theory has provided a simple way of introducing the effect of the electrical field on the rate of ion transfer, though with little justification[57].

The stochastic model of ion transport in liquids emphasizes the role of fast fluctuating forces arising from short (compared to ion transition time) random interactions of the ion with many neighboring particles. Langevin's analysis of this model was reviewed[69] with a focus on aspects important for macroscopic transport theories, namely those based on the Nernst-Planck equation. However, from a microscopic point of view, application of the Fokker-Planck equation is more fruitful[70]. It is noteworthy that an integration of either equation yields the expression for the ion transfer rate, which predicts a nonlinear Tafel plot.

In the treatment[41,42] based on the Fokker-Planck equation, the Gibbs energy of the ion was supposed to be a superposition of the potential energy barrier arising from the short-range repulsive interactions between ion and solvent molecules in the inner layer, and the linear potential connected with the long-range electrostatic interactions, comprising the contribution of the polar solvent around the ion. Although the constant field treatment of long-range interactions might be an oversimplification[34], an estimate of the electrostatic Gibbs energy of finite-size ions near a planar boundary between two dielectric media[71] confirms the absence of a discontinuity on the energy profile, which then can be linearized in a narrow range of the reaction coordinate. It has been argued[41,42] that, owing to the short-range interactions, the top of the barrier is not sharp but smooth and parabolic in shape, which has lead to the introduction of the angular frequency ω^* of the ion motion in the transition state (a harmonic approximation). An expression for the rate constant k_{ft} which has the form of eq. (14),

$$k_{ft} = (R\,T / 2\,\pi\,M)^{1/2}\,(M\,\omega^* / \xi^a)\,\exp(-\,\Delta^*_a\bar{G}^0_i / R\,T) \tag{25}$$

where M is the ion molar mass and ξ^a is the friction coefficient (e.g., in kg s^{-1} mol^{-1}) at the location a. Standard Gibbs energy of activation $\Delta^*_a G^0_i$ is given by eq. (16), with the charge transfer coefficient α being a linear function of $\Delta^b_a\bar{G}^0_i$,

$$\alpha = L^*/L^a + \Delta^b_a\bar{G}^0_i / 2\,M\,(\omega^*\,L^a)^2 \tag{26}$$

where L^* or L^a is the distance between the initial (a) and transition or final (b) locations of the ion, respectively. Obviously, the stochastic approach accounts for the local friction anisotropy or variation of the diffusion coefficient in the interfacial region. Besides, this approach suggests that the ion transfer rate dynamics depends on the local ion mobility, cf. the hydrodynamic factor $(M\omega^*/\xi^a)$ in eq. (25). Provided that the temperature dependencies of the friction coefficient in the bulk of the solution, and at the location a, have equal slopes, a relationship can be derived from eq. (25)[33],

$$E_{tr}^a - E_d^a \approx \Delta\bar{G}^*_i - (RT/2) + \alpha\,(\Delta^O_W H^0_i + z\,F\,\Delta^a_b\varphi) \tag{27}$$

where $E_{tr}^a = -\,R\,\partial \ln k_{ft}/\partial(1/T)$ and $E_d^a = -\,R\,\partial \ln D/\partial(1/T)$. As can be seen from Table 2, the apparent activation energies of the ion transfer and diffusion are almost equal. Nevertheless, the standard Gibbs energy of activation $\Delta\bar{G}^*_i$, which was derived by using eq. (27), has a positive value for all ions studied, though the potential barrier appears to be rather low[33]. Actually, the potential barrier can be effectively lowered when the potential of the ion has a fluctuating contribution, because the particle has more opportunities to escape at times when the barrier is relatively low and need not wait for thermal excitation[72]. After inserting known values of all parameters of the stochastic theory into eq. (25), the values of the hydrodynamic factor $M\omega^*/\xi^a$ are found to be of the order of 10^{-4} [33]. In contrast, an estimate based on the frequency of ion vibration $\omega^* \approx 10^{11}$ s^{-1} and the friction coefficient $\xi = R\,T/D \approx 2.4 \times 10^{15}$ g s^{-1} mol^{-1} in the solution bulk and M = 100 g

mol^{-1} yields $M\omega^*/\xi^a \approx 40 \times 10^{-4}$, a value almost two orders of magnitude greater. Since the estimate of the frequency is corroborated by molecular dynamics calculations[58,59], it appears that the reduction in the hydrodynamic factor is the frictional effect. In a previous communication[34], the standard Gibbs energy of activation $\Delta\bar{G}^*_i$ was necessarily overestimated by using the bulk value of the friction coefficient. Another consequence of these considerations is that the slope of the corrected Tafel plots, i.e., log k_{ft} vs. $\Delta^b_a\bar{G}^0_i$, can vary. Indeed, the denominator $2\,M\,(\omega^*\,L^a)^2$ in eq. (26) can be comparable with $\Delta^b_a\bar{G}^0_i$. For $M \approx 100$ and a characteristic transition time and length of 10 ps (i.e., $\omega^* \approx 10^{11}\ s^{-1}$) and 1 nm[58,59], respectively, the former term would have the value around 2 kJ mol^{-1}. Although this is a very rough estimate, it can explain the curvature of corrected Tafel plots observed[39].

In another treatment[73], the Nernst-Planck equation was integrated by assuming a constant gradient of the electrochemical potential in the inner layer at the ITIES, i.e., between the locations a and b. This layer was not supposed to be necessarily the same entity as the ion-free inner layer at the interface. In the absence of an activation barrier at the interface, the equation for the rate constant k_{ft} can be written as[73]

$$k_{ft} = k_0\, y\, e^y / \sinh y \tag{28}$$

where

$$y = (z\,F / 2\,R\,T)\,(\Delta^a_b\varphi - \Delta^W_O\varphi_i^0) \tag{29}$$

$$k_0 = D / L^a \tag{30}$$

Also in this case the curved corrected Tafel plots are predicted with the charge transfer coefficient at $\Delta^a_b\varphi = \Delta^W_O\varphi_i^0$ being equal to 0.5.

Recently, detailed molecular pictures of the interfacial structure on time and distance scale of the ion crossing event, as well as of ion transfer dynamics have been provided by molecular dynamics computer simulations[58,59,74]. On the long-time scale (hundreds of picoseconds) the water/1,2-dichloroethane interface has been shown to be molecularly sharp[58,59]. The density profile for each solvent varies abruptly over the distance of 0.5 - 1.0 nm, which is roughly the sum of solvent molecule diameters. In this limit also the profile of the Gibbs energy of the ion is a smooth function of the distance, indicating the absence of an activated process. Local diffusion (or friction) coefficient is also a smooth function of the coordinate perpendicular to the interface[59], showing a considerable drop on going from nonpolar to polar solvent. While this result is understandable from a physical point of view[59], it is opposite to an experimentally observed change in the apparent diffusion coefficient. On a shorter time scale (tens of picoseconds), which is actually the time scale of ion crossing the interface[59,74], thermal fluctuations superimpose capillary waves on the sharp interface[58], which play a dynamic role in the ion transfer process[74]. It has been concluded[74] that ion transfer is an activated rather than a simple diffusion process, which is accelerated in the presence of the electrical field. However, the existence of an activation barrier of several kcal mol^{-1} is predicted only in the model, which accounts for the change in the liquid structure near the ion. When the system is treated as two homogeneous dielectric media with the ion as a charged sphere, the Gibbs energy profile is smooth even on the short-time scale.

III. ELECTRON TRANSFER

A. APPARENT KINETIC PARAMETERS

1. Definitions

The reaction (2) can be expected to follow the second-order rate law

$$J_e = k_f c_{R1}{}^w c_{O2}{}^o - k_b c_{O1}{}^w c_{R2}{}^o \tag{31}$$

where J_e is the interfacial electron flux in the direction from water (w) to the organic phase (o). The units of the forward and reverse heterogeneous rate constants, k_f and k_b are seen to be, e.g. $m^4\ mol^{-1}\ s^{-1}$. The relationship between k_f and k_b is analogous to eq. (7)[4]

$$k_f / k_b = \exp(-\Delta^O{}_W\bar{G}^0{}_e /RT) = \exp[-nF(E - E_e{}^0)/RT] \tag{32}$$

where $\Delta^O{}_W\bar{G}^0{}_e = \Delta^O{}_W G^0{}_e + nF\,\Delta^W{}_O\varphi = nF(\Delta^W{}_O\varphi - \Delta^W{}_O\varphi^0{}_e) = nF(E-E_e{}^0)$ is the standard electrochemical Gibbs energy of electron transfer from w to o, and n is the number of electrons transferred in reaction (2). The standard potential difference of electron transfer $\Delta^W{}_O\varphi^0{}_e = E_2{}^{o,0} - E_1{}^{w,0} + \Delta_o{}^w\varphi_{H+}{}^0$, cf. eq. (5). Two apparent kinetic parameters are usually introduced, namely the apparent standard rate constant $k^s{}_0$ at the equilibrium potential $E = E_e{}^0$ defined by eq. (8) and the apparent charge transfer coefficient α_f, cf. eq. (9).

$$\alpha_f = -(RT/nF)(\partial \ln k_f / \partial E) \tag{33}$$

2. Experimental results

Various experimental techniques developed for kinetic measurements of ion transfer are also applicable also to electron transfer. However, in order to make the kinetic analysis feasible, it is necessary to solve the transport problem with the boundary condition given by eq. (31)[75-77]. Alternatively, experimental conditions can be chosen so that the electron transfer occurs as a first-order reaction, for which results inferred for an ion transfer reaction can be used [78].

The first electron transfer reaction was observed [79,80] to occur between ferrocene (Fc) in nitrobenzene and $Fe(CN)_6{}^{3-}$ in water

$$Fe(CN)_6{}^{3-}(w) + Fc(o) = Fe(CN)_6{}^{4-}(w) + Fc^+(o) \tag{34}$$

The overall mechanism of the reaction (34) was corroborated[80] by the predicted[75] dependence of the reversible half-wave potential on the concentrations of reactants, and by an agreement between measured value of the standard potential difference $\Delta^{W}_{O}\varphi^{0}_{e}$, and that calculated with the help of eq. (5)[10]. However, the use of ferrocene presents some problems due to the possible transfer of ferricenium ion, i.e., coupling of electron and ion transfer may occur in this case[81], and due to the limited solubility of ferrocene in water (1.7×10^{-5} mol dm^{-3})[82], owing to which the reaction plane may displaced toward the aqueous phase. Although the transfer of ferricenium ion was found to be well separated from the electron transfer, the question of the mechanism has been left open to evidence based on kinetic analysis[83]. Kinetic parameters of the reaction (34) were evaluated[10] with the help of the convolution potential sweep voltammetry[76]. The apparent rate constant k_b was found to be almost independent of the potential and equal to $k_b \approx 4 \times 10^{-7}$ m^4 s^{-1} mol^{-1} (units to Figs. 5 and 6 in ref. 10 should correctly be read as μm s^{-1} M^{-1}). Some features of the apparent kinetic behavior have been confirmed by a.c. impedance measurements[83a]. In a further study[84], the effect of the nature and concentration of the cation present in the aqueous phase on the apparent rate constant was found to be quite negligible. It is well known that both homogeneous and electrode redox reactions involving $Fe(CN)_6^{3-}/Fe(CN)_6^{4-}$ redox couple depend on the nature and concentration of cation[85-87]. Hence, the absence of such an effect suggests that a mechanism involving homogeneous electron transfer is unlikely.

Several other electron transfer reactions, comprising the redox couple $Fe(CN)_6^{3-}/Fe(CN)_6^{4-}$ in water and Lutetium(III) diphtalocyanine[78], Tin(IV) diphtalocyanine[88,89], bis(pyridine)*meso*-tetraphenylporphyrinato iron(II), bis(pyridine)*meso*-tetraphenylporphyrinatoruthenium (III)[90], ferrocene, dimethyl ferrocene or decamethyl ferrocene[91] in 1,2-dichloroethane, were studied by cyclic voltammetry. An essential advantage of these systems, except for ferrocene and its derivatives, is that none of the reactants or products can cross the interface and interfere with the electron transfer reaction, which could be clearly demonstrated. Owing to a much higher concentration of the aqueous redox couple, the pseudo-first order electron transfer reactions could be analyzed with the help of the Nicholson-Shain theory. However, even though they all appear to be quasi-reversible, kinetic analysis was restricted to an evaluation of the apparent standard rate constant k^{s}_{0}, which was found to be of the order of 10^{-3} cm s^{-1}. [78,90]

A series of redox reactions investigated by the current-scan polarography exhibited a reversible behavior, so that no kinetic data were reported[92]. These systems involved ferrocene and tetrathiafulvalene as electron donors or tetracyanoquinodimethane as electron acceptor in the organic solvent phase, and $Fe(CN)_6^{3-}$, Ce^{4+}, Fe^{3+} and $Cr_2O_7^{2-}$ as electron acceptor, or $Fe(CN)_6^{4-}$ or hydroquinone as electron donors, in the aqueous phase.

B. TRUE KINETIC PARAMETERS

The static[4] and dynamic[94] effects of the electrical double layer on the rate of an electron transfer across an ITIES can be treated in a way that is analogous to the ion transfer case. Thus, the static effect can be accounted for by introducing the true forward rate constant k_{ft} of electron transfer[4].

$$k_f = k_{ft}\,\Phi(1,2) = k_{ft}\exp\left[-F\left(z_{R1}\,\Delta^a_W\varphi + z_{O2}\,\Delta^b_O\varphi\right)/RT\right] \tag{35}$$

where $\Phi(1,2)$ is the two-particle distribution function, which can be approximated by the product of the single-particle distribution functions, with the optimum locations for reactants in each phase being denoted as a and b, cf. also ref. 93.

The role of the electrical double layer in the electron transfer described by eq. (34) seems to be less significant than one would expect for highly charged ions[10,84]. This behavior was interpreted as a consequence of ion association, ion size and the potential of the reaction (34), which is positive to the p.z.c.[10]. Indeed, the ion diameter (0.96 nm) is comparable with the thickness of the space charge region, and because anions are repulsed from the electrical double layer, the optimum location x = a was supposed to be displaced from the outer Helmholtz plane toward the solution bulk by the Debye screening length (e.g. 1.36 nm at ionic strength of 0.05 mol dm^{-3}). The corrected Tafel plots evaluated for $z_{O1} = -2$ are almost independent of the electrolyte concentration and their slopes roughly correspond to $\alpha = 0.5$, with $k_{tt} = 6.6 \times 10^{-6}$ m^4 mol^{-1} s^{-1} at $\Delta^b_a\bar{G}^0_e = 0$ [84].

C. THEORETICAL CONSIDERATIONS

Mechanism of electron transfer across a liquid/liquid interface is probably quite similar to that of a homogeneous electron transfer[65,66]. In either case, changes in the oxidation state of both reactants, in their molecular structure including the valence bond deformation, breaking or formation, and in the polarization state of the solvent must be considered. Because of electrostatic interactions of charged reactants with polar solvent molecules, electron energy levels of the reactants are displaced with respect to their position in vacuum and differ from those in products. However, the energy conservation law requires that electron energy levels in the initial and final states must coincide within the uncertainty limit, before the radiationless electron transfer may occur. In accordance with the Franck-Condon principle, electron transfer occurs at a fixed configuration of heavy particles, and its probability can depend on the overlap of electronic wave functions in the initial and final states, which decreases exponentially with increasing distance between reactants. Consequently, the reactants must first approach each other as closely as possible. Then, thermal fluctuations in orientational vibrations (librations) of solvent molecules and intramolecular vibrations of reactants bring the system to an activated state, in which the radiationless electron transfer can occur. Reorganization of solvent and of intramolecular degrees of freedom represent the main contribution to the Franck-Condon barrier of the process. The electron transfer probability was calculated[95] for the Levich's quantum-mechanical model[66], cf. also a later extension of this approach[96] and the review[68]. Recently, the problem has been addressed by Marcus[97], from the point of view of non-equilibrium thermodynamic theory[65].

On this basis, the semiphenomenological theory of the electron transfer across an ITIES was outlined[4]. The true forward rate constant k_{ft} of the electron transfer was expressed as

$$k_{ft} = Z \exp(-\Delta^{*}_{a}\bar{G}^{0}_{e} / RT) \tag{36}$$

where $\Delta^{*}_{a}\bar{G}^{0}_{e}$ is the standard Gibbs energy of activation. The pre-exponential factor Z was supposed to be proportional to the volume of molecular dimensions V_m (mean molar volume of reactants) and to the thickness of the inner layer d,

$$Z = B\, V_m\, d \tag{37}$$

where the constant B involves the overlap integral of the electronic wave functions in the initial and final states[66]. When the harmonic approximation is used for the classical subsystem, $\Delta^{*}_{a}\bar{G}^{0}_{e}$ can be related to the standard electrochemical Gibbs energy of electron transfer from a to b $\Delta^{b}_{a}\bar{G}^{0}_{e}$ through a quadratic function[65,66]

$$\Delta^{*}_{a}\bar{G}^{0}_{e} = (\lambda + \Delta^{b}_{a}\bar{G}^{0}_{e})^2 / 4\lambda = \lambda / 4 + \alpha\, \Delta^{b}_{a}\bar{G}^{0}_{e} \tag{38}$$

where λ is the sum of contributions from the reorganization of solvent λ_o and reactant λ_i,

$$\lambda = \lambda_o + \lambda_i \tag{39}$$

Solvent reorganization energy λ_o was calculated[95], cf. also[68,69], by taking into account the electrostatic contributions from both ions and their images. The parameters of the system comprise the optical and static dielectric constants, ϵ_{op} and ϵ_s, the radii of the two reactants, a and b, the perpendicular distances from the center of the reactants to the interfacial boundary and center-to-center separation distance between the two reactants. Although the expression derived by Marcus[97] is somewhat different, both approaches[95,97] seem to predict the same correlation between the rates of the heterogeneous and homogeneous electron transfer reactions. A simple correlation holds due to the rather weak effect of the nature of the solvent on the solvent reorganization energy, because typically $\epsilon_{op} \approx 2 << \epsilon_s$. Thus, when the reactants are approximately the same size, and can approach each other to the contact distance in both the heterogeneous and the homogeneous case, the corresponding reorganization energies λ_o and λ_o^{hom} are approximately equal,

$$\lambda_o \approx \lambda_o^{hom} \approx N_A (ne)^2 / 8\pi\epsilon^0 \epsilon_{op}\, a \tag{40}$$

where e is the electronic charge and ϵ^0 is the permittivity of vacuum. A similar relation holds when the two reactants are of the different sizes, as characterized by their radii a and b, but the image forces are practically screened by the supporting electrolyte present in excess,

$$\lambda_o \approx \lambda_o^{hom} \approx N_A (ne)^2 (1/a + 1/b) / 8 \pi \epsilon^0 \epsilon_{op} \tag{41}$$

Since also the reorganization term of the reactant λ_i in eq. (41) is probably not very sensitive to the nature of the solvent, the total reorganization energy for the interfacial and homogeneous electron transfer are approximately equal.

The main difference between the homogeneous and heterogeneous electron transfer rates would be then in the pre-exponential factor Z in eq. (36). When eq. (37) is correct, these rates should differ approximately by the factor equal to the thickness of the inner-layer d, i.e., $Z / Z^{hom} \approx d^4$. Following a rigorous procedure, Marcus[97] derived the expression for Z, which in the case of the sharp liquid-liquid boundary reads

$$Z = 2 \pi \gamma \nu (a + b) (\Delta R)^3 \tag{42}$$

where γ is the Landau-Zener non-adiabacity factor, ν is some relevant frequency for the molecular motion and $\Delta R \approx 0.1$ nm appears in an exponent for the dependence of the electron transfer rate on separation distance R ($\propto \exp(-R/\Delta R)$)[97]. When each reactant can penetrate the other phase, Z was obtained as larger by a factor $(a+b)^2/2(\Delta R)^2$ [97]. However, in this case the expression for λ_o would be more complicated, and was not derived. By applying the same approach to the homogeneous electron transfer an equation for Z^{hom} can be derived,

$$Z^{hom} = 8 \pi \gamma \nu (\Delta R)^3 \tag{43}$$

Hence, $Z / Z^{hom} = (a+b)/4$, a result not very different from the above approximation.

The theoretical relationships were used to compare the kinetic data for the interfacial reaction (34) and for the same reaction occurring in the homogeneous phase[84]. Since experimental data for the homogeneous cross-electron transfer reaction (34) are not available, they were estimated from experimental rate constants 5.7×10^6 dm^3 mol^{-1} s^{-1} in acetonitrile[98] and 26 dm^3 mol^{-1} s^{-1} at zero ionic strength in water[99] for the Fc^+/Fc and $Fe(CN)_6^{3-}/Fe(CN)_6^{4-}$ homogeneous exchange-electron transfer reactions, respectively. When corrected for the work term[99], the former rate constant reaches the value of 1×10^6 dm^3 mol^{-1} s^{-1}, being comparable with the latter one. The homogeneous rate constant at zero corrected standard Gibbs energy can be then estimated as the square root of the product of the exchange rate constants[65], i.e. 2.3×10^6 dm^3 mol^{-1} s^{-1}. The value of this constant, as estimated from the heterogeneous corrected rate constant given above, is not very different, namely $k_{bt} / d \approx 6.6 \times 10^6$ dm^3 mol^{-1} s^{-1} for $d \approx 1$ nm.

Marcus[100] has derived a relationship between the pseudo-first order rate constant for the reaction (2) and the rate constants for the electrode reactions of the redox couples involved, and has concluded that the values of the measured rate constant[78] and those calculated from the electrode kinetic parameters are in reasonable agreement.

ACKNOWLEDGEMENT

The author wishes to acknowledge the financial support from the Grant Agency of the Academy of Sciences of the Czech Republic, Grant No. 440411.

REFERENCES

1. **Nernst, W. and Riesenfeld, E.H.,** Ueber elektrolytische Erscheinnungen an der Grenzfläche zweiter Lösungmittel, *Z. Phys. Chem.*, 9, 137, 1892.
2. **Koryta, J., Vanýsek, P. and Březina, M.,** Electrolysis with an electrolyte dropping electrode II. Basic properties of the system, *J. Electroanal. Chem. Interfacial Electrochem.*, 75, 211, 1977.
3. **Girault, H.H. and Schiffrin, D.J.,** Electrochemistry of Liquid-Liquid Interfaces in *Electroanalytical Chemistry,* Vol. 15, Bard, A.J., Ed., Marcel Dekker, New York, 1989, p.1.
4. **Samec, Z.,** Charge transfer between two immiscible electrolyte solutions. Part I. Basic equation for the rate of the charge transfer across the interface, *J. Electroanal. Chem. Interfacial Electrochem.*, 99, 197, 1979.
5. **Gavach, C. and Henry, F.,** Chronopotentiometric investigation of the diffusion overvoltage at the interface between two non-miscible solutions. I. Aqueous solution - tetrabutylammonium ion specific liquid membrane, *J. Electroanal. Chem. Interfacial Electrochem.*, 54, 361, 1974.
6. **Samec, Z., Mareček, V. and Weber, J.,** Charge between two immiscible electrolyte solutions Part II. The investigation of the Cs^+ ion transfer across the nitrobenzene/ water interface by cyclic voltammetry with IR drop compensation, *J. Electroanal. Chem. Interfacial Electrochem.*, 100, 841, 1979.
7. **Samec, Z. and Mareček, V.,** Charge transfer between two immiscible electrolyte solutions. Part X. Kinetics of tetraalkylammonium ion transfer across the water/nitrobenzene interface, *J. Electroanal. Chem. Interfacial Electrochem.*, 200, 17, 1986.
8. **Gavach, C., d'Epenoux, B. and Henry, F.,** Transfer of tetra-n-alkylammonium ions from water to nitrobenzene. Chronopotentiometric determination of kinetic parameters, *J. Electroanal. Chem. Interfacial Electrochem.*, 64, 107, 1975.
9. **Shao, Y. and Girault, H.H.,** Kinetics of the transfer of acetylcholine across the water + sucrose/ 1,2-dichloroethane interface. A comparison between ion transport and ion transfer, *J. Electroanal. Chem. Interfacial Electrochem.*, 282, 59, 1990.
10. **Samec, Z., Mareček, V., Weber, J. and Homolka, D.,** Charge transfer between two immiscible electrolyte solutions. Part VII. Convolution potential sweep voltammetry of Cs^+ ion transfer and of electron transfer between ferrocene and hexacyanoferrate(III) ion across the water/nitrobenzene interface, *J.Electroanal. Chem. Interfacial Electrochem.*, 126, 105, 1981.
11. **Osakai, T., Kakutani, T. and Senda, M.,** A.c. polarographic study of ion transfer at the water/nitrobenzene interface, *Bull. Chem. Soc. Jpn.*, 57, 370, 1984.
12. **Wandlowski, T., Mareček, V. and Samec, Z.,** Kinetic analysis of the picrate ion transfer across the interface between two immiscible electrolyte solutions from impedance measurements at the equilibrium potential, *J. Electroanal. Chem. Interfacial Electrochem.*,

242, 291, 1988.

13. **Ohkouchi, T., Kakutani, T., Osakai, T. and Senda, M.**, Ion transfer microvoltammetry of acetylcholine, *Rev. Polarogr.*, 31, 179, 1986.
14. **Taylor, G. and Girault, H.H.**, Ion transfer reactions across a liquid-liquid interface supported on a micropipette tip, *J. Electroanal. Chem. Interfacial Electrochem.*, 208, 179, 1986.
15. **Mareček, V., Gratzl, M., Pungor, A. and Janata, J.**, Fluctuation analysis of liquid/ liquid and gel/ liquid interfaces, *J. Electroanal. Chem. Interfacial Electrochem.*, 266, 239, 1989.
16. **Campbell, J.A. and Girault, H.H.**, Steady state current for ion transfer reactions at a micro-liquid/ liquid interface, *J. Electroanal. Chem. Interfacial Electrochem.*, 266, 465, 1989.
17. **Vanýsek, P. and Hernandez, C.**, Ion transport across a microscopic interface between two immiscible electrolytes, *J. Electrochem. Soc.*, 137, 2763, 1990.
18. **Kakiuchi, T., Noguchi, J., Kotani, M. and Senda, M.**, Ac polarographic determination of the rate of ion transfer for a series of alkylammonium ions at the nitrobenzene/ water interface, *J. Electroanal. Chem. Interfacial Electrochem.*, 296, 517, 1990.
19. **Wiles, M.C., Schiffrin, D.J., VanderNoot, T.J. and Silva A.F.**, Experimental artifacts associated with impedance measurements at liquid-liquid interfaces, *J. Electroanal. Chem. Interfacial Electrochem.*, 278, 151, 1990.
20. **Melroy, O.R., Bronner, W.E. and Buck, R.P.**, Chronopotentiometry of one- and two-ion transport at immiscible liquid interfaces: Test of the theory, *J. Electrochem. Soc.*, 130, 373, 1983.
21. **Mareček, V. and Samec, Z.**, Fast performance galvanostatic pulse technique for the evaluation of the ohmic potential drop and capacitance of the interface between two immiscible electrolyte solutions, *J. Electroanal. Chem. Interfacial Electrochem.*, 185, 263, 1985.
22. **VanderNoot, T.J. and Schiffrin, D.J.**, Non-linear regression of impedance data for ion transfer across liquid-liquid interfaces, *Electrochim. Acta*, 35, 1359, 1990.
23. **Boukamp, B.A.**, in *Equivalent Circuit (EQUIVCRT.PAS) Users Manual*, University of Twente, The Netherlands, 1988/89.
24. *Electrochemical Impedance Software, ZView for Windows*. Scribner Associates, Inc., Charlottesville, Virginia, 1993.
25. **Samec, Z., Mareček, V., Koryta, J. and Khalil, M.V.**, Investigation of ion transfer across the interface between two immiscible electrolyte solutions by cyclic voltammetry, *J. Electroanal. Chem. Interfacial Electrochem.*, 83, 393, 1977.
26. **Buck, R.P. and Bronner, W.E.**, Prediction of salts effects on rates of single-ion transfer crossing in ITIES experiments, *J. Electroanal. Chem. Interfacial Electrochem.*, 197, 179, 1986.
27. **Bronner, W.E., Melroy, O.R. and Buck, R.P.**, Apparent transfer coefficients for ion transfer between water and nitrobenzene, *J. Electroanal. Chem. Interfacial Electrochem.*, 162, 263, 1984.
28. **Shao, Y., Campbell, J.A. and Girault, H.H.**, Kinetics of the transfer of acetylcholine across the water/ nitrobenzene-tetrachlormethane interface. The Gibbs energy of transfer dependence of the standard rate constant, *J. Electroanal. Chem. Interfacial Electrochem.*, 300, 415, 1991.
29. **Osakai, T., Kakutani, T. and Senda, M.**, Kinetics of transfer of picrate ion at the water/ nitrobenzene interface, *Bull. Chem. Soc. Jpn.*, 58, 2626, 1985.
30. **Kakiuchi, T., Noguchi, J. and Senda, M.**, Double-layer effect on the transfer of some monovalent ions across the polarized oil-water interface, *J. Electroanal. Chem. Interfacial Electrochem.*, 336, 137, 1992.
31. **Kakiuchi, T., Noguchi, J. and Senda, M.**, Kinetics of the transfer of monovalent anions across the nitrobenzene-water interface, *J. Electroanal. Chem. Interfacial Electrochem.*, 327, 63, 1992.
32. **Kakiuchi, T.**, Mechanism of triethylpropylammonium ion transfer across the nitrobenzene-water interface, *Denki Kagaku*, 61, 932, 1993.
33. **Wandlowski, T.; Mareček, V. ; Samec, Z. and Fuoco, R.**, Effect of temperature on the

ion transfer across an interface between two immiscible electrolyte solutions: Ion transfer dynamics, *J. Electroanal. Chem. Interfacial Electrochem.*, 331, 765, 1992.

34. **Wandlowski, T., Mareček, V., Holub, K. and Samec, Z.**, Ion transfer across liquid-liquid phase boundaries: Electrochemical kinetics by faradaic impedance, *J. Phys. Chem.*, 93, 8204, 1989.
35. **Kakiuchi, T., Takasu, Y. and Senda, M.**, Voltage-scan fluorometry of Rose Bengal ion at the 1,2-dichloroethane- water interface, *Anal. Chem.*, 64, 3096, 1992.
36. **Kakiuchi, T., Takasu, Y.**, Differential cyclic voltfluorometry and chronofluorometry of the transfer of fluorescent ions across the 1,2-dichloroethane- water interface, *Anal. Chem.*, 66, 1853, 1994.
37. **Beattie, P.D., Delay, A. and Girault, H.H.**, Investigation of the kinetics of assisted potassium ion transfer by dibenzo-18-crown-6 at the micro-ITIES by means of steady-state voltammetry, *J. Electroanal. Chem. Interfacial Electrochem.*, 380, 167, 1995.
38. **Holub, K., Lhotský, A. and Mareček, V.**, Fluctuation analysis and faradaic impedance at micro-liquid/liquid interface, *J. Electroanal. Chem. Interfacial Electrochem.*, submitted.
39. **Samec, Z., Kakiuchi, T. and Senda, M.**, Double-layer effects on the Cs^+ ion transfer kinetics at the water/ nitrobenzene interface, *Electrochim. Acta,* submitted.
40. **Samec, Z. and Mareček, V.**, The use of the Frumkin correction in the kinetics of the ion transfer across the interface between two immiscible electrolyte solutions. A comment on the paper by Girault et al., *J. Electroanal. Chem. Interfacial Electrochem.*, 333, 319, 1992.
41. **Gurevich, Yu. Ya. and Kharkats, Yu.I.**, Ion transfer through a phase boundary: A stochastic approach, *J. Electroanal. Chem. Interfacial Electrochem.*, 200, 3, 1986.
42. **Samec, Z., Kharkats, Yu.I. and Gurevich, Yu.Ya.**, Stochastic approach to the ion transfer kinetics across the interface between two immiscible electrolyte solutions. Comparison with the experimental data, *J. Electroanal. Chem. Interfacial Electrochem.*, 204, 257, 1986.
43. **Cunnane, V.J., Schiffrin, D.J., Fleischmann, M., Geblewicz, G. and Williams, D.**, The kinetics of ionic transfer across adsorbed phospholipid layers, *J. Electroanal. Chem. Interfacial Electrochem.*, 243, 455, 1988.
44. **Koryta, J., Hung, L.Q. and Hofmanová, A.**, Biomembrane transport processes at the interface of two immiscible electrolyte solutions with an adsorbed phospholipid monolayer, *Studia Biophys.*, 90, 25, 1982.
45. **Girault, H.H.J. and Schiffrin, D.J.**, Charge transfer through phospolipid monolayers adsorbed at liquid- liquid interfaces, in *Charge and Field Effects in Biosystems*, Allen, M.J. and P.N.R. Usherwood, P.N.R., Eds., Abacus Press, Tunbridge Wells, 1984, p. 171.
46. **Kakiuchi, T., Kondo, T., Kotani, M. and Senda, M.**, Ion permeability of dilauroyl-phosphatidylethanolamine monolayer at the polarized nitrobenzene/ water interface, *Langmuir*, 8, 169, 1992.
47. **Kakiuchi, T., Kotani, M., Noguchi, J., Nakanishi, M. and Senda, M.**, Phase transition and ion permeability of phosphatidylcholine monolayers at the polarized oil/ water interface, *J. Colloid. Interface Sci.*, 149, 279, 1992.
48. **Kakiuchi, T., Kondo, T. and Senda, M.**, Divalent cation induced phase transition of phosphatidylserine monolayer at the polarized oil-water interface and its influence on the ion transfer processes, *Bull. Chem. Soc. Jpn*, 63, 3270, 1990.
49. **Kakutani, T., Nishiwaki, Y., Osakai, T. and Senda, M.**, On the mechanism of transfer of sodium ion across the nitrobenzene/ water interface facilitated by dibenzo-18-crown-6, *Bull. Chem. Soc. Jpn.*, 59, 781, 1986.
50. **Campbell, J.A., Stewart, A.A. and Girault, H.H.**, Determination of the kinetics of facilitated ion transfer reactions across the micro interface between two immiscible electrolyte solutions, *J. Chem. Soc. Faraday Trans. 1*, 85, 843, 1988.
51. **Seno, M., Iwamoto, K. and Chen, Q.**, Kinetic study of ion transport facilitated by crown ethers across water- nitrobenzene interface, *Electrochim. Acta*, 35, 127, 1990.
52. **Samec, Z., Homolka, D. and Mareček, V.**, Charge transfer between two immiscible electrolyte solutions. Part VIII. Transfer of alkali and alkaline earth metal cations across the water/ nitrobenzene interface facilitated by synthetic neutral ion carriers, *J. Electroanal. Chem. Interfacial Electrochem.*, 135, 265, 1982.

53. **d'Epenoux, B.; Seta, P.; Amblard, G. and Gavach, C.,** The transfer mechanism of tetraalkylammonium ions across a water- nitrobenzene interface and the structure of the double layer, *J.Electroanal. Chem. Interfacial Electrochem.*, 99, 77 , 1979.
54. **Buck, R.P.** Electroanalytical chemistry of membranes, *Crit. Rev. Anal. Chem.*, 5, 323 , 1975.
55. **Koryta, J.,** Ion transfer across water/ organic phase boundaries and analytical applications, *Ion-Selec. Electrode Rev.*, 5, 131, 1983.
56. **Melroy, O.R. and Buck, R.P.,** Electrochemical irreversibility of ion transfer at liquid/ liquid interfaces, *J. Electroanal. Chem. Interfacial Electrochem.*, 136, 19 , 1982.
57. **Girault, H.H.J. and Schiffrin, D.J.,** Theory of the kinetics of ion transfer across liquid/ liquid interfaces, *J. Electroanal. Chem. Interfacial Electrochem.*, 195, 213, 1985.
57a. **Girault, H.H.J. and Schiffrin, D.J.,** Thermodynamic surface excess of water and ionic solvation at the interface between immiscible liquids, *J. Electroanal. Chem. Interfacial Electrochem.*, 150, 43, 1983.
58. **Benjamin, I.,** Theoretical study of the water/ 1,2-dichloroethane interface: Structure, dynamics, and conformational equilibria at the liquid- liquid interface, *J. Chem. Phys.*, 97, 1432, 1992.
59. **Benjamin, I.,** Dynamics of ion transfer across a liquid- liquid interface: A comparison between molecular dynamics and a diffusion model, *J. Chem. Phys.*, 96, 577, 1992.
60. **Wandlowski, T., Holub., K., Mareček, V. and Samec, Z.,** The double-layer at the interface between two immiscible electrolyte solutions, *Electrochim. Acta,* submitted.
61. **Senda, M.,** Theory of the double layer effect on the rate of the ion transfer across the oil-water interface, *Anal. Sci*, 7, 585, 1991.
62. **Samec, Z., Mareček, V. and Homolka, D.,** Charge transfer between two immiscible electrolyte solutions. Part IX. Kinetics of the transfer of choline and acetylcholine cations across the water/ nitrobenzene interface, *J. Electroanal. Chem. Interfacial Electrochem.*, 158, 25, 1983.
63. **Dogonadze, R.R. and Kuznetsov, A.M.,** Theory of charge transfer kinetics at solid- polar liquid interfaces, *Progress in Surface Science*, Vol. 6, Davison S.G., Ed., Pergamon Press, Oxford , 1975, pp. 3-41.
64. **Dogonadze, R.R. and Urushadze, Z.D.,** Semi-classical method of calculation of rates of chemical reactions proceeding in polar liquids, *J. Electroanal. Chem. Interfacial Electrochem.*, 32, 235, 1971.
65. **Marcus, R.A.,** On the theory of electron transfer reactions. VI. Unified treatment of homogeneous and electrode reactions, *J. Chem. Phys.*, 43, 679, 1965.
66. **Levich V.G.,** Present state of the theory of oxidation-reduction in solution (bulk and electrode reactions) in *Advances in Electrochemistry and Electrochemical Engineering*, Vol. 4, Delahay, P., Ed., New York , 1966, p. 249.
67. **Eyring, H. and Eyring, E.M.,** Modem Chemical Kinetics, Selected Topics in Modem Chemistry, Reinhold Publ. Corp., New York, 1963, pp. 51-66.
68. **Kuznetsov, A.M. and Kharkats, Yu.I.,** Problems of a quantum theory of charge transfer reactions at the interface between two immiscible liquids, *The Interface Structure and Electrochemical Processes at the Boundary Between Two Immiscible Liquids*, V. E. Kazarinov, Ed., Springer-Verlag, Berlin, 1987, pp. 11-46.
69. **Buck, R.P.,** Kinetics of bulk and interfacial ionic motion: microscopic bases and limits for the Nernst- Planck equation applied to membrane systems, *J. Membrane Sci.*, 17, 1, 1984.
70. **Gardiner, C.W.,** *Hanbook of Stochastic Methods for Physics, Chemistry and Natural Sciences,* Haken, H., Ed., Springer, Berlin, 1985.
71. **Kharkats, Yu.I. and Ulstrup, J.,** The electrostatic Gibbs energy of finite- size ions near a planar boundary between two dielectric media, *J. Electroanal. Chem. Interfacial Electrochem.*, 308, 17, 1991.
72. **Stein, D.L., Doering, C.R., Palmer, R.G., van Hemmen, J.R. and McLaughlin, R.M.,** Escape over a fluctuating barrier: the white noise limit, *J. Phys. A*, 23, L203, 1990.
73. **Kakiuchi, T.,** Current-potential characteristic of ion transfer across the interface between two immiscible electrolyte solutions based on the Nernst- planck equation, *J. Electroanal. Chem. Interfacial Electrochem.*, 322, 55, 1992.

74. **Benjamin, I.**, Mechanism and dynamics of ion transfer across a liquid- liquid interface, *Science*, 261, 1558, 1993.
75. **Samec, Z.**, Charge transfer between two immiscible electrolyte solutions. Part III. Stationary curve of current vs potential of electron transfer across interface, *J. Electroanal. Chem. Interfacial Electrochem.*, 103, 1, 1979.
76. **Samec, Z.**, Charge transfer between two immiscible electrolyte solutions. Part V. Convolution potential sweep voltammetry of ion or electron transfer, *J. Electroanal. Chem. Interfacial Electrochem.*, 111, 211, 1980.
77. **Stewart, A.A., Campbell, J.A., Girault, H.H. and Eddowes, M.**, Cyclic voltammetry for electron transfer reactions at liquid/ liquid interfaces, *Ber. Buns. Phys. Chem.*, 94, 83, 1990.
78. **Geblewicz, G. and Schiffrin, D.J.**, Electron transfer between immiscible solutions. The hexacyanoferrate- lutetium biphtalocyanine system, *J. Electroanal. Chem. Interfacial Electrochem.*, 244, 27, 1988.
79. **Samec, Z., Mareček, V. and Weber, J.**, Detection of an electron transfer across the interface between two immiscible electrolyte solutions by cyclic voltammetry with four-electrode system, *J. Electroanal. Chem. Interfacial Electrochem.*, 96, 245, 1979.
80. **Samec, Z., Mareček, V. and Weber, J.**, Charge transfer between two immiscible electrolyte solutions. Part IV. Electron transfer between hexacyanoferrate(III) in water and ferrocene in nitrobenzene investigated by cyclic voltammetry with four-electrode system, *J. Electroanal. Chem. Interfacial Electrochem.*, 103, 11, 1979.
81. **Kakiuchi, T.**, Free energy coupling of electron transfer and ion transfer in two- immiscible fluid systems, *Electrochim. Acta,* submitted.
82. **Kolthoff, I.M. and Thomas, F.G.**, Electrode potentials in acetonitrile. Estiamtion of the liquid junction potential between acetonitrile solutions and the aqueous saturated calomel electrode, *J. Phys. Chem.*, 69, 3049, 1965.
83. **Hanzlík, J., Samec, Z. and Hovorka, J.**, Transfer of ferricenium cation across the water/ organic solvent interfaces, *J. Electroanal. Chem. Interfacial Electrochem.*, 216, 303, 1987.

83a. **Chen, Q.Z., Iwamoto, K. and Seno, M.**, Kinetic analysis of electron transfer between hexacyanoferrate(III) in water and ferrocene in nitrobenzene by ac impedance measurements, *Electrochim. Acta,* 36, 291, 1991

84. **Hanzlík, J., Mareček, V. and Samec, Z.**, in preparation.
85. **Shporer, M., Ron, G., Loewenstein, A. and Navon, G.**, Study of some cyano-metal complexes by nuclear magnetic resonance. II. Kinetics of electron transfer between ferri- and ferrocyanide ions, *Inorg. Chem.*, 4, 361, 1965.
86. **Marecek, V., Samec, Z. and Weber, J.**, The dependence of the electrochemical charge transfer coefficient on electrode potential. Study of the hexacyanoferrate(III)/ (II) redox system on polycrystalline Au electrode in KF solutions, *J. Electroanal. Chem. Interfacial Electrochem.*, 94, 169, 1978.
87. **Peter, L.M., Durr, W., Bindra, P. and Gerischer, H.**, The influence of alkali metal cations on the rate of the ferrocyanide/ferricyanide electrode peocesses, *J. Electroanal. Chem. Interfacial Electrochem.*, 71, 31, 1976.
88. **Cunnane, V.J., Schiffrin, D.J., Beltran, C., Geblewicz, G.and Solomon, T.**, The role of phase transfer catalysts in two phase redox reactions, *J. Electroanal. Chem. Interfacial Electrochem.*, 247, 203, 1988.
89. **Cunnane, V.J. and Schiffrin, D.J.**, Electron transfer reactions at immiscible electrolyte interfaces: A cause for irreversibility, *Ext. Abstr. 39th ISE Meeting,* Glasgow, 1988, p.246.
90. **Cheng, Y. and Schiffrin, D.J.**, Electron transfer between bis(pyridine)*meso*-tetra-phenylporphyrinato iron(II) and ruthenium(III) and the hexacyanoferrate couple at the 1,2-dichloroethane/ water interface, *J. Electroanal. Chem. Interfacial Electrochem.*, 314, 153, 1991.
91. **Cunnane, V.J., Geblewicz, G. and Schiffrin, D.J.**, Electron and ion transfer potentials of ferrocene and derivatives at a liquid- liquid interface, *Electrochim. Acta,* submitted.
92. **Kihara, S., Suzuki, M., Maeda, K., Ogura, K., Matsui, M. and Yoshida, Z.**, The electron transfer at a liquid/liquid interface studied by current- scan polarography at the

electrolyte dropping electrode, *J. Electroanal. Chem. Interfacial Electrochem.*, 271, 107, 1989.

93. **Girault, H.H.J. and Schiffrin, D.J.,** Electron transfer reactions at the interface between two immiscible electrolyte solutions, J. Electroanal. Chem. Interfacial Electrochem., 244, 15, 1988.
94. **Senda, M.,** Theory of the double layer effect on the rate of the charge transfer across an electrolyte/electrolyte interface, *Electrochim. Acta,* submitted.
95. **Kharkats, Yu.I.,** On the calculation of the rate constant of the charge transfer across the boundary of two dielectric media, *Sov. Electrochem. (Engl.Transl.),* 12, 1257, 1976.
96. **Kharkats, Yu.I. and Volkov, A.G.,** Interfacial Catalysis: Multielectron reactions at the liquid-liquid interface, *J. Electroanal. Chem. Interfacial Electrochem.*, 184, 435, 1985.
97. **Marcus, R.A.,** Reorganization free energy for electron transfers at liquid- liquid and dielectric semiconductor- liquid interfaces, *J. Phys. Chem.,* 94, 1050, 1990.
98. **Yang, E.S., Chan, M.S. and Wahl, A.C.,** Rate of electron exchange between ferrocene and ferricenium ion from nuclear magnetic resonance studies, *J. Phys. Chem.,* 79, 2049, 1975.
99. **Frese Jr., K.W.,** A study of rearrangement energies of redox species, *J. Phys. Chem.,* 85, 3911, 1981.
100. **Marcus, R.A.,** Theory of electron- transfer rates across liquid-liquid interfaces, *J. Phys. Chem.,* 94, 4152, 1990.

Chapter 9

MOLECULAR DYNAMICS OF CHARGE TRANSFER AT THE LIQUID/LIQUID INTERFACE

Ilan Benjamin

I. INTRODUCTION

A. PRELIMINARIES

Charge transfer processes at the interface between two immiscible liquids are of fundamental importance to many areas. Examples include elementary electron transfer reactions at electrochemical liquid/liquid (L/L) interfaces and ion transfer across these interfaces,[1] coupled electron and ion transfer at membrane/liquid interfaces, charge creation and propagation in micelles[2] and processes related to phase transfer catalysis.[3] Thus, it is not surprising that the experimental and theoretical studies of these systems go back at least to the beginning of the century. Until recently, most of our knowledge about charge transfer (and related) processes at the L/L interface has been derived from thermodynamic macroscopic approaches that were ingeniously applied to the study of both the structure of the neat interface and the thermodynamics and dynamics of processes taking place at or across the interface.[4] In recent years, this knowledge has been expanded by the use of experimental[5-11] and theoretical approaches[12-23] that are sensitive to the molecular details of the system. The goal of this chapter is to focus on the new information that has become available about the L/L interface and about charge transfer processes at this interface through the application of molecular dynamics computer simulation techniques. In addition to providing new insight about the systems of interest, this method can be used to test other theoretical models, as will be discussed in detail below.

Since the molecular dynamics method is very widely used and several review articles and books can be found discussing it at length,[24] in the rest of this introductory section we will focus on only those aspects that are important for the study of the interfacial systems. The rest of the chapter includes a discussion of the neat L/L interface followed by the application of the molecular dynamics method to elementary electron transfer and ion transfer processes at the interface.

B. THE MOLECULAR DYNAMICS METHOD

In its simplest form, the molecular dynamics computer simulation technique uses knowledge about forces between atoms and molecules to provide information about the structure of the condensed phases and the dynamics of molecular processes. For the applications discussed in this

0-8493-7694-7/96/$0.00+$.50

chapter, one assumes that the molecular motion can be described using classical mechanics, so that the quantum mechanical nature of the particles is assumed to be taken into account in the formulation of the effective potential energies governing their motion. The use of the classical equations of motion, although approximate, makes it possible to consider the simultaneous positions and velocities of thousands of particles over a time period that is relevant to the systems discussed here. This enables us to view the detailed microscopic structure and dynamics of the system, and to have information about its macroscopic and thermodynamic properties. Thus, connection with experimental observables is possible. Since the actual forces on the atoms are used in determining their velocities and positions, the molecular dynamics method gives information about time-dependent properties such as correlation and relaxation times. If the system is in equilibrium, the time average gives information about the canonical ensemble average when care is taken to insure a wide enough sampling of initial positions and velocities. In the Monte Carlo method, this ensemble average is calculated directly by (properly biased) random moves of the atoms according to the Boltzmann probability distribution, and thus, although the equilibrium structure can be obtained, no information about time-dependent properties is available.[24]

In applying to interfacial liquid/liquid systems care must be taken to insure the stability of the interface. Thus, our discussion below focuses on the issue of boundary conditions in addition to the important subject of the potential energy surfaces. As an example of the type of measurable quantities one can obtain, we discuss the calculation of free energies in general terms, leaving for a more detailed exposition the specific issues involved in its application to the ion transfer and electron transfer reactions.

1. Potential Energy Surfaces

The potential energy surfaces that have typically been employed in the simulations of liquid/liquid interfaces are based on the pair-wise additive approximation. Namely, the total potential energy U of a system composed of N interacting molecules can be written as a sum of interactions of pairs of molecules. The actual many-body character of the forces in the condensed phase is taken into account in an effective way through the proper parameterization of the interaction potential energy between two molecules. These pair interactions are modeled by representing each atom as a "soft" sphere that may include a point charge. Specifically, the pair interaction energy is given by

$$U_{\text{pair}} = \sum_{i,j} \left[\frac{Q_i Q_j}{r_{ij}} + 4\varepsilon_{ij}[(\sigma_{ij}/r_{ij})^{12} - (\sigma_{ij}/r_{ij})^6] \right], \tag{1}$$

where the sum is over all atoms i in one molecule and over all atoms j in a different molecule, and r_{ij} is the distance between the two atoms. The first term in Equation 1 represents the electrostatic interaction between the point charges Q_i and Q_j. These charges are selected to give the approximate effective dipole moment of the molecule in the condensed phase. The second term is the van der Waals non-bonded energy, represented by a Lennard-Jones expression (which includes a dispersion term plus a repulsive term). ε_{ij} is the van der Waals binding energy between atoms i and j, and σ_{ij} is the distance at which the attractive dispersion interaction is exactly balanced by the repulsive core. (This parameter is close to the sum of the van der Waals radii of the two atoms).

The parameters in Equation 1 are normally selected to reasonably reproduce the structural and thermodynamic properties of the individual liquids. A typically employed simplification which helps reduce the number of potential energy parameters is to select a set of "self terms" for each atom, σ_{ii} and ε_{ii}, and to use the "combination rule"[25]

$$\varepsilon_{ij} = (\varepsilon_{ii}\varepsilon_{jj})^{1/2},\ \sigma_{ij} = \tfrac{1}{2}(\sigma_{ii} + \sigma_{jj}) \tag{2}$$

to obtain the parameters for the interactions between different atoms. This approach seems to give reasonable results for both the properties of the individual liquids and for the interface. Table 1 gives typical values used in simulations of water/organic phase interfaces.

Table 1
Typical Potential Energy Parameters (Equations 1,2)

Atom	σ (Å)	ε (kcal/mol)	$Q\,(e)$
CH_2(in dichloroethane)	3.98	0.114	0.227
CH_3(in hydrocarbons)	3.98	0.114	0.0
CH_2(in hydrocarbons)	3.86	0.181	0.0
Cl(in dichloroethane)	3.16	0.5	−0.227
O(in octanol)	3.08	0.175	−0.685
H(in octanol)	2.0	0.1	0.4
α-C (in octanol)	3.98	0.114	0.285
O(in water)	3.17	0.155	−0.82
H(in water)	0	0	0.41

In general, the parameters for a given atom are not transferable across molecules of different types, although they can be used as a reasonable starting point in the refinement process. Note also that, in some cases, hydrogens in CH_2 and CH_3 groups are not treated explicitly. This "united atom" approximation significantly reduces the computational effort without significantly affecting the results, although exceptions have been noted in the literature. In any case, hydrogens bonded to atoms other than carbon must be treated explicitly.

In addition to the intermolecular potential energy, the system's Hamiltonian must include an intramolecular term. The most detailed (and computationally demanding) approach is to include all bond stretching and bending vibrations and torsional motion. In many cases, high frequency vibrational modes are omitted by constraining the bond lengths and bond angles to their equilibrium values, which allows for selecting a larger integration time step. This is a reasonable approximation when the structure and dynamics of the neat liquid/liquid system are concerned, especially if the intermolecular forces are properly adjusted to include the modification in the effective potential due to the molecular flexibility. (For example, flexible water has a slightly larger effective dipole moment than rigid water, and this may be taken into account in simulations of rigid water by means of a slight increase in the equilibrium bond length). When fast charge transfer processes occur in a liquid, it is not clear if the omission of the high frequency modes in the liquid is a reasonable approximation. The results of charge transfer calculations described below have all been obtained with fully flexible molecular geometries.

The inclusion of all the vibrational modes in the molecule also guarantees that the dielectric response of the medium includes the vibrational polarizability in addition to the orientational polarizability. However, the "infinite" frequency response of the medium, which arises from the electronic polarizability of the molecules, has been included in most simulations of interfacial systems only as an additional mean field through the adjustment of the pairwise interaction parameters. The true many-body nature of the electronic polarizability can be approximated by letting the charges on the molecules fluctuate. Several models have been developed,[26-30] most of which have been applied to bulk water and aqueous solutions. In a few cases, the application to neat water surfaces shows that the inclusion of these effects results in only minor changes in the structure of the interface,[31] but the problem of many-body and dynamic polarizability effects in simulations of interfacial systems is still wide open.

2. Boundary Conditions

In simulations of bulk liquids, periodic boundary conditions are used to minimize surface effects. Obviously, care must be taken to insure that in simulations of liquid interfaces and surfaces the boundary conditions are properly treated. The molecular dynamics or Monte Carlo simulations of the flat liquid/vapor interface of a fluid are typically done by starting from a number of molecules enclosed in a rectangular cube whose size is selected to give the correct density of the fluid at the desired temperature. Two opposite faces of the cube are then displaced so as to increase the volume of the system. If the fluid is in the two-phase region, two liquid vapor interfaces parallel to the displaced faces will spontaneously be formed. Experience has shown that these interfaces do not interact with each other and do little to disturb the bulk region.[20]

For simulations of the interface between two liquids, one starts from two separate rectangular boxes containing the two liquids. The two boxes have the same cross sections, but different lengths depending on the number of molecules used and the density of the liquids. The two boxes are brought together face to face to form a long box, and the intermolecular forces between the molecules of the different liquids are slowly increased to their final value. At this point, one could proceed in two different ways that are schematically described in Figure 1.

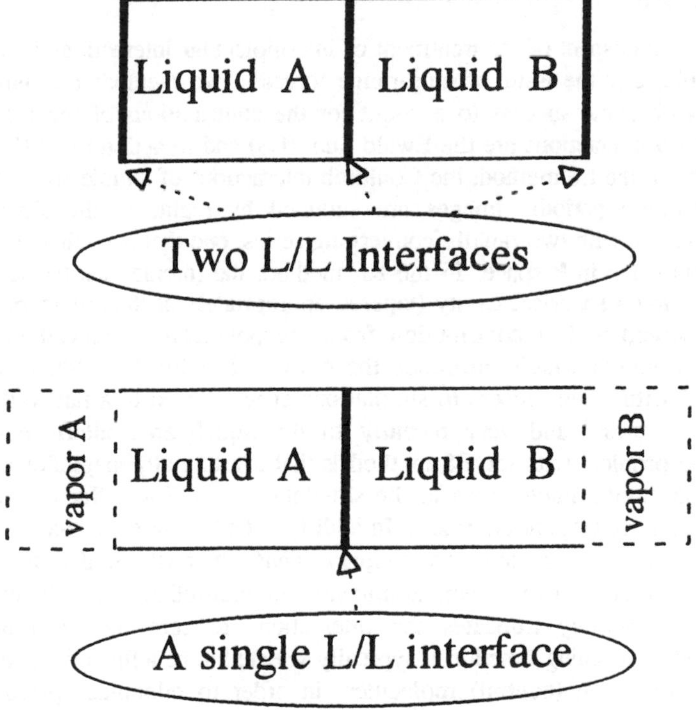

Figure 1. Schematic representation of the type of boundary conditions used in simulations of liquid/liquid interfaces. At the top, periodic boundariesin all three directions give rise to two liquid/liquid interfaces. At the bottom, the two faces normal to the long axis of the box are displaced, allowing for the development of a vapor phase for each liquid and a single liquid/liquid interface.

In the first approach, the periodic boundary conditions in the three directions are maintained. The system has two liquid/liquid interfaces. The pressure of the system must be controlled by continuously adjusting the volume of the new elongated box using a constant pressure molecular dynamics algorithm.[24] In the second approach, after the system is equilibrated, the two faces parallel to the liquid/liquid interface are displaced in order to generate two new liquid/vapor interfaces. Although the periodic boundary conditions are retained in all three directions, the two faces are far enough apart that there is very little or no interaction between the two liquid/vapor interfaces. In this case, there is only one liquid/liquid interface. The advantage of the first approach is that the two liquid/liquid interfaces allow for collecting double the statistics. However, care must be taken to insure that the two interfaces do not interact with each other or with the bulk region. As will be discussed below, the water/1,2-dichloroethane interface exhibits capillary fluctuations that could create a serious problem if this geometry is used.

An important aspect of the treatment of intermolecular interactions in the condensed phase is the issue of long-range forces. Two methods that have been used with some success to account for the contributions of the long-range coulomb interactions are the Ewald Sum (ES) and Reaction Field (RF) techniques.[24] In the ES method, the Coulomb interactions of a molecule with all of its infinite periodic images are summed by replacing the slowly convergent series with two rapidly converging series, one that is evaluated in real space and one in **k** space. In the RF method, the interactions between molecules inside a spherical cavity (tapered appropriately at the boundaries) are supplemented with a contribution from the polarization induced in a dielectric continuum which surrounds the cavity. The Ewald method has been applied with some success to simulations of water next to a flat wall[32] and to membranes[33] and very recently to the liquid/vapor interface of water.[34] One problem with the ES method is that it artificially magnifies the instantaneous dipolar fluctuations in the simulation box. These fluctuations may be particularly large at interfaces. In addition, the two surfaces that must exist in this case may be strongly coupled. Thus, in most simulations of interfaces, the interactions between atomic sites are multiplied by a switching function that smoothly truncates the interactions to zero over a finite distance.[24] The switching function is typically selected to be a function of the distance between two (neutral) molecules, in order to minimize spurious effects at the box boundaries.

3. Free Energy Calculations

Consider a system that is described by a Hamiltonian H which is the sum of the particles kinetic energies and the total potential energy of the system $U(\mathbf{r})$, where $\mathbf{r}$ is the positions of all the particles in the system. In many cases, we are interested in the free energy of the system when a specific property, $X(\mathbf{r})$, has a given value, x. Examples for such a variable include the distance between two atoms in a molecule or solvent polarization that is a function of positions of all atoms in the system, or a given term in the potential energy function U. This free energy is given by the fundamental (classical) statistical mechanical relation:[35]

$$G(x) = -\beta^{-1}\ln\langle\delta[X(\mathbf{r})-x]\rangle = -\beta^{-1}\ln\frac{\int\delta[X(\mathbf{r})-x]e^{-\beta U}d\mathbf{r}}{\int e^{-\beta U}d\mathbf{r}}, \tag{3}$$

where $\beta = 1/kT$, k is the Boltzmann constant, T the temperature, and δ is the Dirac Delta function. A determination of $G(x)$ using the above formula is possible through a sampling of the quantity X. This, however, gives accurate results of $G(x)$ for x that is near the equilibrium value $x_{eq} = \langle X\rangle$. Methods for the determination of $G(x)$ in the region of x far from equilibrium are based on modifying U in a way which increases the sampling statistics of x in this region.[36] In particular, if $U(\mathbf{r})$ is replaced by $U_b(\mathbf{r}) = U(\mathbf{r}) + F[X(\mathbf{r})]$, then from Equation 3 one finds that $G_b(x) = F(x) + G(x) + \text{constant}$. If F is properly selected such that $G_b(x)$ is accurately known in some region, then $G(x)$ can be found from this relation. Specific implementation depends on the system, and examples will be discussed later.

II. THE NEAT INTERFACE

Knowledge about the structure and dynamics of the neat interface between two immiscible liquids is crucial for the interpretation of experimental data which are sensitive to microscopic features of the system, as well as for the development of simplified models of the interface. We summarize below the important information gained from molecular dynamics and Monte Carlo studies of several liquid/liquid interfaces. We stress at the outset that this summary does not include the important subject of the structure of the electric double layer that results from a distribution of a finite concentration of ions. Excellent reviews of this subject are available.[37,38] In addition, although several molecular dynamics calculations have been reported for a model interface between nonpolar liquids,[13,23] we focus here on only those that are relevant to charge transfer processes -- the interface between water and an organic phase.

A. THE WATER/1,2-DICHLOROETHANE INTERFACE

1. General Comments and Density Profiles

The interface between water and 1,2-dichloroethane (DCE) is one of the most common interfacial systems for studies of charge transfer processes. The microscopic structure of the system has recently been examined in detail using a computer simulation that includes 216 DCE molecules and 500 water molecules. The results were found to be very close to the results of an earlier study which uses a smaller system.[39] Figure 2A shows the density profile of the water and the DCE in the system, calculated using a 100 ps trajectory. The water profile is determined by the position of the oxygen atom and the DCE profile by the midpoint of the C-C bond, both being calculated relative to the system's center of mass. The density of each liquid varies smoothly in the interface region, whose total thickness is about 12 Å. In the bulk region, the density of DCE (and of water to a lesser extent) exhibits oscillations about the average value. These oscillations may be an artifact of the small system size and the short simulation, although dampened oscillations extending a few molecular diameters into the bulk region, similar to those observed at the liquid/solid interface, are possible.

It should be stressed that the immiscibility of these two model liquids has been proven only for the time scale of the simulation. A rigorous proof must involve calculations of the free energy difference between the dispersed and the associated states of the two liquids. In general, simple arguments based on nearest-neighbor lattice models[40] show that if the individual pair interaction energy of two liquids A and B are very different, $U_{AA} \gg U_{BB}$, then the associated state is energetically much more favorable than the dispersed state. This energetics factor can overcome the entropic drive toward the dispersed state and lead to immiscibility. The nearly equal enthalpy of vaporization of water and DCE (8.4 kcal/mol) suggests that these pair interaction energies are close to each other. Thus, the immiscibility of water and DCE must be related to the special structure of liquid water. Crudely speaking, the association of organic molecules in liquid water has been referred to as the "hydrophobic effect", a complex phenomenon that remains poorly understood despite numerous studies.[40,41]

Panels B, C of Figure 2 demonstrate the special role that water structure plays in determining the immiscibility of water and DCE. By breaking the hydrogen bond network in liquid water (using a strong constant electric field), the two liquids begin to mix, as is evident from the density profiles in Panel B. The system returns to the initial immiscible state when this perturbation is removed, as reflected by the density profiles shown in Panel C.

2. Other Properties

The structural properties of the interface can be understood through a consideration of the global features of the interface as we have done for the density profiles just discussed, and through the microscopic details obtained by ensemble averages of properties of individual molecules. We limit the discussion here to a summary of the results. More details can be found elsewhere.[39] In this discussion, the "interface region" refers to the region where the density of each liquid is between 10% and 90% of the bulk density.

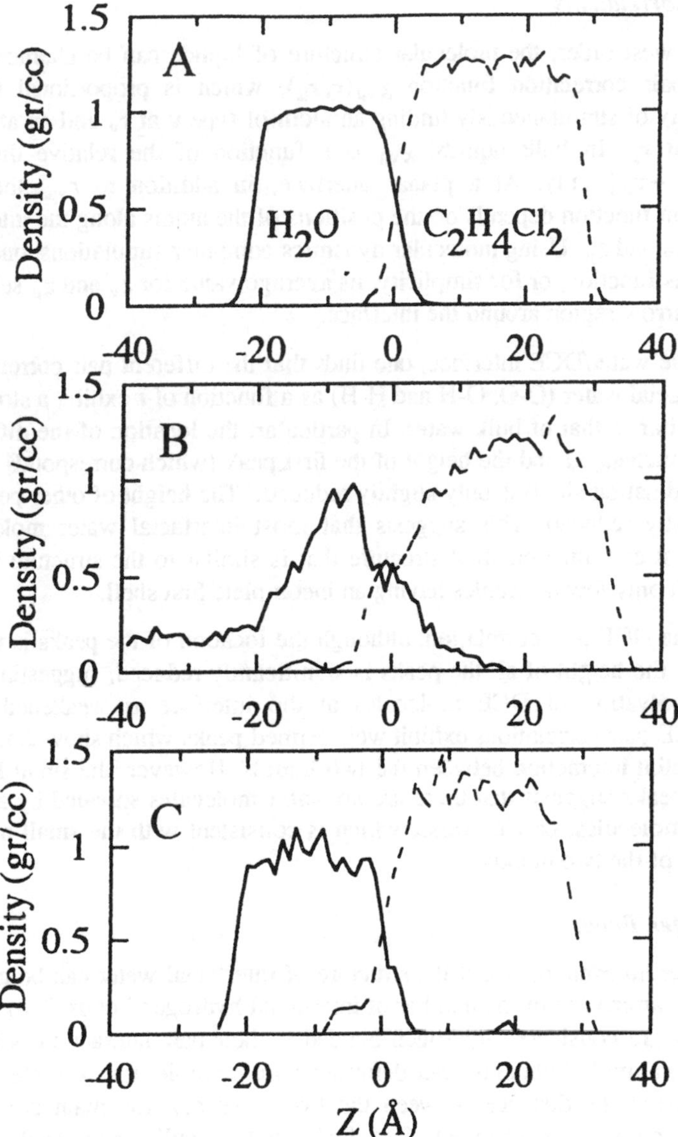

Figure 2. Density profiles of water (solid lines) and of 1,2-dichloroethane (dashed lines) at $T = 300$ K. In panel A, the densities are calculated from a 100 ps trajectory under normal conditions. In panel B, the system is under the influence of an external electric field of intensity 0.5 V/Å. In panel C, the densities are calculated (using a 20 ps trajectory) 100 ps after the external electric field is removed.

a. Pair Correlations

To lowest order, the molecular structure of liquids can be characterized by the pair correlation function $g_{\nu\mu}(\mathbf{r}_\nu \mathbf{r}_\mu)$, which is proportional to the probability of simultaneously finding an atom of type ν at $\mathbf{r}_\nu$ and an atom of type μ at $\mathbf{r}_\mu$. In bulk liquids, $g_{\nu\mu}$ is a function of the relative distance $r_{\nu\mu} = |\mathbf{r}_\nu - \mathbf{r}_\mu|$ only. At a planar interface, in addition to $r_{\nu\mu}$, the pair correlation function depends on the positions of the atoms along the interface normal, z_ν and z_μ. Using molecular dynamics computer simulations, one may obtain this function, or for simplicity, its average value for z_ν and z_μ selected from a narrow region around the interface.

For the water/DCE interface, one finds that the different pair correlations for interfacial water (O-O, O-H and H-H) as a function of r exhibit a structure quite similar to that of bulk water. In particular, the location of the different peaks is unchanged and the height of the first peak (which corresponds to the first coordination shell) is only slightly reduced. The height of other peaks is significantly reduced. This suggests that most interfacial water molecules have a first coordination shell structure that is similar to the structure in the bulk, with only few molecules having an incomplete first shell.

For the DCE pair correlation, although the location of the peaks is nearly invariant, the height of all the peaks is significantly reduced, suggesting that the self-solvation of DCE molecules at the interface is weakened. The water/DCE pair correlations exhibit well-defined peaks which show that there is substantial interaction between the two liquids. However, the small height of these peaks suggests that there are no water molecules solvated by a shell of DCE molecules, or vice versa, which is consistent with the small mutual solubility of the two liquids.

b. Hydrogen Bonds

Further information about the structure of interfacial water can be gained from an examination of the number of interfacial hydrogen bonds. Two water molecules are considered hydrogen bonded if their pair interaction is lower than 2.1 kcal/mol. Although other definitions are possible (for example, using as a criterion the distance between the two oxygens), the main argument discussed below is unchanged. One finds that in bulk water each water molecule is "hydrogen-bonded" to an average of 3.6 water molecules, but at the interface, this number drops to about 2.5. However, taking into account the coordination number of bulk water (4) and of interfacial water (2.9), one finds that a given hydrogen bond exists, on average, in 80% of the configurations in bulk water and in 90% of the configurations in interfacial water. Thus, although there are fewer hydrogen bonds at the interface, they survive longer.

c. Molecular Orientation

The anisotropic nature of the forces in the interfacial region results in the possibility of a specific molecular orientation at the interface. At the water/DCE interface, water dipoles tend to lie parallel to the interface. Thus, the probability distribution for the angle θ between the water dipole and the normal to the interface peaks around 90°. However, this probability distribution is quite broad, and one finds a significant population of water dipoles perpendicular to the interface. This is particularly the case for the water molecules that are bonded by two hydrogen bonds. The specific orientation of water dipoles decays very rapidly as one enters the bulk region, resulting in a totally random orientation for water molecules that are 7Å away from the Gibbs surface (the surface where the water density is about 50% of the bulk value). All this suggests a very small intrinsic surface potential.

d. Dynamics

In general, the dynamical properties of water molecules at the water/DCE interface, such as dipole reorientation time and the diffusion constant, are only mildly different from the properties in the bulk water. Similar behavior was observed for the DCE molecules. One observes a slight decrease in the dipole reorientation times at the interface and a slight decrease in the diffusion rate along the interface normal, due to the more structured interfacial water (consistent with the stronger hydrogen bonds at the interface). In addition to the single-molecule dynamical behavior, the dynamics of surface deformations were also investigated. These dynamics are much slower and may be described as time-dependent surface roughness. One way to characterize this is to examine the decay of transverse surface fluctuations ("fingers") as well as the decay of the fluctuations from the average width. These were found to be on the time-scale of a few tens of picoseconds.

In summary, the above data suggest that the neat water/DCE interface is sharply defined (there is no mixed solvent region) and very rough. This molecular scale roughness can be best described as "fingers" of one liquid protruding into the second liquid. In particular, the water fingers consist of water molecules with one or two hydrogen bonds that strongly interact with a few DCE molecules. An analysis of these "fingers" shows that on the time scale of a few nanoseconds they can reach a size of up to 8Å.

B. OTHER WATER/ORGANIC PHASE INTERFACES

In this section, we briefly review several other molecular dynamics and Monte Carlo simulations of the interface between water and an organic liquid that have been recently published. In general, there are many similarities between these interfaces and the water/DCE interface discussed above.

Linse examined the water/benzene interface using Monte Carlo simulations.[12] The system included 144 benzene molecules and 504 water molecules (MCY potential) at $T = 308$ K and a pressure of 1 atm. He found that the interfacial region was molecularly sharp and broadened by capillary waves. The water dipoles lay parallel to the interface in a region that is only a few molecular diameters wide. In addition, the water-benzene orientation was quite similar to the orientation found in dilute aqueous solutions of benzene. A general enhancement in the water hydrogen bonds at the interface was also found.

Gao and Jorgensen studied the water/1-hexanol interface using Monte Carlo simulations.[14] The system included 40 1-hexanol molecules and 267 water molecules (TIPS2 potential) at $T = 298$ K and a pressure of 1 atm. The system was constructed in monolayer and bilayer arrangements. This simulation also supported the existence of a narrow interfacial region with strong hydrogen bonding across the interface between the water molecules and the hydroxyl group in hexanol.

Carpenter and Hehre[16] studied the interface between water and hexane using 187 hexane molecules and 1200 water molecules (SPC model). Their choice of intermolecular parameters resulted in an interface that was too wide. The system exhibited quite a number of hexane molecules dissolved in water, which is not consistent with the low solubility of hexane in water. No specific molecular orientation at the interface was found.

Berendsen and coworkers[42] examined the sensitivity of the surface properties to the choice of the van der Waals parameters and suggested the parameters that best reproduced the surface tension of the water/hydrocarbon system. The system they studied include 50 decane molecules and 389 water molecules (described using the SPC or the SPC/E models) at $T = 315$ K. They found that at the interface the water showed preferential orientation that got more pronounced as the van der Waals parameters become smaller and the interface sharpened. The decane molecules were found to lie parallel to the interface, which was explained by the fact that this orientation produces a smoother surface.

Michael and Benjamin[22] have similarly studied the water/nonane interface. The system included 500 water molecules and 108 nonane molecules at $T = 300$ K. The structure of the interface was found to be similar to the one between water and decane, with a significant lateral ordering of the hydrocarbon molecules at the interface. The focus of this paper was to examine the effect of the molecular shape of the hydrocarbon liquid on the structure and dynamics of the neat interface and the reorientation dynamics of the solute probe. The interface between water and nonane was compared with the interface between water and a single-atom representation of the nonane molecule whose potential energy function was selected to give properties close to that of nonane. They found that although the thermodynamic properties and relevant structural properties of the two interfaces (such as water orientation) were very similar, the reorientation dynamics of the solute probe were faster by about a factor of two in the water/"spherical"-nonane system due to different molecular packing and shape.

III. ELECTRON TRANSFER

A. OVERVIEW

Electron transfer (ET) at the interface between two immiscible electrolyte solutions is the least understood ET reaction despite the fact that it is an important process in electrochemistry, biophysics and hydrometallurgy. The main reasons for this situation are the lack of experimental data about the rate of the reaction and the factors that influence it, in addition to our insufficient knowledge about the structure of the interface, which is necessary for an interpretation and theoretical modeling of the ET. In recent years, kinetic data are beginning to be available using classical electrochemical techniques,[1,2,7,43-45] and a demonstration of the possibility of detecting ET using the surface-specific, Second Harmonic Generation (SHG) spectroscopic technique has been reported.[9] On the theoretical side, there have been only a few attempts to study this system. Most of the approaches to understanding the basic factors that are involved in interfacial L/L electron transfer have been limited to the use of continuum dielectric model for the liquids and to the calculations of the solvent reorganization free energy and the work terms that are crucial for the rate calculations.[46-48] Our discussion below will thus be limited to an examination of these models in view of the new information available regarding the microscopic structure of the interface (section 1 below) and the molecular dynamics reorganization free energy calculations designed to test these models (section 2).

B. CONTINUUM MODELS

Consider a redox couple which consists of an electron donor (D) and an electron acceptor (A) that are adsorbed at the interface between two immiscible liquids. In order to simplify the discussion and focus on the role of the interface, we assume that the two centers are structurless, and thus the electron transfer between them (according to $D\,A \rightarrow D^{+}\,A^{-}$) involves only outer-sphere solvent reorganization. In practice, the contribution of inner, vibrational modes must be added. This latter part will be only mildly affected by the presence of the interface (for example, by modifying the equilibrium bond length and force constants).

In general, the computation of the rate of an interfacial ET reaction in the limit of small electronic coupling (non-adiabatic limit) requires information about the following ingredients:

1. The position of the activated complex at the interface. In particular, one needs to know if the redox couple is free to rotate in the interfacial region or if each center is confined to one phase. If the latter is the case, can they approach each other through a limited range of angles, or can they take advantage of surface roughness?
2. The solvent reorganization free energy. This quantity depends on the solvents, but also on the location of the redox couple.
3. In addition to the solvent reorganization, the "standard" free energy of the reaction and the work necessary to bring the reactants to the reactive distance and then take them away from the reactive configuration, contribute to the activation free energy for the ET.
4. The geometry of the activated complex is also important for estimating the "frequency factor" - the probability for the reactants to reach the activated complex.
5. In addition to the frequency factor, the electronic coupling between the states involved in the ET determine the pre-exponential factor in the rate expression.

Marcus derived an expression for the rate of ET at the liquid/liquid interface, taking into account the above terms within the local and linear continuum electrostatic model for the liquids and assuming a sharp interfacial boundary and spherical reactants:[48-50]

$$k_r = \kappa \nu V_r e^{-\beta \Delta G^{\#}}, \tag{4}$$

where κ is the Landau-Zener factor for the non-adiabatic transition[51] between the two electronic states near their crossing region, ν is the frequency of the molecular motion that is relevant for the ET process, (which could be best defined using the molecular treatment, as will be discussed below), V_r is the "reaction volume" which accounts for all of the possible configurations of the reactant pair per unit area of the flat and sharp interface. This "reaction volume" is given by

$$V_r = 2\pi(a_1 + a_2)(\delta R)^3, \tag{5}$$

where a_i is the radius of reactant i and δR is a length scale which arises from the weighting of the reactive configuration by the exponential decay ($e^{-R/\delta R}$) of the electronic coupling between the two electronic states as a function of the distance R between the reactants[a]. The activation energy $\Delta G^{\#}$ is given

a. This assumes that the non-adiabatic regime applies to all values of R, which must be incorrect for R small enough, and thus an adiabatic formulation is necessary.

by[48-50, 52]

$$\Delta G^{\#} = W_r + (\lambda + \Delta G^0 + W_p - W_r)^2/(4\lambda), \tag{6}$$

where ΔG^0 is the standard reaction free energy which depends on the standard free energy of formation of the reactants and the products and the potential drop across the interface, W_r is the reversible work required to bring the two reactants from the bulk of each phase to the interface, $-W_p$ is the reversible work required to separate the two products and λ is the reorganization free energy which includes both the solvent λ_s ("outer sphere") and the vibrational λ_i ("inner sphere") contributions. The continuum electrostatic model calculations give:[46, 48, 49]

$$\lambda_s = \tfrac{1}{2}(\Delta q)^2 \left[\frac{a_1^{-1} - \gamma_\infty (2d_1)^{-1}}{\varepsilon_1^\infty} - \frac{a_1^{-1} - \gamma_0 (2d_1)^{-1}}{\varepsilon_1^0} + \frac{a_2^{-1} + \gamma_\infty (2d_2)^{-1}}{\varepsilon_2^\infty} - \frac{a_2^{-1} + \gamma_0 (2d_2)^{-1}}{\varepsilon_2^0} - \frac{4R^{-1}}{\varepsilon_1^\infty + \varepsilon_2^\infty} + \frac{4R^{-1}}{\varepsilon_1^0 + \varepsilon_2^0} \right] \tag{7}$$

$$W_\mu = \frac{\gamma_0}{4} \left[\frac{q_{2\mu}^2}{\varepsilon_2^0 d_2} - \frac{q_{1\mu}^2}{\varepsilon_1^0 d_1} \right] + \frac{2}{R} \frac{q_{1\mu} q_{2\mu}}{\varepsilon_1^0 + \varepsilon_2^0}, \quad \mu = r, p, \tag{8}$$

where reactant i ($i = 1,2$) with charge q_{ri} and radius a_i is located in phase i at a distance d_i from the interface. ε_i^∞ and ε_i^0 are the infinite frequency ("optical") and static dielectric constants of phase i, respectively. The factors $\gamma_0 = (\varepsilon_2^0 - \varepsilon_1^0)/(\varepsilon_2^0 - \varepsilon_1^0)$ and $\gamma_\infty = (\varepsilon_2^\infty - \varepsilon_1^\infty)/(\varepsilon_2^\infty - \varepsilon_1^\infty)$ reflect the contribution of the interfacial image terms to the electrostatic potentials used to compute the λ and the work term W. The work term does not include any specific solvent-solute interaction or the contribution of the potential changes due to the finite concentration of electrolytes.

Marcus showed that λ could be estimated from the reorganization free energy for electron transfer at a metal/solution interface. Application to the reaction between the $Fe(CN)_6^{4-/3-}$ redox couple in the aqueous phase and the $Lu(PC)_2^{+/2+}$ (lutetium biphtalocyanine) couple in DCE gave an "exchange current" rate of 0.01 M^{-1} cm s^{-1},[50] in reasonable agreement with the experimental value of 0.03 M^{-1} cm s^{-1}.[43] Unfortunately, reasonable agreement with the experimental rate constant for this system could be also obtained[b] if one assumes that the interfacial region is a thick homogeneous mixture (rather than a sharp interfacial boundary between the two phases).

C. MICROSCOPIC TREATMENT

Although additional experimental data could be very useful for testing the basic assumptions underlying the continuum model discussed in the previous section, a more detailed test and additional insight into the interfacial ET could be provided by the molecular dynamics calculations. The two main assumptions underlying the continuum model are the linear response approximation necessary for calculating the reorganization free energy and the assumption of a sharp and flat interface. Both of these assumptions can be directly tested by the microscopic treatment. We have already stressed the result that the molecular dynamics calculations suggest that the neat water/DCE interface is molecularly sharp but very rough. This would imply that the continuum model should be doing poorly. However, experience from simulations in bulk liquids shows that despite grossly inaccurate assumptions, continuum models could be useful with proper parameterization of ion sizes and dielectric constants. Calculations of the free energy of adsorption of ions at interfaces indeed show that continuum models could be "fixed" by such parameterization.[53]

Considering the specific problem of ET at the liquid/liquid interface, the major contribution to the rate comes from the reorganization free energy term and we focus here on the microscopic calculation of this quantity and its comparison with the continuum model result. The calculation of the solvent reorganization free energy using molecular dynamics can be best handled using the concept of the solvent coordinate, as this concept is also useful for examining the applicability of the linear response assumption mentioned above.

The electron transfer reaction $DA \rightarrow D^+A^-$ can be viewed as a transition between two localized electronic states, one for the reactants (R) and one for the products (P). A useful definition of a solvent coordinate is based on the energy gap between the Born-Oppenheimer diabatic surfaces for the reactants and products:[54-58]

$$X(\mathbf{r}) = U_R - U_P, \tag{9}$$

where U_P and U_R are the potential energies of the products and the reactants, respectively (including the ground state electronic energy of the solute). X is

---

b. Note an error in the original paper (claiming that there is a two-order of magnitude discrepancy between the calculated and experimental rate). See *J. Phys. Chem.*, 99, 5742, 1995.

a function of the positions of all solvent atoms. If the system is in the ν'th electronic state ($\nu = R,\ P$), then the equilibrium value of X is

$$<x>_\nu = <X(\mathbf{r})>_\nu \equiv \frac{\int X(\mathbf{r}) e^{-\beta H_\nu} d\mathbf{r}}{\int e^{-\beta H_\nu} d\mathbf{r}}, \tag{10}$$

where H_ν is the Hamiltonian of the system in the ν'th state, which includes, in addition to U_ν, a constant term due to the interaction of the solute with an external field. X provided a convenient, one-dimensional representation of the multi-dimensional solvent configuration in the system. For the model discussed in the last section, X is simply the electrostatic interactions between the solvent dipoles (and higher order terms) and a pair of opposite atomic charges located on the "A" and "D" sites. If the liquid molecules are isotropically distributed around the pair DA, then $<X>_{DA} = 0$, but $<X>D^+A^- \ll 0$ due to the stabilization of the ion pair by the solvent's dipoles.

Due to thermal motion, X fluctuates around the equilibrium value. Electron transfer occurs with high probability when the energy of the two electronic states is the same (i.e. $H_R = H_P$). Depending on the difference in the ground electronic state energy of the reactants and products and the external potential, the two electronic states will be nearly degenerate for solvent configurations characterized by an $x^{\#}$ value very different from the equilibrium value. Thus, the rate of electron transfer will be (in part) determined by the probability that X will be close to $x^{\#}$. Specifically, the free energy associated with the fluctuations in X when the system is in the ν'th electronic state is given by an expression similar to that in Equation 3:

$$G_\nu(x) = -\beta^{-1} \ln\left\{ <\delta(X(\mathbf{r}) - x)>_\nu \right\} \tag{11}$$

gives a quantitative measure for the rareness of these fluctuations. On the other hand, the standard reaction free energy is given by:

$$\Delta G_r = -\beta^{-1} \ln \frac{\int e^{-\beta H_P} d\mathbf{r}}{\int e^{-\beta H_R} d\mathbf{r}}. \tag{12}$$

If one considers $G_R(x)$ as the free energy surface for the reactants, and $G_P(x) + \Delta G_r$ the free energy surface for the products, then it is straightforward to show that the intersection between these surfaces occurs at a value of x that corresponds to $H_R = H_P$. At this value of x, $G_R(x) = \Delta G^{\#}$ is the activation free energy for the ET transfer reaction. The functions $G_R(x)$ and $G_P(x)$ are not independent. It can be shown that:

$$G_P(x) + \Delta G_r - \Delta E_0 = -x + G_R(x), \tag{13}$$

where ΔE_0 is an energy difference between the products and the reactants due to a constant external field.[17,58,59]

Marcus' linear response theory corresponds to the approximation:

$$G_v(x) - G_v(<X>_v) = \tfrac{1}{2}k(x - <X>_R)^2 \tag{14}$$

Thus, the free energy surfaces for the reactants and products are paraboli of equal curvature. They are shifted vertically relative to each other by the amount $\Delta G_r + \Delta E_0$. The horizontal displacement $<x>_P - <x>_R$ is given by k^{-1}, as can be obtained from Equation 13. The reorganization free energy λ is defined as the difference $G_R(<x>_P) - G_R(<x>_R)$, which for the linear model is just $(2k)^{-1}$. The intersection of these two paraboli gives rise to an activation energy formula that is identical to Equation 6 without the work terms. The different terms discussed above are schematically depicted in Figure 3.

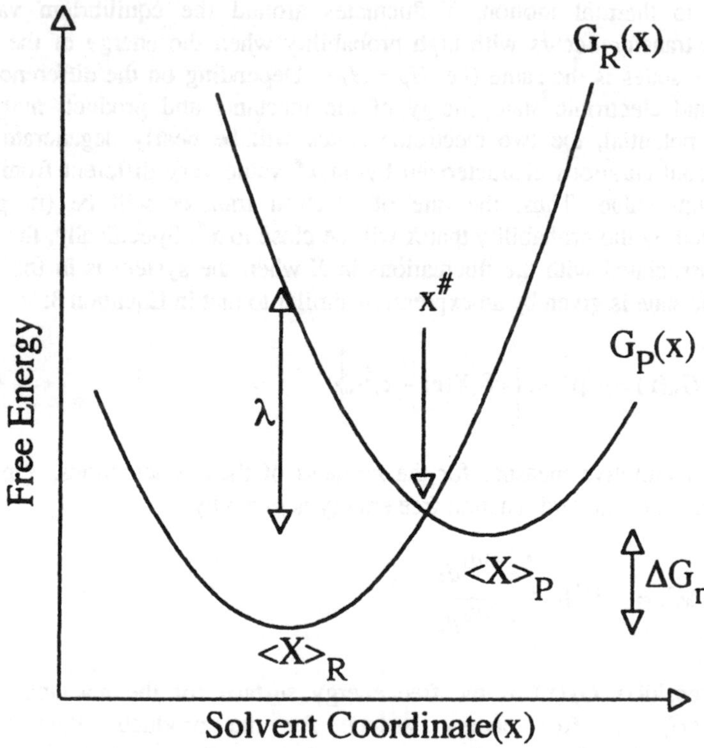

Figure 3. Schematic representation of the solvent free energy functions for an electron transfer reaction. λ is the reorganization free energy and $x^{\#}$ is the value of the solvent coordinate at the transition state. Other quantities are defined in the text.

Using equilibrium molecular dynamics calculations with the Hamiltonian H_R or H_P, one can efficiently and accurately obtain the "force constants" k_R and k_P. The assumption of equal curvature can thus be immediately checked. In order to determine to what extent the curves $G_R(x)$ and $G_P(x)$ can be approximated by paraboli, one needs to use preferential sampling techniques to obtain the free energy associated with large fluctuations from the most probable values of x. A simple way to accomplish this for the ET problem, following the general discussion in section B.3, is to add a biasing potential linear in X to the Hamiltonian. This shifts the minimum of the free energy curve to a new value close to the region where sampling is required. Because of the relation given in Equation 13, this modification can be exactly accounted for in reconstructing the original free energy curve. In practice, one can show that the addition of a linear term in X is equivalent to transferring the electron from the D to the A site in small fractions of an atomic unit. More details can be found elsewhere.[17,56,58]

The results of the molecular dynamics calculations for a model redox pair at the water/DCE interface are shown in Figure 4 using a total of 500 ps trajectories. The redox couple is modeled using two spherical sites, each of which interacts with the two liquids via a Lennard-Jones potential. The Lennard-Jones parameters of each site are $\sigma = 5Å$ and $\varepsilon = 0.1$ kcal/mol. The distance between the two sites is held fixed at $R = 6Å$, while the center of the line connecting the two sites is restricted to being at the Gibbs dividing surface. Otherwise, they are free to rotate. The calculations are repeated for the same system in bulk water under the same conditions, except that the translation of the pair of sites does not need to be restricted. In each case, the full free energy curves (thick lines) for zero reaction free energy are compared with the parabolic fit based on the curvature near the equilibrium reactants and products (thin lines). The assumption of equal curvature and parabolic dependence seems to be excellent for the ET reaction at the interface. This is somewhat different from the situation in bulk water, where the full free energy curves are not very well approximated by paraboli, and in addition, the curvatures near the reactants and the products minima are significantly different. The results in bulk water are consistent with other calculations of charge separation/recombination processes in water.[58] The smaller solvent "force constant" near the ion pair in water reflects the "structure breaking" effect of the ions, which makes the solvation shell more "fluid-like". Nevertheless, note that the activation free energies predicted by the full calculations and the quadratic approximation are nearly the same for the case where the net free energy of the reaction is near zero, a region where most ET rate measurements are performed.

The activation free energy (or the reorganization free energy) can be compared with the prediction of the continuum electrostatic model. To do this, the dielectric constant of each liquid is calculated via standard methods[24] using molecular dynamics simulations of the independent bulk liquids. We find $\varepsilon^0_{H_2O} = 82$ and $\varepsilon^0_{DCE} = 10$. We take the infinite frequency dielectric constants to be 1 for each liquid (consistent with the electronically non-polarizable model). The diameter of each center is taken to be equal to the Lennard-Jones parameter σ. The distances of each center from the interface is taken to be the average distance from the Gibbs surface, calculated from the molecular dynamics trajectories. Inserting all of these parameters into Equation 7 gives $\lambda = 74$ kcal/mol, compared with the value of 80 ± 2 kcal/mol determined from the molecular dynamics free energy calculations, as shown in Figure 4.

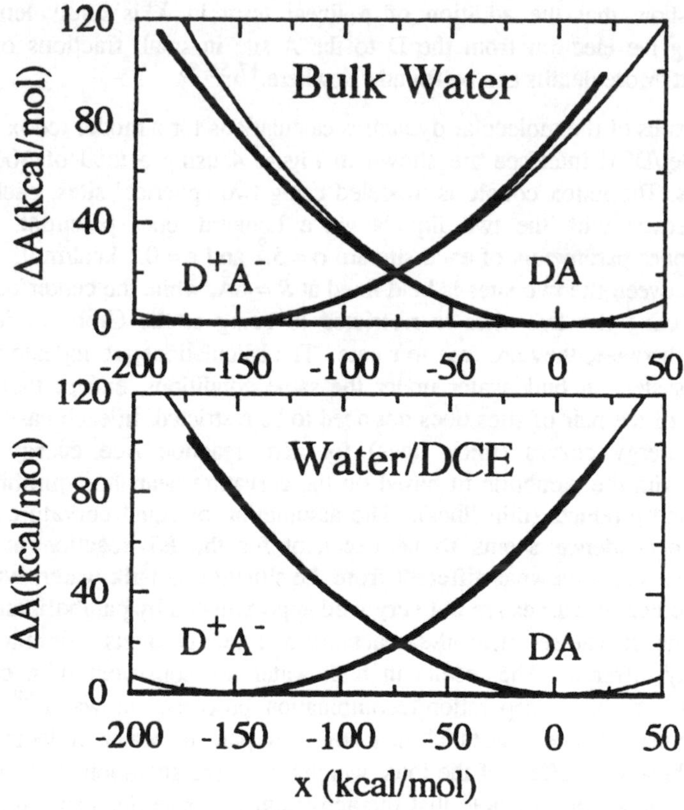

Figure 4. Solvent free energy functions for a model outer-sphere electrontransfer reaction in bulk water (top panel) and at the water/1,2-dichloroethane interface (bottom panel). The thick lines give the results of the molecular dynamics free energy sampling.The thin lines correspond to a parabolic fit. The curvature of the paraboli in bulk water is 0.0026 $(\text{kcal/mol})^{-1}$ for the ion pair and 0.0038 $(\text{kcal/mol})^{-1}$ for the neutral pair. In DCE it is 0.0032 $(\text{kcal/mol})^{-1}$ for the ion pair and 0.0034 $(\text{kcal/mol})^{-1}$ for the neutral pair.

The reasonably close agreement between the molecular dynamics calculations and the continuum model results is surprising in light of the fact that the interface between water and DCE is quite rough. One clear demonstration of this is provided by examining the angle that the two charge centers can approach each other relative to the interface normal. The sharp model puts a limit of $\theta_{max} = \cos^{-1}[(a_1 + a_2)/R]$ on this value, which for our specific example should be about 34°. In the molecular dynamics trajectories, the angular distribution is broad and can be as big as 120° for the case where the charges on the two centers are ±½ (the "transition state").[60] However, one should note that the average value of θ from the molecular dynamics calculations used in Equation 7 (45°) is not far from θ_{max}. More interesting is an examination of the electric potentials induced by each liquid at the location of the charge transfer centers. These potentials are used in the continuum model to compute the free energy of the reversible "charging up" of the ion pair, an important step in the derivation of the continuum model expression for the reorganization free energy. Linear response theory predicts that these potentials are linear in the charge on the ion. An examination of the molecular dynamics results shows that the continuum model underestimates the contribution of the water to the potential at the location of the ion pair, but overestimates the contribution of the DCE. However, the total potential is nearly linear in the charge of the ion, which is consistent with the nearly perfect quadratic dependence of the free energy curves, as shown in Figure 4.

D. SOLVENT DYNAMICAL EFFECTS

Our discussion thus far has focused on the calculation of the free energy, and thus, the corresponding probability that the redox couple will reach the transition state where coupling between the two electronic states is substantial, resulting in the electron transfer reaction. In recent years, it has become clear that the rate of very fast electron transfer reactions may be influenced by the time scale of solvent motion, in particular, the dynamics of solvent dipole reorientation.[61-64] As new experimental techniques are beginning to be applied to liquid/liquid interfacial ET,[9,65,66] the issue of the solvent dynamical response to fast charge transfer processes at the liquid/liquid interface may become relevant. Because there are no fast, time-resolved data on liquid/liquid interfacial charge transfer to date, we only briefly make some comments about this issue, based on several molecular dynamics studies.

The effect of solvent dynamics on electron transfer reactions belongs to the more general class of a solvent response to a change in the solute's charge distribution. This process has been intensively investigated in recent years theoretically[67] (using molecular dynamics, analytical statistical mechanical models and continuum models) and experimentally.[62,68] The solvent response may be studied by following the time-dependent shift in the emission spectra from a photochemically excited solute. The advantages of this approach are that solvent response can be directly probed instead of indirectly inferred from the ET measurements and that simulations of this process are straightforward[67,69] and can be directly compared with experiments.

Studies of solvent dynamics in bulk solutions have revealed that the solvent response can be qualitatively accounted for at long times using continuum models, and that these models may be improved by taking into account the finite size of the solvent molecules.[70-72] At early time, deviation from continuum models due to inertial solvent motion has been noted.[63,73] An important conclusion of these studies has been that most of the contribution to the solvent response comes from the first solvation shell.[74]

Simulations of the solvent response at liquid/vapor interfaces[53,75,76] and liquid/metal interfaces[77] have shown that the tendency of ions to keep their solvation shell is reflected by a small change in the solvent dynamical response at these interfaces relative to the response in the bulk.

A different picture has emerged from simulations of the solvent dynamical response to photochemical charge transfer at the liquid/liquid interface.[21,60] If the solvents have significantly different response times, then a solute probe at the interface will have components from both liquids, which will result in a decay which cannot be described by a single exponential. The contribution of each liquid can be directly related to the degree of solvation of the probe by each liquid, and it thus gives valuable information about the structure of the interface and the position of the solute probe at the interface. This has been demonstrated for charge jump computer simulations at the water/DCE interface.[60]

IV. ION TRANSFER

A. OVERVIEW

Understanding the process of ion transfer across the L/L interface is of fundamental importance to many areas, including electrochemical charge transfer,[1] phase transfer catalysis,[3] drug delivery problems in pharmacology[78] and membrane biophysics.[79] In particular, the process of ion transfer across the interface between two immiscible electrolyte solution has been extensively studied using a variety of experimental and theoretical methods.[1,44,80-89]

Most of the experimental techniques used to date, although having significantly contributed to an understanding of this process, lack the sensitivity necessary for probing it at a microscopic level. The theoretical methods used, which are based on continuum level descriptions of the liquids,[47,90-93] had to be developed with an incomplete knowledge of the interface structure. Thus, it is not surprising that the mechanism of the ion transfer process is not very well understood. Some of the fundamental questions which are yet to be fully resolved include: Does the process of ion transfer from the organic phase to the aqueous phase involve a barrier? If so, what is the molecular nature of this barrier? How does it relate to the process of switching the solvation shell members? What are the molecular factors that influence the rate of the transfer? Does the process of ion transfer into the organic phase involve a significant dragging of the aqueous shell?

Recent progress in experimental techniques that are sensitive to the microscopic details of the system is beginning to provide information about the structure and dynamics at the L/L interface.[6,8-11] These techniques have not been applied yet to the problem of ion transfer, and thus most of the new microscopic insight into this problem has been obtained by molecular dynamics computer simulations. Hayoun *et. al*[23,94] have studied the problem of a neutral solute transfer across a model liquid/liquid interface using Lennard-Jones potentials for the liquids and the solute. They have shown that the process can be understood as a problem of an activated crossing of a well-defined barrier. This barrier was attributed to the process of switching solvation shell members, but it is not clear if this system is relevant to the process of ion transfer across the aqueous/organic phase.

We have studied the process of ion transfer across the interface between model polar/non-polar Lennard-Jones liquids[18] and across the interface between water and DCE.[19,95] These studies shed some light on the mechanism of the transfer of small ions across the electrochemical interface, and they provide partial answers to the questions mentioned above. The main results of these studies are discussed below.

In typical electrochemical experiments, the ion transfer is studied under reversible equilibrium conditions, using techniques such as cyclic voltammetry.[96] The process is analyzed using the classical approaches developed for processes at metallic electrodes.[96] Depending on the polarity of the external potential, ion current is set up from the aqueous to the organic phase, or vice verse. A microscopic analysis under these conditions is extremely complicated because of the necessity to consider double layer effects, ion atmosphere interactions, ion-pairing and other phenomena. In order to gain an insight into the microscopic events that accompany the ion transfer, we have to simplify the system considerably. We thus consider the behavior of a single ion at the interface, under an external electric field which may have either polarity. Under these conditions, the ion transfer is a non-equilibrium process, because the equilibrium condition of a constant chemical potential requires a finite concentration of ions to be distributed across the interface.

B. NON-EQUILIBRIUM CALCULATIONS OF ION TRANSFER

We first consider the process of ion transfer under non-equilibrium conditions. This process is studied using the molecular dynamics method by initiating trajectories with the ion initially in the bulk phase, and letting the ion cross the interface under a condition of zero electric field, as well as with the help of an external electric field. Both the down-hill transfer (from the organic to the aqueous phase, which involves a negative free energy change) and the reverse process have been studied under the influence of several electric field values. In each case, an average over 20 trajectories allows for the elucidation of some general features about the process. These calculations have been described in detail elsewhere,[95] and here we summarize the main points.

1. Transfer From the DCE to the Aqueous Phase

The left panels of Figure 5 describe a rapid transfer of the Cl^- from the DCE to the water phase. The crossing of the interface region, which is 10-20 Å wide, is accomplished in a few tens of picoseconds, under the condition of an external electric field of 0.2V/Å. On average, a full water hydration shell is formed during this period. The rapid rise in the build-up of the hydration shell is accompanied by an almost concerted "shelling off" of the DCE coordination shell. An examination of the animated individual trajectories shows that the actual process of the build-up of the hydration shell is very rapid, and the 20 ps time-scale for the replacements of the solvation shell corresponds to the fact that different ions (different members of the ensemble of trajectories) reach the interface at different times. This is consistent with the information conveyed in the bottom panel, where the first peak of the water oxygen-ion radial distribution function remains narrow and at a fixed O-Cl^- distance, while its height increases as more members of the ensemble are hydrated. The appearance of the second peak toward the end of the trajectories corresponds to a full second hydration shell being formed as the ion continues its motion toward the bulk water phase.

An examination of the individual trajectories reveals that the process of the transfer begins with a deformation of the DCE solvation shell, which allows for a water molecule that is loosely connected with the bulk water phase to interact with the ion. This water molecule is bonded to the other water molecules with an average of 1.5 hydrogen bonds, whereas a typical interfacial water molecule is bonded via 2.5 bonds on average. This is also reflected by the fact that the initial approach of this water molecule to the negatively charged chloride ion is with both hydrogens pointing toward the ion. However, the equilibrium structure of the water-Cl^- hydration shell (in which Cl^---H-O is nearly collinear) is very rapidly formed. It is found that, on average, ions that cross the interface very rapidly interact very early with a water "finger" that has at its end such a loosely bonded water molecule.

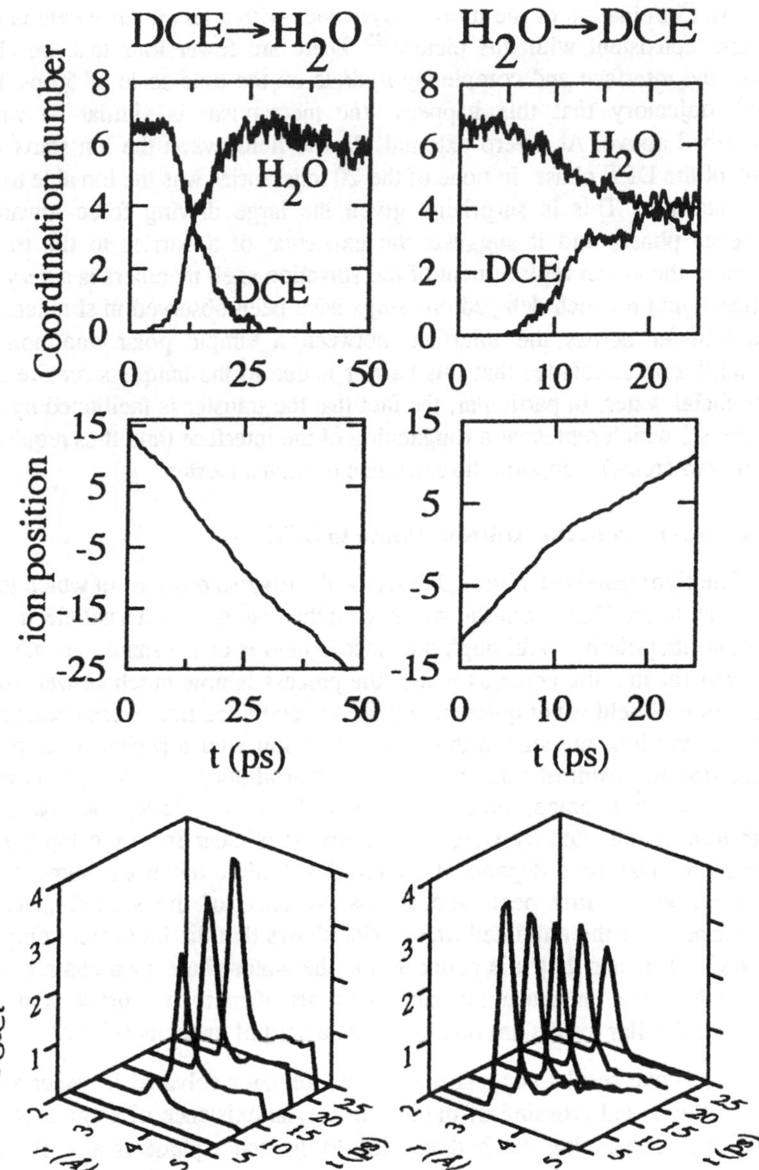

Figure 5. Time-dependent ensemble averages of several properties associated with the transfer of a chloride ion across the water/1,2-dichloroethane interface. Left panels: transfer from the DCE to the aqueous phase under the influence of an external electric field of 0.2 V/Å. Right panels are for the reverse process. Top panels give the coordination number of the ion, center panels describe the position of the ion relative to the interface (located at zero) and the bottom panels show the oxygen-ion radial distribution function.

An examination of the transfer dynamics with a less intense external field is also consistent with this picture.[95] There are fewer ions that are able to cross the interface and completely hydrate on the time-scale of 50 ps, but in each trajectory that this happens, the mechanism is similar to what is described above. At a zero external electric field, when the ion starts at the bulk of the DCE phase, in none of the 20 trajectories was the ion able to cross the interface. This is surprising given the large driving force toward the aqueous phase, and it suggests the existence of a barrier to the transfer. Because the actual replacement of the solvation shell members is a very rapid process, and no such delayed crossings have been observed in simulations of ion transfer across the interface between a simple polar and non-polar liquid,[18] one concludes that this barrier is due to the unique structure of the interfacial water. In particular, the fact that the transfer is facilitated by water "fingers", which represent a roughening of the interface (and thus require free energy to create), supports the existence of such a barrier.

2. Transfer From the Aqueous Phase to DCE

The right panels of Figure 5 describe the reverse process, in which the ion is driven to the DCE from the water, with the help of an external electric field of opposite polarity. Although the electric field is of the same strength as for the transfer into the aqueous phase, the process is now much slower. In fact, this external field is not quite enough to overcome the free energy barrier, and most of the ions are still in the interface region after a period of 25 ps. The most striking result of this calculation is that although the ion position after 25 ps is, on average, near 10 Å *into the DCE phase*, the ion is still significantly solvated by water molecules, as is clear from the top panel of Figure 5. The time-dependent radial distribution functions show a slow decrease in the first peak and a disappearance of the second peak. An examination of the animated trajectories shows that the ion/water complex is in the DCE phase, but it is connected to the water phase by a chain of water molecules. The interface appears to be significantly perturbed and much broader. Similar results are obtained with a field of intensity 0.3 V/Å.

The above results suggest that the ion remains solvated in water at least during the actual crossing of the interface. The existence of a chain of water molecules connecting the hydrated ion to the water phase is also consistent with the time-reversal of the events that take place during the spontaneous transfer of the ion from the DCE to the water phase. The fact that the ion tends to keep its hydration shell is found to be a general feature of the behavior of small ions at water surfaces and interfaces.[76]

C. FREE ENERGY PROFILE FOR ION TRANSFER

The molecular dynamics calculations described in the previous section give direct, microscopically detailed information about the mechanism of the ion transfer. However, experimental measurements of ion transfer rate are done under conditions of steady-state ion current. To make direct comparison with such measurements, the free energy profile for the ion transfer, which is an equilibrium property of the system, needs to be calculated. This quantity will also give the net free energy of transfer of ions between the two bulk liquids. Despite the importance of this quantity, very little is known about it.

The molecular dynamics calculation of the free energy profile is simple in principle, and it is based on the direct application of Equation 3 with X now standing for the position Z of the ion along the interface normal. Calculations of the solute free energy profile in an inhomogeneous liquid environment have been reported for several systems, and the results have been compared with continuum electrostatic models.[18,20,97-100] In general, any continuum model which includes a dielectric discontinuity (the dielectric constant of each bulk phase is constant up to the interface) results in a free energy profile which varies too quickly at the interface as compared with the molecular dynamics results. Although this situation can be improved by considering inhomogeneous dielectric models, very little work has been done on applications of such models to liquid interfaces.[101]

Most of the molecular dynamics calculations have been for one-component systems. Free energy profiles for solute and ion transfer across the liquid/liquid interface have been determined in only a few cases. Hayoun *et al* [23] have calculated the free energy surface for atom transfer across the interface between two Lennard-Jones liquids by integrating the average force on the atom. They use it to demonstrate that the transfer of atoms across this interface can be described using a transition state theory formalism. Benjamin has calculated [18] the free energy surface for the transfer of an ion from a model non-polar diatomic liquid to a polar diatomic liquid, using biased sampling molecular dynamics. A comparison with a continuum dielectric model (utilizing dielectric constants derived from independent molecular dynamics calculations of the bulk liquids) was made.[76] It was found that although qualitatively reasonable, the continuum model gives rise to a free energy profile that changes too rapidly as the ion crosses the interface.

The free energy profile for the transfer of a Cl^- ion across the water/DCE interface includes, in addition to the electrostatic contribution (reflecting the different dielectric constants of water and DCE), a term due to the different amount of work necessary to create a cavity in the water and the DCE phase. Although this term is automatically included in the free energy calculated using the molecular dynamics free energy sampling procedure, it is useful to consider it separately. The electrostatic and cavity terms are shown in Figure 6. These profiles have been calculated by an approximate procedure discussed in detail elsewhere.[95] Briefly, the cavity term is estimated by generalizing the scale particle theory[102-104] (developed for bulk liquids) to the interface between two liquids. Specifically, the work of cavity formation is calculated by determining the probability of inserting a hard sphere into the interface region, which is assumed to be made of two different hard-sphere liquids, each of which is restricted to being on one side of the interface. The insertion probability is written as a product of the probability of inserting the appropriate fractions of the cavity in each liquid. Each of these probabilities is obtained from the (bulk) scale particle theory. The electrostatic contribution is estimated by the Gaussian model for the electrostatic potential fluctuations.[105] This model has been compared with the exact free energy calculations for a model ion transfer across a simpler liquid/liquid interface, and it has been found to be very accurate.[18]

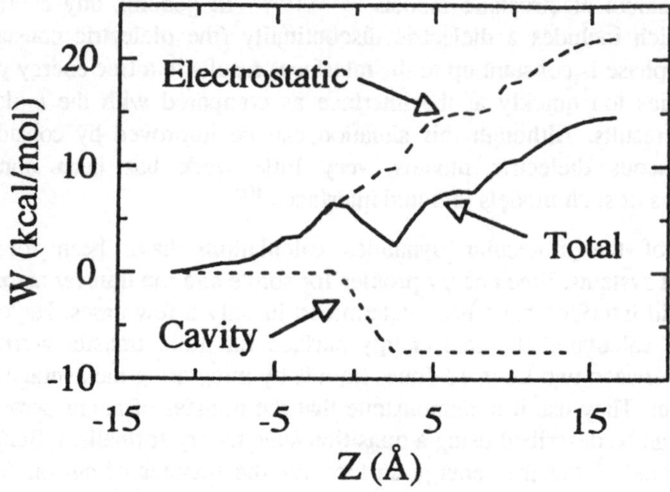

Figure 6. Free energy profile for the transfer of a chloride ion across the water/1,2-dichloroethane interface. The water occupies, on average, the region $Z < 0$. The contribution of the cavity and the electrostatic terms to the total free energy are shown.

As is shown in Figure 6, the electrostatic contribution monotonically decreases as the chloride ion is transferred from the DCE to the water. This just reflects the favorable solvation of small ions in water compared with their solvation in DCE. On the other hand, the work of cavity formation monotonically increases as the chloride ion is transferred from the DCE to the water. This is consistent with the larger solubility of inert gases in DCE than in water.[106, 107] From the total free energy profile, one sees that the net free energy of transfer of Cl^- from water to DCE is about 15 kcal/mol, in reasonable agreement with the experimental value of 12.4 kcal/mol.[106] The free energy profile exhibits a significant barrier of about 3 kcal/mol for the transfer of Cl^- from DCE to water. This is consistent with the trajectory calculations presented earlier, which show transfer rates slower than one would expect based on the diffusion constant of the ion and the significant driving force. As the simple model suggests, the origin of the barrier is in the special structure of interfacial water. As demonstrated earlier, the transfer of ions is assisted by surface roughness. This roughness (water "fingers") consists of water molecules with fewer hydrogen bonds than "typical" surface water molecules, which require free energy to create. The actual process of switching the solvation shell members is too fast to account for the barrier.

V. CONCLUSIONS AND OUTLOOK

In this chapter we have considered the insight that molecular dynamics trajectory calculations provide about charge transfer processes at the liquid/liquid interface. The ability to study the behavior of the solute and the neat interface at the microscopic level and on the picosecond time-scale provides new information that helps in the elucidation of mechanisms and is able to provide tests of simpler models.

The molecular dynamics (and Monte Carlo) studies of the interface between two immiscible liquids show, at least for liquids that are relevant to charge transfer processes, that the interface is molecularly sharp but very rough. The roughness at the water/1,2-dichloroethane interface can be described as the protrusion of a few water molecules, hydrogen-bonded to each other, into the organic phase. This roughness plays an important role in the ability of two ions to approach each other enroute to an electron transfer reaction and in assisting the transfer of ions across the interface.

The unique dielectric properties of the interface can sometimes be qualitatively described using continuum dielectric models. However, a quantitative assessment of some specific applications to charge transfer processes at the interface shows that these models may be misleading. In some cases, the molecular structure of the liquid at the interface plays a role that cannot be properly accounted for using these models.

The applications of microscopic models to liquid/liquid interfacial problems are only in their infancy. The study of the transfer of large hydrophobic ions and of neutral solutes, as well as the incorporation of finite ionic concentration into the molecular dynamics calculations, are feasible and important. Another important area where little work has been done to date is the development of approximate statistical mechanical approaches to the problem of interfacial charge transfer where the molecular structure of the liquid is explicitly taken into account. Progress in this area will complement the simulational studies in a way similar to the progress made in the understanding of solvation and charge transfer in bulk liquids.

VI. REFERENCES

1. **Girault, H. H. J. and Schiffrin, D. J.**, Electrochemistry of liquid-liquid interfaces, in *Electroanalytical Chemistry*, A. J. Bard, Eds., Dekker, NewYork, 1989, p 1.
2. *The Interface Structure and Electrochemical Processes at the Boundary Between Two Immiscible Liquids*, V. E. Kazarinov, Ed., Springer, Berlin, 1987.
3. **Starks, C. M., Liotta, C. L. and Halpern, M.,** *Phase Transfer Catalysis*, Chapman & Hall, New York, 1994.
4. **Adamson, A. W.**, *Physical Chemistry of Surfaces*, Wiley, New York, Fifth edition, 1990.
5. **Grubb, S. G., Kim, M. W., Raising, T. and Shen, Y. R.,** Orientation of molecular monolayers at the liquid-liquid interface as studied by optical second harmonic generation, *Langmuir*, 4, 452, 1988.
6. **Lee, L. T., Langevin, D. and Farnoux, B.**, Neutron reflectivity of an oil-water interface, *Phys. Rev. Lett.*, 67, 2678, 1991.
7. **Cheng, Y. F. and Schiffrin, D. J.**, Electron transfer between bis(pyridine)meso-tetraphenylporphyrinato iron(II) and ruthenium(III) and the hexacyanoferrate couple at the 1,2-dichloroethane water interface, *J. Electroanal. Chem.*, 314, 153, 1991.
8. **Wirth, M. J. and Burbage, J. D.**, Reorientation of acridine orange at liquid alkane water interfaces, *J. Phys. Chem.* , 96, 9022, 1992.
9. **Kott, K. L., Higgins, D. A., McMahon, R. J. and Corn, R. M.**, Observation of photoinduced electron transfer at a liquid-liquid interface by optical second harmonic generation, *J. Am. Chem. Soc.,* 115, 5342.
10. **Higgins, D. A. and Corn, R. M.**, 2nd harmonic generation studies of adsorption at a liquid-liquid electrochemical interface , *J. Phys. Chem.*, 97, 489, 1993.
11. **Conboy, J. C., Daschbach, J. L. and Richmond, G. L.**, Studies of alkane/water interfaces by total internal reflection second harmonic generation, *J. Phys. Chem.*, 98, 9688, 1994.
12. **Linse, P.**, Monte Carlo simulation of liquid-liquid benzene-water interface, *J. Chem. Phys.*, 86, 4177, 1987.
13. **Meyer, M., Mareschal, M. and Hayoun, M.,** Computer modeling of a liquid-liquid interface, *J. Chem. Phys.*, 89, 1067, 1988.
14. **Gao, J. and Jorgensen, W. L.**, Theoretical examination of hexanol-water interfaces, *J. Phys. Chem.,* 92, 5813, 1988.
15. **Smit, B.**, Molecular dynamics simulation of amphiphilic molecules at a liquid-liquid interface, *Phys. Rev. A.*, 37, 3431, 1988.
16. **Carpenter, I. L. and Hehre, W. J.,** A Molecular dynamics study of the hexane/water interface, *J. Phys. Chem.*, 94, 531, 1990.
17. **Benjamin, I.**, Molecular dynamics study of the free energy functions for electron transfer reactions at the liquid-liquid interface, *J. Phys. Chem.*, 95, 6675, 1991.
18. **Benjamin, I.**, Dynamics of ion transfer across a liquid-liquid interface: A comparison between molecular dynamics and a diffusion model., *J. Chem. Phys.* , 96, 577, 1992.
19. **Benjamin, I.**, Mechanism and dynamics of ion transfer across a liquid-liquid interface, *Science*, 261, 1558, 1993.
20. **Pohorille, A. and Wilson, M. A.**, Molecular structure of aqueous interfaces, *J. Mol. Struct. (Theochem)*, 284, 271, 1993.
21. **Benjamin, I.**, Solvent dynamics following charge transfer at the liquid-liquid interface, *Chem. Phys.*, 180, 287, 1994.
22. **Michael, D. and Benjamin,** I., Solute orientational dynamics and surface roughness of water/hydrocarbon interfaces, *J. Phys. Chem.*, 99, 1530, 1995.
23. **Hayoun, M., Meyer, M. and Turq, P.**, Molecular dynamics study of a solute-transfer reaction across a liquid-liquid interface, *J. Phys. Chem.*, 98, 6626, 1994.
24. **Allen, M. P. and Tildesley, D. J.,** *Computer Simulation of Liquids*, Clarendon, Oxford, 1987.
25. **Hansen, J. -P. and McDonald, I. R.**, *Theory of Simple Liquids*, Academic Press, London, 2nd edition, 1986. p 179.
26. **Sprik, M. and Klein, M. L.**, A polarizable model for water using distributed charge sites, *J. Chem. Phys.*, 89, 7556, 1988.
27. **Ahlstrom, P., Wallqvist, A., Engstrom, S. and Jonsson, B.,** A molecular dynamics study of polarizable water, *Mol. Phys.,* 68, 563, 1989.

28. **Dang, L. X., Rice, J. E., Caldwell, J. and Kollman, P. A.,** Ion solvation in polarizable water -molecular dynamics simulations, *J. Am. Chem. Soc.*, 113, 2481, 1991.
29. **Dang, L. X.**, The nonadditive intermolecular potential for water revised, *Chem. Phys.*, 97, 2659, 1992.
30. **Rick, S. W., Stuart, S. J. and Berne, B. J.,** Dynamical fluctuating charge force fields. Application to liquid water, *J. Chem. Phys.*, 101, 6141, 1994.
31. **Motakabbir, K. and Berkowitz, M.**, Liquid vapor interface of TIP4P water: Comparison between a polarizable and a nonpolarizable model, *Chem. Phys. Lett.*, 176, 61, 1991.
32. **Hautman, J., Halley, J. W. and Rhee, Y.-J.,** Molecular dynamics simulation of water between two ideal classical metal walls, *J. Chem. Phys.*, 91, 467, 1989.
33. **Hautman, J. and Klein, M. L.,** An Ewald summation method for planar surfaces and interfaces, *Mol. Phys.*, 75, 379, 1992.
34. **Alejandre, J., Tildesley, D. J. and Chapels, G. A.,** Molecular dynamics simulation of the orthobaric densities and surface tension of water, *J. Chem. Phys.*, 102, 4574, 1995.
35. **Chandler, D.,** *Introduction to Modern Statistical Mechanics*, Oxford University Press, Oxford, 1987.
36. **Bennett, C. H.**, Molecular dynamics and transition state theory: the simulation of infrequent events, in *Algorithms for Chemical Computations*: ACS Symposium Series 46, E. Christofferson, R., Ed., American Chemical Society, Washington, D. C., 1977.
37. **Torrie, G. M., Kusalik, P. G. and Patey, G. N.**, Theory of the electric double layer: Ion size effects in a molecular solvent *J. Chem. Phys.*, 91, 6367, 1989.
38. **Blum, L.**, Structure of the electric double layer, *Adv. Chem. Phys.*, 78, 171, 1990.
39. **Benjamin, I.**, Theoretical study of the water/1,2-dichloroethane interface: Structure, dynamics and conformational equilibria at the liquid-liquid interface, *J Chem. Phys.*, 97, 1432, 1992.
40. **Israelachvili, J. N.,** *Intermolecular and Surfaces Forces*, Academic Press, London, 1992.
41. **Tanford, C.**, *The Hydrophobic Effect*, Wiley, New York, 1981.
42. **Vanbuuren, A. R., Marrink, S. J. and Berendsen, H. J. C.,** A molecular dynamics study of the decane water interface, *J Phys. Chem.*, 97, 9206, 1993.
43. **Geblewicz, G. and Schiffrin, D. J.,** Electron transfer between immiscible solutions. The hexacyanoferrate-lutetium biphthalocyanine system, *J. Electroanal. Chem.*, 244, 27, 1988.
44. **Maeda, K., Kihara, S., Suzuki, M. and Matsui, M.,** Voltammetric interpretation of ion transfer coupled with electron transfer at a liquid liquid interface, *J Electroanal. Chem.*, 303, 171, 1991.
45. **Brown, A. R, Yellowlees, L. J. and Girault, H. H.,** Photoinduced electron-transfer across the interface between 2 immiscible electrolyte solutions., *J Chem. Soc. Faraday Trans.*, 89, 207, 1993.
46. **Kharkats, Yu. I. and Volkov, A. G.,** Interfacial catalysis: Multielectron reactions at the liquid-liquid interface, *J. Electroanal. Chem.*, 184 , 435, 1985.
47. **Kuznetsov, A. M. and Kharkats, Y. I.,** Problems of a quantum theory of charge transfer reactions, in *The Interface Structure and Electrochemical Processes at the Boundary Between Two Immiscible Liquids*, Kazarinov, V. E., Ed., Springer, Berlin, 1987, p. 11.
48. **Marcus, R. A.**, Reorganization free energy for electron transfers at liquid-liquid and dielectric semiconductor-liquid interfaces, *J. Phys. Chem.*, 94, 1050, 1990.
49. **Marcus, R. A.,** Theory of electron-transfer rates across liquid-liquid interfaces, *J Phys. Chem.*, 94, 4152, 1990.
50. **Marcus, R. A.,** Theory of electron-transfer rates across liquid-liquid interfaces. 2. Relationships and Application, *J. Phys. Chem.*, 95, 2010, 1991.
51. **Zener, C.**, Non-adiabatic crossing of energy levels, *Proc. R. Soc.London, Ser. A*, 137, 696, 1932.
52. **Marcus, R. A.**, On the theory of electron-transfer reactions. VI. Unified treatment for homogeneous and electrode reactions, *J. Chem. Phys.*, 43, 679, 1965.
53. **Benjamin, I.,** Theory and Computer Simulations of Solvation and Chemical Reactions at Liquid Interfaces, *Acc. Chem. Res.*, 28, 233, 1995.
54. **Warshel, A.,** Dynamics of reactions in polar solvents. Semiclassical trajectory studies of electron-transfer and proton-transfer reactions, *J. Phys. Chem.*, 86, 2218, 1982.
55. **Hwang, J. K. and Warshel, A.,** Microscopic examination of free-energy relationships for electron transfer in pola solvents, *J. Am. Chem. Soc.*, 109, 715, 1987.

56. **Kuharski, R. A, Bader, J. S, Chandler, D., Sprik, M., Klein, M. L. and Impey, R. W.**, Molecular model for aqueous ferrous-ferric electron transfer, *J. Chem. Phys.*, 89, 3248, 1988.
57. **Carter, E. A. and Hynes, J. T.**, Solute-dependent solvent force constants for ion pairs and neutral pairs in polar solvent, *J. Phys. Chem.*, 93, 2184, 1989.
58. **King, G. and Warshel, A.**, Investigation of the free energy functions for electron transfer reactions, *J. Chem. Phys.*, 93, 8682, 1990.
59. **Tachiya, M.**, Relation between the electron-transfer rate and the free energy change of reaction, *J. Phys. Chem.*, 93, 7050, 1989.
60. **Benjamin, I.**, A molecular model for an electron transfer reaction at the water/1,2-dichloroethane interface., in *Structure and Reactivity in Aqueous Solution*: ACS Symposium series 568, Cramer, C. J. and Truhlar, D. G., Eds., American Chemical Society, Washington, D. C., 1994, p. 409.
61. **Maroncelli, M, MacInnis, J. and Fleming, G. R.**, Polar solvent dynamics and electron-transfer reactions, *Science*, 243, 1674, 1989.
62. **Barbara, P. F. and Jarzeba, W.**, Ultrafast photochemical intramolecular charge and excited state solvation, *Adv. Photochem.*, 15, 1, 1990.
63. **Carter, E. A. and Hynes, J. T.**, Solvation dynamics for an ion pair in a polar solvent: Time dependent fluorescence and photochemical charge transfer, *J. Chem. Phys.*, 94, 5961, 1991.
64. **Weaver, M. J.**, Dynamical solvent effects on activated electron-transfer reactions: principles, pitfalls, and progress, *Chem. Rev.*, 92, 463, 1992.
65. **Marecek, V., DeArmond, A. H. and DeArmond, M. K.**, Photochemical electron transfer in liquid/liquid solvent systems, *J. Am. Chem. Soc.*, 11 1, 2561, 1989.
66. **Dvorak, O., DeArmond, A. H. and DeArmond, M. K.**, Photoprocesses at the liquid-liquid interface. 4. Photooxidative transfer with $[Ru(BPZ)_3]^{2+}$ complexes, *Langmuir*, 8, 955, 1992.
67. **Bagchi, B.**, Dynamics of solvation and charge transfer reactions in dipolar liquids, *Annu. Rev. Phys. Chem.*, 40, 115, 1989.
68. **Simon, J. D.**, Time-resolved studies of solvation in polar media, *Acc. Chem. Res.*, 21, 128, 1988.
69. **Maroncelli, M.**, Computer simulations of solvation dynamics in acetonitrile, *J. Chem. Phys.*, 94, 2084, 1991.
70. **Wolynes, P. G.**, Linearized microscopic theories of nonequilibrium solvation, *J. Chem. Phys.*, 86, 5133, 1987.
71. **Rips, I., Klafter, J. and Jortner**, J., Solvation dynamics in polar liquids, *J. Chem. Phys.*, 89, 4288, 1988.
72. **Nichols, A. L. and Calef, D. F.**, Polar solvent relaxation: The mean spherical approximation approach, *J. Chem. Phys.*, 89, 3783, 1988.
73. **Chandra, A. and Bagchi, B.**, Inertial effects in solvation dynamics, *J. Chem. Phys.*, 94, 3177, 1991.
74. **Maroncelli, M. and Fleming, G. R.**, Computer simulation of the dynamics of aqueous solvation, *J. Chem. Phys.*, 89, 5044, 1988.
75. **Benjamin, I.**, Theoretical study of ion solvation at the water liquid-vapor interface, *J. Chem. Phys.* , 95, 3698, 1991.
76. **Benjamin, I.**, Solvation and charge transfer at liquid interfaces, in *Reaction Dynamics in Clusters and Condensed Phases*, Jortner, J., Levine, R. D. and Pullman, B., Eds., Kluwer, Dordrecht, The Netherlands, 1994, p 179.
77. **Rose, D. A. and Benjamin, I.**, Solvation of Na^+ and Cl^- at the water-platinum (100) interface, *J. Chem. Phys.*, 95, 6856, 1991.
78. **Arai, K., Ohsawa, M., Kusu, F. and Takamura, K.**, Drug ion transfer across an oil-water interface and pharmacological activity, *Bioelectrochem. Bioenerg.*, 31, 65, 1993.
79. **Gennis, R. B.**, *Biomembranes*, Springer, New York, 1989.
80. **Gavach, C. and Henry, F.**, Chronopotentiometry at the liquid membrane-aqueous solution interface, *C. R. Acad. Sci.*, C274, 1545, 1972.
81. **Kakiuchi, T. and Senda, M.**, Structure of the electrical double layer at the interface between nitrobenzene solution of tetrabutylammonium tetraphenylborate and aqueous solution of lithium chloride, *Bull. Chem. Soc. Jpn.*, 56, 1753, 1983.
82. **Hanna, G. J. and Noble, R. D.**, Measurement of liquid-liquid interfacial kinetics, *Chem. Rev.*, 85, 583, 1985.

83. **Wandlowski, T., Marecek, V., Holub, K. and Samec, Z.**, Ion transfer across liquid-liquid phase boundaries - electrochemical kinetics by faradaic impedance, *J. Phys. Chem.*, 93, 8204, 1989.
84. **Sabela, A., Marecek, V, Samec, Z. and Fuoco, R.**, Standard Gibbs energies of transfer of univalent ions from water to 1,2-dichloroethane, *Electrochim. Acta,* 37, 231, 1992.
85. **Wandlowski, T., Marecek, V., Samec, Z. and Fuoco, R.**, Effect of temperature on the ion transfer across an interface between two immiscible electrolyte solutions - ion transfer dynamics, *J. Electroanal. Chem.*, 331, 765, 1992.
86. **Samec, Z. and Marecek, V.**, The use of Frumkin correction in the kinetics of the ion transfer across the interface between two immiscible electrolyte solutions - comment, *J. Electroanal. Chem.*, 333, 319, 1992.
87. **Kakiuchi, T.**, DC and AC response of ion transfer across an oil water interface with a Goldman-type current potential characteristic, *J. ElectroanaL Chem.*, 344, 1, 1993.
88. **Kakiuchi, T. and Takasu,** Y., Differenfial cyclic voltfluorometry and chronofluorometry of the transfer of fluorescent ions across the 1,2- dichloroethane-water interface, *Analytical Chem.*, 66, 1853, 1994.
89. **Kakiuchi, T. and Takasu, Y.**, Potential-step chronofluorometric response of fluorescent-ion transfer across a liquid-vertical-bar-liquid interface, *J. Electroanal. Chem.*, 381, 5, 1995.
90. **Gavach, C. and D'Epenoux, B.**, Chronopotentiometric investigation of the diffusion overvoltage at the interface between two nonmiscible solutions. II. Potassium halide aqueous solution-hexadecyltrimethylammonium picrate nitrobenzene solution, *J. Electroanal. Chem.*, 55, 59, 1974.
91. **Kornyshev, A. A. and Volkov, A. G.**, On the evaluation of standard Gibbs free energies of ion transfer between two solvents, *J. Electroanal. Chem.*, 180, 363, 1984.
92. **Gurevich, Y. Y. and Kharkats, Y. I.**, Ion transfer through a phase boundary: A stochastic approach, *J. Electroanal. Chem.*, 200, 3, 1986.
93. **Samec, Z., Kharkats, Y. I. and Gurevich,** Y. Y., Stochastic approach to the ion transfer kinetics across the interface between two immiscible electrolyte solutions. Comparison with the experimental data, *J. Electroanal. Chem.*, 204, 257, 1986.
94. **Hayoun, M., Meyer, M. and Mareschal, M.**, Molecular dynamics simulation of a liquid-liquid interface, in *Chemical Reactivity in Liquids*, Ciccotti, G. and Turq, P., Eds., Plenum, New York, 1987.
95. **Schweighofer, K. J. and Benjamin, I.**, Transfer of small ions across the water/1,2-dichloroethane interface, *J. Phys. Chem.*, 99, in press, 1995.
96. **Bard, A. J. and Faulkner, L. R.**, *Electrochemical methods: fundamentals and applications*, Wiley, New York, 1980.
97. **Wilson, M. A. and Pohorille, A.**, Interaction of monovalent ions with the water liquid-vapor interface. A molecular dynamics study, *J. Chem. Phys.*, 95, 6005, 1991.
98. **Pohorille, A. and Benjamin, I.**, Molecular dynamics of phenol at the lquid-vapor interface of water, *J. Chem. Phys.*, 94, 5599, 1991.
99. **Schweighofer, K. J. and Benjamin, I.**, Dynamics of ion desorption from the liquid-vapor interface of water, *Chem. Phys. Lett.*, 202, 379,
100. **Pohorille, A. and Benjamin, I.**, Structure and energetics of model amphiphilic molecules at the water liquid-vapor interface. A molecular dynamics study, *J. Phys. Chem.*, 97, 2664, 1993.
101. **Stillinger, F. H. and Ben-Naim, A.**, Liquid-vapor interface potential for water, *J. Chem. Phys.*, 47, 4431, 1967.
102. **Reiss, H., Frisch, H. L. and Lebowitz, J. L.**, Statistical mechanics of rigid spheres, *J. Chem. Phys.*, 31, 369, 1959.
103. **Stillinger, F. H.**, Structure in aqueous solutions of nonpolar solutes from the standpoint of scaled-particle theory, *J. Solution Chem.*, 2, 141, 1973.
104. **Pierotti, R. A.**, A scaled particle theory of aqueous and nonaqueous solutions, *Chem. Rev.*, 76, 717, 1976.
105. **Levy, R. M, Belhadj, M. and Kitchen, D. B.**, Gaussian fluctuation formula for electrostatic free-energy changes in solution, *J Chem. Phys.*, 95, 3627.
106. **Marcus, Y.**, *Ion Solvation*, Wiley, New York, 1985. Ch. 6.
107. **Pohorille, A. and Pratt, L. R.**, Cavities in molecular liquids and the theory of hydrophobic solubilities, *J. Am. Chem. Soc.*, 112, 5066, 1990.

Chapter 10

PHOTOELECTROCHEMICAL EFFECT AT THE INTERFACE BETWEEN TWO IMMISCIBLE ELECTROLYTE SOLUTIONS

Nicholas A. Kotov and Michael G. Kuzmin

I. INTRODUCTION

Charge transfer reactions at liquid-liquid (L-L) interfaces have considerable significance in the real world. In fact, the very process of reading the previous sentence required a series of L-L charge transfer reactions. This chapter will focus on the process of photoinduced ion transfer across macroscopic L-L interfaces. Such interfacial ion transfer reveals itself in various phenomena and particularly in the photoelectrochemical effect at the interface between two immiscible electrolyte solutions (ITIES), which was detected about ten years ago. We will also briefly consider similar processes in colloidal particles to point out a number of features in macro- and microheterogeneous systems that are relevant to photoinduced ion transfer. The mechanism of this process at the interface of two immiscible electrolyte solutions is considered in detail with the emphasis on its kinetic features.

For the last two decades the study of photoinduced charge separation at liquid-liquid interfaces, and in nonhomogeneous systems in general, has become a popular area of research. Initially, the motivation for investigating such systems was centered on the possibility of mimicking the process of natural photosynthesis for the collection and storage of solar energy[1-6]. The border between two liquids of different polarities facilitates the separation of initially formed products of intermolecular charge transfer and prevents their subsequent recombination. A variety of systems based primarily on micro-heterogeneous aggregates like micelles, vesicles (liposomes), and microemulsions for photoinduced decomposition of water have been designed[1-10].

Recently photoelectrochemical cells based on TiO_2 and WS_2 with quantum efficiencies close to unity have been discovered[11, 12]. This is only a single example of a tremendous progress in semiconductor photochemistry[13-15]. These and other discoveries resulted in the shift of attention of L-L interface researchers toward the investigation and modeling of biological systems. In fact, solar light is one of the most important environmental factors and its effects on various aspects of life are still at a rather primitive level of understanding. Even photosynthesis in plants poses a number of challenging questions[16], despite vigorous long-term investigation. Apart from that there are numerous other processes in living organisms triggered by absorption of photons which involve charge

0-8493-7694-7/96/$0.00+$.50

separation at aqueous-organic interfaces: examples include vision, light-dependent movements and rhythms of plants and animals, and photomorphogenesis.[17]. Solar radiation can be both a healing and a damaging environmental agent. For instance, UV light is known to cause serious injuries to membranes, DNA, and proteins[18, 19]. Selective activation of these processes would afford the creation of environmentally friendly herbicides, pesticides and other chemicals for agriculture. Medicinal aspects of photobiology are attracting increasing attention as well. Photoinduced ion and electron transfer through organic membrane-electrolyte interface plays a key role in photodynamic therapy of cancer[20] and a number of other diseases such as arthritis[21], atherosclerosis[22], psoriasis[23] and others.[24] Pretreatment of tissues by laser light was also found to be useful in transplantation of organs[25]. The mechanism of photodynamic therapy has been discussed in several recent review articles[26]. It was discovered that special photosensizers can selectively accumulate in malignant cells[27]. Upon laser irradiation they produce singlet oxygen and/or other active species which eventually kill cancerous tissue. This direction of photobiology has undergone a stage of rapid development since laser light causes almost no side effects compared to radiation therapy or anticancer drugs[28].

In recent years processes at interfaces of immiscible liquids have been the focus of intense research interest[29]. Photoinduced processes have been studied at nonpolarizable interfaces starting in the sixties by E. Rabinovitch *et al*[30] and then by L. I. Boguslavsky, A. G. Volkov *et al*[31]. The generation of photopotential has also been observed for bacteriorhodopsin proton pumps adsorbed at the nonpolarizable L-L interfaces by R. N. Robertson *et al*[32]. Although several mechanisms of the photopotential generation have been proposed[30-32], the lack of control over interfacial potential does not allow many other possibilities to be ruled out.

The majority of papers dealing with photoinduced charge transfer across polarizable liquid-liquid interfaces (ITIES), have appeared during the last 10 years[33-46]. Generally, ITIES is a more convenient and controllable system for the observation of photoeffects at L-L interface compared to simple alkane/water or ether/water interfaces. The first communication was published by N. Zaitsev, M. G. Kuzmin *et al.* in 1985[33]. The authors observed the interfacial potential induced by illumination of the border between an aqueous solution of NaCl and a solution of protoporphyrin and quinones in 1,2-dichloroethane, and for several other redox pairs. Quantitative results on the formation and diffusion of charge carriers were obtained later by monitoring the photocurrent under a constant interfacial potential[34-37, 39-45]. Z. Samec, V. Marecek, H. H. Girault, and K. Dearmond reported on the observation of comparable effects, attributing them to both ion and electron transfer across the water/organic interface[35-40].

Analogous processes have been extensively studied in microheterogeneous colloidal systems such as micelles, vesicles (liposomes), microemulsions and others. It would be beneficial for further development of this field to compare various possibilities in both macro- and microheterogeneous systems.

II. REACTIONS OF CHARGE TRANSFER AT LIQUID-LIQUID INTERFACES IN MICROHETEROGENEOUS SYSTEMS

A. INTERFACIAL EFFECTS ON THE CHARGE TRANSFER IN MICROHETEROGENEOUS LIQUID-LIQUID SYSTEMS

Photoinduced charge transfer across a liquid-liquid interface has been thoroughly investigated in micelles, vesicles (liposomes), microemulsions [1, 3-10, 15], and bilayer lipid membranes[47]. The processes occurring at the contact of aqueous solutions with organic media in proteins, polymers, Langmuir-Blodgett films and conducting organic films are similar to the ones in organic colloidal systems. The reactions of photoinduced charge transfer in these systems have been reviewed by several authors[3-9, 48, 49]. However, the effect of the interfacial potential ΔE_o^w on the path and efficiency of photoinduced charge separation in micro-heterogeneous systems as well as for immiscible liquid phases in general, has not been given sufficient attention, probably because of experimental difficulties with measurements and control of electric potential. Although the effect of potential on charge separation may look rather straightforward[50], recent investigations have revealed many unexpected phenomena connecting ΔE_o^w and reactions at interfaces. For instance, one of the most important features of cell membranes is the ability to control the ion flow into and out of an organelle. Ion channels embedded in membranes react to small changes of the composition of intracellular fluid, maintaining the necessary balance of components on both sides of the membrane. The gating function of ion channels is controlled by the interfacial potential and a few millivolts difference is enough to "switch" the open-closed modes for a particular ion[51].

For simpler chemical systems the interfacial potential brings about many effects that cannot be observed in homogeneous media. For instance, the photoionization potential I_p of various organic molecules drastically decreases in micellar and vesicular systems[49, 52, 53].

Alterations of ΔE_o^w are believed to cause transformations in the morphology of the interface. The extended study by L. Kevan and coworkers[54] showed that not only the interfacial potential but also the structure of the interface plays a role in the photoionization of solubilized phenothiazines and porphyrins. The interplay of interfacial potential and environment has been observed experimentally for many other charge-transfer reactions[55] as well as considered theoretically by Y. Dakhnovskii[56].

In vesicles the transmembrane potential creates dramatic differences in the translocation and binding of hydrophobic ions by altering free energy barriers in the middle of the bilayer and the depth of the free energy minima at the interfaces. In fact, otherwise similar cations and anions were observed to have as much as 1000000 times difference in their transport rate constants[57, 58]. In the case of photoinduced reactions this difference is expected to be even larger due to the effect of potential on both primary charge separation and following recombination steps. The influence of electric field on photoinduced electron transfer was studied by several groups headed by R. Marcus, S. Boxer, P. Dutton, G. Tollin and others. Electric fields can both elevate and diminish the yield free charge carriers[59] depending on susceptibility of various rate constants to the electrostatic field.

Y. Shchipunov and A. Kolpakov demonstrated by electric measurements that the change in the interface potential can cause reorganization of phospholipid headgroups[60], while J. M. Leenhouts et al. found that membrane potential has no detectable effect on the phosphocholine conformation in vesicles as determined by H^2-NMR[61].

Thus, the effect of the interfacial potential should be considered far from being trivial and well understood. The macroscopic L-L interface opens unique possibilities for further study of this complex phenomenon.

B. WHAT IS THE INTERFACIAL POTENTIAL?

In a timely methodological review V. S. Markin and A. G. Volkov[62] discussed several types of potentials at L-L interfaces. To avoid any confusion with terminology we would like to dwell briefly on the physical meaning of the interfacial potential ΔE_o^w.

The potential drop at a L-L interface arises from the presence of a layer of oriented molecular dipoles, from the ionization of surfactant headgroups and from the adsorption of ions present in the environment. Potential difference in the compact layer of oriented molecular dipoles is almost independent of electrolyte composition, while the potential in the diffuse Gouy-Chapman layer is strongly affected by the ionic strength of the medium (for a detailed description see the chapter by T. J. VanderNoot). At the potential of zero charge condition the potential drop in the compact layer is about 5-50 mV[63, 64]. However the specific adsorption, observed even for inorganic ions can substantially elevate the potential difference in the compact layer[65]. It is noteworthy that in small microheterogeneous aggregates like micelles or vesicles (liposomes) the dipole potential is larger than at a macroscopic interface and may reach 100 mV[66] while the compact layer spans a significant part of the organic phase.

The diffusion layer is formed by dissolved ions from the ambient solution which are attracted to the intrinsically charged interface. The potential difference in it may be as high as 300 mV[67]. The sum of the potential drops in both dipole and diffusion layers can be referred to as the interfacial potential (the so-called Galvani potential) which by definition cannot be measured experimentally[62]. For a macroscopic interface this problem is solved by an extrathermodynamic assumption, i.e., by the postulate of equality of transfer energies (the energy required for the transfer of an ion from one phase to another) for two reference ions: a tetraphenylborate anion and tetraphenylarsonium cation. The validity of this assumption had been established in a number of works by A. J. Parker and O. Popovich and used by hundreds of scientists[68]. For microheterogeneous systems like micelles, vesicles, microemulsions and others this problem has not yet been solved. Usually researchers operate with a change of ΔE_o^w in a certain chemical process with an arbitrary reference point. For many cases such measurements are quite valuable and carry a substantial amount of information regardless of some inconsistency in methodological background.

C. MEASUREMENT OF THE INTERFACIAL POTENTIAL AT THE MICROHETEROGENEOUS LIQUID-LIQUID INTERFACES

Usually the interfacial potential in microheterogeneous systems is estimated by the degree of ionization of acid/base indicators. This was initially proposed by G. S. Hartley and J. W. Roe in 1940[69]. The basis of this technique is the dependence of the apparent pK_a of a weak acid adsorbed at the liquid-liquid interface on the interfacial potential[70]:

$$pK_a^{obs} = pK_a^0 - (\Delta E_o^w F/2.3RT) \qquad (1)$$

where pK_a^{obs} is the apparent pK of an indicator at the interface, pK_a^0 is interfacial pK in the absence of the electric field, ΔE_o^w is the interfacial potential, and F, R, and T are Faraday constant, gas constant and absolute temperature respectively. The titration of the indicator for various surface potentials will give different values of pK_a^{obs} and then ΔE_o^w can be calculated. This method has been widely used in micelles, vesicles and microemulsions for the determination of the potential difference at the L-L interface[71]. All scientific groups dealing with this problem have used neutral micelles for the determination of pK_a^0 assuming that the properties of an indicator are similar in different micelles[48, 71]. This assumption is fairly broad, and those who work with microheterogeneous liquid systems must understand its limitations, which were discussed in the extensive review by F. Griezer and C. J. Hummond[72]. In the context of the present work, it is important that even so called "uncharged" or "neutral" L-L interfaces in microheterogeneous systems formed by nonionic surfactants do have a substantial potential drop of at least 50 mV [64-66]. Fortunately this potential is expected to be little affected by the ambient conditions because it is formed by oriented dipoles. Consequently, it can be included in pK_a^0 for a series of similar measurements. However, in the scale of absolute potential this unknown constant represents the error of ΔE_o^w measurements. While recognizing the convenience and simplicity of this method, it should be understood that a calculated potential of, say, 150 mV actually refers to the real potential somewhere between 100 and 200 mV. This makes the comparison of the ΔE_o^w data acquired by means of indicator ionization with figures obtained by independent techniques a rather difficult endeavor.

An idea similar to the use of acid/base indicators for the determination of ΔE_o^w was the basis of two other methods for the evaluation of interfacial potential employing spin-labels[73] and electrochemical probes[74]. The former makes use of a difference in ESR spectra between spin label bound to micelle and an unbound spin label. The equilibrium between these two forms depends on the interfacial potential at the micelle surface. Thus, ΔE_o^w can be determined from the intensity of ESR signals corresponding to these two states of the spin-label. A detailed description of this technique first proposed by Franklin at al. is given in their recent publication[73].

Interfacial potential also affects the thermodynamic characteristics of oxidation/reduction processes of solubilized molecules[75]. In particular, this has been demonstrated for the half-wave potential of ferrocene derivatives embedded in micelles[74]. Taking advantage of the Gouy-Chapman theory one can finally construct an equation similar to Equation (1) that can be used for the determination of the interfacial potential.

The same reservations regarding the use of acid/base indicators apply to spin-labeled and electrochemical probes as well as for a number of other techniques making use of voltage dependent changes in UV absorption, fluorescence, circular dichroism, and birefringence[76]. None of these can be singled out for best performance, so one may employ a method that appears to be the most convenient. However, one should also be aware of problems arising from the use of arbitrarily chosen reference zero points.

Some dyes were found to be sensitive to the surrounding electrical field and polarity of the medium, showing attractions in UV absorption or fluorescent spectra[76, 77]. When embedded in microheterogeneous systems or adsorbed at the L-L interface they could be used to monitor changes caused by an increasing interface potential[78]. This method is very attractive for some applications due to its simplicity. However, we note that it can be used only for the determination of the *direction* of the potential changes and requires that the probe molecule does not change its adsorption site.

Micelles, vesicles and microemulsions form stable colloidal solutions that can also be characterized by zeta-potential or electrokinetic potentials. Application of various theories of electrical double layer and electric-field-assisted diffusion permits an estimate of the total interfacial potential from an experimentally available zeta-potential. This method is rather sensitive and even slight variations in interface characteristics (area, charge density, ionic strength etc.) can be reliably detected[79]. Importantly, this technique does not require any involvement of probe molecules which can cause a noticeable disturbance[80]. On the other hand, it does need relatively complicated laboratory equipment. The underlying theory requires knowledge of such parameters as mobility of ions and their size, which are rarely available with better than 20% error even for simple organic ions. Additionally, several reports indicated that Gouy-Chapman theory is not always applicable to the microscopic liquid-liquid interface[81], which limits the use of zeta-potential monitoring of ΔE_o^w. Nevertheless, under favorable conditions this method can provide very important kinetic as well as thermodynamic data for photochemical processes at interfaces, as demonstrated by Boxall and Kelsall[82].

D. METHODS FOR INTERFACIAL POTENTIAL CONTROL IN MICROHETEROGENEOUS SYSTEMS

Currently only two ways of changing the interfacial potential of the microscopic L-L interface are used: alternation of ionic strength of the medium and surfactant substitution. The large variety of available surfactants can be divided into three major groups: cationic, anionic and nonionic. Obviously the replacement of a cationic surfactant with an anionic one will result in the opposite sign of the interfacial potential. Mixtures of nonionic and ionic surfactants can be used for more gradual ΔE_o^w variation. This approach has been used in many studies dealing with photoinduced charge separation, ion partitioning, solubilization, and drug targeting[49, 50, 54, 58, 72, 83]. In nonionic surfactants the interfacial potential is smaller than in ionic surfactants and can be estimated to be about ± 50 mV[64,66]; the sign of ΔE_o^w in nonionic colloids is difficult to predict especially for zwitterionic surfactants. For polyethylenoxide derivatives the organic phase (micelle) is likely to be negatively charged.

A more accurate way to change the interfacial potential is by modifying the ionic strength of the ambient electrolyte, which varies the potential over a range of 200 mV[84]. Calculations of potential-distance profiles based on the numerical solution of the Poisson-Boltzman equation for spherical particles are also available[66, 67, 79, 84]. The disadvantage of this method is the gradual decline of the stability of the microheterogeneous systems with increased electrolyte concentration[84, 85]. The strong point of this procedure is the simplicity and convenience of potential variation. It has often been used in conjunction with the acid/base indicators acting as "interfacial voltmeters"[86].

E. COMPARISON OF MACRO- AND MICROSCOPIC LIQUID-LIQUID INTERFACES

The processes which occur between aqueous and organic phases represent a very important class of reactions responsible for many functions of living organisms. Microheterogeneous systems such as micelles, vesicles (liposomes), and microemulsions have been widely used for modeling interfacial reactions. However, further understanding of the mechanism of these processes relation to the interfacial potential requires new methods of investigation. The macroscopic interface and particularly ITIES opens new perspectives for the investigation of processes at an L-L interface. Here we list several possibilities which merit at least some attention:

1. The process of charge transfer accompanying various chemical reactions, can be observed directly at a macroscopic interface as a current flow. This provides a simple and accurate way to follow the course of a reaction in a two-phase system. For most other liquid-liquid systems (except BLM) secondary effects on spectroscopic, electrochemical, and magnetic properties of solutes must be employed.
2. The nature of microheterogeneous systems makes it rather difficult to monitor and to control the potential between two phases. For the macroscopic border between organic and aqueous phases the precision of potential measurements is incomparably higher and is determined only by the validity of TBATPB assumption.
3. The macroscopic liquid-liquid interface offers a much easier way to observe and to control the structure and properties of the interfacial layer. Measurements of impedance and capacitance of the interface can monitor conformations in surfactant headgroups as well as adsorbed substances (proteins, surfactants etc.). In fact, even an ultrathin polymer membrane can be positioned at the interface[87]. The macroscopic interface between two immiscible electrolytes can be an excellent test system for the creation of artificial cellular membranes.
4. A new set of methods previously used in solid state physics can be employed. Recent reports about second harmonic generation at the macroscopic L-L interface[40, 88, 89], measurements of absorption spectra at liquid-liquid interfaces[90] and other methods are expected to be of increasing importance for the investigation of interfacial processes. For instance, T. Kakiuchi and Y. Takasu recently reported on the application of fluorescent spectroscopy to the investigation of the charge-transfer process at ITIES[91].

At the same time several experimental limitations of the macroscopic L-L interface must be mentioned:

1. A polarizable macroscopic interface requires the presence of an electrolyte which may interfere with processes under investigation. Particularly, the effect of $B(Ph)_4^-$ a very common supporting-electrolyte

counterion on the photochemical process at the ITIES will be discussed in the course of this paper.

2. The choice of solvents used for the organic phase is rather limited. Currently chlorinated hydrocarbons or nitrobenzenes are used for this purpose. Despite the similarity to the apparent dielectric constant of hydrocarbon tails in membranes, which is higher than in corresponding bulk solvents, even subtle changes in dielectric permittivity may effect the mechanism of an interfacial reaction[92]. Last, but certainly not least, a large variety of organic phases are desirable to adjust the solubility of redox reagents.

Despite these inconveniences the macroscopic interface has considerable promise. A perfect example is the successful modeling of photosynthesis at a nonpolarizable hydrocarbon/water interface where a great number of unique features of this process have been demonstrated and a close resemblance with the native mechanism has been achieved[93]. As one of the active future areas of research the investigation of natural oscillations of the interfacial potential in biomembranes can be noted. These oscillations were proven to play an important role in performance of many organs and especially that of brain cells[94]. Being rather small in amplitude, these oscillations are difficult to model anywhere else but at a macroscopic boundary. Recently it was demonstrated that the oscillating[95] and coupled[96] processes can be successfully transferred to the interface between immiscible electrolyte solutions.

III. PHOTOELECTROCHEMICAL EFFECT AT THE INTERFACE OF IMMISCIBLE ELECTROLYTE SOLUTIONS

A. PHOTOINDUCED CHARGE TRANSFER AT THE INTERFACE OF IMMISCIBLE ELECTROLYTE SOLUTIONS

Photoinduced charge transfer at the interface of immiscible electrolyte solutions (ITIES) can be observed in many systems and experimental arrangements[33-46]. Generally, the experimental cell has to provide the opportunity of working in an oxygen free environment in order to avoid the quenching of excited states (Figure 1). However, for some applications such as interfacial reactions of a photogenerated superoxide anion, which are of great importance for photodynamic therapy, the presence of O_2 is desirable. Normally, photoeffects at ITIES are monitored under potentiostatic conditions[33-36, 39-46], in which the interfacial potential is maintained constant while the change in dc current through the interface is monitored. The open circuit photopotential[33, 40] and ac photocurrent transients[37, 38, 40] have proven to be quite informative too. The ac mode of the photocurrent is achieved by chopping the light beam with a certain frequency. Both methods may be especially helpful since they allow measurements of the photoeffect when the interface is nonpolarizable.

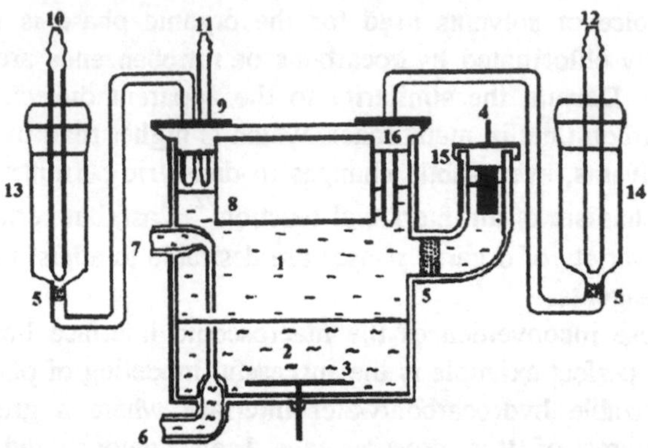

Figure 1. A photoelectrochemical cell. 1 - an aqueous phase, 2 - an organic phase, 3, 4 - counter electrodes, 5 - fused glass, 6, 7 - reference electrodes, 8 - a quartz window, 9 - ring aperture, 10, 11, 12 - inlets for argon purging, 13, 14 - vessels for argon bubbling prior to phase contact, 15, 16 - Teflon stoppers[46]. Reproduced with permission from Elsevier Sequoia S.A.

Theoretically, charge transport reactions at the interface can proceed as electron, proton or ion relocation across the water/organic border. E. Rabinovitch *et al.* experimentally observed the transfer of dye photoproducts across the water/ether interface in 1962[30]. They also proposed to use this reaction for solar energy storage. The first observation of photoinduced ion transfer at ITIES was reported by N. Zaitsev, M. Kuzmin *et al.* in 1985 [33]. Later this process was extensively studied in a number of publications by N. A. Kotov and M. G. Kuzmin[34, 41-46]. Z. Samec and H. H. Girault observed photoinduced ion transfer across ITIES upon photoexcitation and subsequent decomposition of ions of the supporting electrolyte[35, 36, 39]. Photoinduced proton transfer across the boundary between immiscible nonelectrolytes, such as water and hydrocarbons, has been studied by E. Rabinovitch *et al.*[30], by L. I. Boguslavsky, A. G. Volkov *et al* [31] and by R. N. Robertson *et al.*[32] N. Kotov and M. Kuzmin observed pH-dependent photocurrent upon excitation of 2-hydroxynaphthaline adsorbed at polarized ITIES, which can be attributed to the transport of a protons from the hydroxy group of this organic molecule to a proton acceptor in aqueous phase[97]. Interestingly, all processes at the surface of biomembranes occur at almost potentiostatic conditions (ΔE_o^w variations do not exceed 50 mV) due to various compensation mechanisms. From this point of view, conditions at ITIES are, in fact, closer to really biological systems than the nonpolarizable alkane/water interface where ΔE_o^w can change by several hundred millivolts[31].

There have been multiple attempts to register *photoinduced electron transfer* across ITIES. In 1988 H. H. Girault and coworkers[35] reported photocurrents across the interface of an organic solution of heptylviologen and an aqueous solution of $Ru(bpy)_3^{2+}$ (bpy - bipyridyl). In the same year V. Marecek, A. Dearmond, and K. Dearmond[37,38] investigated a similar photoreaction at the interface between $Ru(bpy)_3^{2+}$ and methylviologen by using the original technique of monitoring ac photocurrent amplitude and phase shift. In both cases the observed photocurrent was ascribed to interfacial electron transfer.

Recently R. M. Corn *et al* [88], K. Dearmond *et al* [38], and J. Conboy *et al* [89] utilized a light beam reflected at the interface to monitor second harmonic generation (SHG). An increase in the SHG signal was observed upon illumination of the interface and was attributed to electron transport from organic to an aqueous phase.

One should exercise extreme caution assigning an observed photocurrent or SHG signal to photoinduced electron-transfer processes, especially taking into consideration the unexpectedly lengthy decay signals[37, 38, 88, 89] that may correspond to the diffusion of stable charge carriers. Stable ions may form in various secondary reactions with both supporting electrolyte and water molecules present in an equilibrium concentration of ca. 10^{-3} M. This amount of water is more than sufficient to partake in photoinduced reactions and to produce large amounts of secondary charged particles. A convenient way to determine the contribution of photogenerated species crossing the interface is by observation of a photocurrent - potential dependence, similar to the one presented below (Figure 5), which can be regarded as an analogue of traditional polarography. It is noteworthy that H_3O^+ or OH^- ions that are likely to accumulate in the organic phase under irradiation, should not have S-shaped i-ΔE_o^w plots in the available at an ITIES polarization window.

O. Dvorak, A. Dearmond, and K. Dearmond observed the effect of interfacial potential on ac photocurrent monitored with lock-in technique upon continuous scanning of ΔE_o^w [40]. This method can be related to cyclic voltamperometry often used for monitoring processes at the interface of two immiscible electrolyte solutions[29, 104, 108, 111]. The position of the maximum on the ac-photocurrent-ΔE_o^w curve was found to depend on redox properties of compounds present both in aqueous and in organic phases. However, further thermodynamic analysis of the dependence was hindered by multiple side effects.

B. IONS AT THE INTERFACE. WHY DO THEY CROSS IT?

Interfacial transfer of photogenerated ions is a key step in the photoelectrochemical effect at ITIES. The thermodynamics of this transfer can be characterized by the distribution coefficient B of an ion between the two phases. The interfacial potential ΔE_o^w between organic and water phases also influences the Gibbs energy ΔG_o^w of the transfer of a charged particle from organic into a water phase:

$$\Delta G_o^w = RT\ln B + zF\Delta E_o^w \qquad (2)$$

where z is the charge of the particle and F is the Faraday constant.

The kinetics of the interfacial ion transfer was studied earlier by luminescent methods in micellar solutions and microemulsions[1, 2-9, 17, 47, 49, 70]. By monitoring fluorescence quenching, a linear relationship between the exit rate constants from the micellar phase and distribution coefficient of the substance between micellar and bulk aqueous phases ($\log k_{ex}$ vs. $\ln B$ ΔG_s of solubilization) has been established for SDS micelles. Such correlations were observed for some alkyliodates[98] and other organic species[99], but no correlation between $\log k_{ex}$ and $\log \rho$ was observed for inorganic ions[101]. Various kinetic data have also indicated the absence of a substantial potential barrier for diffusion of these substances across the interface.

A more detailed consideration of the kinetics of ion transfer is necessary for quantitative discussion of the behavior of the photoelectrochemical effect at ITIES. Theoretical examination of the mechanism of ion transfer from one liquid phase into another has been done using different approaches - classical, diffusional, stochastic and quantum (theory of charge transfer in polar media)[102-110]. Consequently a number of expressions for k_{tr} have been derived, all similar to the classical Brönsted equation, despite different sets of physical parameters. The classical approach was developed by C. Gavach *et al.*[103] and J. Koryta *et al.*[104, 105] They considered the liquid-liquid interface as an analogue of a metal-liquid junction. Yu. I. Kharkats and A. G. Volkov applied Marcus theory to charge transfer at ITIES and discussed catalytic properties of the L-L boundary[106], while R. Marcus extended his general theory of charge transfer to the description of reactions at liquid-liquid interfaces later in 1991[107]. The Levich-Dogonadze theory of reactions in polar media was applied to the processes at ITIES by Z. Samec[108]. The stochastic approach of ion transfer was developed by Z. Samec[109], Yu. Kharkats and M. Gurevich[110]. The application of these approaches to experimental data has been also considered[107, 109, 111].

H. Girault and D. Schiffrin[112] described the interfacial ion transfer as a sequence of diffusional jumps. This approach yielded the following expression for k_{tr}:

$$k_{tr} = L(kT/h)\cdot \exp(-zF(E^A-E^O)/RT\cdot \exp(-\Delta G^{\neq}{}_A/RT)\cdot \exp(-\alpha_e zF\Delta_B{}^A E/RT)\cdot$$
$$\cdot \exp(\alpha_n \Delta G_{tr}{}^{\rho, A\rightarrow B}/RT) \qquad (3)$$

where $\Delta G^{\neq}{}_A$ is the activation energy of the diffusional jump from a starting position A of to a final position B, L is the length of the diffusional jump,

E^{A}, E^{B} are potentials at the points A and B, E^{O} and $E^{\neq}$ are potentials in the bulk of the organic phase and at the point of an activated state respectively, $\Delta_{B}{}^{A}E = E^{A} - E^{B}$,

$$\alpha_{n} = \Delta G_{tr}{}^{\rho, A \rightarrow \neq} / \Delta G_{tr}{}^{\rho, A \rightarrow B} \quad (4)$$

$$\alpha_{e} = (E^{\neq} - E^{A})/(E^{B} - E^{\neq}) \quad (5)$$

It was implicitly assumed that the border between two immiscible liquids is rather abrupt and can be almost completely spanned by one diffusion jump. However, the majority of data show that the transitional region stretches for several molecular diameters into either phase and thus several diffusional jumps are likely to be necessary to cross the interface. Other theories provide more accurate representations of molecular events, but this approach has one significant advantage: most of the physical parameters of the Equation 3 can be estimated in contrast to the other methods where this cannot be done with satisfactory precision [102-110]. Regardless of the inaccuracy this method provided a satisfactory explanation of the kinetic features of photoinduced ion transfer [43].

Equation 3 can regrouped as

$$\ln k_{tr} = \ln(LkT/h) - zF(E^{A} - E^{O})/RT - \Delta G^{\neq}{}_{A}/RT) - \alpha_{e} zF\Delta_{B}{}^{A}E/RT) + \alpha_{n}\Delta G_{tr}{}^{\rho, A \rightarrow B}/RT \quad (6)$$

All addends of Equation (6), excluding $- zF(E^{A} - E^{O})/RT$, are independent of the interfacial potential. The equation relating the potential difference in the diffuse part of the double electric layer from the organic phase side $E^{A} - E^{O}$ and the overall interfacial potential $\Delta_{o}{}^{w}E$ was derived from the main correlations of the Gouy-Chapman theory:

$$\tanh(F(E^{A}-E^{O})/2RT) = (\epsilon_{aq}C_{aq})^{0.5}\sinh(F\Delta_{o}{}^{w}E/2RT)/\{(\epsilon_{aq}C_{aq})^{0.5}\cosh(F\Delta_{o}{}^{w}E/2RT) + (\epsilon_{org}C_{org})^{0.5}\} \quad (7)$$

The following approximated equation is valid for rather small values of interfacial potential ($\Delta_{o}{}^{w}E < 0.5$ V):

$$E^{A} - E^{O} \approx 0.736\Delta_{o}{}^{w}E \quad (8)$$

Thus Equation 6 can be simplified:

$$\ln k_{tr} = \ln(LkT/h) - \Delta G^{\neq}{}_{A}/RT - \alpha_{e} zF\Delta_{B}{}^{A}E/RT + \alpha_{n}\Delta G_{tr}{}^{\rho, A \rightarrow B}/RT + 28.5\Delta_{o}{}^{w}E = \ln k_{tr}{}^{0} + 28.5\Delta_{o}{}^{w}E \quad (9)$$

where $\ln k_{tr}^{0} = \ln(LkT/h) - \Delta G^{\neq}_{A}/RT - \alpha_{e} zF\Delta_{B}^{A}E/RT + \alpha_{n}\Delta G_{tr}^{\rho,\ A\to B}/RT$. Therefore the slope of the dependence $\ln k_{tr}$ vs. $\Delta_{o}^{w}E$ is expected to be 28.5 V^{-1}. It was shown for benzoquinone and toluquinone radical-anions that the slope of the experimentally observed $\ln k_{tr}$ vs. $\Delta_{o}^{w}E$ dependence is indeed very close to the calculated theoretical value[43].

C. DIFFUSIONAL KINETICS OF PHOTOINDUCED ION TRANSPORT ACROSS ITIES. A GENERAL EQUATION.

For not very complex systems the photocurrent through ITIES rises steeply at the start of illumination and eventually reaches a steady-state value that depends on light intensity, photoreaction quantum yield, a lifetime of charge carriers, thickness of the light absorbing layer, interfacial potential, and other factors. Once the illumination is terminated, the photocurrent gradually decays with a rate depending on the same factors. More complex kinetics of the photocurrent may be observed due to chemical transformations of charge carriers during their diffusion to and across the interface, consumption of reactants or formation of side products, photoinduced adsorption or desorption of solutes at the interface, *etc.*

Equation (6) and similar ones[101-109] allow the assessment of current density through a L-L interface provided that electroactive ions are stable and their concentration is known. The generation of charge carriers as a result of the interaction of light with molecules in one of the phases establishes a new set of conditions. The kinetics of the *photocurrent* is to be obtained as the solution of a general diffusion equation describing the movement of photogenerated ions. Interestingly, similar conditions arise for monocrystalline semiconductor electrodes, where electrons and holes undergo an identical process of diffusion to the electrode/electrolyte interface[113]. Because of a substantially greater length of the space charge region and an inherently high absorption coefficient of semiconductors, the interfacial electric field directly influences the photogeneration of charge carriers. The equations describing the dependence of the photocurrent on various parameters are usually solved in the stationary approach $\delta i/\delta t=0$ and the initial stages of the photocurrent have not been investigated yet.

Assuming the photon flux is homogeneous and perpendicular to the interface we can consider one-dimensional diffusion in the direction x orthogonal to the interface. The region of space charge is limited by the interfacial double layer and does not exceed 1 μm[114] even for extremely low electrolyte concentrations. Thus, one may consider that the diffusion of photogenerated charged particles within the volume of the organic phase occurs in a quasi-neutral medium. In this case, a diffusion equation for charge carriers can be expressed as:

$$\delta c/\delta t = D(\delta^2 c/\delta x^2) + w(x) + v(c) \qquad (10)$$

where c is the concentration of the charge carriers in a point x at a moment of time t; D is their diffusion coefficient; w(x) and v(c) are the rates of their formation and decay in the bulk phase. Region $x>0$ involves the organic phase containing light-absorbing reactant and point $x=0$ corresponds to the outer Helmholtz surface of the interfacial double layer.

New ions are generated in the light-absorbing layer. Its thickness depends on the absorption coefficient of the solution, α, and can vary from microns (at $\alpha=10^5$ dm^{-1}) to the full depth of the cell (a few cm)

$$\mathrm{w}(x) = I_0 \phi \alpha \exp(-\alpha x) \tag{11}$$

where I_0 is the incident photon flux (Einstein s^{-1} dm^{-2}); ϕ is the quantum yield of the photogeneration of charged particles; $\alpha=23\epsilon C_0$ (dm^{-1}); ϵ and C_0 are the molar decimal absorption coefficient and the concentration of the light-absorbing reactant. To produce a photocurrent, the newly formed ions must diffuse to the interface. During the experiment (about 10^3 s) only the conditions in a thin boundary layer with the thickness of about $(Dt)^{0.5}$ <1 mm are substantial for the production of photocurrent.

There are two boundary conditions which permit the solution of the diffusion Equation 10. The first one is the absence of photogenerated species prior to illumination

$$c(\mathrm{x}) = 0 \tag{12}$$

The effect of interfacial potential on the volume concentration of charge carriers is taken into consideration by the second boundary condition at the point $x=0$. For the irreversible diffusion of ions from the organic phase into the aqueous one

$$D(\delta c/\delta x)|_{x=0} = k_{tr}\, c|_{x=0} \tag{13}$$

where k_{tr} is the rate constant of the transfer of charge carriers from organic to an aqueous phase which is exponentially dependent on $\Delta E^{w}{}_{o}$ [102-110]. The effect of $\Delta E^{w}{}_{o}$ on k_{tr} may be expressed by the equation

$$k_{tr} = k_{tr}^{o} \exp(-0.736 \Delta E^{w}{}_{o} /RT) \tag{14}$$

where k_{tr}^{o} and the coefficient 0.736 were discussed in the Section 2.2.

The photocurrent is

$$i = zFDS(\delta c/\delta x)|_{x=0} \tag{15}$$

where S is illuminated area.

In a general case Equation 10 becomes nonlinear and no exact solution of this equation in the form of a finite sequence of elementary functions was

shown to exist[45]. If photogenerated particles disappear mainly by diffusion to the interface rather than by some bulk reactions, Equation 10 may be solved by using the Fourier and Laplace transforms[45] in the form of

$$c = (I_0\, \alpha\phi_0 /(2(\pi D)^{0.5}) \int_0^t P(\xi, \tau)dt, \qquad (16)$$

where

$$P(x,t) = \int_0^{\infty} \{\exp[-(x - \xi)^2/(4D(t-\tau)] - \exp[-(x + \xi)^2/4D(t-\tau)]\} \cdot$$

$$\cdot\ [\exp(-a\xi)/(t-\tau)^{0.5}]\, d\xi \qquad (16a)$$

The function $P(\xi, \tau)$ may be presented as a combination of standard integrals such as

$$\mathrm{erf}(y) = (2/(\pi)^{0.5}) \int_0^t \exp(-y^2)dy.$$

Thus, the solution of Equation 10 is both intricate and cumbersome. Below we will show that for particular photochemical systems, Equation 10 may be further simplified. Eventually, the diffusion equation of virtually any level of difficulty can be solved by numerical means.

D. ANALYTICAL APPROXIMATION

The analytical approximation is convenient for the demonstration of major regularities of photocurrent kinetics. In the case of the first order decay of charge carriers in an organic phase ($v(c) = -k_1 c$) Equation 10 may be written as follows:

$$\delta c/\delta t = D(\delta^2 c/\delta x^2) + I_0\, \phi\alpha \exp(-\alpha x) - k_1 c \qquad (17)$$

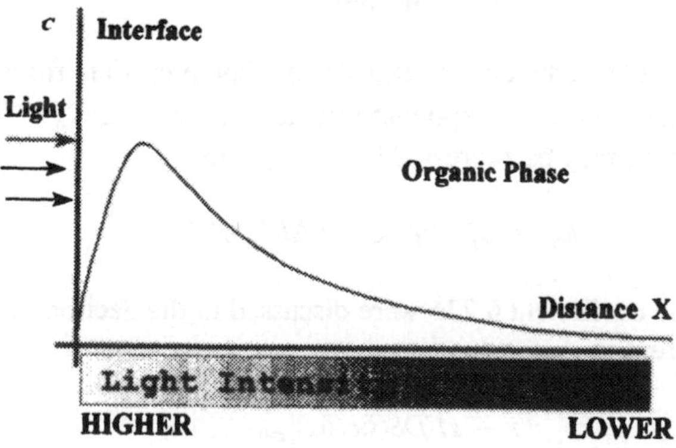

Figure 2. Typical spatial distribution of photogenerated ions for fast interfacial transfer.

If the thickness of the complete-absorption layer does not exceed 1 mm and is much smaller than the total thickness of the organic phase (about 0.5 cm), the diffusion of photogenerated ions can be considered to occur in an infinite volume i.e. $c(\infty,t)=0$. For a photocurrent independent of the interfacial potential, $c(0,t) = 0$ can be chosen as the second boundary condition. The latter expression is equivalent to the assumption that the transfer of photogenerated ions is controlled by the diffusion in the organic phase rather than across the interface. For many ions it was shown that this premise is, indeed, valid provided that $\pm\Delta E^{w}{}_{o}$ is relatively high or the photogenerated ions are rather hydrophilic[115].

For a fast interfacial transfer ($k_{tr} >> (Dk_1)^{0.5}$) the spacial distribution of the photo-generated ions may be represented by the difference of two exponential functions with the same amplitudes

$$c(x,t) = \gamma(t)\{\exp(-\alpha x) - \exp[-\beta(t)x]\}\,, \tag{18}$$

where $\alpha(t)$ and $\beta(t)$ are time-dependent functions. Equation 18 describes a bell-shaped $c(x,t)$ function (Figure 2) with two fixed points $c(0,t) = 0$ and $c(\infty, t) = 0$, while the point of maximum changes with time. The highest concentration of photogenerated ions for time t grows accordingly to the function $\gamma(t)$. An explicit equation for the photocurrent and an analytical expression for $\gamma(t)$ and $\beta(t)$ can be obtained by substituting Equation 18 into Equation 10. For a thin front layer $x < (Dt)^{0.5}$ and for not very high values of absorption coefficient $\alpha << 1/(Dt)^{0.5} \approx 10\ \text{cm}^{-1}$

$$c=(I_0\alpha\phi/k_1)[1-\exp(-k_1t)]\{\exp(-\alpha x)-\exp(-x(k_1/D[1-\exp(-k_1t)])^{0.5})\} \tag{19}$$

The first exponent in the braces is related to the light flux decay along the x axis and does not depend on time. The second exponent is related to the rate of diffusion of photogenerated ions to the interface. The maximum concentration of charge carriers (the top point of the bell) rises with a time constant equal to $1/k_1$, i.e. the lifetime of photogenerated species. In a steady state, that is when the photocurrent ceases changing, the position of max(c) will be determined by

$$x = \ln(\alpha/(k_1/D)^{0.5})/(\alpha - (k_1/D)^{0.5}) \tag{20}$$

The corresponding spacial distribution of photogenerated ions in the steady state ($k_1t > 3$) can be found from

$$c = (I_0\alpha\phi/k_1)\{\exp(-\alpha x) - \exp(-x(k_1/D)^{0.5})\} \tag{21}$$

For small $k_1 t < 0.3$ and relatively stable charge carriers Equation 21 can be transformed into

$$c = I_0\,\alpha\,\phi t[\exp(-\alpha x) - \exp(-x(Dt)^{0.5})]. \qquad (22)$$

Thus, the photocurrent is equal to

$$i = zFDS(\delta c/\delta x)|_{x=0} =$$
$$= (I_0 \alpha\,\phi_0\, zFDS/k_1)[1-\exp(-k_1 t)] \cdot \{(k_1/D)^{0.5}[1-\exp(-k_1 t)] - \alpha\} \qquad (23)$$

For small $k_1 t < 0.3$

$$i = I_0 \alpha\,\phi\, zFDSt(1/(Dt)^{0.5} - \alpha) \qquad (24)$$

If $\alpha << 1/(Dt)^{0.5}$, then

$$i \approx I_0\,\alpha\,\phi\, zFS(Dt)^{0.5} \qquad (25)$$

For a large α the steady state is achieved quite quickly in $t > 3/\alpha^2 D$ and the photocurrent can be represented as

$$i_0 = I_0 \alpha\,\phi\, zFS/(\alpha + (k_1/D)^{0.5}), \qquad (26)$$

while the photocurrent quantum yield in the steady state is

$$\phi_i = i/zFSI_0 = \phi/(1 + 1/\alpha(D/k_1)^{0.5}) \qquad (27)$$

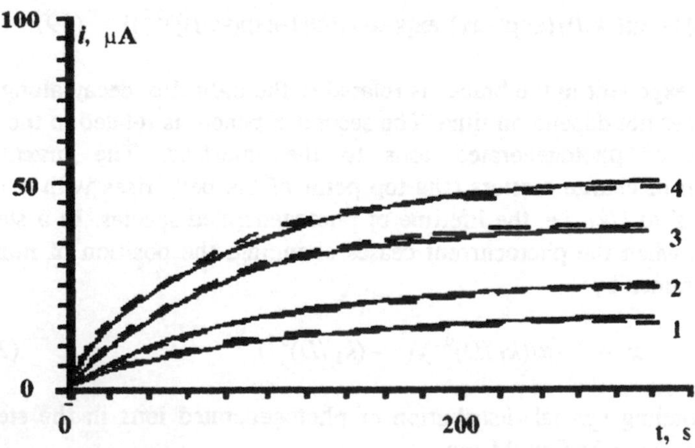

Figure 3. Experimental (solid lines) and calculated (dashed lines) photocurrent kinetics for relatively stable charge carriers[43] and various α: 1 - 1.5 cm^{-1}, 2 - 2.3 cm^{-1}, 3 - 3.13 cm^{-1}, 4 - 3.95 cm^{-1}. Reproduced with permission from Elsevier Sequoia S. A.

We have shown[45] that Equations 25 and 26 describe the kinetics of photocurrent quite well for short durations of illumination when the current was caused mainly by the interfacial transfer of semiquinone radical anions. Comparison of the results obtained by numerical methods[45] and by biexponential approximation[44] revealed that the spacial distribution of the semiquinone ion radicals were, indeed, very similar. Note, however, that the effect of potential cannot be described within the limits of this approximation because for slow transfer the concentration of charge carriers at the boundary of two liquids is not equal to zero, which is necessary for the validity of Equation 18. Consequently, despite the elegance of Equations 18 and 21 especially with respect to Equation 16, we would like to dwell mostly on the computer assisted solution of diffusion equations, which permits discrimination of very complex processes at the interface.

E. A COMPUTER SIMULATION OF THE PHOTOCURRENT KINETICS

A numerical solution of Equation 10 may be used to simulate the photocurrent kinetics. It has none of the disadvantages of the approximation methods and makes it possible to consider miscellaneous processes taking place in two-phase systems such as adsorption at the interface, variation of the interfacial potential, and formation of the new light adsorbing species.

The observed photocurrent can be calculated as $i = zFDS\, dc/dx|_{x=0}$, while $dc/dx|_{x=0}$ can be found as a numerical solution of Equation 10. Both spacial distribution of photogenerated ions and photocurrent kinetics can be quite easily obtained by this method. The photocurrent decay curve after turning out the light can also be calculated.

Several physical parameters are necessary to solve Equations 10-15. I_0 and α can be measured experimentally. An average value of D=$1.0{\cdot}10^{-5}$ cm^2/s may be used for calculations since it is rather difficult to find the values of diffusion coefficients D for particular organic ions or radical ions. Actually, the diffusion coefficients for various species in 1,2-dichloroethane vary only from $0.7{\cdot}10^{-5}$ [116, 117] to $1.1{\cdot}10^{-5}$ cm^2/s[118]. It can be demonstrated that if any particular value of D within these limits is used, it will not change the principal inferences of the computer analysis.

Numerical solution of Equation 10 was shown to be a very powerful method for the description of photocurrent kinetics. Figure 3 presents the results obtained for a system of benzoquinone and $B(Ph)_4^-$. It can be clearly seen that the calculated and experimental kinetics of the photocurrent coincide very well. Importantly, no additional assumptions of any kind were necessary. All curves in Figure 3 were calculated on the basis of I_0, α, D, and ϕ obtained from independent experiments.

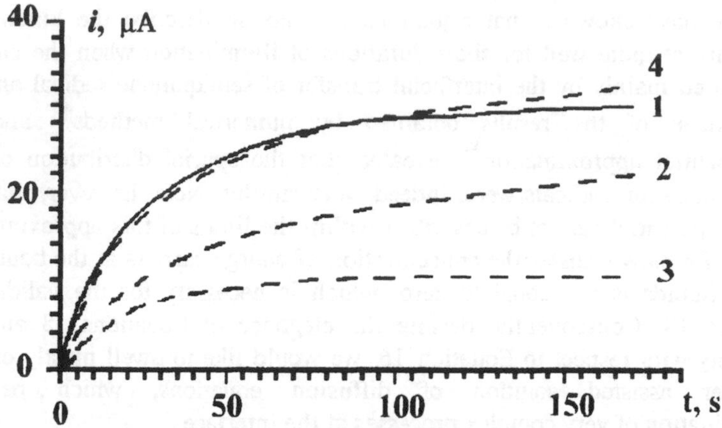

Figure 4. Computer calculation of the photocurrent from multiple charge carriers. 1 - experimental photocurrent; 2 - calculated photocurrent from stable photogenerated ions; 3 - calculated photocurrent from benzoquinone radical-anions; 4 - the sum of 2 and 3. An organic phase: protoporphyrin IX 0.5 mM, benzoquinone 10 mM. Interfacial potential 0.35 V, illumination wavelength 530 nm[43]. Reproduced with permission from Elsevier Sequoia S. A.

The photocurrent kinetics in the protoporphyrin IX - quinone system (Figure 4) significantly differed from curves that were obtained from the numerical[43] or analytical solutions[45]. The discrepancy indicated the simultaneous formation of two types of photogenerated charged particles, namely, semiquinone radical anions with lifetimes of several milliseconds and long-lived negatively charged products of $B(Ph)_4^{\bullet}$ radicals formed in the reaction of protoporphyrin radical cations with the supporting electrolyte. The presence of two types of charge carriers became apparent from the decay kinetics of the current after irradiation[43]. A rather fast decay of the photocurrent observed in the initial part of the curve corresponded to the decay of semiquinone radical anions in the bulk of the organic phase. Later the rate of the current decay significantly decreased. This part of the curve was assigned to a slow equilibration of the concentration of relatively stable charge carriers originating from $B(Ph)_4^{\bullet}$ in the bulk of an organic phase.

The computer simulation allowed evaluation of the contribution of each charge carrier to the total photocurrent[43]. Initially, semiquinone radical-ions were responsible for approximately 40% of the photocurrent (Figure 4). Their contribution slowly decreased upon accumulation of more stable charge carriers and was about 30% in 200 s of illumination.

For interfacial transfer of semiquinone radical-ions the dependence of photocurrent on the interfacial potential has been observed (Figure 5). If the interfacial potential is high enough (+ in water, - in an organic phase), benzo- and toluquinone radical-ions can cross the interface. Consequently, significant increase of the photocurrent upon sweeping the available range of interfacial potentials was observed (Figure 5). The shift between the curves for benzo- and toluquinone radical-ions was about 0.06 V and corresponded to the presence of an additional methyl group. This value coincides very well with the difference in solubilization energy for these two radical-ions as determined by independent means[43]. Thus, the influence of ΔE_o^w on the rate of interfacial transport of ions can be easily observed at a macroscopic L-L interface. Moreover, i-ΔE_o^w plots (Figure 5) may be used for the characterization of species participating in interfacial reactions. The S-shaped i vs. ΔE_o^w dependence reflects thermodynamic parameters of the interfacial transfer; it is, in fact, quite specific for a particular charge carrier. Note that the kinetics of photocurrent rise and decay contain information about the lifetime of charged particles crossing the interface. The combination of these two parameters can be very helpful for the identification of a mechanism and participants of interfacial reactions.

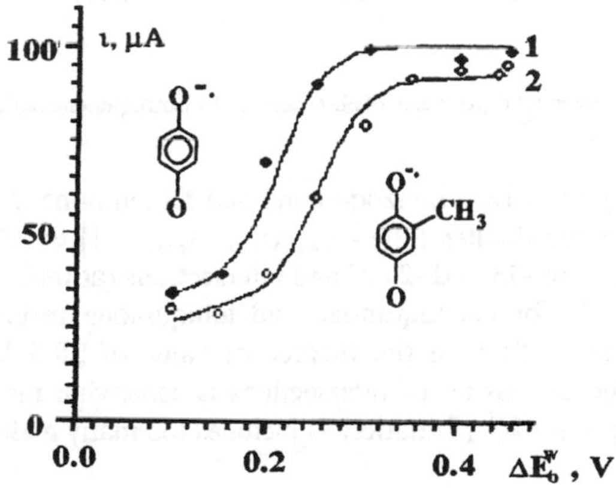

Figure 5. ITIES photopolarography. The effect of interfacial potential on photocurrent for the transfer of similar photogenerated species: 1 - benzoquinone radical-anion; 2 - toluquinone radical-anion[43]. Reproduced with permission from Elsevier Sequoia S. A.

The dependence of the steady state photocurrent on the interfacial potential (Figure 5) can be expressed by the equation

$$(i - i_{min})/(i_{max} - i_{min}) = k_{tr}/(k_{tr} + k_d), \quad (28)$$

which is typical for the relative rate of a process consisting of two consecutive steps with the rate constants k_{tr} and k_d, where k_d is, in fact, a one-dimensional diffusion rate constant along the x axis perpendicular to the interface; i_{max}

corresponds to a maximum photocurrent when it is limited by the transport through the bulk phase; i_{min} is a limiting value of the photocurrent at a small ΔE_o^w being attributed to secondary charge carriers as well as to nonfaradaic current.

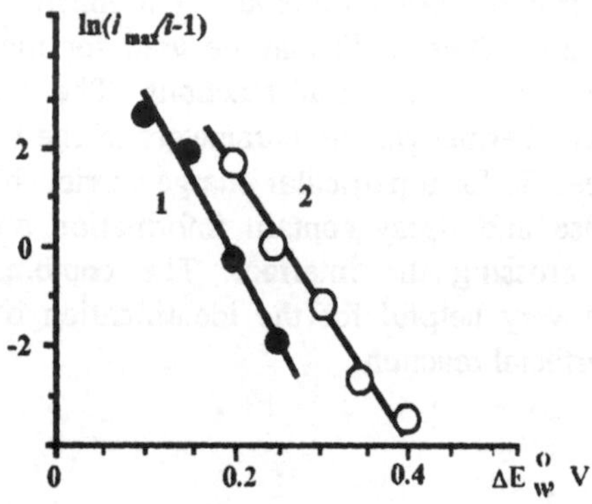

Figure 6. Linearized potential dependence of photocurrent: 1 - benzoquinone radical-anion; 2 - toluquinone radical-anion.

For protoporphyrin IX - benzoquinone and toluquinone, i vs. ΔE_o^w plots were linearized in coordinates $\ln[(i - i_{min})/(i_{max} - i_{min}) - 1]$ vs. ΔE_o^w (Figure 6) giving a slope equal to -33 and -27 V and intersections (at $\ln(k_d/k_{tr}) = 0$) equal to 0.19 and 0.26 V for benzoquinone and toluquinone respectively. These slopes are reasonably close to the theoretical value of 28.5 V discussed in Section III. B. The discussion of intersections is somewhat more problematic since the expression for k_{tr}^0 (Equation 9) includes too many addends.

F. AN INVERSE PROBLEM: DETERMINATION OF THE RATE CONSTANTS AND OTHER PARAMETERS FROM THE PHOTOCURRENT

The inverse problem, or how to find kinetic and diffusion parameters of Equation 10 from the experimental data on the photocurrent kinetics, is important for the description of the investigated systems. An optimization method maybe applied for the determination of unknown parameters. Usually, the minimization of the sum of squares of standard deviations G:

$$G = \sum_{n=1}^{N} [(i_n^c - i_n^{ex})/i_n^{ex}] , \tag{29}$$

is used as a standard procedure. i_n^c and i_n^{ex} denote the calculated and experimental values of the photocurrent respectively at the point of time $n \cdot \Delta t$. The maximization of $1/G$ instead of minimization of G may turn out to be more advantageous because of faster convergence of the search procedure.

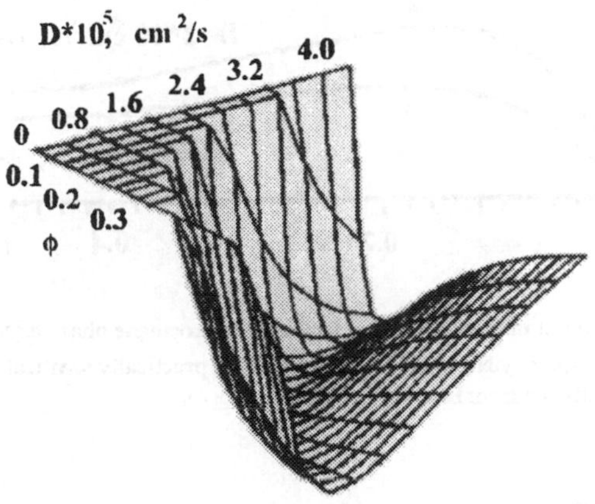

Figure 7. G-surface for the optimization of D and ϕ on the basis of calculated photocurrent kinetics with D=10^{-5} cm/s^2, ϕ=0.3 and a random 5% experimental error[44]. Reproduced with permission from Elsevier Sequoia S. A.

When the charge carriers are quite stable, four physical parameters determine the photo-current kinetics: α, I_0, D, and ϕ. α and I_0 can easily be measured experimentally but D and ϕ can be obtained independently only in rather labor-consuming experiments. First of all, the dependence of G (Equation 29) on the fitting parameters has to be considered. The accuracy of the obtained quantities depends directly on the sensitivity of G to the parameters of interest. The variation of either D or ϕ alone produced significant changes in the photocurrent kinetics[44], i.e. the $G(D)$ and $G(\phi)$ functions had clear minima. Therefore, if only one of these parameters were unknown, it could easily be obtained within the accuracy of the experimental data. Moreover, random errors of experimental points as high as 15% were found to have no significant influence on the values of D or ϕ in the minima of the functions $G(D)$ and $G(\phi)$, respectively. However, rather high sensitivity of the solution to the variation of D or ϕ did not mean that a similar optimization procedure for a two-variable system would also provide a clear minimum. This problem always has to be taken into account when searching extremum points of a multiparameter function[44, 46].

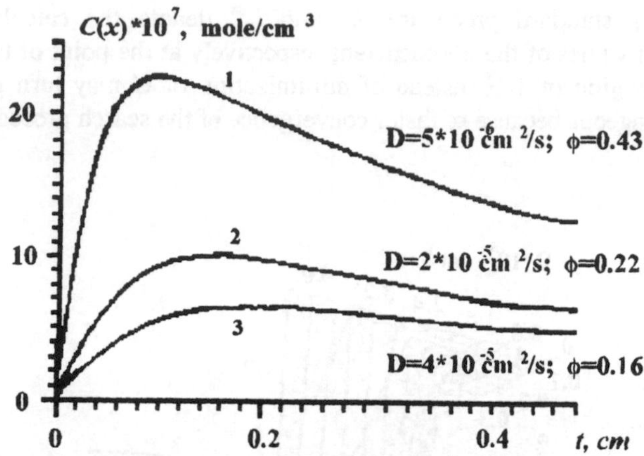

Figure 8. The distribution of photogenerated ions in dichloroethane phase after 300 s of illumination and corresponding *D*-ϕ pairs yielding photocurrent kinetics practically identical to curve 1, Figure 3[44]. Reproduced with permission from Elsevier Sequoia S. A.

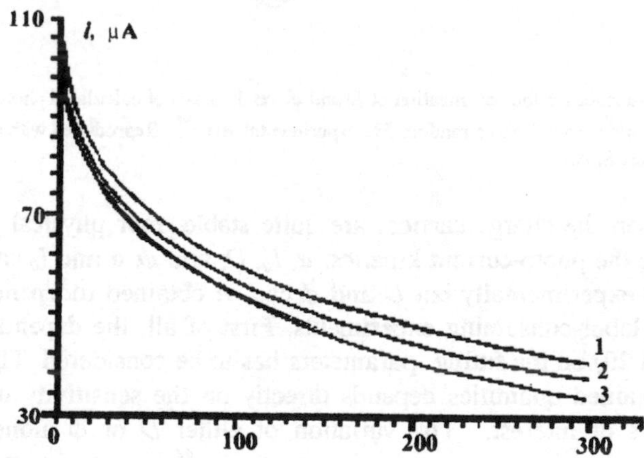

Figure 9. Decay kinetics of the photocurrent for charge carrier distribution 1, 2, and 3 presented in Figure 8 [44]. Reproduced with permission from Elsevier Sequoia S. A.

The variations of both D and ϕ had similar effects on the photocurrent. Neither D nor ϕ had a specific influence on a selected part of the curve. Hence, any deviation of calculated photocurrent kinetics could result from the alteration of either D or ϕ. Consequently, various pairs of these parameters can describe an experimental curve with similar accuracy. To prove this uncertainty in the determination of D and ϕ, the surface of the G

values vs. D and ϕ as variables were calculated (Figure 7). There was a long valley in the resulting graph with an essentially flat bottom. The larger the experimental error of the kinetics, the broader this valley became. A wide range of pairs ($4\cdot10^{-6} < D < 4\cdot10^{-5}$ cm^{2}s^{-1} and $0.15 < \phi < 0.5$) can be assigned to an experimental kinetics and the true D-ϕ pair cannot be determined by the optimization procedure. Therefore, values of D and ϕ formally estimated by the optimization program can vary and may depend on starting values and on details of the numerical algorithm. Significantly, unlike the photocurrent, the concentration distribution of the photogenerated ions was always different for assorted pairs of D and ϕ. For all distribution functions $c(x)$ presented in Figure 8 the photocurrent kinetics were the same as curve 1 in Figure 3. In spite of constantly changing derivatives $\delta c/\delta x|_{x=0}$, the products $D(\delta c/\delta x|_{x=0})$ were identical for all $c(x)$ and so were the photocurrent kinetics. Nevertheless, as long as $c(x)$ after the irradiation is different for each D - ϕ pair, then the decay curves should be unique. Theoretically, D and ϕ may be determined by running the optimization procedure for the rise and decay kinetics at once. Figure 9 shows that the decay curves were, indeed, separate but the displacement was too small demanding practically unachievable accuracy of the experimental results.

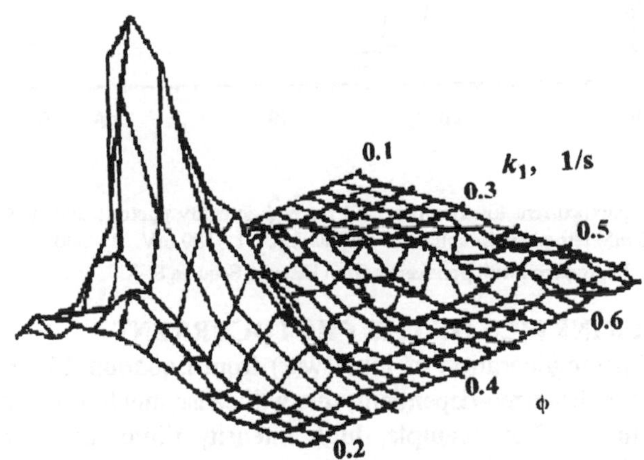

Figure 10. G-surface for the optimization of k_1 and ϕ on the basis of calculated photocurrent kinetics with a random 5% experimental error[44]. Reproduced with permission from Elsevier Sequoia S. A.

Unlike D-ϕ pairs, the simultaneous optimization of D - k_1 or ϕ - k_1 pairs were much more accurate. The effect of k_1 variation on the photocurrent kinetics was quite different from that of D or ϕ, because k_1 influenced both magnitude and rise-time of the photocurrent. Therefore, the kinetic consequences of various k_1 and D (k_1 and ϕ) could not compensate each other. G-surfaces in coordinates D-k_1 and ϕ-k_1 had a crater (or a peak in 1/G scale) rather than a valley and these variables could be determined by using a two-parameter optimization with good resulting accuracy (Figure 10).

It is important to note that the uncertainty in the determination of D and ϕ pairs, which can be obtained by the proposed technique, is not a result of the calculation method or poor experimental data. This is an intrinsic feature of the phenomenon.

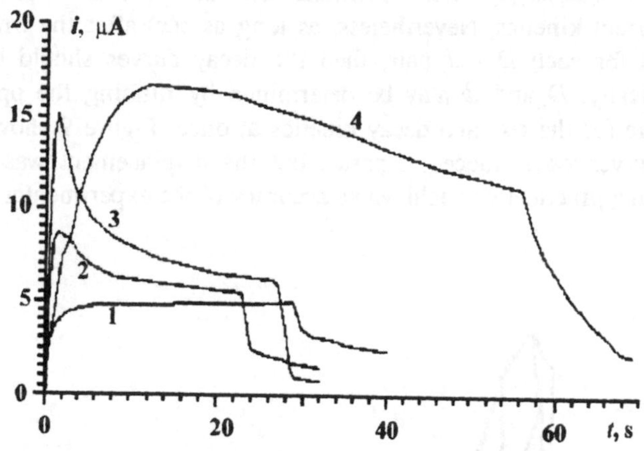

Figure 11. Typical photocurrent kinetics observed for high-intensity photoexcitation of organic phase containing 10 mM tetraphenylporphine at various ΔE_o^w: 1 - 100 mV, 2 - 300 mV, 3 - 450 mV, 4 - 550 mV [46]. Reproduced with permission from Elsevier Sequoia S. A.

G. COMPLEX KINETICS OF THE PHOTOCURRENT

The rate of photogeneration of ions (w(x) from Equation 10) in many cases may be implicitly time-dependent; this will cause much more complex photocurrent kinetics. For example, high intensity illumination prompts rapid consumption of the light-absorbing species in the vicinity of the interface which can be substantially faster than the restoration of its concentration by diffusion and convection. Consequently, the function w(x) becomes time dependent. Similar complications may be caused by the phototransformations of the light-absorbing reactant, secondary reactions, inner filter effect etc. The rate of carrier generation may decrease or accelerate in the course of the experiment depending on the particular chemical system. It is possible to take these effects into account using numerical solutions of Equation 10. The consumption of the light-absorbing reactant causes a gradual shift of the light-absorbing layer from the interface deeper into the organic phase, with a rate proportional to the consumption quantum yield ϕ and the light flux I_0

$$\delta x/\delta t = I_0\, \phi / C_c \tag{30}$$

This shift will result in an elongation of the diffusion pathway of photogenerated ions from the point of origin to the interface, and in a decrease of the photocurrent. A similar $i(t)$ dependence may be also brought about by consumption of another reactant which participates in the photogeneration of charged particles. In both cases w(x), which follows the exponential Beer-Lambert law during the initial time period, becomes bell-shaped in the course of illumination.

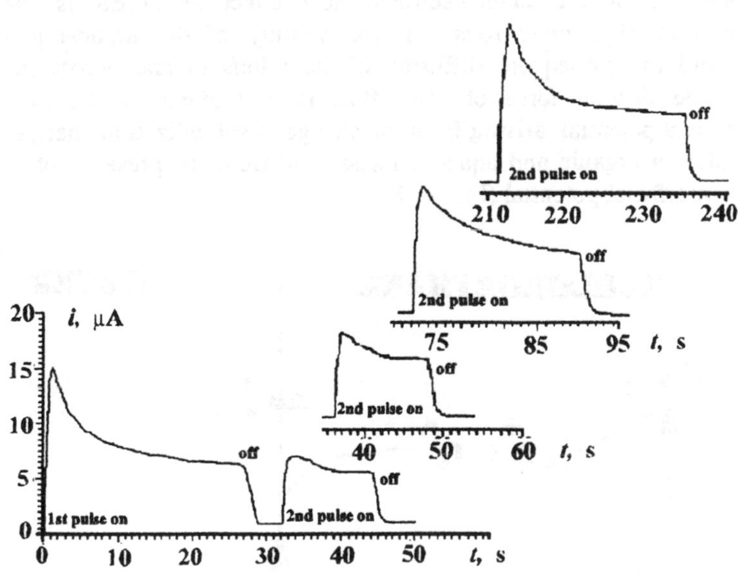

Figure 12. Recovery of the photocurrent from photoexcitated tetraphenylporphine after 25 s period of illumination. Please, note the difference in the time scale corresponding to the second light pulse.

Here we will consider some examples of systems where similar effects were observed. For tetraphenylporphine or protoporphyrin in the absence of quinones, a high-intensity light source (1000 W) was used due to the rather small quantum yield of the photocurrent. Very interesting photocurrent kinetics was observed: under illumination the photocurrent quickly rose and then dropped to a steady-state value (Figure 11). It was found that this effect was caused by the fast consumption of some impurity which was present in the initial porphyrins (probably a product of their oxidation or photodecomposition) which provided a greater photogeneration quantum yield than the porphyrin alone. When we repeated the experiment with a sufficient time interval, convection recovered the concentration of the impurity in the vicinity of the interface (Figure 12) and a gradual restoration of the original photocurrent kinetics could be observed. It was shown[46] that the processes of formation, consumption, recombination, diffusion of porphyrin and its radical cations and anions, and the reaction of the radical cations with $B(Ph)_4^-$ yielding long-living anions could be incorporated into a system of differential equations. The numerical solution of the latter provided a satisfactory description of the experimental results.

IV. CONCLUSION

The essence of the photoelectrochemical effect at ITIES is the photogeneration of organic ions in the vicinity of the liquid-liquid boundary and the subsequent diffusion of these ions to and across the interface. The driving force of this effect is a gradient of the ions' electrochemical potential arising from the change of solubilization energies of molecules in organic and aqueous phases and from the presence of a controlled interfacial potential (Figure 13).

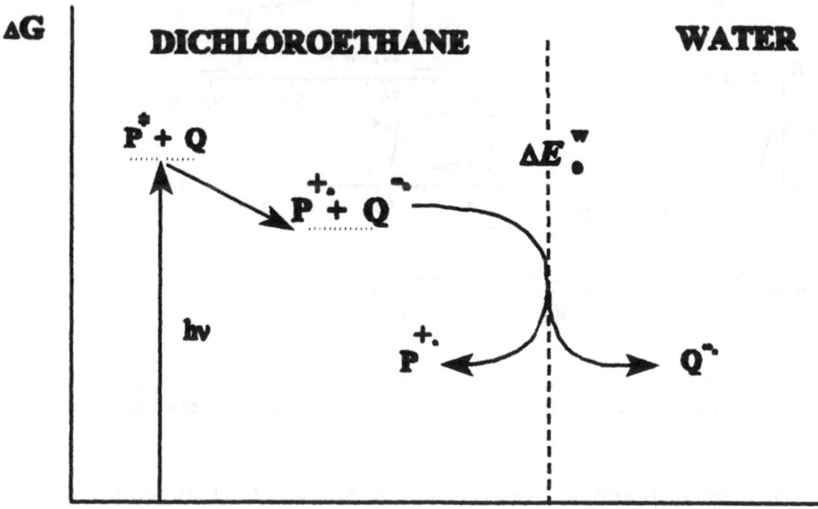

Figure 13. Gibbs energy diagram for interface diffusion of photogenerated semiquinone radical-anions.

Photogeneration of charge carriers may proceed as electron or proton transfer reactions between an excited state of the light-absorbing reactant and other components of the solution including the supporting electrolyte. It was shown that stable ionic species may form in secondary reactions of primary charge carriers.

The interface region plays a critical role in the observed effect. The interfacial potential actually gates the passage of organic ions: a change of ΔE_o^w equal to 0.2 V can switch the process from the diffusion controlled mode to an almost complete blockage of the interface.

The kinetics of the photocurrent is quite sensitive to the properties of the interface and, therefore, they may be used for the investigation of the liquid-liquid boundary. Extreme care should be taken when attributing observed effects to a particular interfacial process. The complex dependence of the photocurrent on the interface properties and many other factors should always be taken into consideration. Scanning of the interfacial potential allows determination of the type of photo-generated species and should be regarded as the most essential step in discriminating the mechanism of the interfacial charge transfer.

Computer simulation proved to be a powerful method for modeling various events at a L-L interface. It was shown that transport, diffusion, decay, transformations, and many other possible processes going on at the liquid-liquid interface may be taken into account and quantitative results describing the effect of each process can be obtained. These findings can serve as a mathematical background for further investigation of similar systems.

Phenomena comparable to the ones observed at macroscopic liquid-liquid interfaces are expected to proceed in intracellular membranes, in particular for conjugated reactions such as photosynthesis. They are likely be of considerable importance for many biochemical systems and should be taken into account when discussing mechanisms and kinetics.

REFERENCES

1. **Sutin, N. and Creutz, C.**, Light induced electron transfer reactions of metal complexes, *Pure Appl. Chem.*, 52, 2717, 1980; **Gratzel, M.**, Artificial photosynthesis: water cleavage into hydrogen and oxygen by visible light, *Acc. Chem. Res.*, 14, 276, 1981; **Kalyanasundaram, K.**, Photophysics, photochemistry and solar energy conversion with tris(bipyridyl)ruthenium (II) and its analogues, *Coord. Chem. Rev.*, 46, 159, 1982; **Whitten, D. C., Russel, J. C. and Schnell, R. H.**, Photo-chemical reactions in organized assemblies: environmental effects on reactions occurring in micelles, vesicles, films and multilayer assemblies at interfaces, *Tetrahedron*, 38, 2455, 1982; Photo-induced electron transfer reactions of metal complexes in solutions, *Acc. Chem. Res.*, 13, 83, 1980; **Calvin, M.**, Simulating photosynthetic quantum

conversion, *Acc. Chem. Res.*, 11, 369, 1978; **Porter, G.**, In vitro models for photosynthesis, *Proc. R. Soc. London Ser. A.*, 362, 281, 1978.
2. **Kiwi, J. and Gratzel, M.**, Hydrogen evolution from water induced by visible light mediated by redox catalysis, *Nature*, 281, 657, 1979.
3. *Energy resources through photochemistry and catalysis*, Gratzel, M., Ed., Academic Press, New York, 1983.
4. *Kinetics and Catalysis in Microheterogeneous Systems. Surfactant Science Series*, Vol. 38, Gratzel, M. and Kalyanasundaram, K., Eds., Marcel Dekker Inc., New York, 1991.
5. **Kuhn, E. R. and Hurst, J. K.**, Mechanism of vectorial transmembrane reduction of viologens across phosphatidylcholone bilayer membranes, *J. Phys. Chem.*, 97, 1712, 1993.
6. **Kalyanosundaram, K.**, *Photochemistry in Organized Systems*, Academic Press, Orlando, 1987.
7. *Organic Phototransformations in Nonhomogenious Media., ACS symposium series*, Vol. 278, Fox, M. A., Ed., American Chemical Society, Washington, 1985.
8. **Almgren, M.**, Kinetics of Excited Processes in Micellar Media, in *Kinetics and Catalysis in Microheterogeneous Systems. Surfactant Science Series*, Vol. 38, Gratzel, M. and Kalyanasundaram, K., Eds., Marcel Dekker, New York, 1991, p. 63.
9. **Turro, N. J., Cox, G. S., and Paczkowski, M. A.**, Photochemistry in Micelles, in *Photochemistry and Organic Synthesis. Topics in Current Chemistry*, Vol. 129., Springer-Verlag, Berlin, 1985, p. 57.
10. **Khramov, M., Lazarev, G. G., Garcia, F. and Zentella, A.**, Photochemical transfer of an electron and a proton across the interface in microemulsions, *J. Am Chem. Soc.*, 116(14), 6447, 1994.
11. **O'Reagan, B. and Gratzel, M.**, A low-cost high-efficiency solar cell based on dye sensitized colloidal TiO_2 films, *Nature*, 353, 737, 1991.
12. **Spitler, M. T. and Parkinson, B. A.**, Efficient infrared dye sensitization of Van-der-Waals surfaces of semiconductor electrodes, *Langmuir*, 2, 549, 1986.; **Parkinson, B. A. and Spitler, M.**, Efficient infrared sensitization of Van-der-Waals surfaces of semiconductor electrodes, *J. Electrochem. Soc.*, 133, (3), C110, 1986.
13. *Homogeneous and Heterogeneous Photocatalysis, NATO ASI Series, Series C: Mathematical and Physical Sciences*, Vol. 174, Pelizzetti, E. and Serpone, N., Eds, D. Reidel Publishing Company, Dodrecht, 1986.
14. *Photocatalysis and Environment. Trends and Applications, NATO ASI Series, Series C: Mathematical and Physical Sciences*, Vol. 237, Schiavello, M., Ed., Kluwer Academic Publishers, Dortrecht, 1988.
15. **Fujishima, A. and Honda, K.**, Electrochemical photolysis of water at a semiconductor electrode, *Nature*, 238, 37, 1972.
16. **Steffen, M. A., Lao K. and Boxer, S. G.**, Dielectric asymmetry in the photosynthetic reaction center, *Science*, 264, 810, 1994; **Nisbet, E. G., Cann, J. R. and Van Dover, C. L.**, Origin of photosynthesis, *Nature*, 373(6514), 479, 1995.
17. **Mathis, P.**, Photosynthesis: Biological Conversion of light into Chemical Energy, in *Photoprocesses in Transition Metal Complexes, Biosystems and Other Molecules. Experiment and Theory., NATO ASI Series, Series C: Mathematical and Physical Sciences*, Vol. 376, Kochanski, E., Ed., Kluwer Academic Publishers, Dortrecht, 1992, p. 333.
18. **Musser, D. A. and Oseroff, A. R.**, The use of tetrazolium salts to determine sites of damage to the mitochondrial electron-transport chain in intact cells following in vitro photodynamic therapy with photofrin-II, *Photochem. Photobiol.*, 59(6), 621, 1994; **Vasvari, G. and Elzemzam, S. D.** Physicochemical modeling of the role of free radicals in photodynamic therapy. 2. Interactions of ground state sensitizers with free radicals studied by chemiluminescence spectrometry, *Biochem. Biophys. Res. Commun.*, 197(3), 1536, 1993; **Deahl, J. T., Oleinick, N. L. and Evans, H. H.**, Large mutagenic lesions are induced by photodynamic therapy in murine L5178Y lymphoblasts, *Photochem. Photobiol.*, 58(2), 259, 1993.
19. **Reimannphilipp, U., Schafer, E., Batschauer A., Behnke, S. and Apel, K.**, The effect of light on the biosynthesis of leaf specific thionins in barley *hordeum vulgare*, *Europ. J.*

Biochem., 182(2), 283, 1989; **Arena, V.**, *Ionizing radiation and life*, The C. V. Mosby Company, Saint Louis, 1971.

20. **Regula, J., Ravi, B., Bedwell, J., Macrobert, A. J. and Bown, S. G.**, Photodynamic therapy using 5-aminolevulinic acid for experimental pancreatic cancer prolonged animal survival, *Brit. J. Cancer*, 70 (2), 248, 1994; **Marcus, J., Glassberg, E., Diminoemme, L., Yamamoto, R., Moy, R. L., Vari, S. G., Papaioannou, T., Pergadia, V. R., Snyder, W. J., Grundfest, W. S. and Lask G. P.**, Photodynamic therapy for the treatment of squamous-cell carcinoma using benzoporphyrin derivative, *J. of Dermatologic Surgery and Oncology*, 20(6), 375, 1994; **Purkiss, S. F., Grahn, M. F., Abulafi, A. M., Dean, R., Allardice, J. T. and Williams, N. S.**, Multiple fiber interstitial photodynamic therapy of patients with colorectal liver metastases, *Lasers in Med. Sci.*, 9(1), 27, 1994; **Brasseur, N., Nguyen, T. L., Langlois, R., Ouellet, R., Marengo, S., Houde, D. and Vanlier, J. E.**, Biological potential of silicon 2,3-naphthalocyanine derivatives as sensitizers for photodynamic therapy of cancer, *J. de Chimie Physique et de Physico-Chimie Biologique*, 91(7), 1011, 1994; **Kriegmair, M., Waidelich, R., Baumgartner R., Lumper W., Ehsan A. and Hofstetter A.**, Photodynamic therapy (PDT) for superficial bladder cancer. An alternative to radical cystectomy, *Urologe-Ausgabe A*, 33(4), 276, 1994; **Cairnduff, F., Stringer, M. R., Hudson, E. J., Ash, D. V. and Brown, S. B.**, Superficial photodynamic therapy with topical 5-aminolevulinic acid for superficial primary and secondary skin cancer, *Brit. J. Cancer*, 69(3), 605, 1994; **Dolphin, D.**, Syntex award lecture. Photomedicine and photodynamic therapy, *Can. J. Chem.*, 72(4), 1005, 1994.
21. **Ratkay, L. G., Chowdhary, R. K., Neyndorff, H. C., Tonzetich, J., Waterfield, J. D. and Levy J. G.**, Photodynamic Therapy Treatments of Arthritis, *Clinical and Experimental Immunology*, 95(3), 373, 1994; **Ratkay, L. G., Chowdhary, R. K., Tonzetich, J., Waterfield, D. and Levy, J.**, Photodynamic therapy and conventional immunomodulatory treatments of adjuvant enhanced arthritis in MRL/Lpr mice, *Arthritis and Rheumatism*, 36(5), R37, 1993.
22. **Tang, G., Hyman, S., Schneider, J. H., Giannotta, S. L. and Laws, E. R.**, Application of photodynamic therapy to the treatment of atherosclerotic plaques, *Neurosurgery*, 32(3), 438, 1993.
23. **Boehncke, W. H., Konig, K., Kaufmann, R., Scheffold, W., Prummer, O. and Sterry, W.**, Photodynamic therapy in psoriasis, *Arch. Dermatological Res.*, 286(6), 300, 1994; **Boehncke, W. H., Sterry, W. and Kaufmann, R.**, Treatment of psoriasis by topical photodynamic therapy with polychromatic light, *Lancet*, 343(8900), 801, 1994.
24. **Abramson, A. L., Shikowitz, M. J., Mullooly, V. M., Steinberg, B. M. and Hyman, R. B.**, Photo-dynamic therapy for laryngeal papillomas, *Arch. Otolaryngology - Head & Neck Surgery*, 120(8), 852, 1994; **Bown, S. G.**, Photodynamic therapy in gastroenterology - current status and future-prospects, *Endoscopy*, 25(9), 683, 1993; **Lamuraglia, G. M., Chandrasekar, N. R., Flotte, T. J., Abbott, W. M., Michaud, N. and Hasan, T.**, Photodynamic therapy inhibition of experimental intimal hyperplasia, *J. Vascular Surgery*, 19(2), 321, 1994; **Biel, M. A.**, Photodynamic therapy and the treatment of neoplastic diseases of the larynx, *Laryngoscope*, 104(4), 399, 1994; **Origitano, T. C., Caron, M. J. and Reichman, O. H.**, Photodynamic therapy for intracranial neoplasms. Literature review and institutional experience, *Mol. Chem. Neurapothology*, 21(2-3), 337, 1994; **Wang, K. K., Gutta, K. and Laukka, M. A.**, A prospective randomized trial of low dose photodynamic therapy in the treatment of *barretts esophagus*, *Gastroenterology*, 106(4), A208, 1994; **Garza, O., Abati, A., Sindelar, W., Pass, H. and Hijazi, Y.**, Cytologic effects of photodynamic therapy (PDT) in body fluids, *Laboratory Investigation*, 70(1), A36, 1994; **Tang, G. and Giannotta, S. L.**, Treatment of atheromas with photodynamic therapy, *Stroke*, 25(1), 256, 1994; **Hourigan, A. J., Kells, A. F. and Schwartz, H. S.**, In vitro photodynamic therapy of musculoskeletal neoplasms, *J. of Orthopaedic Res.*, 1(5), 633, 1993; **Abramson, A. L., Alvi, A. and Mullooly, V. M.**, Clinical exacerbation of systemic lupus erythematosus after photodynamic therapy of laryngotracheal papillomatosis, *Lasers in Surgery and Medicine*, 13(6), 677, 1993; **Dartsch, P. C., Coppenrath, E., Coppenrath, K. and Ischinger, T.**, Photodynamic therapy of vascular stenosis. Results from cell culture studies on

human endothelial cells, *Coronary Artery Disease*, 4(2), 207, 1993; **Laukka, M. A., Wang, K. K., Cameron, A. J. and Alexander, G. L.**, The use of photodynamic therapy in the treatment of *Barretts Esophagus*. Preliminary results, *Gastrointestinal Endoscopy*, 39(2), 291, 1993; **Evrard, S., Aprahamian M. and Marescaux, J.**, Intraabdominal photodynamic therapy. From theory to feasibility, *Brit. J. of Surgery*, 80(3), 298, 1993.

25. **Qin, B. S., Selman, S. H., Payne, K. M., Keck, R. W. and Metzger, D. W.**, Enhanced skin allograft survival after photodynamic therapy. Association with lymphocyte inactivation and macrophage stimulation, *Transplantation*, 56(6), 1481, 1993.
26. **Guillemin, F., Patrice, T., Brault, D., Dhallewin, M. A., Leroy, M., Meunier, A. and Lignon, D.**, Photodynamic Therapy, Pathologie Biologie, 41(1), 110, 1993; **Nseyo, U. O.**, Photodynamic therapy, *Urologic Clinics of North America*, 19(3),591, 1992; **Photodynamic** therapy. Shining light where it is needed, *J. Clinical Oncology*, 11(10), 1844, 1993; **Vanhillegersberg, R., Kort, W. J. and Wilson, J. H. P.**, Current status of photodynamic therapy in oncology, *Drugs*, 48(4), 510, 1994; **Hampton, J. A., Goldblatt, P. J. and Selman, S. H.**, Photodynamic therapy. A new modality for the treatment of cancer, *Annals of Clinical and Lab. Sci.*, 24(3), 203, 1994; **Penning, L. C. and Dubbelman, T. M.**, Fundamentals of photodynamic therapy. Cellular and biochemical aspects, *Anti-cancer Drugs*, 5(2), 139, 1994; **Dougherty, T. J.**, Photodynamic therapy, *Photochem. Photobiol.*, 58(6), 895, 1993.
27. **Teuchner, K., Pfarrherr, A., Stiel, H., Freyer, W. and Leupold, D.**, Spectroscopic properties of potential sensitizers for new photodynamic therapy start mechanisms via two step excited electronic states, *Photochem. Photobiol.*, 57(3), 465, 1993; **Lipshutz, G. S., Castro, D. J., Saxton, R. E., Haugland, R. P. and Soudant, J.**, Evaluation of four new carbocyanine dyes for photodynamic therapy with lasers, *Laringoscope*, 104(8), 996, 1994; **Vidoczy, T.**, On the feasibility of the modified mechanism of photodynamic therapy proposed by Leupold and Freyer, *J. Photochem. Photobiol. B: Biology*, 17(1), 83-84, 1993; **Schiwon, K., Brauer, H. D., Gerlach, B., Muller, C. M. and Montforts, F. P.**, Potential photosensitizers for photodynamic therapy, *J. Photochem. Photobiol. B: Biology*, 23(2-3), 239, 1994; **Schmidt, S.**, Antibody targeted photodynamic therapy, *Hybrydoma*, 12(5), 539, 1993.
28. **Kato, H., Horai, T., Furuse, K., Fukuoka, M., Suzuki, S., Hiki, Y., Ito, Y., Mimura, S., Tenjin, Y., Hisazumi, H. and Hayata, Y.**, Photodynamic therapy for cancers. A clinical trial of porfimer sodium in Japan, *Jap. J. Cancer Research*, 84(11), 1209, 1993.
29. **Samec, Z., Marecek, V. and Weber, J.**, Detection of an electron transfer across the interface between two immiscible electrolyte solutions by cyclic voltammetry with four electrode system, *J. Electroanal. Chem.*, 96, 245, 1977; **Senda, M.**, Theory of the double layer effect on the rate of ion transfer across an oil-water interface, *Anal. Sci.*, 10(4), 649, 1994; **Benjamin, I.**, Mechanism and dynamics of ion transfer across a liquid-liquid interface, *Science*, 261(5128), 1558, 1993; **Schweighofer,, K. J. and Benjamin I.**, Dynamics of ion transfer across the liquid-liquid interface, *Abst. Papers Am. Chem. Soc.*, 207, 199-Phys, 1994; **Kakiuchi, T., Noguchi, J., and Senda, M.**, Double-layer effect on the transfer of some monovalent ions across the polarized oil-water interface, *J. Electroanal. Chem.*, 336(1-2), 137, 1992; **Lin, S., Shen, D. Z. Nie, L. H. and Yao, S. Z.**, The transfer mechanisms and analytical properties of the variable valency drug cinchonidine across the liquid-liquid interface, *Electrochim. Acta*, 38(18), 2707, 1993; **Kakiuchi, T., Noguchi, J. and Senda, M.**, Kinetics of the transfer of monovalent anions across the nitrobenzene-water interface, **J. Electroanal. Chem.**, 327, 63, 1992; **Markin, V. S. and Volkov, A. G.**, The Gibbs free-energy of ion transfer between two immiscible liquids, *Electrochim. Acta*, 34(2), 93, 1989.
30. **Mathai, K. G. and Rabinowith, E.**, Studies of the thionine-ferrous iron reaction in a heterogeneous system, *J. Phys. Chem.* 66, 663, 1962; **Frankowiak, D. J. and Rabinowitch, E.**, The methyl blue ferrous iron reaction in a two-phase system, *J. Phys. Chem.* 70, 3012, 1966.
31. **Boguslavsky, L. I., Kondrashin, A. A., Kozlov, I. A., Metelsky, S. T., Skulachev, V. P. and Volkov, A. G.**, Charge transfer between water and octane phases by soluble mitochondrial H^+-ATPase, bacteriorhodopsin and respiratory chain enzymes, *FEBS Letters*, 50, 223, 1975; **Boguslavsky, L. I. and Volkov, A. G.**, Photoinduced proton transfer across decane/water interface in the presence of chlorophyll, *Doklady AN SSSR*, 224, 1201, 1975; **Yaguzhinsky,**

L. S., Boguslavsky, L. I., Volkov, A. G. and Rakhmaninova, A., Synthesis of ATP coupled with action of membrane protonic pumps at the octane-water interface, *Nature*, 259, 494, 1976; **Boguslavsky, L. I., Volkov, A. G., Kandelaki, M. D. and Nizhnikovsky, E. A.**, Photooxidation of water and proton transport through the interface between two immiscible liquids in the presence of chlorophyll, *Doklady AN SSSR*, 227, 727, 1976; **Volkov, A. G., Kolev, V. D., Levin, A. L. and Boguslavsky, L. I.**, Oxygen photoevolution at the octane/water interface in the presence of β–carotene and chlorophyll *a*, *Photobiochem. Photobiophys.*, 10, 105, 1985.

32. **Post, A., Young, S. E. and Robertson, R. N.**, Bacteriorhodopsin proton pump at oil/water boundary, *Photobiochem. Photobiophys.*, 8, 153, 1984.
33. **Zaitsev, N. K., Kulakov, I. I. and Kuzmin, M. G.**, Photoelectrochemical effect at the interface between immiscible liquid electrolyte solutions, *Soviet Electrochemistry (Engl. Ed.)*, 21(10), 1293, 1985.
34. **Zaitsev, N. K., Gorelik, N. F., Kotov, N. A. and Kuzmin M. G.**, A photoelectrochemical effect at the polarizable interface between liquid electrolyte solutions in protoporphyrin-quinone systems, *Soviet Electrochemistry (Engl. Ed.)*, 24, 1346, 1988.
35. **Thompson, F. L., Yellowlees, L. J. and Girault, H. H.**, Photocurrent measurements at the interface between two immiscible electrolyte-solutions, *J. Chem. Soc. Chem. Commun.*, 1547, 1988.
36. **Samec, Z., Brown, A. R., Yellowlees, L. J., Girault, H. H. and Base, K.**, Photochemical ion transfer across the interface between two immiscible electrolyte solutions, *J. Electroanal. Chem.*, 259, 309, 1989.
37. **Marecek, V., Dearmond, A. and Dearmond, K.**, Photoinduced polarization of the interface between two immiscible electrolyte solutions, *J. Electroanal. Chem.*, 261, 287, 1989.
38. **Marecek, V., Dearmond, A. and Dearmond, K.**, Photochemical electron transfer in liquid-liquid solvent systems, *J. Am. Chem. Soc.*, 111, 2561, 1989.
39. **Samec, Z., Brown, A. R., Yellowlees, L. J. and Girault, H. H.**, Photochemical transfer of tetraaryl ions across the interface between two immiscible electrolyte solutions, *J. Electroanal. Chem.*, 288, 245, 1990.
40. **Dvorak, O., Dearmond, A. H. and Dearmond, M. K.**, Photoprocesses at the liquid-liquid interface. 4. Photooxidative transfer with $Ru(Bpz)_3^{2+}$ complexes, *Langmuir*, 8(3), 955, 1992; **Dvorak, O., Dearmond, A. H. and Dearmond, M. K.**, Photoprocesses at the liquid-liquid interface. 3. Charge transfer details for photoactive metal complexes, *Langmuir*, 8(2), 508, 1992.
41. **Kotov, N. A. and Kuzmin, M. G.**, The photocurrent kinetics across the polarizable interface of immiscible electrolyte solutions in the protoporphyrine-quinone system, *Soviet Electrochemistry (Engl. Ed.)*, 26(12), 1484, 1990.
42. **Kotov, N. A. and Kuzmin, M. G.**, Analysis of photocurrent kinetics in photoelectrochemical effect at polarizable interface between electrolyte solutions by mathematical modeling method, *Soviet Electrochemistry (Engl. Ed.)*, 27(1), 76, 1991.
43. **Kotov, N. A. and Kuzmin, M. G.**, Computer analysis of photoinduced charge transfer at the ITIES in protoporphyrin-quinone system, *J. Electroanal. Chem.*, 341, 47, 1992.
44. **Kotov, N. A. and Kuzmin, M. G.**, Computer analysis of photoinduced charge transfer at the ITIES and potential of optimization technique, *J. Electroanal. Chem.*, 327, 47, 1992.
45. **Kotov, N. A. and Kuzmin, M. G.**, A photoelectrochemical effect at the interface of immiscible electrolyte solutions, *J. Electroanal. Chem.*, 285, 223, 1990.
46. **Kotov, N. A. and Kuzmin, M. G.**, Nature of the processes of charge-carrier generation at ITIES by the photoexcitation of porphirins, *J. Electroanal. Chem.*, 338, 99, 1992.
47. **Tricot, Y.-M., Rafaeloff, R., Emeren, Å. and Fendler, J.**, Photosensitized water reduction mediated by semiconductors dispersed in membrane mimetic systems, in *Organic Phototransformations in Nonhomogenious Media., ACS symposium series,* Vol. 278, Fox, M. A., Ed., American Chemical Society, Washington, 1985, p. 99.
48. **Hurst, J. K.**, Dynamics of charge separation across vesicle membranes, in *Kinetics and Catalysis in Microheterogeneous Systems. Surfactant Science Series*, Vol. 38, Gratzel, M. and Kalyanasundaram, K., Eds., Marcel Dekker, New York, 1991, p. 183; **Willner, I.**,

Photosensitized electron-transfer reactions in organized systems. The role of synthetic catalysts and natural enzymes in fixation processes in *Organic Phototransformations in Nonhomogenious Media., ACS symposium series*, Vol. 278, Fox, M. A., Ed., American Chemical Society, Washington, 1985, p. 191.

49. **Kalyanosundaram, K.**, *Photochemistry in Organized Systems*, Academic Press, Orlando, 1987, p. 104.

50. **Beckman, L. S. and Brown, D. G.**, The interaction between vitamin B-12 and micelles in aqueous solutions, *Biochim. Biophys. Acta.*, 428, 720, 1976; **James, A. D. and Robinson, B. H.**, Micellar catalysis of metal-complex formation. Kinetics of the reaction between Ni(II) and pyridine-2-azo-p-dimethylaniline (PADA) in the presence of sodium dodecyl sulfate micelles: A model system for the study of metal ion reactivity at charged interfaces, *J. Chem. Soc. Farad. 1*, 74, 10, 1978, **Pileni, M. P. and Gratzel, M.**, Light-induced redox reactions of proflavin in aqueous and micellar solutions, *J. Phys. Chem.*, 84, 2403, 1980; **Usui, Y. and Saga, K.**, The photo-reduction and photosensitized reduction of dyes bound to a surfactant micellar surface, *Bull. Chem. Soc. Jpn.*, 55, 3302, 1982; **Frank, A. J. and Gratzel, M.**, Sensitized photoreduction of nitrate in homogeneous and micellar solutions, *Inorg. Chem.*, 21, 3834, 1982; **Kalyanasundaram, K.**, Photoredox reactions in micellar solutions sensitized by surfactant derivatives of tris(2,2'-bipyridyl)ruthenium (II), *J. Chem. Soc. Chem. Commun.*, 628, 1978; **Wilner, I., Ford, W. E., Otvos, J. W. and Calvin, M.**, Photoinduced electron transfer across a water-oil boundary as a model for redox reaction separation, *Nature*, 280, 823, 1979; **Furois, J. M., Brochette, P. and Pileni, M. P.**, Photoelectron transfer in reverse micelles: 2-photooxidation of magnesium porphyrin, *J. Colloid Inter. Sci.*, 97, 552, 1984.

51. **Stein, W. D.**, Ed., *Current topics in membranes and transport. v. 21., Ion channels: molecular and physicochemical aspects.*, Academic Press Inc., Orlando, 1984; **Yeagle, P.**, Ed., *The structure of biological membranes*, CRC Press, Boca Raton, 1992.

52. **Thomas, J. K. and Piciulo, P.**, Photoionization by green light, *J. Am. Chem. Soc.*, 101, 2502, 1979; **Thomas, J. K. and Piciulo, P.**, Photoionization by green light in micellar solution, *J. Am. Chem. Soc.*, 100, 3239, 1978.

53. **Hall.**, E., Comment on the Communication "Photoionization by green light", *J. Am. Chem. Soc.*, 100, 8260, 1978.

54. **Baglioni, P., Rivaraminten, E., Stenland, C. and Kevan, L.**, Photoionization of N,N,N',N'-tetramethylbenzidine in a mixed micelle of ionic and nonionic surfactants. Electron spin-echo modulation and electron-spin resonance studies, *J. Phys. Chem.*, 95(24), 169, 1991; **Kang, Y. S., Baglioni, P., Mcmanus, H. J. D. and Kevan L.**, Alkyl chain-length effects on the photoionization of N-alkylphenothiazines and sulfonated alkylphenothiazines in anionic alkyl sulfate and cationic alkyltrimeyhylammonium bromide micelles, *J. Phys. Chem.*, 95(20), 7944, 1991; **Decastaing, E. C. and Kevan, L.**, Location and photoionization studies of a series of alkylporphyrin derivatives solubilized in dioctadecylmethylammonium chloride and dihexadecyl phosphate vesicles, *J. Phys. Chem.*, 95(24), 178, 1991; **Bratt, P., Kang, Y. S., Kevan, L., Nakamura, H. and Matsuo, T.**, Photoionization of neutral and positively charged alkylphenothiazines in positive, neutral, and negatively charged vesicles. Effect of the alkyl chain length, *J. Phys. Chem.*, 95(17), 6399, 1991; **Bratt, P. J., Kang, Y. S. and Kevan, L.**, Photoionization of neutral alkylphenothiazines in positive, neutral, and negative charged vesicles. Effect of the addition of cholesterol and alkyl chain length, *J. Phys. Chem.*, 96(13), 5629, 1992; **Kang, Y. S., Mcmanus, H. J. D. and Kevan, L.**, Comparative electron magnetic resonance, electron spin echo modulation, and electron nuclear double-resonance studies of the photoionization of N-alkylphenothiazines in variously charged micelles and vesicles, *J. Phys. Chem.*, 96(18), 7473, 1992; **Kang, Y. S., Mcmanus, H. J. D. and Kevan, L.**, An electron magnetic-resonance study of the photoionization of a series of nalkylphenothiazines in AOT reverse micelles, *J. Phys. Chem.*, 96(21), 8647, 1992; **Stetland, C. and Kevan, L.**, *J. Phys. Chem.*, 97(19), 5177, 1993; **Kang, Y. S. and Kevan, L.**, Photoinduced electron-transfer from (alkoxyphenyl)triphenylporphyrins to interface water of dihexadecyl phosphate, dipalmitoyl-phosphatidylcholine, and dioctadecyldimethylammonium chloride vesicles, *J. Phys. Chem.*, 98(16), 4389, 1994; **Kang, Y. S. and Kevan, L.**, Photoinduced electron-transfer from N-alkylphenothiazines to interface of sodium dodecylsulfate micelles as a function of

poly(ethylene oxide) interaction with the interface, *J. Phys. Chem.*, 98(9), 2478, 1994; **Kang, Y. S., Mcmanus, H. J. D., Liang, K. N. and Kevan, L.**, Photoinduced electron transfer from (alkoxyphenyl)-triphenylporphyrins to interface water of aerosol dioctyl- and cetyltrimethyl-ammonium bromide/alcohol reverse micelles at 77 K, *J. Phys. Chem.*, 98(3), 1044, 1994; **Stenland, C. and Kevan, L.**, Electron-spin resonance and electron-spin echo modulation studies of photoionization of N,N,N',N'-tetramethylbenzidine in anionic, zwitterionic, and cationic vesicles. Correlation of photoreduced cation location with the photoyield., *Langmuir*, 10(4), 1129, 1994.

55. **Claudemontigny, B. and Tondre, C.**, Microenvironment effects on the kinetics of electron-transfer reactions involving dithionite ions and viologens. 3. Comparison between micelles and some other microheterogeneous systems, *New J. Chem.*, 18(5), 597, 1994; **Grand, D.**, Photoionization in cationic micelles -Effect of alcohol or salt addition, *J. Phys. Chem.*, 94(19), 7585, 1990; **Ilichev, Y. V., Demyashkevich, A. B. and Kuzmin, M. G.**, Protolitic photodissociation of hydroxyaromatic compounds in micelles and lipid bilayer membranes of vesicles, *J. Phys. Chem.*, 95(8), 3438, 1991; **Solntsev, K. M., Ilichev, Y. V., Demyashkevich, A. B. and Kuzmin, M. G.**, Excited-state, proton-transfer reactions of substituted naphthols in micelles. Comparative study of reactions of 2-naphtol and its long-chain alkyl derivatives in micellar solutions of cetyltrimethylammonium bromide, *J. Photochem. Photobiol.*, 78(1), 39, 1994.
56. **Dakhnovskii, Y.**, Nonadiabatic chemical reactions in a strong time dependent electric field. An electron-transfer reaction in a polar solvent, *J. Chem. Phys.*, 100(9), 6492, 1994.
57. **Flewelling, R. F. and Hubbel, W. L.**, Hydrophobic ion interactions with membranes - thermo-dynamic analysis of tetraphenylphosphonium binding to vesicles, *Biophys J.*, 49, 531, 1986.
58. **Deamer, D. W. and Volkov, A. G.**, Proton permeation of lipid bilayers, in *Permeability and Stability of Lipid Bilayers*, Disalvo, E. A. and Simon, S. A., Eds., CRC Press, Boca Raton, 1995, p. 161.
59. **Lockhart, D. J., Goldstein, S. G. and Boxer, S.**, Structure based analysis of the initial electron transfer step in bacterial photosynthesis. Electric field induced fluorescence anisotropy, *J. Phys. Chem.*, 89, 1408, 1988; **Lockhart, D. J. and Boxer, S.**, Electric field modulation of the fluorescence from rhodobacterum-sphaeroides reaction centers, *Chem. Phys. Lett.*, 144, 243, 1988; **Boxer, S., Goldstein, R. A. and Franzen, S.**, The use of magnetic and electric fields to probe electron transfer reactions., in *Photoinduced Electron Transfer. Part B. Experimental Techniques and Medium Effects.*, Fox, M. A. and Chanon, M., Eds., Elsevier, Amsterdam, 1988, p. 163 and references therein; **Lao, K. Q., Franzen, S., Stanley, R. J., Lambright, D. G. and Boxer, S. G.**, Effects of applied electric-fields on the quantum yields of the initial electron-transfer steps in bacterial photosynthesis .1. Quantum yield failure, *J. Phys. Chem.*, 97(50), 13165, 1993; **Franzen, S. and Boxer, S. G.**, Temperature dependence of the electric field modulation of electron transfer rates: charge recombination in photosynthetic reaction centers, *J. Phys. Chem.*, 97(10), 6304, 1993; **Marcus, R. A. and Sutin, N.**, Electron transfers in chemistry and biology, *Biochem. Biophys. Acta*, 811, 265, 1985; **Gunner, M. R., Robertson, D. E. and Dutton, P. L.**, Kinetic studies on the reaction center protein from rhodo-pseudomonas-sphaeroides - the temperature and free energy dependence of electron-transfer between various quinones in the Q_a site and the oxidized bacteriochlorophyll dimer, *J. Phys. Chem.*, 90(16), 3783, 1986; **Ogorodnic, A. and Michel-Beyerle, M. E.**, Testing primary charge separation in photosynthetic reaction centers with external electric fields, *Photoprocesses in Transition Metal Complexes, Biosystems and Other Molecules. Experiment and Theory., NATO ASI Series, Series C: Mathematical and Physical Sciences*, Vol. 376, Kochanski, E., Ed., Kluwer Academic Publishers, Dortrecht, 1992, p. 349 and the references therein; **Cheddar, G. and Tollin, G.**, Electrostatic effects on the kinetics of electron-transfer reactions of cytochrome-C caused by binding to negatively charged lipid bilayer vesicles, *Arch. Biochem. Biophys.*, 286(1), 201, 1991; **Suga, K., Fujita, S., Yamada, H. and Fujihira, M.**, Comparison between intramolecular and intermolecular photoinduced electron-transfer reactions of micelle solubilized substances, *Bull. Chem. Soc. Jpn.*, 63(12), 3369, 1990.

60. **Shchipunov, Y. A. and Kolpakov, A. F.**, Phospholipids at the oil-water interface. Adsorption and interfacial phenomena in electric field, *Adv. Coll. Inter. Sci.* , 35, 31, 1991.

61. **Leenhouts, J. M., Chupin, V., Degier, J. and Dekruijff, B.**, The membrane potential has no detectable effect on the phosphocholine headgroup conformation in large unilamellar phosphatidylcholine vesicles as determined by H^2 NMR, *Biochim. Biophys. Acta*, 1153(2), 257, 1993.

62. **Markin, V. S. and Volkov, A. G.**, Potentials at the interface between two immiscible electrolyte solutions, *Adv. Coll. Inter. Sci.*, 31(1-2), 111, 1990.

63. **Benjamin, I.**, Theoretical study of the water 1,2-dichloroethane interface. Structure, dynamics, and conformational equilibria at the liquid/liquid interface, *J. Chem. Phys.*, 97(2), 1432, 1992; **Benjamin, I.**, Dynamics of ion transfer across a liquid/liquid interface. A comparison between molecular dynamics and a diffusional model, *J. Chem. Phys.*, 96(1), 577, 1992; **Benjamin, I.**, Charge transfer across the liquid-liquid interface. Molecular dynamics and continuum models, *Abst. Papers Am. Chem. Soc.*, 204 98, 1992; **Benjamin, I.**, Solvent dynamics following charge-transfer at the liquid-liquid interface, *J. Chem. Phys.*, 180(2-3), 287, 1994.

64. **Franklin, J. C. and Cafiso, D. S.**, Internal electrostatic potentials in bilayers. Measuring and controlling dipole potentials in lipid vesicles, *Biophys. J.*, 64(2) A297, 1993; **Maitra, A., Jain, T. K. and Shervani, Z.**, Interfacial water structure in lecithin-oil-water reverse micelles, *Coll. Surf.*, 47, 255, 1990; **Thompson, T. E.**, Phosphatidylcholine vesicles - structure and formation, *Hepatology*, 12(3), S51, 1990; **Rao, K. S., Goyal, P. S., Dasannacharya, B. A., Menon, S. V. G., Kelkar, V. K., Manohar, C., and Mishra, B. K.**, Application of Baxter sticky hard-sphere model to nonionic micelles, *Physica B*, 174(1-4), 170, 1991; **Flewelling, R. F. and Hubbell, W. L.**, The membrane dipole potential in a total membrane potential model - applications to hydrophobic ion interactions with membranes, *Biophys. J.*, 49(2) 541, 1986.

65. **Hajkova, P., Volkov, A. G., Samec, Z., Marecek, V. and Homolka, D.**, Measurement of electric double layer capacity at the water dichloroethane interface in the presence of metal-porphyrin complexes, *Soviet Electrochemistry (Engl. Ed)*, 21(2), 190, 1985; **Schiffrin, D. J., Calde,r M. R. and Wiles, M. C.**, The adsorption of modified affinity ligands at polarized liquid-liquid interfaces, *J. Electrochem. Soc.*, 133(3), C134, 1986.

66. **Franklin, J. C. and Cafiso, D. S.**, Internal electrostatic potentials in lipid vesicles, *Biophys. J.*, 65(1) 289, 1993.

67. **Tomic, M. and Kallay, N.**, Effect of charge distribution within a droplet on the electrical conductivity of water-in-oil microemulsions, *J. Phys. Chem.*, 96(9), 3874; **Carmona-Ribeiro, A. M. and Midmore, B. R.**, Surface potential in charged synthetic amphiphile vesicles, *J. Phys. Chem.*, 96(8), 3542, 1992; **Feitoza, E., Neto, A. A. and Chaimovich, H.**, Integration of the nonlinear Poisson-Boltzmann equation for charged vesicles in electrolytic solutions, *Langmuir*, 9(3), 702, 1993.

68. **Parker, A. J.**, *Chem. Rev.*, Protic-dipolar aprotic solvent effects on rates of bimolecular reactions, 69 (1), 1, 1969; **Popovich, O.**, Physical significance of transfer activity coefficients for single ions, *Anal. Chem.*, 46, 2009, 1974; **Koryta, J.**, *Ion-selective Electrodes*, Cambridge University Press, Cambridge, 1975; **Koryta, J.**, Electrochemical polarization phenomena at the interface of two immiscible electrolyte solutions, *Electrochim. Acta*, 24, 293, 1979; **Koryta, J. and Vanysek, P.** in *Advances in Electrochemistry and Electrochemical Engineering*, vol. 12, Gerisher, H. and Tobias, C. W., Eds., Wiley, New York, 1981, p. 113; **Girault, H. H. and Schiffrin, D. J.**, A new approach for the definition of Galvani potential scales and ionic Gibbs energies of transfer across liquid-liquid interfaces, *Electrochim Acta.*, Vol. 31, (10) 1341, 1986.

69. **Hartley, G. S. and Roe, J. W.**, Solubilization sites of aromatic optical probes in micelles, *Trans Farad. Soc.*, 36, 101, 1940.

70. **Kalyanosundaram, K.**, *Photochemistry in Organized Systems*, Academic Press, Orlando, 1987, 187; **Fernandez, M. S.**, *Biochim. Biophys. Acta*, 601, 152, 1980.

71. **Fernandez, M. S. and Fromhertz, P. J.**, Lipoid pH indicators as probes of electrical potential and polarity in micelles, *J. Phys. Chem.*, 81(18), 1755, 1977; **Murray, B. S., Drummond, C. J., Gale, L., Grieser, F. and White, L. R.**, Electrostatic surface-potentials of cationic and anionic oil-in-water microemulsion droplets free from added electrolyte, *Coll. Surf.*, 52(3-4),

287, 1991; **Drummond, C. J., Grieser, F. and Healy, T. W.**, Interfacial properties of a novel group of solvatochromic acid-base indicators in self-assembled surfactant aggregates, *J. Phys. Chem.*. 92, 2604, 1988; **Alexiev, U., Scherrer, P., Otto, H., Marti, T. and Khorana, H. G.**, Surface charge of bacteriorhodopsin micelles measured with an optical pH-sensitive dye bound to specific sites on the extracellular and cytoplasmic side of the protein, *FASEB J.*, 6(1), A529, 1992; **Scherrer, P., Alexiev, U., Otto, H., Marti, T. and Khorana, H. G.**, Measurements of light induced proton movements. Enhanced velocity of proton movement along the micelle surface, *FASEB J.*, 6(1), A529, 1992; **Lovelock, B., Grieser, F. and Healy, T. W.**, Properties of 4-octadecyloxy-1- naphthoic acid in micellar solutions and in monolayer films adsorbed onto silica attenuated total reflectance plates, *J. Phys. Chem.*, 85, 501, 1985; **Murray, B. S., Godfrey, J. S., Grieser, F., Healy, T. W., Lovelock, B. and Scales, P. J.**, Spectroscopic and electrokinetic study of pH-dependent ionization of Langmuir-Blodgett films, *Langmuir*, 7, 3057, 1991: **Ganesh, K. N., Mitra, P. and Balasubramanian, D.**, Solubilization sites of aromatic optical probes in micelles, *J. Phys. Chem.*, 86, 4291, 1982; **Hazarika, R., Dutta, R. K. and Bhat, S. N.**, Effect of cationic micelles on pKa of acridine. A spectroscopic study., *Ind. J. Chem. A: Inorg. Bioinorg. Phys. Theor. Anal Chem.*, 32(3), 239, 1993; **Hobson, R. A., Grieser, F. and Healy, T. W.**, Surface potential measurements in mixed micelle systems, *J. Phys. Chem.*, 98(1), 274, 1994.

72. **Grieser, F. and Drummond, C. J.**, The physicochemical properties of selfassembled surfactant aggregates as determined by some molecular spectroscopic probe techniques, *J. Phys. Chem.*, 92, 5580, 1988 and references therein.
73. **Franklin, J. C., Cafiso, D. S., Flewelling, R. F. and Hubbell, W. L.**, Probes of membrane electrostatics. Synthesis and voltage dependent partitioning of negative hydrophobic ion spin labels in lipid vesicles, *Biophys. J.*, 64(3), 642, 1993.
74. **Fujihira, M., Yanagisawa, M. and Kondo, T.**, Investigation of electron-transfer through the interfacial double-layers of various micelles, *Bull. Chem. Soc. Jpn.*, 66(12), 3600, 1993.
75. **Lee, C. W. and Oh, M. K.**, Redox potential of N-hexadecyl-N'-methyl viologen (2+/+) solubilized in cetiltrimethylammonium chloride micelle, *Bull. Korean Chem. Soc.* , 12(6), 593, 1991; **Lei, Y. and Hurst, J. K.**, Reduction potential of vesicle bound viologens, *J. Phys. Chem.*, 95(20), 7918, 1991; **Myers, S. A., Mackay, R. A. and Brajetorth, A.**, Solution microstructure and electrochemical reactivity. Effect of probe partitioning on electrochemical formal potentials in microheterogeneous solutions, *Anal. Chem.*, 65(23), 3447, 1993; **Lee, C. W., Oh, M. K. and Jang, J. M.**, Reduction potentials of N-Hexadecyl-N'-Methyl viologen(2+/+) solubilized in cationic, nonionic, and anionic micelles, *Langmuir*, 9(7), 1934, 1993.
76. **Ross, W. N, Salzberg, B. M., Cohen, L. B. and Davaila, H. V.**, A large change in dye absorption during the action of potential, *Biophys J.*, 14, 983, 1974; **Ross, W. N, Salzberg, B. M., Cohen, L. B., Grinvald, A., Davaila, H. V., Waggoner, A. S. and Wang, C. H.**, Changes in adsorption, fluorescence, dichroism, and birefrigence in stained giant axons: optical measurement of membrane potential, *J. Membr. Biol.*, 33, 141, 1977.
77. **Borsarelli, C. D., Cosa, J. J. and Previtali, C. M.**, The interface effect on the properties of exciplexs formed between pyrene derivatives and N.N-dimethylalanine in reverse micelles, *Langmuir*, 9(11), 2895, 1993; **Ueda, M., Kimura, A., Wakida, T., Yoshimura, Y. and Schelly, Z. A.**, Investigation of the micropolarity of reverse micelles using quinolinium betaine compounds as probes, *J. Coll. Inter. Sci.*, 163(2), 515, 1994; **Martic, P. A. and Nair, M.**, Microenvironment sensing of block-copolymer micelles by fluorescence spectroscopy, *J. Coll. Inter. Sci.*, 163(2), 517, 1994; **Zouni, A., Clarke, R. J., Visser, A. J. W. G., Visser, N. V. and Holzwarth, J. F.**, Static and dynamic studies of the potential sensitive membrane probe Rh421 in dimyristoyl-phosphatidylcholine vesicles, *Biochim. Biophys Acta*, 1153(2), 203, 1993.
78. **Nishimoto, J., Iwamoto, E., Fujiwara, T. and Kumamaru, T.**, Strongly polarized water at the interfacial region in reversed micelles containing 1,4,8,11-tetramethyl-1,4,8,11-tetraaza-cyclotetradecanenickel as a probe, *J. Chem. Soc. Faraday Trans.*, 89(3), 535, 1993; **Clarke, R. J.**, Binding and diffusion kinetics of the interaction of a hydrophobic potential-sensitive dye with lipid vesicles, *Biophys. Chem.*, 39(1), 91, 1991; **Waggoner, A. S.** in *The Enzymes of*

Biological Membranes, 2nd edn., Hartonosi, A. N., Ed., Plenum Press, New York, Vol. 3, 1985, 313.

79. **Carmona-Ribeiro, A. M. and Midmore, B. R.**, Surface potential in charged synthetic amphiphile vesicles, *J. Phys. Chem.*, 96(8), 3542, 1992.
80. **Hobson, R. A., Grieser, F., and Healy, T. W.**, Surface potential measurements in mixed micelle systems, *J. Phys. Chem.*, 98(1), 274, 1994; **Drummond, C. J., Griezer, F. and Healy, T. W.**, Interfacial properties of a novel group of solvatochromic acid-base indicators in selfassembled surfactant aggregates, *J. Phys. Chem.*, 92(9), 2604, 1988; **Warr, G. G. and Griezer, F.**, The effect of long-chain fluorescence probes on the size of sodium dodecyl-sulfate micelles, *Chem. Phys. Lett.*, 116, 505, 1985; **Turro, N. J. and Yekta, A.**, Luminescent probes for detergent solutions. A simple procedure for determination of the mean aggregation number of micelles, *J. Am. Chem. Soc.*, 100, 5951, 1978; **Zaitsev, A. K., Zaitsev, N. K., Kuzmin, M. G. and Iliichev Y. V.**, Increase of the proton phototransfer reaction efficiency in the micellar solution via a base-carrier, *Doklady Acad. Nauk SSSR.*, 283(4), 900, 1985.
81. **Loew, L. M.**, Electrical properties of Biomembranes, in *Biomembranes. Physical Aspects*, Shinitzky M. Ed., VCH Publishers, Weinheim, 1993, 341; **Simon, S. A. and McIntosh, T. J.**, *Proc. Natl. Acad. Sci. USA.*, 86, 9263, 1989; **Lei, Y. and Hurst, J. K.**, Reduction potential of vesicle bound viologens, *J. Phys. Chem.*, 95(20), 7918, 1991; **McLaughlin, S. G. A., Szabo, G., Eiseman G. and Ciani, S. M.**, Surface charge and the conductance of phospholipid membranes, *Proc. Natl. Acad. Sci. USA.*, 67(3), 1268, 1970; **Mosior, M. and McLaughlin, S.**, Electrostatic and reduction of dimentionality produce apparent cooperativity when basic peptide bind to acidic lipids in membrane, *Biochem. Biophys. Acta*, 1105, 185, 1992.
82. **Boxall, C.**, The electrophoresis of semiconductor particles, *Chem. Soc. Rev.*, 137, 1994; **Boxall, C. and Kelsall, G. H.**; Photoelectrophoresis of colloidal semiconductors, *J. Electroanal. Chem.*, 328, 75, 1992; **Boxall, C. and Kelsall, G. H.**, Photoelectrophoresis of colloidal semiconductors; **Boxall, C. and Kelsall, G. H.**, Photoelectrophoresis of colloidal semiconductors. Part 1. The technique and its applications, *J. Chem. Soc. Faraday. Trans.*, 87(21), 3537, 1991; **Boxall, C. and Kelsall, G. H.**, Photoelectrophoresis of colloidal semiconductors. Part 2. Transient experiments on TiO_2 particles, *J. Chem. Soc. Faraday. Trans.*, 87(21), 3547, 1991.
83. **Bilski, P. and Chignell, C. F.**, Properties of differently charged micelles containing Rose Bengal. Application in photosynthesitization studies, *J. Photochem. Photobiol.*, 77(1), 49, 1994; **Lee, C. W., Oh, M. K., and Jang, J. M.**, Reduction potentials of N-hexadecyl-N'-methyl viologen (2+/+) solubilized in cationic, nonionic, and anionic micelles, *Langmuir*, 9(7), 1934, 1993; **Resch, U., Hubig, S. M. and Fox, M. A.**, Photoinduced electron transfer from surfactant zinc porphyrins to dialkylviologens in water-in-oil microemulsions - effect of interfacial charge, *Langmuir*, 7(12), 2923, 1991; **Gehlen, M. H., Fo, P. B. and Neumann, M. G.**, Fluorescence quenching of acridine-orange by aromatic amines in cationic, anionic and nonionic micelles, *J. Photochem. Photobiol. A: Chemistry*, 59(3), 335, 1991.
84. **Feitosa, E., Neto, A. A. and Chaimovich, H.**, Integration of the nonlinear Poisson-Boltzmann equation for charged vesicles in electrolytic solutions, *Langmuir*, 9(3), 702, 1993.
85. **Carrion, F. J., Delamaza, A, and Parra, J. L.**, The influence of the ionic strength and lipid bilayer charge on the stability of liposomes, *J. Coll. Inter. Sci.*, 164(1), 78, 1994.
86. **Ilichev, Y. V. and Shapovalov, V. L.**, Effect of the electrostatic potential of microemulsion droplets on photoprotolytic dissociation of 1-Naphthol, *Bull. Russ., Acad. Sci. Division of Chem. Sci.*, 41(10), 1762, 1992; **Shapovalov, V. L.**, New charged microheterogeneous system. A microemulsion with droplets of variable electrostatic potential, *Bull. Russ., Acad. Sci. Division of Chem. Sci.*, 41(10) 1756, 1992; **Zaitsev, A. K., Zaitsev, N. K., Pavlov, A. A. and Kuzmin, M. G.**, Damping of fluorescence of acridinium cations in solutions of sodium dodecyl sulfate. Effect of the ionic solution strength, *Khimicheskaya Fizika (Russ. J. Chem. Phys.)*, 4(2), 182, 1985; **Miki, T., Miki, M. and Orii, Y.**, Membrane potential-linked reversed electron-transfer in the beef-heart cytochrome-BC(1) complex reconstituted into potassium-loaded phospholipid vesicles, *J. Biol. Chem.*, 269(3) 1827, 1994.
87. **Hundhammer, B. and Wilke, S.**, Investigation of ion transfer across the membrane stabilized interface of two immiscible electrolyte solutions .2. Analytical application, *J. Electroanal.*

Chem., 266(1), 133 1989; **Albery, W. J., Choudhery, R. A. and Fisk, P. R.**, Kinetics and mechanism of interfacial reactions in the solvent extraction of copper, *Faraday Discuss. Chem. Soc.*, 77, 53, 1984; **Hundhammer, B., Solomon, T., Zerihun, T., Abegar, M., Bekele, A. and Graichen, K.**, Investigation of ion transfer across the membrane-stabilized interface of two immiscible electrolyte solutions. 3. Facilitated ion transfer, *J. Electroanal. Chem.*, 371, 1, 1994; **Kakiuchi, T., Kotani, M., Noguchi, J., Nakanishi, M. and Senda, M.**, Phase transition and ion permeability of phosphatidylcholine monolayers at the polarized oil/water interface, *J. Coll. Inter. Sci.*, 149(1), 279, 1992.

88. **Corn, R. M.**, Optical second harmonic generation studies of molecular orientation and order at liquid-liquid surfaces, *Abst. Papers Am. Chem. Soc.*, 204, 104, 1992; **Higgins, D. A. and Corn, R. M.**, Second harmonic generation studies of adsorption at a liquid/liquid electrochemical interface, *J. Phys. Chem.*, 97(2), 489, 1993; **Kott, K. L., Higgins, D. A., Mcmahon, R. J. and Corn, R. M.**, Observation of photoinduced electron transfer at a liquid-liquid interface by optical second harmonic generation, *J. Am. Chem. Soc.*, 115(12), 5342, 1993.
89. **Conboy, J. C., Daschbach, J. L. and Richmond, G. L.**, Second harmonic generation studies of the neat liquid-liquid interface, *Abstr. Papers Am. Chem. Soc.*, 207, 123-Phys, 1994.
90. **Watarai, H. and Chida, Y.**, Simple devices for the measurements of absorption spectra at liquid-liquid interfaces. *Anal. Sci.*, 10(1), 105, 1994.
91. **Kakiuchi, T., and Takasu, Y.**, Ion-selectivity of voltage-scan fluorometry at the 1,2-dichloroethane water surface, *J. Electroanal. Chem.*, 365(1-2), 293, 1994; **Kakiuchi, T. and Takasu, Y.**, Potential-step chronofluorometric response of fluorescent-ion transfer across a liquid-liquid interface, *J. Electroanal. Chem.*, 381, 5, 1995.
92. **Kandelaki, M. D. and Volkov, A. G.**, The influence of dielectric permittivity of the nonaqueous phase on the photooxidation of water at the interface of two immiscible liquids in the presence of a hydrated oligomer of chlorophyll. The role of a proton acceptor, *Can. J. Chem.*, 69(1), 151, 1991.
93. **Volkov, A. G., Gugeshashvili, M. I. and Deamer, D. W.**, Energy conversion at liquid-liquid interfaces: artificial photosynthetic systems, *Electrochim. Acta*, 1995 (in press); **Boguslavsky, L. I. and Volkov, A. G.**, in *The Interface Structure and Electrochemical Processes at the Boundary Between Two Immiscible Liquids*, Kazarinov, V. E., Ed., Springer Verlag, Berlin, 1987, p. 143; **Volkov, A. G.**, Oxygen evolution in the course of photosynthesis. *Bioelectrochem. Bioenerg.*, 21(1), 3, 1989; **Volkov, A. G.**, Molecular mechanism of the photooxidation of water during photosynthesis - cluster catalysis of synchronous multielectron reactions, *Mol. Biol.*, 20(3), 584, 1986.
94. **Bhattacharyya, M. L., Sarker, S. and Seth, K.**, Modulations of membrane-potential oscillations with drive, calcium overload, ryanodine, and caffeine , *J. Electrocardiology*, 27(2), 105, 1994; **Bleasel, A. F. and Pettigrew, A. G.**, The effect of bicarbonate free artificial cerebrospinal fluid on spontaneous oscillations of the membrane potential in inferior olivary neurons of the rat, *Brain Res.*, 639(1), 8, 1994; **Kononenko, N. I.**, Dissection of a model for membrane potential oscillations in bursting neuron of snail, *Helix Pomatia, Comparative Biochem. Physiol. A: Physiol.*, 107(2), 323, 1994; **Garciamunoz, A., Barrio, L. C. and Buno, W.**, Membrane potential oscillations in Ca1 hippocampal pyramidal neurons *in vitro.* Intrinsic rhythms and fluctuations entrained by sinusoidal injected current, *Exp. Brain Res.*, 97(2), 325, 1993.
95. **Maeda, K., Kihara, S., Suzuki, M. and Matsui, M.**, Voltammetric study on the oscillation of the potential difference at a liquid-liquid or liquid-membrane interface accompanied by ion transfer, *J. Electroanal. Chem.*, 295(1-2), 183, 1990.; **Kihara, S., Maeda, K., Shirai, O., Suzuki, M., Ogura, K. and Matsui, M.**, Elucidation of the oscillation of the potential difference accompanied by ion transfer at a liquid/liquid membrane interface using ion-transfer voltammetry, *Bunseki Kagaku*, 40(11), 767, 1991; **Arai, K.**, Electroanalytical study of the electrical potential oscillation across a liquid membrane and drug transfer at an oil-water interface, *Bunseki Kagaku* , 43(9) 729, 1994; **Arai, K., Fukuyama, S., Kusu, F. and Takamura, K.**, Effects of biologically important substances on spontaneous electrical potential

oscillation across a liquid membrane of a water/octanol/water system, *Bioelectrochem. Bioenerg.*, 33(2), 159, 1994.

96. **Maeda, K., Kihara, S., Suzuki, M. and Matsui, M.**, Voltammetric interpretation of ion transfer coupled with electron-transfer at a liquid-liquid interface, *J. Electroanal. Chem.*, 303(1-2), 171, 1991.
97. **Kotov, N. A. and Kuzmin, M. G.**, unpublished results, 1991.
98. **Lofroth, J. E., Almgren, M.**, Quenching of pyrene fluorescence by alkyl iodides in sodium dodecyl sulfide micelles *J. Phys. Chem.*, 86, 1636, 1982.
99. **Miyashita, T., Murakata, T. and Matsuda, M.**, Kinetic studies of the quenching reactions of photoexcited ruthenium(II) complexes by dialkylviologens in sodium dodecylsulfate micellar solutions, *J. Phys. Chem.*, 87, 4529, 1983.
100. **Miyashita, T., Murakata, T., Jamaquchi, J. and Matsuda, M.**, Kinetic studies of the emission quenching of photoexcited ruthenium(II) complexes by univalent and bivalent pyridinium cations in sodium dodecylsulfate solutions, *J. Phys. Chem.*, 89, 497, 1985.
101. **Dederen, J. C., Van der Auweraer, M. and De Schryver, F. C.**, Fluorescence quenching of solubilized pyrene and pyrene derivatives by metal ions in SDS micelles, *J. Phys. Chem.*, 85, 1198, 1981.
102. **Melroy, O. R. and Buck, R. P.**, Electrochemical irreversibility of ion transfer at liquid/liquid interfaces. Part II. Quasithermodynamic analysis and time dependencies for single ion transfer, *J. Electroanal. Chem.*, 99, 77, 1977.
103. **Gavach, C., D'Epenoux, B. and Henry, F.**, Transfer of tetraalkylammonium ions from water to nitrobenzene. Chronopotentiometric determination of kinetic parameters, *J. Electroanal. Chem.*, 64, 107, 1975.
104. **Koryta, J., Vanysek, P. and Brezina, M.**, Electrolysis with electrolyte dropping electrode. Part II. Basic properties of the system, *J. Electroanal. Chem.*, 75, 211, 1977.
105. **Koryta, J.**, Ion transfer across water organic-phase boundaries and analytical applications. 2., *Selective Electrode Rev.*, 13(2), 133, 1991; **Koryta, J.**, Electrochemical polarization phenomena at the interface of two immiscible electrolyte solutions. 3. Progress since 1983, *Electrochim. Acta*, 33(2), 189, 1988.
106. **Kharkats, Yu. I. and Volkov, A. G.**, Interfacial catalysis: multilectron reactions at liquid/liquid interface, *J. Electroanal. Chem.*, 184, 435 , 1985; **Kharkats, Yu. I. and Volkov, A. G.**, Membrane catalysis: synchronous multielectron reactions at the liquid/liquid interface. Bioenergetical mechanism, *Biochim. Biophys. Acta*, 891, 56, 1987; **Volkov, A. G. and Kharkats, Yu. I.**, Catalytic properties of the interface between two immiscible liquids during redox reaction, *Kinetica i Kataliz*, 26, 1322, 1985.
107. **Marcus, R. A.**, Theory of electron transfer rates across liquid/liquid interfaces. 2. Relationships and applications, *J. Phys. Chem.*, 95(5), 2010, 1991.
108. **Samec, Z., and Marecek, V.**, Charge-transfer between two immiscible electrolyte solutions. 10. Kinetics of tetraalkylammonium ion transfer across the water nitrobenzene interface, *J. Electroanal. Chem.*, 200, 17, 1986; **Wandlowski, T., Marecek, V., Samec, Z. and Holub, K.**, Ion transfer across liquid/liquid phase boundaries. Electrochemical kinetics by Faradaic impedance, *J. Phys. Chem.*, 93, 8204, 1989.
109. **Samec, Z., I., Gurevich, Yu. Ya. and Kharkats, Yu.**, Stochastic approach to the ion transfer kinetics across the interface between two immiscible electrolyte solutions. Comparison with the experimental data, *J. Electroanal. Chem.*, 204, 257, 1986.
110. **Kharkats, Yu. I. and Gurevich, Yu. Ya.**, Theory of ion transfer across interfaces between two media, *Soviet Electrochemistry*, 22(4), 463, 1986; **Kharkats, Yu. I. and Gurevich, Yu. Ya.**, Ion transfer through a phase boundary. A stochastic approach, *J. Electroanal. Chem.*, 200(1-2) 3, 1986.
111. **Samec, Z. and Marecek, V.**, Charge transfer between two immiscible electrolyte solutions. Part X. Kinetics of tetraalkylammonium ion transfer across the water-nitrobenzene interface, *J. Electroanal. Chem.*, 200, 17, 1986; **Shao, Y., Campebell, J. A., and Girault, H. H.**, Kinetics of the transfer of acetylcholine across the water nitro-benzene-tetrachloromethane interface. The Gibbs energy of transfer dependence of the standard rate-constant, *J. Electroanal. Chem.*, 300, 415, 1991; **Shao, Y. and Girault, H. H.**, Kinetics of the transfer of acetylcholine across the

water/1,2-dichloroethane interface. A comparison between ion transport and ion transfer, *J. Electroanal. Chem.*, 282, 59, 1990; **Kakiuchi, T., Noguchi, J. and Senda, M.**, Double layer effect on the transfer of some monovalent ions across the polarized oil/water interface, *J. Electroanal. Chem.*, 336(1-2), 137, 1992; **Wang, E. and Liu, Y.**, A study of proton transfer extracted by 2,2'-bipyridine from water to nitrobenzene using cyclic voltammetry, *J. Electrochem. Soc.*, 133(3), C134, 1986.

112. **Girault, H. H. and Schiffrin, D. J.**, Theory of the kinetics of ion transfer across liquid/liquid interfaces, *J. Electroanal. Chem.*, 195, 213, 1985.
113. **Memming, R.**, Kinetic Aspects in Photoelectrochemical Solar Cells, in *Photoelectrochemistry, Photocatalysis and Photoreactors. Fundamentals and Developments, NATO ASI Series, Series C: Mathematical and Physical Sciences*, Vol. 146, Schiavello, M., Ed., D. Reidel Publishing Company, Dodrecht, 1985, 107; **Peter, L. M.**, Dynamic aspects of semiconductor photoelectrochemistry, in *Homogeneous and Heterogeneous Photocatalysis, NATO ASI Series, Series C: Mathematical and Physical Sciences*, Vol. 174, Pelizzetti, E. and Serpone, N., Eds., D. Reidel Publishing Company, Dodrecht, 1989, 243; **Fox, M. A.**, Charge Injection into Semiconductor Particles - Importance in Photocatalysis, *ibid*, 363.
114. **Hiemenz, P. C.**, *Principles of Colloid and Surface Chemistry*, Marcel Dekker Inc., New York, 1993.
115. **Ogawa, N. and Freiser, H.**, Study of ion transfer at a liquid/liquid interface by current linear sweep voltammetry. 1. The 1,10-phenantroline phenantrolinium system, *Anal. Chem.*, 65(5), 517, 1993; **Sabela, A., Marecek, V., Koryta J. and Samec, Z**, Mechanism of the facilitated ion transfer across a liquid-liquid interface, *Collect. Czech. Chem. Comm.*, 59(6), 1287, 1994; **Hayoun, M., Meyer, M. and Turq, P.**, Molecular dynamics study of a solute-transfer reaction across liquid-liquid interface, *J. Phys. Chem.*, 98(26), 6626, 1994; **Stewart, A. A., Campebel, J. A., Girault, H. H. and Edowes, M.**, Cyclic voltammetry for electron-transfer reactions at liquid -liquid interfaces, *Ber. Bunzen. Ges. Phys. Chem.*, 94(1), 83, 1990.
116. **Homolka, D. and Marecek, V.**, Charge transfer between two immiscible electrolyte solutions. Part VI. Polarographic and voltammetric study of picrate ion transfer across the water/nitrobenzene interface, *J. Electroanal. Chem.*, 112, 91, 1979 and references therein.
117. **Samec, Z., Marecek, V. and Weber, J.**, Detection of an electron transfer across the interface between two immiscible electrolyte solutions by cyclic voltammetry with four electrode system, *J. Electroanal. Chem.*, 100, 841, 1979 and references therein.
118. *Tables of Physical Values*, Kikoin, I. K., Ed., Atomizdat, Moscow, 1976.

ACKNOWLEDGEMENTS

M. G. K. would like to acknowledge financial support from ISF (grant MDW000) and INTAS (grant 93-0751).

Chapter 11

EXCITED STATE ELECTRON TRANSFER AT THE INTERFACE OF TWO IMMISCIBLE ELECTROLYTE SOLUTIONS

M. Keith De Armond and Anna H. De Armond

I. INTRODUCTION

In discussing excited state electron transfer at the interface between two immiscible electrolyte solutions we necessarily must bring together the theory and practice of two distinct, even disparate, areas. The first topic, the Interface between Two Immiscible Electrolyte Solutions (ITIES), was initially developed in the laboratories of Gavach[1,2] and Czech electrochemistry community[3-7] (Koryta, Marecek and Samec) and did focus upon electrochemical methods to examine charge transfer at a polarized interface. Simultaneous with the report of these experimental methods and data, a qualitative model of the interface was developed by Marecek and Samec[8-11], with some important contributions and perspectives from the laboratory of Schiffrin[12-14]. Only in the recent years have the "pure" theoreticians[15-18] begun to examine this interface between the two liquid phases.

Contrasting this situation is the extensive photochemical literature of d^6 transition metal complexes as $[Ru(bpy)_3]^{2+}$ (bpy is 2,2-bipyridine) initiated in the 70's and continuing through the 80's until the present[19-21]. Much of the huge volume of literature was motivated by the desire to photochemically split water into H_2 and O_2 (eqn. 1)

$$H_2O \xrightarrow[\text{catalyst}]{h\nu} H_2(g) + O_2(g) \tag{1}$$

Two key problems, the need for a multielectron transfer reagent and the requirement to block energy loss have frustrated much of this effort.

From the overview of the two distinct topic areas, we focus on the topics to be elaborated for the ITIES. These include a discussion of the electrochemical and the ground state electron transfer experiments using metal complexes. A description of the contrasting models deriving from the experiments of the Prague group[8-11] and the Schiffrin group[12-14] will follow. A brief elaboration of the theoretical work of Marcus[15,16] and Benjamin[17,18] and how it may relate to electron transfer results will conclude the first section. The second section will deal with the use of the

0-8493-7694-7/96/$0.00+$.50

ITIES to block the back reaction, presenting some experimental results with some suggestions for future effort.

II. ELECTROCHEMICAL PROBING OF THE ITIES

A primary purpose of the early Prague experiments was the proper description of the interface region, so in a 1985 contribution from the Heyrovsky Institute[8], galvanostatic pulse measurements at 25°C were performed for the water/nitrobenzene interface enabling the evaluation of the capacitance as a function of the interfacial potential difference for a series of electrolytes in water and in nitrobenzene. From the data presented, the authors described the double layer in terms of the modified Verwey-Niessen (MVN) first suggested by Gavach and co-workers[2]. In this model a diffuse double layer, where one phase contains an excess of the positive charge and the other an equal excess of negative charge, is separated by a compact layer of one or two solvent molecules. The authors[8] assume that the electrolyte ions would penetrate into the inner layer.

In 1987, the Heyrovsky workers[9] used impedance and galvanostatic pulse measurements for the water/dichloroethane (DCE) system with LiCl in H_20 and tetrabutylammonium tetraphenylborate (TBATPB) in the DCE. They concluded that the interface structure is quite similar to that of water/nitrobenzene and that potential drop is mainly within the diffuse double layer.

Later, in 1987, these authors[22] summarized the importance of the measurement techniques required to calculate the interfacial capacitance, indicating that the Gouy-Chapman theory underestimated the interfacial capacitance. They noted that this discrepancy is larger for larger ions (organic layer) and when the solvent dielectric permittivity increases.

III. ELECTRON TRANSFER KINETICS

However, a conclusive statement of the interface model (from the Czech workers) occurs in a 1989 study[10] of the electrochemical kinetics of ions across the water-nitrobenzene interface at equilibrium potentials. The measurements of the rate constants for a series of mono- and divalent cations with perchlorate anions were done using an equilibrium impedance technique. The measured rate constants were substantially larger (10^2-10^3) than the previous ones. Using a three step transition state model originally proposed by Buck[23], they calculate an activation energy of 14-17 kJ mol^{-1}, which is associated with the existence of a compact solvent layer at the interface.

Ground state electron transfer at the liquid-liquid interface provides another view of this interface and a baseline for the photoelectron transfer measurement. Samec, Marecek and Weber[4] in 1979 presented the first example of an electron transfer between a species in the aqueous and one in the organic phase. Cyclic voltammetry with a four electrode potentiostat

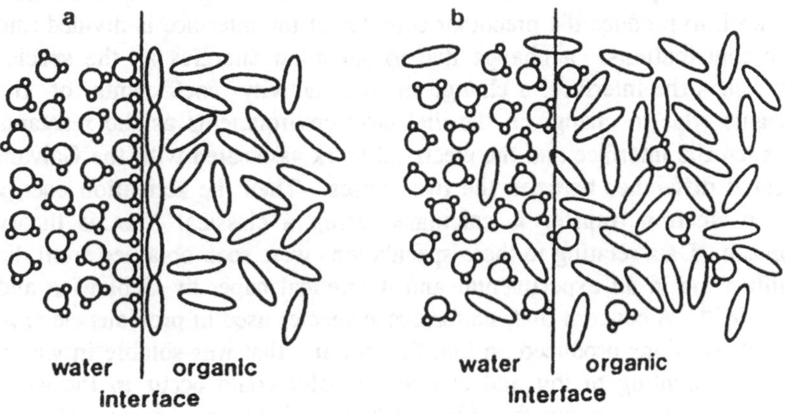

Figure 1. Model of sharp (a) and diffuse (b) boundary between two immiscible solvent.

was used to examine the electron transfer between hexacyanoferrate in the aqueous phase and ferrocene in the nitrobenzene phase (eqn. 2)

$$[Fe(CN)_6]^{3-}(w) + (C_5H_5)_2Fe(n) \,/\, [Fe(CN)_6]^{4-}(w) + [(C_5H_5)^2Fe]^+(n) \quad (2)$$

In a later paper[6], these authors used the convolution analyses procedure of Imbeaux and Saveant to obtain rate constants from the cyclic voltammogram data but were not successful, in part due to the association of the $[Fe(CN)_6]^{3-}$ ion with the alkali metal ion (Li^+ or K^+).

An alternative point of view of ground state electron transfer at the ITIES is that provided by the Schiffrin lab in South Hampton and the Girault lab in Edinburgh. In a 1987 discussion of the results of the Schiffrin-Girault cooperation and the Czechs, Girault[24] concludes that "no inner layer" exists, indeed that the potential difference appears unlikely for the two back to back double layers and that the interface region can be considered to be a "mixed solvent" region. While a part of the difference between the sharp inner layer model and the "diffuse mixed solvent" model may be semantics, it would appear that these two models do describe the limiting cases possible for the liquid-liquid interface (Figure 1).

The kinetics of ion and electron transport across the ITIES was the vehicle used by Schiffrin and Girault to argue in 1985[5,12] and 1988 articles[26] that the interface region is best described by "the diffuse mixed solvent layer" model. These authors suggest that the rate constant for transfer across the immiscible electrolyte interface measured at the potential of zero charge is most useful for elaboration of electron transfer theory. Subsequently, the authors model the electron transfer process using the homogeneous approach of Newton and Sutin[27] in which a reactive precursor complex is followed by the rate determining electron transfer. The work to produce the precursor complex at the interface is divided into three contributions: a change due to solvation energies as the species approaches the interface, a change in the activity coefficients of the reactants due to change in the dielectric environments as the reactants approach the interface and the electrical work associated with the Galvani potential difference between the two phases. Then the activation energy for the electron transfer is calculated using a classical Marcus theory approach. Data relating to these speculations were soon obtained from the Schiffrin lab in an experimental and theoretical paper by Geblewicz and Schiffrin[14]. A concern that the ferrocene species used in previous electron transfer reactions produced an ion, ferricinium, that was soluble in water, (hence a coupling of ion and electron transfer could occur in the same phase) was the impetus for this Schiffrin - Geblewicz work. Results reported simultaneous with the initiation of this work indicate that the ferrocene and ferrociniuim ion interface crossover potential occur independently of one another. Nevertheless, the Lutetium bipthalocyanine, Lu $(PC)_2$ was substituted for ferrocene since neither the Lutetium complex nor its oxidation product is “soluble” in water. Consequently electron transfer is sure to be the only process observed. Moreover the authors chose a large excess of the $[Fe(CN)_6]^{3-/4-}$ redox couple so that only the diffusion of the Lutetium complex had to be considered. Such conditions enabled them to analyze the voltammetry results using the classical (Marcus) theory for metal electrodes.

The authors determined that the electron transfer was quasi-reversible and using the Nicholson calculation method[28] they obtained a value of 0.9×10^{-3} ms^{-1} for the electron transfer process. For the theoretical calculations of the rate constant, the rate constant for each of these redox couples with a metal electrode was utilized. For the Lutetium complex, no data was available, therefore an estimated $k'^{o} = 0.04$ cms^{-1} was used, that had been obtained for porphyrins. The $k'^{o} = 0.02$ cms^{-1} for $[Fe(CN)_6]^{3-}$ was obtained from the work of Peter and co-workers[29]. Geblewicz and Schiffrin used an impedance method to calculate a $k' = 0.035$ cms^{-1}. The electron transfer constant is at least a factor of 10 smaller than the rate constants of the redox couples. The authors assume the "mixed solvent" (diffuse) interface model in an attempt to "correct" the measured k^{o}, therefore presuming that the applied potential will appear across the two diffuse double layers. Moreover, the large excess of the aqueous phase concentration enables them to reduce the problem to a calculation of the potential drop that occurs across the organic phase only. They measured a lower value of k^o than on the metal electrode and rationalized this as resulting from differences in the solvent reorganization for the liquid-liquid interface from that of the metal electrode. An alternative rationale is that the distance between the redox centers in the liquid-liquid interface differ from the distances of the metal electrodes.

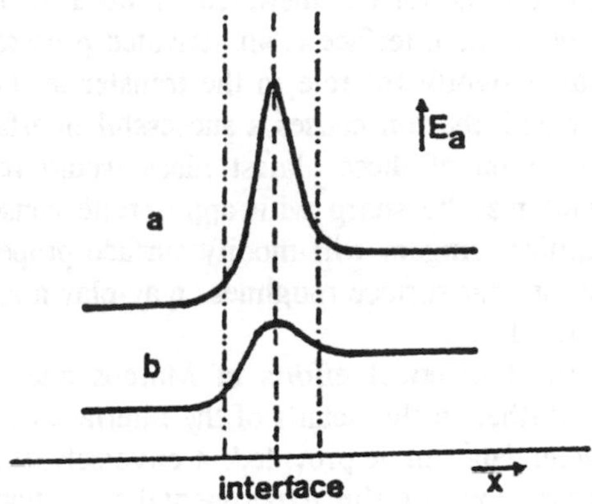

Figure 2. Model of activation energy barrier of the sharp (a) and diffuse (b) interface between two immiscible electrolyte solutions.

IV. THEORY OF ELECTRON TRANSFER RATES ACROSS LIQUID-LIQUID INTERFACES

The Marcus work of 1990[17] makes an improvement upon the Geblewicz-Schiffrin model by avoiding the assumption that one phase containing the high concentration of reactant behaves as a metal interface. Here Marcus used the expression for the exchange rate constant k''_{12} for an electron transfer between the two redox species in the separate phases. From this assumption he obtained a calculated value of 0.01 M cm s^{-1} for a sharp boundary and 1 M cm s^{-1} for the diffuse boundary, these to be compared with the experimental value of 0.03 M cm s^{-1} from the Geblewicz and Schiffrin data. However, in view of the uncertainties in the experimental data and the assumptions of the theory, the data do not enable conclusions about the diffuse or sharp nature of the interface to be made.

The ability of theory to discriminate between the two limiting models of the interface was tested by the molecular dynamics contributions of Ilan Benjamin[15,16]. In the first paper, Benjamin concludes that the calculations indicate a molecularly sharp interface with "capillary wavelength distortions" at the interface. Some of this distortion would result in fingers as long as 8Å, thus resulting in a rough surface. Benjamin also suggests that ordered water molecules would exist at the interface, as would be expected for a sharp interface, however, he suggests that this orientation would not contribute more than a few kJ to any interface barrier (Figure 2). In his most recent contribution[16], Benjamin concedes that this activation barrier question is not yet answered. Indeed, he does conclude that ion transfer through the interface is an activated process and that the capillary fingers play a significant role in the transfer of the ion, i.e. the contact of the finger with the ion causes a successful interface transition. So, a useful interpretation of these latest ideas would recognize that, although the interface may be sharp with appropriate consequences, the existence of the capillary fingers will modify surface properties. A key result is the recognition that surface roughness may play a substantial role in ion and electron transfer.

At this stage, the theoretical efforts of Marcus and Benjamin are unlikely to progress further in the details of the interface description until additional rate constant data can be provided. Conversely, the utility of the interface model description for the experimentalist is that the role of energy barriers and solvent or electrolyte effects may be limited. The current situation is in limbo and awaits a series of precise redox rate constant measurements with a systematic and significant variation of solution parameters so that, at least, a correct pragmatic interface model can be produced.

V. THE PHOTOCHEMICAL REDOX PROCESS

While the lack of a correct detailed description of the interface model may slow the systematic utilization of the ITIES, an empirical approach can continue. The appearance of a unique interface result by I. Willner and coworkers[30] in 1984 did stimulate our interest in the use of the ITIES system for photoredox systems. In a two-phase water organic system excluding supporting electrolyte species, these workers did produce a photoinduced one electron reduction product of N,N'-dioctylbipyridiniium (C_8V^{2+}) that does result in a disproportion due to an additional electron reduction. The two phase system also served to separate the products of the disproportionation in the two phases. This result, together with the prior experience that one of us had with electrochemical ITIES methods, did provide motivation for the initiation of discussions and assembly of appropriate equipment for the combined liquid-liquid electrochemistry and photochemistry effort. The other relevant preliminary experimental results to this ITIES photochemistry effort derive from two papers dealing with the ITIES cyclic voltammetry (CV) of the compound, tris-bipyridine

Ruthenium(II), in which Marecek and coworkers[31] reported the ion transfer of the Ru(II) complex across the interface. An extension[32] of the CV results to other bipyridine complexes indicated that the transfer of $[M(bpy)_3]^{2+}$ ions from water to 1,2-dichloroethane resulted in the simple ion transfer of the intact metal complex for $M^{2+} = Ru^{2+}$, Os^{2+} and Fe^{2+}, but that the charge transfer for $M^{2+} = Zn^{2+}$, Co^{2+} and Cu^{2+} resulted in accompanying chemical changes to the chemical species[34]. To date, no other simple transport across an ITIES for these metal complexes appears to have been reported.

In contrast, the photochemistry of metal complexes, in particular Ru(II) photocomplexes, has received an immense amount of attention dating from the late seventies and diminishing only recently. The quantity of the work and the variety of metal complexes, mostly (Ru(II) complexes is immense as suggested by the comprehensive review articles[19-21], dealing with the photochemical and photophysical properties of these materials. A major fraction of the studies have been concerned with the creation of a useful high energy catalysis products as, for example, hydrogen and oxygen from water or electric power light absorbing Ru(II) complex systems. In all of these different processes, homogeneous and heterogeneous alike, one key problem is the blocking of the so called "back reaction".

Using the $[Ru(bpy)_3]^{2+}$ species, the basic thermodynamics of the photocharge transfer can be illustrated (eqns. 3 and 4).

$$*[Ru(bpy)_3]^{2+} + Q \,/\, [Ru(bpy)_3]^{3+} + Q^- \text{ (oxidative quenching)}, \quad (3)$$

$$*[Ru(bpy)_3]^{2+} + Q \,/\, [Ru(bpy)_3]^{+} + Q^+ \text{ (reductive quenching)}, \quad (4)$$

Q is an electron transfer quencher and $*[Ru(bpy)_3]^{2+}$ is the excited state reactant. A problem in the production of such high energy photoproducts as $[Ru(bpy)_3]^{3+}$ and Q^+ is the so called "back reaction", e.g. (5).

$$Q^- + [Ru(bpy)_3]^{3+} \,/\, [Ru(bpy)_3]^{2+} + Q, \quad (5)$$

A majority of the electron transfer studies attempting to solve this back reaction problem have utilized <u>homogeneous</u> media in which both donor and acceptor are in the same liquid phase. Typifying this approach is the detailed and precise work of Hoffman and coworkers[33,34], who used sacrificial reagents to block the endoergonic back reaction of the photoproducts. Another approach to blocking the back reaction is the use of <u>heterogeneous</u> media, as illustrated by the electron transfer experiments of the Calvin[35,36] and Matsuo[37,38] groups, who utilized lipid vesicle and membrane media to provide charge separation capable of blocking the back reaction. Typically, the charge transfer efficiency was small because the media used were insulating. Also Fendler[39] and Gratzel[40] have utilized vesicles to produce electron transfer and charge separation. Contrasting these liquid phase heterogeneous media are porous vicor glass media of Gafney and coworkers[41,42] and the clay and the silica gel media of Kerry Thomas[43,44]. In these systems, a liquid - solid interface typically blocks the back reaction. One of the charge transfer species, often a donor metal complex, is bound at a site in the solid medium resulting in a static quenching of the excited state by the electron transfer. The heterogeneous approach was our original motivation for use of the liquid-liquid system to separate the charged transfer products.

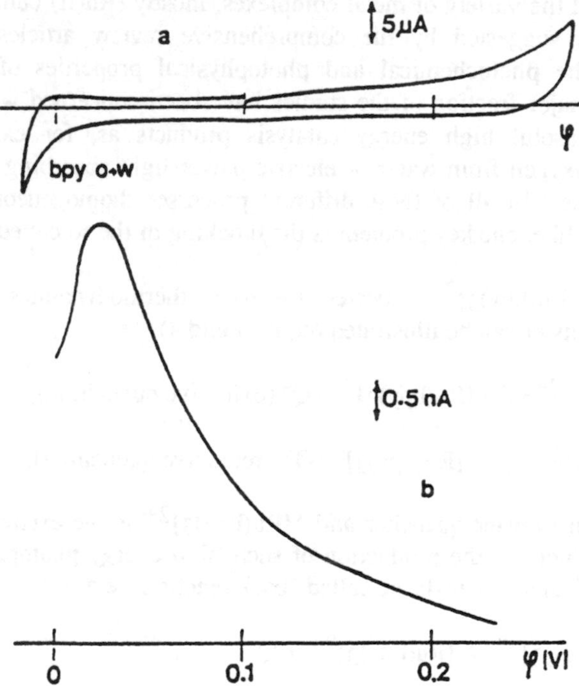

Figure 3. Cyclic voltammogram (a) and dc potential dependence of the system containing 10^{-2} M $Ru(bpy)_3(CBB)_2$ in 1,2-dichloroethane. For galvanic cell see a diagram above. Polarization rate was 20 mV/s, chopper frequency 10.4 Hz, light intensity 100 mW/cm^2.

The use of the ITIES technique to separate charge transfer products of photoexcitation is an unusual and novel heterogeneous liquid technique for solving the back reaction problem using the donor (D) - acceptor (A) electron transfer system, because these products are present in the different phases (contrary to the homogeneous media). In the ITIES photosystem, the heterogeneous liquid media avoid use of a sacrificial reagent. Since the two immiscible solvents with dissolved salts are electrolyte media, a controlling potential can enrich the phases at the interface, with properly chosen reactants. These heterogeneous liquid media differ from the heterogeneous solid media described above and are able to produce high charge transfer yields.

VI. PHOTOEFFECTS AT THE POLARIZED LIQUID-LIQUID INTERFACE

The initial photochemical electron transfer system examined was the $[Ru(bpy)_3]^{2+}$/methyl viologen system and was reported nearly simultaneously in the DeArmond[45] and Girault[46] labs, however the details of the experiments were different. The reaction in the DeArmond lab utilized the $[Ru(bpy)_3]^{2+}$ donor in the form of a CBB^- salt (CBB^- is hexabromomonocarbadodecaborane(6) - $[CB_{11}Br_6H_6]^-$) and it was dissolved in the dichloroethane (1,2-DCE) or the benzonitrile (BN) phase while the methylviologen chloride, the more hydrophilic substance, was dissolved in the aqueous phase. Thus the galvanic cell used was:

Ag | AgCl | 0.025 M LiCl, H_2O || 0.001 M TPAsCBB, 1,2-DCE or BN | 0.01 M TPAsCl, H_2O | AgCl | Ag

Particularly significant are the supporting electrolyte species, with LiCl used for the aqueous and tetraphenylarsonium hexabromomonocarbadodecacaborane(6) (TPAsCBB) used in the organic phase.

The Girault experiment dissolved the donor $[Ru(bpy)_3]^{2+}$ cation in the aqueous phase and used hexadecyl-4,4'-bipyridinium chloride as the acceptor in the organic (toluene or DCE) phase. While the DeArmond group used the colored TPAsCBB species as the organic supporting electrolyte, the Girault experiment used the photosensitive[47] tetraphenylborate as the supporting electrolyte. Further, the irradiation of the Pt electrode in the cell construction could produce another complication since irradiated Pt electrodes in aqueous solution are known to produce a photocurrent[48]. Nevertheless, the likelihood is that the photocurrent measured did contain some contribution from the donor-acceptor pair. Typical Marecek-DeArmond results with Pt electrodes (shielded from light) are shown in Figure 3 where the cyclic voltammetry curves demonstrate how the DC polarizing potential is used to bring the donor and acceptor ions to the interface permitting charge transfer.

The Marecek-DeArmond results[45] could be analyzed by one or more of three mechanisms, each differing in the microscopic location of the electron transfer process:

$$[Ru(bpy)_3]^{2+}(o) + [MV]^{2+}(w) / [Ru(bpy)_3]^{3+}(o) + [MV]^{+}(w) \qquad (a)$$

$$[Ru(bpy)_3]^{2+}(o) / [Ru(bpy)_3]^{2+}(w) \qquad (b)$$

$$[Ru(bpy)_3]^{2+}(w) + [MV]^{2+}(w) / [Ru(bpy)_3]^{3+}(w) + [MV]^{+}(w)$$

$$[MV]^{2+}(w) / [MV]^{2+}(o) \qquad (c)$$

$$[Ru(bpy)_3]^{2+}(o) + [MV]^{2+}(o) / [Ru(bpy)_3]^{3+}(o) + [MV]^{+}(o)$$

Reaction (a) is a photoinduced electron transfer occurring at the interface (the interface is used to block the back reaction) while equation (b) involves transfer of the metal complex to the aqueous phase and the subsequent homogeneous reaction. This was excluded as the dominant process on the basis of the phase shift of the current from the applied potential. The homogeneous phase reaction in the organic phase (c) as a major source of the photocurrent was discounted since the concentration of the MV^{2+} at the interface was decreasing in the potential range of the maximum photocurrent.

To verify these results from the Marecek-DeArmond collaboration, the experimental system was modified (see Experimental section) and the experiment for the $[Ru(bpy)_3]^{2+}/MV^{2+}$ system repeated[49]. To determine if the photocurrent of the $[Ru(bpy)]_3{}^{2+}/MV^{2+}$ could result from a bulk solution reaction both donor and quencher were dissolved in the same phase. No photocurrent was measurable even with the new more sensitive detection system. Further, it was not possible to detect transfer of reaction products ($[Ru(bpy)_3]^{3+}$ and MV^{+}) across the interface, and both products are known to be stable under these reaction conditions.

To ascertain the generality of the electron transfer across the polarized liquid-liquid interface, another photoactive Ru(II) complex, $[Ru(bpz)_3]^{2+}$ (where bpz is 2,2'-bipyrazine) was used with ferrocene or dppd (where dppd is N,N'-diphenyl-1,4-phenylenediamine) as the excited state quencher[50].

The electrochemical cell for the photoeffect measurements was

Ag	AgCl	0.1M LiCl	0.01M $MgSO_4$ or $Ru(bpz)_3(NO_3$	0.01M TBACBB	0.01M TBACl	AgCl	Ag
			H_2O	1,2-DCE	H_2O		

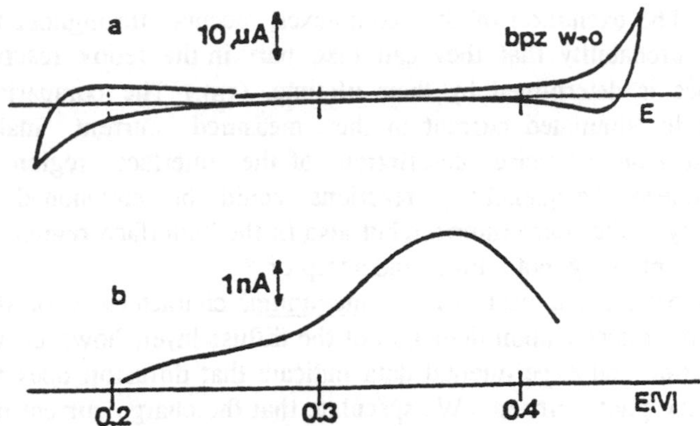

Figure 4. Cyclic voltammetry (a) and dc potential dependence of the interfacial quenching photoreaction (b) of the system containing $5x10^{-3}$ M $Ru(bpz)_3(NO_3)_2$ in the aqueous phase and 10^{-4}M ferrocene in 1,2-dichloroethane. For the reaction and the galvanic cell see above. Polarization rate was 20 mV/s, chopper frequency 10.4 Hz, light intensity 100 mW/cm^2.

The $[Ru(bpz)_3]^{2+}$ complex is more hydrophilic than $[Ru(bpy)_3]^{2+}$ but has comparable excited state energy and lifetime properties to the $[Ru(bpy)_3]^{2+}$. However the ground state electrochemical properties of $[Ru(bpz)_3]^{2+}$ are shifted ~0.5V positive relative to the oxidation and redox potentials of the $[Ru(bpy)_3]^{2+}$. Thus, the $[Ru(bpz)_3]^{2+}$ reduction potential occurs at E° = - 0.7V as SCE. Consequently the excited state of the bpz complex, $*[Ru(bpz)_3]^{2+}$, now becomes a strong oxidizing agent, rather than a reducing agent as $*[Ru(bpy)_3]^{2+}$. The reaction for the ferrocene quencher would be:

$$*[Ru(bpz)_3]^{2+}(w)+Fe(C_5H_5)^2(o) / [Ru(bpz)_3]^+(w)+[Fe(C_5H_5)_2]^+(o) \quad (6)$$

An analogous photoreaction takes place for the dppd species.

Both photocurrent and photopotential measurements were done and a typical photocurrent and photopotential measurement is shown in Figure 4. The amplitudes of the photopotential and the photocurrent were proportional to the light intensity (λ_{max} = 443 nm) and the concentration of the $[Ru(bpz)_3]^{2+}$ species.

Here, as for the $[Ru(bpy)_3]^{2+}$, the contribution of bulk reaction to the photocurrent was estimated to be negligible, although the steady state current is controlled by the creation of the excited state species at the "interface." (The excitation of the complexes occurs throughout the phase but the probability that they can take part in the redox reaction on the interface is determined by their lifetime, (τ_p).) The comparison of the digitally simulated current to the measured current makes apparent that a more precise description of the interface region is necessary. Indeed, the quenching reactions could be envisioned to occur not only at the sharp interface but also in the "interface region" in a thin layer containing both donor and acceptor.

Figure 4 produces a peak with a maximum, characteristic of that observed in voltammetry upon depletion of the diffuse layer, however, the digital simulation and experimental data indicate that diffusion does not contribute to the photo current. We speculate that the charge current due to the Ru(II) complex transfer across the interface cancels some portion of the photocurrent resulting in the photocurrent peak shape.

VII. ANOMALOUS PHOTOEFFECTS

The observation of a photopotential for light absorbing species at the liquid-liquid interface was ascribed to a photothermal effect that is this amplified by the liquid-liquid interface[51]. Subsequently two experiments[49] were done that corrected this description of the effect. First, the $[Fe(bpy)_3]^{2+}$ complex was excited in the liquid-liquid cell and no photoinduced potential was observed. The $[Fe(bpy)_3]^{2+}$ has an absorption spectrum virtually identical to that of $[Ru(bpy)_3]^{2+}$, however, the Fe(II) complex does not produce a long lived MLCT excited state due to a low lying d-d* excited state for the Fe complex. This result suggested that the MLCT state and not a photothermal effect must play a key role in the occurrence of the photopotential for the $[Ru(bpy)_3)^{2+}$. Subsequently, examination of the O_2 effect in experiment demonstrated that a bimolecular quenching process in which O_2 quenches the $*[Ru(bpy)_3]^{2+}$ is the source of the photopotential.[47] The absence of a photopotential for the aerated $[Ru(bpz)_3]^{2+}$ is consistent with this mechanism since $[Ru(bpz)_3]^{2+}$ is not quenched by O_2.

VIII. KINETICS OF CHARGE TRANSFER

The impedance measurements[49] were done with the same experimental arrangement as the photoeffect measurements and with a 4 $MHzs^{-1}$ sine wave source used to modulate the signal. The photocurrent and photopotential are measured simultaneously for the interface region which we consider to be the photochemical source of electricity. The photocurrent and photovoltage are related by the impedance of the system and this impedance behavior can be modeled by the Randles

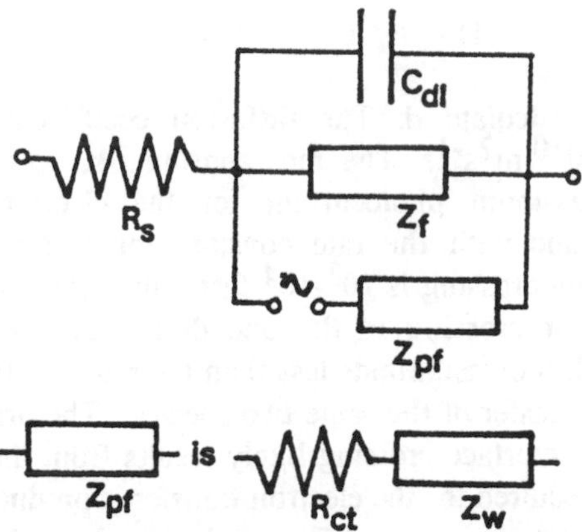

Figure 5. Equivalent circuit for ITIES system in the dark (Randles) and under illumination (including branch with photoelectrochemical source and Z_{pf}). R_S - electrolyte resistance, Z_f - faradaic impedance in the dark (comprising of supporting electrolytes and nonphotoprocesses impedance), C_{dl} - double layer capacity, Z_{pf} - faradaic impedance of the photoprocess, R_{ct}- charge transfer resistance, Z_W - Wartburg impedance.

equivalent circuit (Figure 5). The amplitudes of the photocurrent and photopotential and the phase shift between them enable calculation of the real impedance, Z_r, and the imaginary impedance, Z_i. The impedance, Z, of the system in the dark was measured by a standard technique. The resistance, $R_{S,}$ unaffected by light, determined the high frequency limit of the real part of the "dark" impedance. Then R_S was subtracted from both the "dark" and "light" real impedance. After converting these data to admittances, the Faradaic admittances (real and imaginary) were calculated by subtracting "dark" admittances (real and imaginary). The resultant admittance data were then converted to impedance, Z_{pf}. Since accurate measurements were done only for frequencies below 80 Hz, k is calculated from the difference between the Z_r and Z_i part of Z_{pf} ($Z_{pf} = Z_r - Z_i$). This difference, equal to R_{ct}, enables use of eqn. (7)

$$R_{ct} = RTnFi_o. \tag{7}$$

to calculate the exchange current, i_o. Then eqn. (8) can be used to calculate k for this one dimensional electron transfer, process

$$i_o = nFAkc \tag{8}$$

where A is the interfacial area and c is the concentration of the excited state of the Ruthenium complex. The area, A, is estimated by determining the distance, d, from which the excited state Ru(II) complex can diffuse before the excited state decays. The Einstein-Smoluchowski equation

$$D = d^2/2t \tag{9}$$

can then be used to calculate d. The diffusion coefficient[32], D, of $[Ru(bpy)_3]^{2+}$ is 2.51×10^{10} m^2s^{-1}. The rate constant, k, was estimated to be 10^2-10^3 at maximum photocurrent for the electron transfer. Comparison of this value with the rate constant for crossing of <u>ions</u> indicates that the electron crossing is 10^3-10^4 faster than the ion crossing, but the rate constant for crossing of the one dimensional interface is approximately three orders of magnitude less than the rate constant for the homogeneous electron transfer of the same two species. The origin of the much smaller k for the interface crossing likely results from the fact that the precursor complex required for the electron transfer is produced only at the interface since the particles are in different phases. In such a process occurring at the sharp boundary of the heterogeneous interface, the electron likely must traverse a larger barrier than the electron involved in the transfer between donor and acceptor for the homogeneous reaction. This restriction (of the forward reaction rate constant) may provide significant overall advantage since it apparently effectively prevents the back electron transfer and, consequently, permits efficient charge separation.

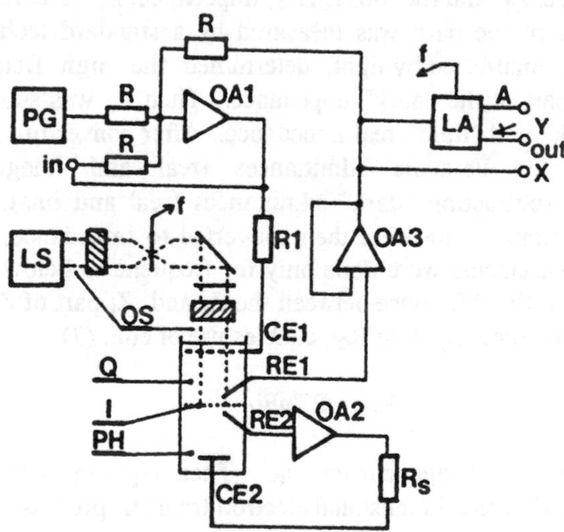

Figure 6. Galvanostatic experimental setup: PG - pulse generator, LS - light source, LA - lock-in amplifier, OS - optical system (for the details see Ref. 51), Q - quencher containing phase, I - ITIES, PH - photosensitive compound containing phase, CE_1, RE_1, CE_2, RE_2 - counter and reference electrodes of the phase 1 and 2, OA - operational amplifiers, R - 100 kW resistor, R_1 - 200 kW resistor.

IX. THE INSTRUMENTAL SYSTEM

The measurement system (Figure 6) used for the standard electrochemical measurements (cyclic voltammetry) has remained approximately constant. The optical system has evolved and the one currently used is indicated in Figure 7. A 500 W Xe lamp used with fiber

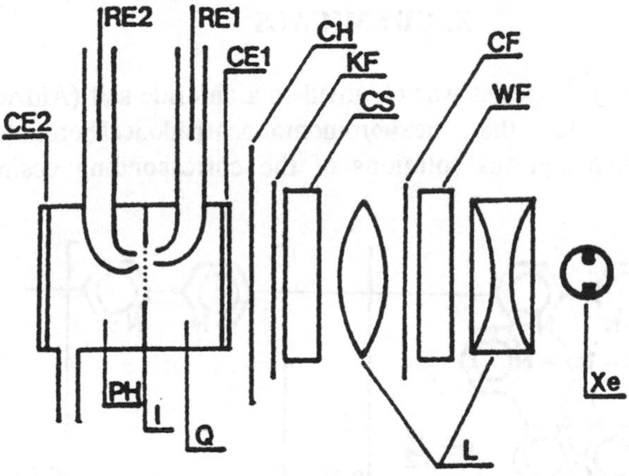

Figure 7. Optical setup with vertical interface: CE_1, RE_1, CE_2, RE_2 - counter (from transparent ITO slides) and reference electrodes of the phase 1 and 2, PH - photosensitive compound containing phase, I - glass septum with vertical interface (dotted line), Q - quencher containing phase, CH - chopper, KF - Kodak gelatin filter No. 2C, Cs - cuvette with saturated solution of $CuSO_4$, WF - cuvette filled with water, Xe - Xe lamp.

optic cable to focus the filtered broad band radiation that was then chopped. The modulated excitation was focused upon the vertically oriented interface with transparent Tin doped Indium oxide current electrodes and Luggin capillaries now replacing the Pt electrodes of the earlier cell. The galvanic cell used in the measurements was described previously in the text.

The four electrode potentiostat connected to the all glass electrochemical cell is shown in Fig. 6. The photoinduced potential difference was measured by a two-phase lock-in amplifier (Stanford Research System 530). The dc potential was varied using a small current in the galvanostatic mode. The four electrode potentiostat provided the galvanostatic function by connecting the output of the operational amplifier, OA1, to the second program input (in) through which the resistor R_1 at the counter electrode, CE1, was connected. The other potentiostat connections were not changed so the reference electrode, RE2, is connected to the virtual ground. Therefore, the output of the voltage follower, OA3, that provides both the ac and the dc components of the potential difference across the interface could be recorded. The lock-in amplifier and the X input of an X-Y recorder were connected to the output of OA3. The Y output of the recorder could be connected to the amplitude or phase shift output of the lock-in amplifier. Impedance measurements were done with the same system as above but with the addition of a signal generator, a 4 MHz sine wave generator, Wavetech Model 182 A.

X. CHEMICALS

The $Ru(bpy)_3^{2+}$ species was obtained as a chloride salt (Aldrich) and was converted to the hexabromomonocarbadodecaborane(6) by precipitation from aqueous solutions of the corresponding cesium salt dissolved in a

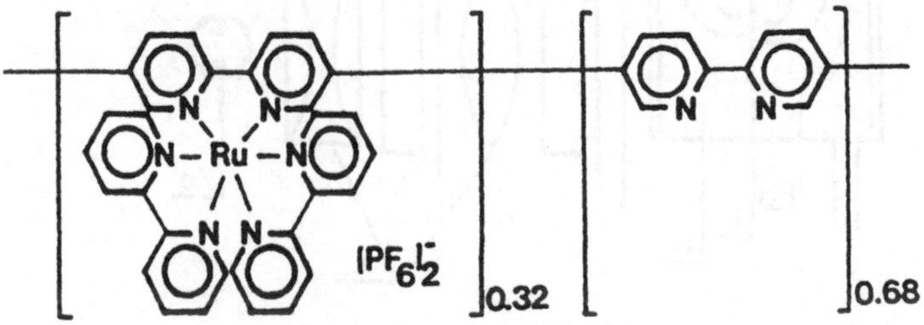

Figure 8. Structure of Ruthenium (II) Polybipyridine complex.

mixture of ethanol and water. The $Ru(bpz)_3Cl_2$ salt was prepared and purified by a literature procedure[52]. Since the chloride salt resulted in spurious photochemistry upon irradiation, this complex salt was converted to the nitrate salt using an aqueous solution of silver nitrate (precipitation of AgCl and subsequent separation of the $[Ru(bpz)_3](NO_3)_2$). Ferrocene and $FeCl_3$ (for preparation of $[Fe(bpy)_3]Cl_2$) were Aldrich products. The $[Fe(bpy)_3]Cl_2$ was prepared by mixing an ethanol water solution of the ligand with $FeCl_3$. The cesium hexabromomonocarbadodecaborane(6) was a gift from Karel Base, currently with Boron Biologicals, Inc., Research Triangle, NC.

Tetrabutylammonium chloride (Aldrich) and tetraheptylammonium bromide (Aldrich) were used with the cesium hexabromocarbadodecaborane(6) to produce tetraalkylammonium salts of the hexabromomonocarbadodecaborane(6) by a procedure similar to that used to produce the metal complex salts. Lithium chloride was an Aldrich product.

The organic materials, as methylviologen dichloride (Aldrich), and N,N'-diphenyl-1,4-phenylenediamine (dppd) were obtained form Aldrich.

Extensive purification was required for the latter material[50], and the dppda was stored in the dark in an oxygen and water free environment.

The solvent dichloroethane (HPLC grade) was used. The benzonitrile solvent (Aldrich) was fractionally distilled and only the middle portion of the distillate used.

XI. THE FUTURE OF ITIES PHOTOEFFECTS

The results obtained for the photo processes with $[Ru(bpy)_3]^{2+}$ and $[Ru(bpz)_3]^{2+}$ do suggest that efficient charge separation is accomplished with the liquid-liquid interface. However, a question remains whether the methodology can be generalized and the efficiency improved. To this purpose additional photoexcited Ru(II) complexes with various donors and acceptors should be examined for the DCE/H_2O system and the benzonitrile/H_2O system. The earlier results suggest that, although the efficiency may be as high as 40% for some systems, the choice of Ru(II) complexes (or other photoexcited species) that are adsorbed at the liquid-liquid interface could increase the efficiency close to 100%. Therefore, very hydrophobic species as $[Ru(biq)_3]^{2+}$, where biq is 2,2'-biquinoline, should be examined. Another type of metal complex that could result in adsorption at the water-organic interface is a mixed ligand complex molecule as, for example, the $[Ru(bpz)_2\ biq]^{2+}$ complex, in which the bpz ligands would produce a hydrophilic portion of the molecule and the biq ligand would provide a hydrophobic portion of the molecule. One of the most intriguing possibilities for adsorption at the interface with subsequent enhancement of the charge separation efficiency is the oligomeric $Ru(bpy)_2Pbpy^{n+}$ (Figure 8), in which Pbpy is 5,5'-diyl-2,2'-bipyridine ligand. The rigid rod-like structure of the Pbpy ligand has produced ESR results for the reduced species suggesting that this covalently bonded bpy backbone is conducting[53].

"Media manipulation" to vary and, perhaps, enhance the charge separation efficiency can also be attempted. Thus, stirring of the photochemical layer to keep the diffusion layer thin and constant will be attempted to avoid the depletion of the photochemically active species.

A second method could utilize the sol-gel methodology in combination with the Langmuir-Blodgett method. In these experiments, the water layer of the water/DCE system would be replaced by a siloxane sol-gel system. This could mimic the $[Ru(bpy)_3]^{2+}$/methylviologen liquid-liquid experiment. The goal of such experiments would be the stabilization and isolation of the reduced MV^+ in the siloxane and the oxidized $[Ru(bpy)_3]^{3+}$ product in the dichloroethane layer. As in the previous liquid-liquid study, the photocurrent measurements can be done for these sol-gel systems. The ability to monitor the paramagnetic redox products via ESR spectroscopy could provide a quantitative measure of the product concentration that could be correlated with the photocurrent measured.

A desire to characterize the liquid-liquid interface, both to provide a fundamental understanding of the interface and to enable improvement of the charge separation efficiency suggests spectroscopic experiments. A spectroscopic probe could, if properly exploited, distinguish the continuous mixed solvent interface model from the sharp boundary (Verwey-Niessen) model. Early in this article, the modeling efforts of Benjamin favoring the sharp boundary method were described. Benjamin's theory and the experimental work of Mary Wirth[54,55] point up the role of "surface roughness" in describing a liquid-liquid interface. The use of evanescent wave excitation to probe the interface by monitoring the luminescence decay

$$r(t) = \frac{I_{II}(t) - I\wedge(t)}{I_{II}(t) - 2I\wedge(t)} \tag{10}$$

Where I_{II} is the intensity of emission polarized parallel to the absorption polarization and $I\wedge$ is emission polarized perpendicular at time (t). The theory for hindered motion at an interface has been developed[55] and applied to a liquid-liquid interface of an alkane with water, not an ITIES media, but pertinent to the polarized liquid-liquid interface since water and an organic solvent were used.

A final topic area that may ultimately contribute to the utility of the ITIES are the experiments using an interface to obtain second harmonic generation. Several years ago we proposed laser probing of the ITIES interface to obtain nonlinear optical effects. Now three research groups have programs that ultimately could use an ITIES system to produce a SHG signal, (second harmonic generation). Among these, the group of R. Corn at the University of Wisconsin has succeeded in producing a photoinduced electron transfer[56] at the interface using second harmonic generation method. However extension of this technique to obtain electron transfer for a variety of redox couples is limited by the requirement for an adsorption of the nonlinear probe at the interface and this group's use of the photoactive tetraphenylborate ion[47] The groups of Eisenthal (Columbia)[57] and Richmond (Oregon)[58] have used the second harmonic generation technique to examine a variety of phenomena at solid-air interfaces including polarization of water at the air-liquid interface, adsorption of molecules, and surface structure of a variety of solid electrochemical surface. To date, no publication of a SHG effort probing an ITIES system has appeared.

XII. REFERENCES

1. **Gavach, C. and Henry, F. J.**, Chronopotentiometric investigation of the diffusion overvoltage at the interface between two non-miscible solutions, *J. Electroanal. Chem.*, 54, 361, 1974.
2. **Gavach, C., Seta, P. and d'Epenoux, B.**, The double layer and ion adsorption at the interface between two non-miscible solutions Part I Interfacial tension measurements for the water-nitrobenzene, *J. Electroanal. Chem.* , *83*, 225, 1977.
3. **Samec, Z., Marecek, V., Weber, J. and Homolka, D.**, Investigation of ion transfer across the interface between two immiscible electrolyte solutions by cyclic voltammetry, *J. Electroanal. Chem.*, 126, 105, 1981.
4. **Samec, Z., Marecek, V. and Weber, J.**, Charge transfer between two immiscible electrolyte solutions. II. The investigation of Cesium ion transfer across the nitrobenzene/water interface by cyclic voltammetry with IR compensation, *J. Electroanal. Chem.*, 100, 841, 1971.
5. **Homolka, D., Hung, L. Q., Hofmanova, A., Khalil, J., Koryta, J., Marecek, V., Samec, Z., Sen, S. K., Vanysek, P., Weber, J. and Brezina, M.**, Faradaic ion transfer across the interface of two immiscible electrolyte solutions: Chronopotentiometry and cyclic voltammetry, *Anal. Chem.*, 52, 1606, 1980.
6. **Samec, Z., Marecek, V., Weber, J., Homolka, D., Samec, Z., Marecek, V., Weber, J. and Homolka, D.**, Charge transfer between two immiscible electrolyte solutions. Part VII. Convolution potential sweep voltammetry of ion transfer and of electron transfer between ferrocene and hexacyanoferrate ion across the water-nitrobenzene interface, *J. Electroanal. Chem.*, 126, 105, 1981.
7. **Marecek, V. and Samec, Z.**, Fast performance galvanostatic pulse technique for evaluation of the ohmic potential drop and capacitance of the interface between two immiscible electrolyte solutions, *J. Electroanal. Chem.*, 185, 263, 1985.
8. **Samec, Z., Marecek, V. and Homolka, D.**, The double layer at the interface between two immiscible electrolyte solutions. Part II. Structure of the water/nitrobenzene interface, *J. Electroanal Chem.*, 187, 31, 1985.
9. **Samec, Z., Marecek, V., Holub, K., Racinsky, S., and Hajkova, P.**, The double layer at the interface between two immiscible electrolyte solutions Part III Capacitance of the water/1,2-dichloroethane interface, *J. Electroanal Chem.*, 225, 65, 1987.
10. **Wandlowski, T., Marecek, V., Holub, K. and Samec, Z.**, Ion transfer across liquid-liquid phase boundaries: Electrochemical kinetics by faradaic impedance, *J. Phys. Chem.*, 93, 8204, 1989.
11. **Samec, Z., Marecek, V. and Homolka, D.**, The double layer at the interface between two immiscible electrolyte solutions. Part II. The water/nitrobenzene interface in the presence of 1:1 and 2:2 electrolytes, *J. Electroanal. Chem.*, 187, 31, 1987.
12. **Girault, H. H. and Schiffrin, D. J.**, Thermodynamics of a polarized interface between two immiscible electrolyte solutions, *J. Electroanal. Chem.*, 170, 127, 1984.

13. **Girault, H. H. and Schiffrin, D. J.**, Electron transfer reactions at the interface between two immiscible electrolyte solutions, *J. Electroanal. Chem.*, 244, 15, 1988.
14. **Geblewicz, G. and Schiffrin, D. J.**, Electron transfer between immiscible solutions the hexacyanoferrate-Lutetium biphthalocyanine system, *J. Electroanal Chem.*, 244, 27, 1988.
15. **Benjamin, I.**, Theoretical study of the water/1,2-dichloroethane interface: Structure, dynamics and conformation equilibrium at the liquid-liquid interface, *J. Chem. Phys.*, 97, 1432, 1992.
16. **Benjamin, I.**, Mechanism and dynamics of ion transfer across a liquid-liquid interface, *Science*, 261, 1558, 1993.
17. **Marcus, R. A.**, Theory of electron transfer rates across liquid-liquid interfaces *J. Phys. Chem.*, 94, 4152, 1990.
18. **Marcus, R. A.**, Theory of electron transfer rates across liquid-liquid interfaces. 2 Relationships and application, *J. Phys. Chem.*, 95, 2010, 1991.
19. **Kalyanasundaram, K.**, Photophysics, photochemistry and solar energy conversion with tris (bipyridyl) Ruthenium(II) and its analogues, *Coord. Chem. Rev.*, 46, 159, 1982.
20. **Juris, A., Balzani, V., Bariglletti, F., Campagna, S., Belser, P., and Zelewsky, A.**, Ru(II) polypyridine complexes: Photophysics, photochemistry, electrochemistry and chemiluminescence, *Coord. Chem. Rev.*, 84, 85, 1988.
21. **Hoffman, M. Z., Bolletta, F., Moggi, L. and Hug, G. L.**, Rate constants for the quenching of excited states of metal complexes in fluid solution, *J. Phys. Chem. Ref. Data*, 18, 219, 1989.
22. **Samec, Z. and Marecek, V.**, A Study of the electrical double layer at the interface between two immiscible electrolyte solutions by impedance measurements, in *The Interface Structure and Electrochemical Processes at the Boundary Between Two Immiscible Liquids*, V. E. Kazarinov, Ed., Springer-Verlag, Berlin, 1987, p. 123 .
23. **Buck, R. P.**, Electroanalytical chemistry of membranes, *Crit. Rev. Anal. Chem.*, 5, 323, 1975.
24. **Girault, H. H.**, Electrochemistry at the interface between two immiscible electrolyte solutions, *J. Electrochim. Acta*, 132, 383, 1987.
25. **Girault, H. H. and Schiffrin, D. J.**, Theory of the kinetics of ion transfer across liquid/liquid interfaces, *J. Electroanal. Chem.*, 195, 213, 1985.
26. **Girault, H. H., Schiffrin, D. J.**, Electron transfer reactions at the interface between two immiscible electrolyte solutions, *J. Electroanal. Chem.*, 244, 15, 1988.
27. **Newton, M. D. and Suit, N.**, Electron transfer reactions in condensed phases, *Ann. Rev. Phys. Chem.*, 35, 1091, 1984.
28. **Nicholson, R. S.**, Theory and application of cyclic voltammetry for measurement of electrode reaction kinetics, *Anal. Chem.*, 37, 1351, 1965,
29. **Peter, L. M., Dour, W., Binder, P. and Gerischer, H.**, The influence of alkali metal cations on the rate of the $Fe(CN)_6^{4-}/Fe(CN)_6^{3-}$ electrode process. *J. Electroanal Chem.*, 71, 31, 1976.
30. **Maiden, R., Goren, Z., Becker, J. Y. and Wilner, I.**, Application of multielectron charge relays in chemical and photochemical debromination

processes. The role of induced disproportionation of N,N′-dioctyl-4,4′-bipyridinium radical cation in two-phase systems, *J. Amer. Chem. Soc.*, 106, 6217, 1984.

31. **Samec, Z., Homolka, D., Marecek, V. and Kavan, L.**, Charge transfer between two immiscible electrolyte solutions. Transfer of 2,2′-bipyridine Ruthenium(II) and alkyl viologen dications across the water/nitrobenzene interface, *J. Electroanal. Chem.*, 145, 213, 1983.
32. **Hanzlik, J., Hovorka, J. and Camus, A. M.**, Transfer of trisbipyridine transition metal complexes across the water-dichloroethane interface, *Coll. Czech. Chem. Commun.*, 52, 838, 1987.
33. **Geogopoulos, M. and Hoffman, M. Z.**, Cage escape yields in the quenching of $Ru(bpy)_3^{2+}$ by methylviologen. Presence of ethanolamine as a sacrificial donor, *J. Phys. Chem.*, 95, 7717, 1991.
34. **Ohno, T., Yoshimura, A., Prasad, D. R. and Hoffman, M. Z.**, Weak G° dependence of back electron transfer within the geminate redox pairs formed in the quenching of excited Ruthenium(II) complexes by methylviologen, *J. Phys. Chem.*, 95, 4723, 1991.
35. **Ford, W. E., Otvos, J. W. and Calvin, M.**, Photosensitized electron transport across lipid vesicle walls: Quantum yield dependence on sensitizer concentration, *Proc. Natl. Acad. Sci. U.S.A.*, 76, 3590, 1979.
36. **Laune, C., Ford, W. E., Otvos, J. W. and Calvin, M.**, Photosensitized electron transport across lipid vesicle walls: Enhancement of quantum yield by ionophores and transmembrane potentials, *Proc. Natl. Acad. Sci. U.S.A.*, 2017, 1981.
37. **Nagamura, T., Takuma, K., Tsutsui, Y. and Matsuo, T.**, Photo induced electron transfer between amphipathic Ruthenium(II) complex and N,N′-dimethylaniline synthetic bilayer membranes and phospholipid liposomes, *Chem. Letters*, 503, 1980.
38. **Matsuo, T., Itoh, K., Takuma, K., Hashimoto, K. and Nagamura, T.**, A concerted two-step activation of photo induced electron-transport across lipid membrane, *Chem. Letters*, 1009, 1980.
39. **Tunuli, M. and Fendler, J. H.**, Aspects of artificial photosynthesis, photosensitized electron transfer across bilayers, charge separation, and hydrogen production in anionic surfactant vesicles, *J. Am. Chem. Soc.*, 103, 2507, 1981.
40. **Infelta, P., Gratzel, M. and Fendler, J. H.**, Aspects of artificial photosynthesis, photosensitized electron transfer and charge separation in cationic surfactant vesicles, *J. Am. Chem. Soc.*, 102, 1479, 1980.
41. **Kenelly, T., Gafney, H. D. and Braun, M.**, Photo induced disproportionation of $Ru(Bpy)_3^{2+}$ on porous Vycor glass, *J. Am. Chem. Soc.*, 107, 4431, 1985.
42. **Gafney, H. D.**, Spectral, photophysical and photochemical properties of $Ru(bpy)_3^{2+}$ on porous Vycor glass, *Coord. Chem. Rev.*, 104, 113, 1990.
43. **Thomas, J. K.**, Characterization of surfaces by excited states, *J. Phys. Chem.*, 91, 267, 1987.
44. **Liu, X. and Thomas, J. K.**, Study of surface properties of clay laponite using pyrene as a photo physical probe molecule, *Langmuir*, 7, 808, 1991.

45. **Marecek, V., DeArmond, A. H. and DeArmond, M. K.**, Photochemical electron transfer in liquid/liquid solvent, *J. Am. Chem. Soc.*, 111, 2561, 1989.
46. **Thomson, F. L., Yellowlees, L. J. and Girault, H. J.**, Photocurrent measurements at the interface between two immiscible electrolyte solutions, *J. Chem. Soc., Chem. Comm.*, 1547, 1988.
47. **Wilkey, J. D., Schuster, G. B.**, Irradiation of tetraphenylborate does not generate borene anion, *J. Org. Chem.*, 52, 2117, 1987.
48. **Delahay, P.**, Photoelectron emission spectroscopy of aqueous solutions, *Accts. Chem. Research*, 15, 40, 1982.
49. **Dvorak, O., DeArmond, A. H. and DeArmond, M. K.**, Photoprocesses at the liquid-liquid interface, 3. Charge transfer details for photoactive metal complexes, *Langmuir*, 8, 508, 1992.
50. **Dvorak, O., DeArmond, A. H., and DeArmond, M. K.**, Photoprocesses at the liquid-liquid interface, 4. Photo oxidative transfer with $[Ru(bpz)_3]^{2+}$ complexes, *Langmuir*, 8, 955, 1992.
51. **Marecek, V., DeArmond, A. H. and DeArmond, M. K.**, Photoinduced polarization of the interface between two immiscible electrolyte solutions, *J. Electroanal. Chem.*, 261, 287, 1989.
52. **Haga, M., Dodsworth, E. S., Eryarec, G., Seymours, E. and Lever A. B. P.**, Luminescence quenching of the tris (2,2′-bipyrazine) Ruthenium(II) cation and its monoprotonated complex, *Inorg. Chem.*, 24, 1901, 1985.
53. **Sun, Y. and DeArmond, M. K.**, ESR Study of the reduction products of a pendant complex with an oligomeric bipyridine backbone, *J. Phys. Chem.*, 97, 8549, 1993.
54. **Burbage, J. D. and Wirth, M. H.**, Effect of wetting on the reorientation of acridine orange at the interface of water on a hydrophobic surface, *J. Phys. Chem.*, 96, 5943, 1992.
55. **Burbage, J. D. and Wirth, M. H.**, Reorientation of acridine orange at liquid alkane - water interfaces, *J. Phys. Chem.*, 96, 9022, 1992.
56 **Kott, K. L., Higgins, D. A., McMahon, R. J. and Corn, R. M.**, Observation of photoinduced electron transfer at a liquid-liquid interface by optical second harmonic generation, *J. Am. Chem. Soc.*, 115, 5342, 1993.
57. **Conboy, J. C., Daschbach, J. L. and Richmond, G. L.**, Studies of alkane/water interfaces by total internal reflection. Second harmonic generation, *J. Phys. Chem.*, 98, 9688, 1994.
58. **Eisenthal, K. B.**, Liquid interfaces, *Acc. Chem. Res.*, 26, 636, 1993.

Chapter 12

AMPEROMETRIC ION-SELECTIVE ELECTRODE SENSORS

Mitsugi Senda and Yukitaka Yamamoto

I. INTRODUCTION

Recent electrochemical studies on ion transfer reactions across oil/water (O/W) interfaces, such as nitrobenzene/water or 1,2-dichloroethane/water, have shown that the O/W interface can be electrochemically polarized. Furthermore, ion transfer across the interface within the polarizable potential range or what is called the potential window can be studied by use of voltammetric or polarographic techniques. Thus, the polarizable O/W interface can function as an ion selective electrode that responds voltammetrically to specified ions that are transferable across the interface. Two types of ion-selective electrodes are possible: amperometric and potentiometric. The former gives a current response that is proportional to the concentration of analyte ion, whereas the latter gives a potential response that changes linearly with the logarithm of the activity of analyte ion[1-3]. In this chapter, the electrochemical principle of the ion-selective electrodes based on the polarizable o/w interface is briefly described and electrochemical sensors and biosensors based on them, particularly, those on amperometric ion-selective electrodes are discussed in some detail.

II. ELECTROCHEMICAL PRINCIPLE OF ION-SELECTIVE ELECTRODES (ISE). AMPEROMETRIC ISE *VS.* POTENTIOMETRIC ISE

First, we consider an electrochemical cell:

$$R_1 \,\Big|\, B_1^+, A_1^-(O) \,\overset{*}{\Big|}\, B_2^+, A_2^-\,(W) \,\Big|\, R_2 \qquad \text{(I)}$$

where (O) represents the organic or oil phase and (W) the aqueous or water phase, and the interface marked by * is the O/W interface to be polarized. B_1^+ and B_2^+, and A_1^- and A_2^- are the supporting electrolyte cations and anions, respectively, and R_1 and R_2 the reference electrodes. An electric field is applied across the O/W interface by the two reference electrodes. The cell potential, E, is defined as the terminal potential of the reference electrode R_2 referred to reference electrode R_1, and is related to the potential difference across the O/W interface, $\Delta\phi$ ($= \Delta_o^w\phi = \phi^w - \phi^o$, ϕ^α being the Galvani potential of α-phase (α = o,w)), by

$$E = \Delta\phi - \Delta E_{ref} \qquad (1)$$

0-8493-7694-7/96/$0.00+$.50

where ΔE_{ref} is determined by the composition of the reference electrode system of the electrochemical cell. When the ions B_1^+ and A_1^- are extremely hydrophobic, like tetrabutylammonium (TBA^+) and tetraphenylborate (TPB^-) ions, while the ions B_2^+ and A_2^- are extremely hydrophilic, like Li^+ and Cl^- ions, as long as the potential difference across the O/W interface does not exceed a certain range of positive and negative magnitudes, the transfer of B_1^+ and A_1^- from O to W and that of B_2^+ and A_2^- in the opposite direction should be negligible, so that no current will flow across the interface. This is illustrated in Figure 1A, where the positive (or anodic) current stands for the transfer of cations from W to O and of anions from O to W and the negative (or cathodic) current for the transfer of ions in the opposite direction. Thus, the O/W interface behaves as an ideal-polarized interface in this range of potential difference, which we call the polarizable potential range or the potential window of the O/W interface.

We consider the second case when a moderately hydrophilic or semi-hydrophilic ion j is present in one of the two phases, *e.g.*, a semi-hydrophilic cation B_3^+, like tetramethylammonium (TMA^+) ion, in aqueous phase (W),

$$\mathrm{R_1} \left| \mathrm{B_1^+, A_1^-(O)} \overset{*}{\left|} \mathrm{B_3^+, B_2^+, A_2^-\,(W)} \right| \mathrm{R_2} \qquad \text{(II)}$$

(amperometric ISE) (test solution)

Then, the transfer of the j-ion (B_3^+) ion, across the interface will take place at an intermediate potential within the polarizable potential range of cell I and the current, i, associated with the transfer of j-ion will be observed in this polarizable potential range. Kinetics of the ion transfer at the interface can be expressed, in analogy with the ordinary electrode kinetics, by [1]

$$i = z_j FA(k_f c_j^{w,s} - k_b c_j^{o,s}) \qquad (2)$$

where z_j is the number, including the sign, of the charge of j-ion, F the Faraday constant, A the interface area, $c_j^{\alpha,s}$ the surface concentration of j-ion in α-phase (α = o,w), and k_f and k_b are the rate constants for the transfer from W to O and from O to W, respectively. The rate constants are functions of $\Delta\phi$ and may be expressed by a Butler-Volmer type equation as given by

$$k_f = k_s \exp[(\alpha z_j F/RT)(\Delta\phi - \Delta\phi^0)]$$
$$(3)$$
$$k_b = k_s \exp[(-\beta z_j F/RT)(\Delta\phi - \Delta\phi^0)]$$

where k_s is the standard rate constant, that is, the rate constant when $\Delta\phi = \Delta\phi_j^0$, $\Delta\phi_j^0$ being the standard potential of j-ion transfer at the O/W interface, α and β ($\alpha + \beta = 1$) are the transfer coefficients, and R and T have their usual meanings. The standard potential is related to the standard Gibbs energy of transfer of j-ion from O to W, $\Delta_o^w G_{tr,j}^0$, by

$$\Delta\phi_j^0 = -\Delta_o^w G_{tr,j}^0 / z_j F \tag{4}$$

Thus, the ion transfer current across the O/W interface will be observed at about the standard potential or the half-wave potential within the polarizable potential range (Figure 1B, where the ion transfer current *vs.* potential (i - $\Delta\phi$) curve is represented by a polarographic wave with the half-wave potential, $\Delta\phi_{1/2}$, and the limiting current, i_l). In cell II, the left-hand half-cell R_1 / B_1^+, A_1^- (O) / constitutes an amperometric ISE which is immersed in an external or test solution B_2^+, A_2^- (W) containing an analyte B_3^+ with a reference electrode R_2. The voltammetric current, usually observed as the limiting current in polarography or the peak current in potential sweep voltammetry etc., is proportional to the concentration of analyte ion.

We consider the third case when a semi-hydrophilic (or -hydrophobic) j-ion, here B_3^+ ion, is present in both phases:

$$R_1 \left| B_1^+, A_1^-, B_3^+ \text{ (O)} \right|^{*} B_3^+, B_2^+, A_2^- \text{(W)} \left| R_2 \right. \tag{III}$$

(potentiometric ISE) (test solution)

Here the composite positive-negative current wave of the transfer of j-ion from W to O and from O to W (Figure 1C) and the zero current potential or the equilibrium potential, $\Delta\phi_{j,eq}$ (at i=0 in eq. 2), should be given by the Nernst equation:

$$\Delta\phi_{j,eq} = \Delta\phi_j^0 + (RT/z_j F)\ln[c_j^o / c_j^w] \tag{5}$$

Therefore, the EMF, that is, the cell potential of cell III at $i = 0$, E_{eq}, is given by $E_{eq} = \Delta\phi_{j,eq} + \Delta E_{ref}$ (see Eq. 1). In cell III, the left-hand half-cell R_1 / B_1^+, A_1^-, B_3^+ (O) / constitutes a potentiometric ISE which is immersed in an external or test solution B_2^+, A_2^- (W) containing an analyte B_3^+ with a reference electrode R_2. Thus, the potentiometric ISE gives the potential response at the zero-current control which changes linearly with the logarithm of the concentration of the analyte ion, here B_3^+ ion, in the organic phase of the ISE. In this chapter, for the sake of simplicity, the activity of ions is equated to their concentration, unless otherwise stated.

In many cases, in order to make the O/W interface selectively responsive to a specified ion M, a hydrophobic ionophore L which associates with the specified ion M to form a hydrophobic complex LM is added in the organic phase. Usually, the formation constant of the complex, K^o, defined by $K^o = c_{LM}^o / c_L^o c_M^o$, is set to be much larger than unity that the concentration of the free M-ion in organic phase is negligibly small compared with that of the complex ML, that is, $c_{ML}^o >> c_M^o$. Then, the standard potential of the transfer of M-ion at the O(containing L)/W interface should be replaced, when $c_L^o >> c_M^o$ (and usually also $c_L^o >> c_M^w$), by [1]

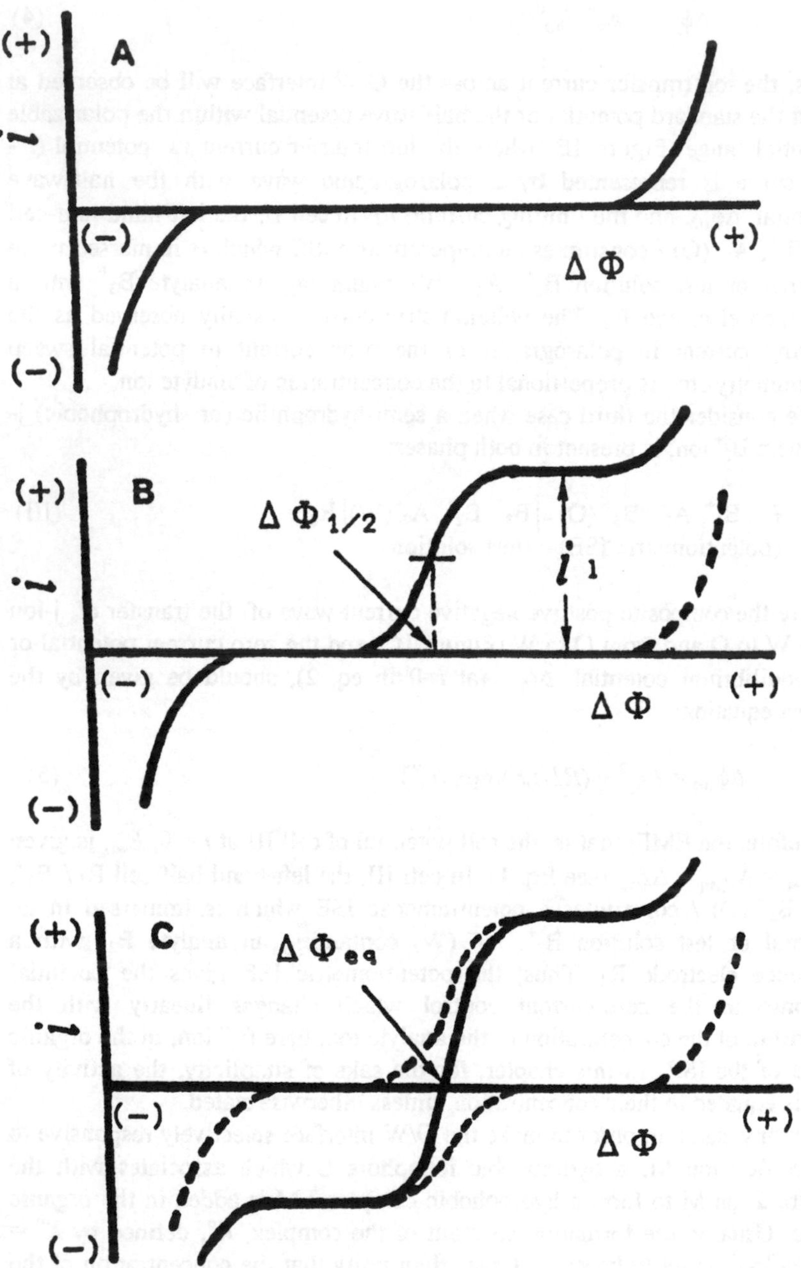

Figure 1. A: Ideal-polarized O/W interface. B: Voltammetric (polarographic) current vs potential curve. C: Composite positive-negative (or anodic-cathodic) current vs. potential curve and equilibrium potential at zero current.

$$\Delta\phi_M^{0'} = \Delta\phi_M^0 + (RT/z_M F)\ln[1/(c_L^{\circ} K^{\circ})] \tag{6}$$

Consequently, the standard potential (and also the half-wave potential) of M-ion transfer at the O (containing L)/W interface is selectively shifted to less positive (when $z_M > 0$, or less negative when $z_M < 0$) potential to make the interface the electrode surface selectively responsive to M-ion present in aqueous phase.

As stated above, the amperometric ISE gives the current response, I, which is proportional to the concentration of analyte ion(s) in test solution, c_M. The current response is measured under the control of the potential applied to the electrode interface, E_{app}, which may conventionally be represented by the half-wave potential, $E_{1/2}$, in polarography or the peak potential, E_p, in potential sweep voltammetry:

$$I = k_{amp} c_M \quad \text{at } E = E_{app} \text{ (or } E_{1/2}, E_p) \tag{7}$$

where k_{amp} is the constant which depends on the mode of potential control, current measurement and experimental conditions, such as the cell and electrode design. On the other hand the potentiometric ISE gives the potential response, E, which changes linearly with the logarithm of the concentration (activity) of analyte ion in test solution, c_M, where the current flowing across the electrode interface, I, is controlled usually at zero;

$$E = k_{pot}\log[c_M] + b \quad \text{at } I = 0 \tag{8}$$

where k_{pot} and b are the constants and $k_{pot} = 2.303RT/z_M F$ for Nernstian response. Accordingly, we have the following two equations for the variation of the response with the variation of analyte concentration ($k_{pot}' = k_{pot}/2.303$);

$$\Delta I = k_{amp}\Delta c_M \tag{9}$$

$$\Delta E = k_{pot}'\Delta c_M/c_M \tag{10}$$

that is, the response of amperometric ISE sensors indicates directly the change of analyte concentration, whereas that of potentiometric ISE sensors gives the relative change of analyte concentration. The former may advantageously be used for sensitive determination of concentration within limited ranges, and the latter for concentration varying over wide ranges.

Potentiometric ion-selective electrodes have a long history and their analytical applications are well developed, while the amperometric ion-selective electrodes based on the polarizable O/W interface are rather new types of ISE. Some important properties of sensors and biosensors based on the amperometric ISE, as studied by the authors and their coworkers, will now be discussed.

III. AMPEROMETRIC ISE SENSORS

The left-hand half-cell of cell II represents an amperometric ISE that consists of an organic phase (O) and can be used for monitoring an analyte, here B_3^+, in an aqueous phase (W). Likewise, an amperometric ISE that consists of an aqueous phase (W) for monitoring an analyte in organic phase (O) can be constructed[4]. The former is occasionally called an organic solvent electrode, like a nitrobenzene electrode, and the latter a water electrode. For practical purposes organic solvents of low vapor pressure, such as o-nitrophenyloctylether, o-nitrophenylphenylether, and 2-fluoro-2'-nitrodiphenylether[5], can be used in place of nitrobenzene, though at the cost of lowering the conductivity of organic solvent by about one tenth at the same supporting electrolyte concentration. Also, it is common to stabilize the liquid electrode by gelation; a nitrobenzene poly(vinylchloride) gel electrode and a water agar gel electrode have been studied[4]. Stabilization of the liquid electrode interface by placing a thin, hydrophilic membrane at the interface has proved very useful for constructing amperometric ISE sensors (see below)[6,7,8]. Some important properties of the ion sensors based on the amperometric ISE will be discussed by taking a laboratory-made potassium and sodium ion sensor[8] as an example.

A. POTASSIUM AND SODIUM ION SENSOR

1. Electrochemical cell

The electrochemical cell for amperometric determination of potassium and sodium ions with this sensor is represented by[8]

$$\begin{array}{l|l|l|l||l|l|l} \text{Ag} & \text{AgCl} & \begin{array}{c}\text{0.02M TPenACl}\\ \text{0.1 M MgSO}_4\\ \text{(W)}\end{array} & \begin{array}{c}\text{0.1 M TPenATPB}\\ \text{0.02M BB15C5}\\ \text{(NB)}\end{array} & \begin{array}{c}\text{0.01M MgCl}_2\\ \text{(test sol.)}\\ \text{(W)}\end{array} & \text{AgCl} & \text{Ag} \end{array} \qquad \text{(IV)}$$

(the polarized interface between (NB) and (W) is marked * and stabilized by HSM)

(amperometric K^+ and Na^+ ion sensor)

In this cell TPenACl, TPenATPB and BB15C5 are tetrapentylammonium chloride, tetrapentylammonium tetraphenylborate and bis[(benzo-15-crown-5)-4'-ilmethyl]-pimelate (an ionophore), respectively. The polarized nitrobenzene(NB)/water(W) interface is marked by *. In the presence of an ionophore BB15C5 at 0.02M in NB the transfer of potassium and sodium ions across the NB/W interface is observed at $E_{1/2}$ = 0.198 and 0.381 V, respectively, when these ions are present in W (test solution). The polarized NB/W interface is stabilized by placing a hydrophilic semipermeable membrane (HSM, a dialysis membrane 20 μm in thickness, Visking Co.) at the interface. Since a usable reference electrode for organic phase (R_1 in cell II) is not available, it is a common practice to use an $Ag/AgCl/Cl^-(W)$ electrode with $TPenA^-(W)/TPenA^-(NB)$ interface, making a reference electrode reversible to $TPenA^-$ ion in NB phase. Thus, the left-hand half-cell, Ag/AgCl/0.02M TPenACl, 0.1M $MgSO_4$(W)/0.1M TPenATPB, 0.02M

BB15C5(NB)// represents the potassium and sodium ion sensor, which is immersed in a test solution that may contain 0.01M $MgCl_2$ as the supporting electrolyte. The presence of HSM at the interface gives the sensor physical strength in handling. It also protects the electroactive or ion-sensing o/w interface from contaminants such as by colloidal particles in test solutions. The laboratory-made potassium and sodium ion sensor is illustrated in Figure 2[8].

2. Pulse amperometry

In the amperometric ISE the flow of current across the interface changes the electrolyte distribution at and near the electrode interface. This is a disadvantage of amperometric ISE sensors especially when the sensors are used for a long period. However, such changes can be eliminated by the pulse amperometric technique (Figure 3); the electrode potential is controlled first at the initial potential E_i at which negligible ion-transfer current flows. After a fixed time interval, for instance, 5 seconds, the potential is changed abruptly to E_{app} (= $\Delta E + E_i$) at which an ion-transfer current will flow for approxination 100 ms. The potential pulse is ended by a return to the initial potential E_i and the electrode is kept at E_i until the next potential pulse is applied. Since the ion transfer reaction at the O/W interface is generally reversible, the electrode interface returns to its original state at the end of the waiting time; and highly reproducible current response can be obtained for long term measurements. The current is sampled usually at a time near the end of the pulse, and a signal proportional to this sampled value is recorded. Thus, the recorded current *vs.* potential curve is equivalent to a normal-pulse polarogram in polarography with a dropping mercury electrode. When the applied potential E_{app} is sufficiently large to give the limiting current, the current signal is directly proportional to the concentration of analyte ion M in test solution (W):

$$i = z_M FAD^{1/2} c_M / (\pi\tau)^{1/2} \quad (11)$$

when the current is sampled at the end of the pulse, D being the diffusion coefficient of M ion (here, in HSM(W) since the W-side of the O/W interface is coated by HSM).

The pulse amperometry technique appears essential to obtain reproducible results with amperometric ISE sensors. The life time of the present laboratory-made amperometric potassium and sodium ion sensor was more than four weeks.

3. Current sensitivity and response time

Calibration curves for the ion selective electrode desired above were linear for sodium and potassium ions up to 0.7 mM, beyond which the curves deviated downward from linearity. The upper concentration limit of linearity should be improved by elevating the concentration of ionophore in the

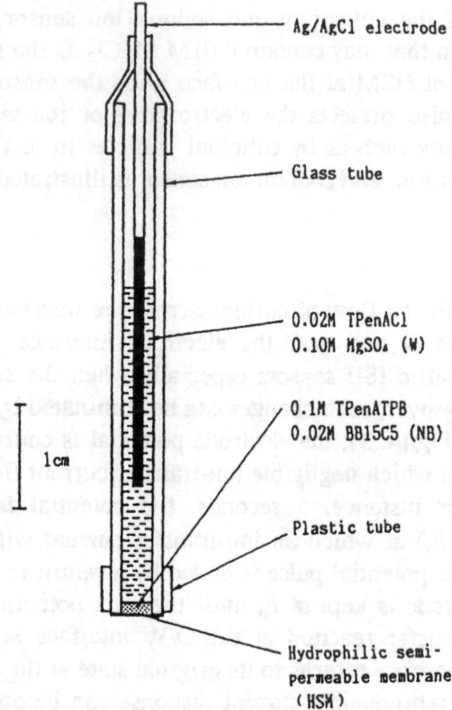

Figure 2. Cross-sectional view of a laboratory-made amperometric potassium and sodium sensor. (From Ref .8, after modification, with permission).

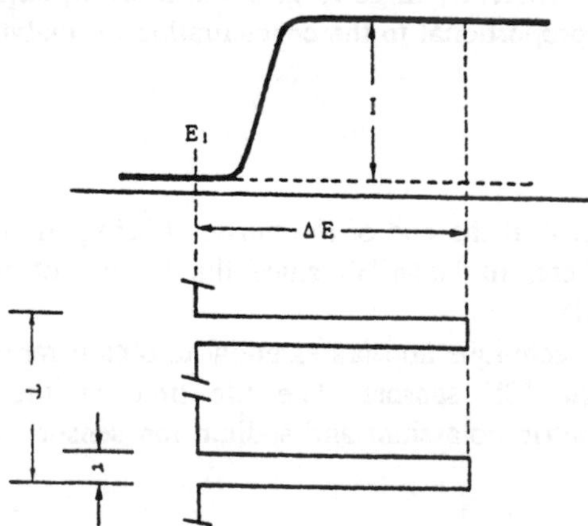

Figure 3. The pulse amperometry.

organic phase since the condition to realize linearity is that the ionophore concentration is higher than the analyte concentration. The relative standard deviation was 1.84 % (n = 5, at 0.3 mM) and the detection limit was 3σ = 0.02 mM.

The response time of electrodes in which the ion-selective O/W interface is stabilized by placing a hydrophilic semipermeable membrane (HSM) at the interface, is determined by the transient change of the surface concentration of analyte ion on the W-side of the O/W interface. Surface concentration is controlled by diffusion of analyte ion within the HSM (of the thickness of d_m) when the concentration of analyte ion at the surface of HSM facing to test solution is abruptly changed, for instance, from $c^w{}_1$ to $c^w{}_2$ at the time $t = 0$. The diffusion equation for the surface concentration $c^{w,s}$ as a function of time as given by (Figure 4[8])

$$(c^{w,s} - c^w{}_1)/(c^w{}_2 - c^w{}_1) = 1 - (4/\pi)\exp[-(\pi^2 D/4d_m{}^2)t] + ... \quad (12)$$

The calculated response time for the current response of this sensor to reach 95% of the final equilibrium value, $t_{95} = 3.25 \times 4d_m{}^2/\pi^2 D = 1.8$ s (when d_m (swollen) = 37 μm and $D = 1 \times 10^{-5}$ cm^2/s). Experimentally it was determined to be about 20 s, when a sample solution containing potassium ion was added to the test solution under stirring. This may be considered to be a reasonable value, taking into account the presence of an unstired layer on the HSM surface.

4. Simultaneous determination of two or more components

When two or more ionic are present the ISE electrode response reflects the sum of their independent contributions at their half-wave potentials. Therefore, if the half-wave potentials are reasonably separated, the concentration of these components can simultaneously be determined with the same ion sensor. As stated above, the difference in half-wave potentials of potassium and sodium ions is reasonably large ($E_{1/2,Na} - E_{1/2,K} = 0.183$ V). For simultaneous determination of two analytes the dual pulse amperometry technique can be used.[8] The voltage pulses (τ = 100 ms) of different amplitudes (here, $\Delta E_1 = 0.29$ V and $\Delta E_2 = 0.47$ V on $E_i = 0.12$ V), each corresponding to the limiting current of the first (potassium ion) and second (sodium ion) steps of the two ions, are applied alternatively to the electrode at a fixed time interval (T=5 s). The current response of the first pulse gives the concentration of the first ion, and the current response of the second pulse represents the sum of the current responses of the two ions, so that the second response minus the first gives the concentration of the second ion. Table 1 shows the analytical results of potassium and sodium contents in a soft drink sample obtained by use of dual pulse amperometry with a laboratory-made sensor. Analytical application of the potassium and sodium ion sensor to food chemistry as well as clinical chemistry have been explored[8,10,11].

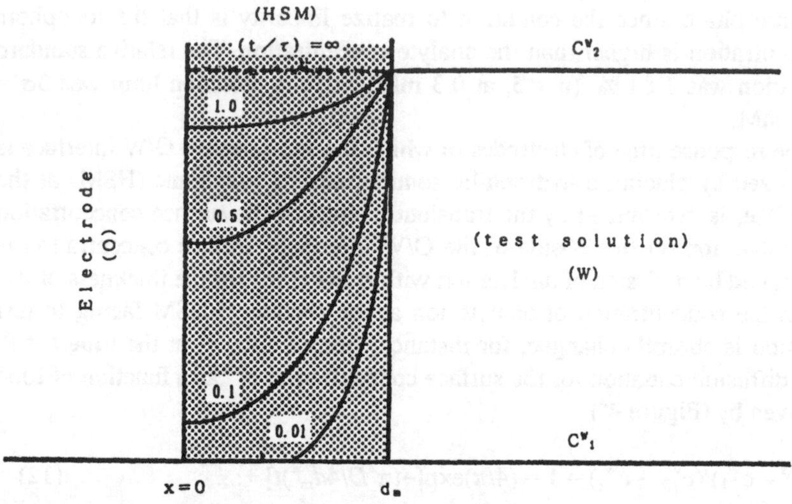

Figure 4. The concentration profile of an ion as a function of time t in a hydrophilic semipermeable membrane (HSM) coating the ion-selective electrode surface when the outside ion concentration is changed from c_1^w to c_2^w at t=0. The figures on the curves indicate t/τ, $\tau = 4d_m^2/\pi^2D$ (see text). (From Ref.8, after modification, with permission.)

Table 1. Potassium and sodium contents in foods and drinks determined by the amperometric ISE Sensor method.

Sample	Dilution	Potassium Ion		Sodium Ion	
		$c^{a)}$ /mM	Content/mg/100g	$c^{a)}$ /mM	Content/mg/100g
Pepperbush (NIES No.1)	x833	0.48	1560 (1510+60)$^{b)}$	-	-
Soft drinks	x50	0.098	19.2 (18,9)$^{c)}$	0.23	26.4 (26.8)$^{c)}$
Soy	x10,000	-	-	0.20	4560
	x 1,000	0.38	1490	-	-
Miso	x2,000	-	-	0.30	1380
	x 400	0.30	469	-	-
Condiment	x2,000	-	-	0.47	2160
	x 400	0.26	407	-	-

a) Concentration in test solution.
b) The certified value of the standard material by NIES.
c) The indicated values.

The additivity of response in the amperometric ISE is also advantageous in other applications of such sensors (see below).

B. AMMONIUM ION AND VOLATILE AMINE SENSORS

1. Electrochemical Cell

An amperometric ammonium ion sensor can be constructed by adding an ionophore of ammonium ion in the organic phase on the same principle as in the potassium and sodium ion sensor discussed above. Here, an ionophore dibenzo-18-crown-6 ether (DB18C6) was used. Because potassium and sodium ions interfere with the response of the sensor to ammonium ion, the ammonium ISE surface was covered by a thin, gas permeable membrane to eliminate the interference. The electrochemical cell for amperometric determination of ammonium ion or ammonia gas with this sensor is represented by[7]

				*		
Ag	AgCl	0.1M TBACl	0.1M TBATPB 0.02M DB18C6		0.05M $MgCl_2$ 0.05M L-Lys	Test Sol. (pH 9.0)
		(W)	(NB)	HSM ↑	(W)	GPM

Ag | AgCl (V)

(amperometric NH_4^+ ion and NH_3 sensor)

where TBACl and TBATPB are tetrabutylammonium chloride and tetrabutylammonium tetraphenylborate, respectively. The polarizable o/w interface (marked by *) is stabilized by placing a hydrophilic semipermeable membrane (HSM, a dialysis membrane of 20μm thickness) at the o/w interface and the ammonium-ISE surface is covered by a gas permeable membrane(GPM, a Teflon membrane 50μm in thickness, Sumitomo Denko FP-200) with the inner solution of 0.05M $MgCl_2$, 0.05M L-lysine (pH 8.5) between the GPM and the polarized NB/W(HSM) interface. The counter reference electrode Ag/AgCl(W) is connected to the cell through the inner solution. The GPM-covered sensor is immersed in test solution, usually of pH 9.0, into which an aliquot of sample solution is added. The pulse amperometric technique can be used to record the current response of the sensor. The laboratory-made GPM-covered ion sensor gave a linear current response to the concentration of ammonium ion in test solution. The response time was about 60 s. The large value of the response time reflects a slow diffusion process through the GPM and inner solution layer.

2. Volatile Amine Sensor

The sensor discussed above also gives a current response to the ions of other volatile amines like trimethylamine or trimethylammonium ion. Therefore, the GPM-covered volatile amine sensor can be used to quantify the volatile amine content in foods. Since trimethylammonium ion also produces the ion transfer current at the NB(without ionophore)/W interface, separate determination of ammonia and trimethylamine in foods can be made by use of two sensors, one based on the NB(with ionophore)/W interface and the other on the NB(without ionophore)/W interface. The former gives the sum of the current responses of two amines and the latter that of trimethylamine only[7,10].

C. AMPEROMETRIC ULTRAMICRO ISE SENSORS

It may be possible to fabricate of an amperometric ultramicro ISE sensors by constructing the polarizable o/w interface at the tip of a micro glass micropipette[12,13]. However in vivo application of an amperometric ultramicro acetylcholine sensor was unsuccessful due to lack of sensitivity[14]. Amperometric micro-hole ISE sensors also appear promising[15].

IV. AMPEROMETRIC ISE BIOSENSORS

Enzyme sensors or biosensors based on the amperometric ISE can be based on other electrochemical devices that have been extensively developed in recent years [16,17]. These applications involve enzymatic reactions, usually taking place in the immobilized-enzyme layer on an electrode surface, with rates proportional to the concentration of analyte (substrate). The reaction is monitored by measuring the rate of formation of a product or the disappearance of a reactant. If the product or reactant gives a response on the amperometric ISE, then its concentration may be monitored directly. Some important features of biosensors based on the amperometric ISE will be discussed by taking a urea biosensor[18,19,20] as an example.

A. UREA BIOSENSOR

1. Electrochemical Cell

The principle of a urea biosensor is shown in Figure 5. Urease is immobilized on the surface of the GPM-covered ammonium ion sensor (cell V, above). Urea is transported by diffusion through the immobilized-enzyme layer while it is enzymatically hydrolyzed by

$$NH_2CONH_2 + H_2O \xrightarrow{urease} CO_2 + 2NH_3 \qquad (13)$$

The product NH_3 is in reversible equilibrium with its dissociated ionic form NH_4^+ and these decomposition products are also transported by diffusion through the immobilized-enzyme layer. The rate of the enzymatic reaction may be expressed by Michaelis-Menten equation and, when the substrate concentration, c_{urea}, is so low that $c_{urea} << K_M$, K_M being the Michaelis constant, the rate is proportional to the substrate concentration. Then, as a result of the diffusion process associated with the enzymatic reaction, the concentration of the products (that is, $NH_3 + NH_4^+$) on the GPM surface of the ammonium ion sensor is proportional to the concentration of urea on the surface of the immobilized-urease layer facing toward the test solution. Consequently, the current response of the urease-immobilized GPM-covered ammonium ion sensor is proportional to the concentration of urea[19].

The electrochemical cell for amperometric determination of urea with a laboratory-made urea biosensor immersed in a test solution is represented by

Ag | AgCl | 0.1M TBACl | 0.1M TBATPB, 0.02M DB18C6 || * | 0.05M $MgCl_2$, 0.05M L-Lys | Urease | Test Soln. (pH 9.0)

(W) (NB) HSM ↑ (W) GPM HSM

Ag|AgCl

(amperometric urea biosensor) (VI)

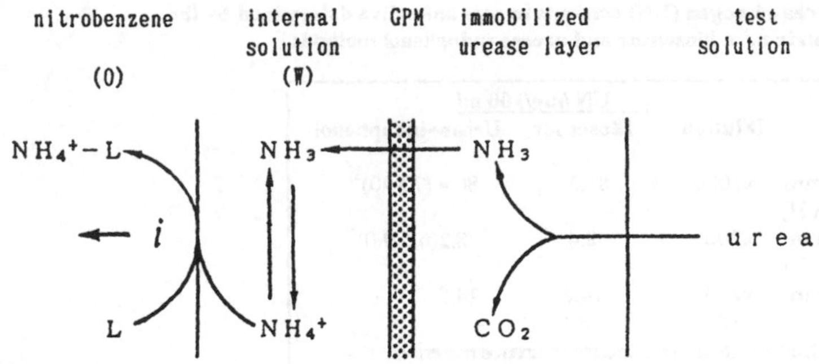

Figure 5. Principle of the amperometric urea biosensor.

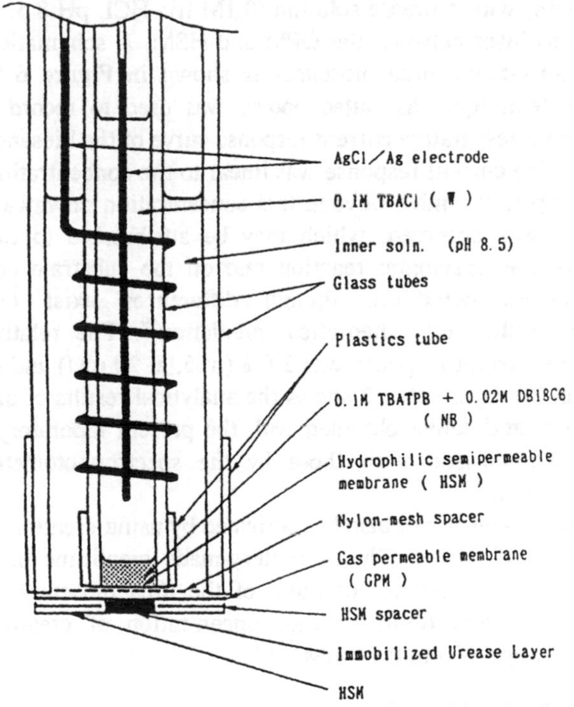

Figure 6. Schematic cross-section of a laboratory-made amperometric urea biosensor. (From Ref. [18], after modification, with permission.)

Table 2. Urea-nitrogen (UN) contents in sera and saliva determined by the amperometric u. : a biosensor and urease-indophenol methods.

Sample	Dilution	UN /mg/100 ml Biosensor	Urease-indophenol
Animal Serum (Pathonorm H)	x1000	81.2	80.4 (70-90)[a)]
Animal serum (Pathonorm L)	x200	8.4	8.2(6.5-9.0)[a)]
Human serum	x200	14.6	14.0
Saliva	x100	8.1	-

a) The certified value of the standard reference materials.

The electrochemical cell of the GPM-covered ammonium ion sensor is the same as cell V discussed above. Urease (jack bean urease, usually, 100 U) was immobilized by cover˙ g the GPM surface of the ammonium ion sensor by a hydrophilic semipermeable membrane (HSM, a dialysis membrane 20 μm in thickness) with a urease solution (0.1M tris-HCl, pH 8.5, 15% bovine serum albumin) layer between the GPM and HSM. A schematic illustration of the laboratory-made urea biosensor is shown in Figure 6[18] The pulse amperometric technique, as stated above, was used to record the current response. The representative current response curve of the biosensor is shown in Figure 7[19]. The current response was linear to the concentration of urea in test solutions up to 0.1 mM. Beyond this concentration downward deviation from linearity was observed, which may be attributable to the parabolic dependence of the enzymatic reaction rate on the substrate concentration (Michaelis-Menten equation), though differences exist between the experimental results and theoretical prediction[19]. The relative standard deviation of the current response was 3.8% (n=5, at 20 μM) and the life time was more than 20 days. Table 2 shows the analytical results of urea-nitrogen contents in sera and saliva obtained with the present laboratory-made urea biosensor in comparison with those by the spectrophotometric (urease-indophenol) method[18].

A creatinine biosensor can also be fabricated by using creatinine deiminase (50 U) in place of urease. The laboratory-made creatinine biosensor also showed similar characteristics to those of the urea biosensor and gave a current response proportional to the concentration of creatinine in test solution in the range of 0 to 0.14 mM [18,20].

2. Correction for Residual Current

An advantage of the amperometric urea biosensor stated above is that the correction for the current due to the residual ammonium ion that may be present in test solution can relatively easily be achieved with the amperometric ISE biosensor compared with the potentiometric ISE biosensor. For this purpose, a sensor of the same structure as the urea biosensor, but without urease in the immobilized-enzyme layer was fabricated. This sensor gave a current response proportional to the concentration of ammonium ion present in the test solution but no current response to urea. The urea biosensor, gives the sum of the current responses, each proportional to their concentrations when both urea and ammonium ion are present in test solution. The current sensitivities to ammonium ions of the two sensors coincided within experimental error less than 5%. Therefore, the concentration of urea corrected for the residual ammonium ion can be computed from the difference between the current response of the (urease-immobilized) urea biosensor and that of the urease-removed urea sensor[19].

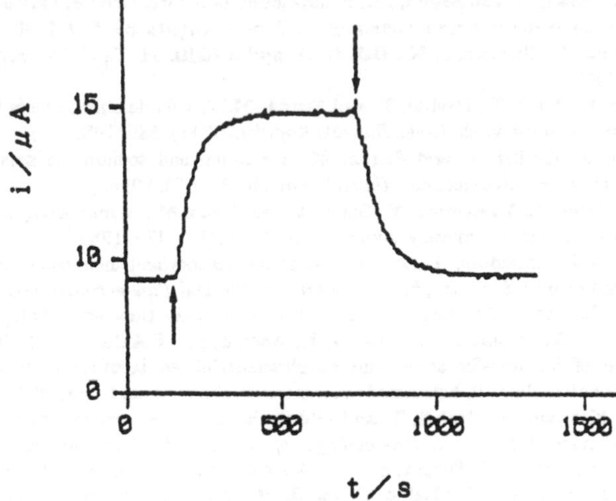

Figure 7. A pulse amperometric current vs. time curve obtained with a laboratory-made urea biosensor immersed in a test solution (see cell B). A 0.2 mM urea solution was added to the test solution at the time indicated by a upward arrow followed by washing the sensor by the base solution at the time indicated by a downward arrow. $E_i = 0.25$ V, $\Delta E = 100$ mV, $\tau = 100$ms, T = 5 s. (From Ref. [19], with permission.

V. ELECTROANALYTICAL CHEMISTRY AT LIQUID/LIQUID INTERFACES

A number of other analytes are accessible by ion-transfer voltammetry at the polarizable O/W interface. Among these are the organic compounds of biological importance such as drugs (including local anesthetic, hypnotic, cholinergic and anti-cholinergic agents) [20,21] and uncouplers of mitochondrial oxidative phosphorylation[22,23] with pharmacological and biological activity, phospholipid monolayers on the polarized o/w interface and determination of hydrolytic activity of phospholipase D as a function of the surface potential.[24,25] Spectroelectrochemical approaches to ion transfer reactions[26] and electron-transfer voltammetry at the polarizable O/W interface[27] also appears interesting and promising.

REFERENCES

1. **Senda, M., Kakiuchi, T. and Osakai, T.** , Electrochemistry at the interface between two immiscible electrolyte solutions, *Electrochim. Acta*, 36(2), 253, 1991, and papers cited therein.
2. **Senda, M.**, Ion-selective electrodes based on polarizable electrolyte/electrolyte solutions interface, *Anal. Sci.*, 7(S), 585, 1991.
3. **Senda, M., Kakiuchi, T., Osakai, T., Nuno, T. and Kakutani, T.**, Theory of ion-selective electrodes; amperometric ISE and potentiometric ISE, in *Proceedings of the 5th Symposium on Ion-Selective Electrodes*, Matrafured, Hungary, 1988, Pungor, E., Ed., Akademiai Kiado, Budapest, 1990, p.559.
4. **Osakai, T., Kakutani, T. and Senda, M.**, Ion transfer voltammetry with the interface between polymer-electrolyte gel and electrolyte solution, *Bunseki Kagaku*, 33(9), E371, 1984
5. **Sawada, S., Osakai, T. and Senda, M.**, Polarizability of o-nitrophenyl ethers/water interfaces and its applicability to ion-transfer voltammetry, *Bunseki Kagaku*, 39, 539, 1990.
6. **Hundhammer, B., Dhawan, S. K., Bekele, A. and Seidlitz, H. T.**, *J. Electroanal. Chem.*, 217, 253, 1987,
7. **Yamamoto, Y., Nuno, T., Osakai, T. and Senda, M.**, A volatile amine sensor based on the amperometric ion-selective electrode, *Bunseki Kagaku*, 38(11), 589, 1989.
8. **Yamamoto, Y., Osakai, T. and Senda, M.**, Potassium and sodium ion sensor based on amperometric ion-selective electrode, *Bunseki Kagaku*, 39, 655, 1990.
9. **Osakai, T., Nuno, T., Yamamoto, Y., Saito, A. and Senda, M.**, A microcomputer-controlled system for ion-transfer voltammetry, *Bunseki Kagaku*, 38(10), 479, 1989.
10. **Senda, M. and Yamamoto, Y.**, Amperometric ion sensors and their applications in food chemistry and clinical chemistry, in *Proceedings of the 2nd Bioelectroanalysis Symposium*, Matrafured, Hungary, 1992, Pungor, E., Ed., Akademiai Kiado, Budapest, 1993, p.139.
11. **Hundhammer, B., Solomon, T., Zerihun, T., Abegaz, M., Bekele, A. and Graichen, K.**, Investigation of ion transfer across the membrane-stabilized interface of two immiscible electrolyte solutions. Part III. Facilitated ion transfer, *J. Electroanal. Chem.*, 371, 1, 1994.
12. **Senda, M., Kakutani, T, Osakai, T. and Ohkouchi, T.**, A new amperometric acetylcholine ion-selective microelectrode, in *Proceedings of the 1st Bioelectroanalysis Symposium*, Matrafured, Hungary, 1986, Pungor, E., Ed., Akademiai Kiado, Budapest. 1987, p.353.
13. **Ohkouchi, T., Kakutani, T., Osakai, T. and Senda, M.**, Voltammetry with an ion-selective microelectrode based on polarizable oil/water interface, *Anal. Sci.*, 7(3), 371, 1991.
14. **Miyazaki, H.**, personal communication, 1990.
15. **Osborn, M. C., Shao, Y., Pereira, C. M. and Girault, H. H.**, Micro-hole interface for the amperometric determination of ionic species in aqueous solutions, *J. Electroanal. Chem.*, 364, 155, 1994.
16. **Turner, A. P. F., Karube, I. and Wilson, G. S.**, Eds., *Biosensor; Fundamentals and Applications*, Oxford Univ. Press, Oxford, 1987, p. 770.
17. **Wise, D. L.**, Ed., *Bioinstrumentation: Research, Developments and Applications*, Butterworths, Boston, 1990, p. 1563.
18. **Yamamoto, Y. and Senda, M.**, Amperometric ammonium ion sensor and its application to biosensors, *Sensors and Actuators b*, 13/14, 57, 1993.
19. **Senda, M. and Yamamoto, Y.**, Urea biosensor based on amperometric ammonium ion electrode, *Electroanalysis*, 5, 775, 1993.
20. **Yamamoto, Y.**, Study on amperometric ion-selective electrode sensors, *Ph.D. Thesis*. Kyoto University, 1991, p. 81.
21. **Arai, K., Ohsawa, M., Kusu, F. and Takamura, K.**, Drug ion transfer across oil-water interface and pharmacological activity, *Bioelectrochem. Bioenerg.*, 31, 65, 1993.
22. **Ohkouchi, T., Kakutani, T. and Senda, M.**, Electrochemical study of the transfer of uncouplers across the organic/aqueous interface, *Bioelectrochem. Bioenerg.*, 25, 71, 1991.
23. **Ohkouchi, T., Kakutani, T. and Senda, M.**, Electrochemical theory of the transfer of protons across a biological membrane facilitated by weak acid uncouplers added to the medium, *Bioelectrochem. Bioenerg.*, 25, 81, 1991.
24. **Kondo, T., Kakiuchi, T. and Senda, M.**, Hydrolysis of phospholipid monolayers by phospholipase D at the oil/water interface under the control of the potential drop across the monolayer, *Biochim. Biophys. Acta*, 1124, 1, 1992.

25. **Kondo, T., Kakiuchi, T. and Senda, M.**, Hydrolytic activity of phospholipase D from plants and *Strptomyces* spp. against phosphatidylcholine monolayers at the polarized oil/water interface. *Bioelectrochem. Bioenerg.*, 34, 93, 1994.
26. **Kakiuchi, T. and Takasu, Y.**, Differential cyclic voltfluorometry and chronofluorometry of the transfer of fluorescent ions across the 1,2-dichloroethane-water interface, *Anal. Chem.*, 66(11), 1853, 1994.
27. **Cheng, Y. and Schiffrin, D. J.**, A. C. impedance study of rate constants for two-phase electron-transfer reactions, *J. Chem. Soc. Faraday Trans.*, 89(2), 199, 1993.

Chapter 13

LIQUID/ LIQUID INTERFACES AND SELF-ORGANIZED ASSEMBLIES OF LECITHIN

Yurii A. Shchipunov

I. INTRODUCTION

The commonly accepted model for adsorption of amphiphiles at interfacial boundaries between gas and water or between two immiscible liquids, tracing back to Langmuir [1], is molecular filling of the interface by adsorbed substances. This model is based on experimental observations of monomolecular films, summarized in monographs by Adam, Davies and Rideal, and Gaines. [2-4] The monomolecular film can become multimolecular if collapse occurs during compression or if excess amphiphile is spread on the dividing surface.[2,5-8] Soluble amphiphile will transfer into the solution bulk and produce monomolecular films at interfacial boundaries.

Numerous experimental observations in the literature suggest that these views are simplified. Thus, water soluble surfactants are capable of forming multimolecular layers, termed admicelles, on solid supports owing to unrestricted adsorption.[9-11] Similar filling of an interface by adsorbed amphiphiles occurs in liquid/liquid systems.[12-16] The formation of thick interfacial films is often observed in extraction processes.[17] The stabilization of emulsions by phospholipids is due to three-dimensional liquid-crystalline shells of droplets.[18-24] The thinning of nonaqueous and aqueous films to stratified films consisting of several bimolecular lamellae, has been reported in [16,24-27]. These observations show that the amphiphiles can self-assemble at the interfacial boundaries between immiscible liquids into more complex structures than the monomolecular layer.

Phospholipids in particular are very prone to self-organization into different supramolecular assemblies and polymorphic transformations.[29-32] The aim of this chapter is to demonstrate that this noteworthy feature is revealed during adsorption at the oil/water interface and in unusual properties of the adsorption layer when it is exposed to external electric fields. This will be exemplified by data obtained mainly for egg yolk and soybean lecithin (phosphatidylcholine).

II. LECITHIN SELF-ASSEMBLY AND SELF-ORGANIZATION AT THE INTERFACE

A. DILUTE SOLUTIONS

Phospholipids at interfacial boundaries have been studied extensively in the form of monomolecular films on air/water interfaces.[2-8] Among these should be mentioned classical works of Pethica, Mingins and Taylor with

0-8493-7694-7/96/$0.00+$.50

coauthors.[33-35] They performed exhaustive studying of properties, behavior, and phase transitions of phospholipid monolayers.

The adsorption of surface-active agents is described in the framework of thermodynamic approach advanced by Gibbs. The corresponding equation may be represented as follows:

$$d\Pi = RT\,\Gamma\, d\ln C \tag{1}$$

where Π is the interfacial pressure equal to an interfacial tension difference in the absence and presence of an amphiphile in the system, R the gas constant, T the temperature, Γ the surface excess, and C the concentration of substance in the solution bulk. As seen from the Gibbs equation, the concentration of an amphiphile at the interface Γ, expressed in mole/m^2, may be obtained from the experimental dependence of interfacial pressure on bulk concentration. There is a limitation on its use, lying in the fact that surfactant exerts influence on the interfacial tension until micelles start forming in the system.[36] The critical micelle concentrations of phospholipids in nonaqueous media are 10^{-6}-10^{-5} mM,[16,37] in water, 10^{-10}-10^{-9} M.[36] For this reason, it is essential to study phospholipid adsorption in very dilute solutions.

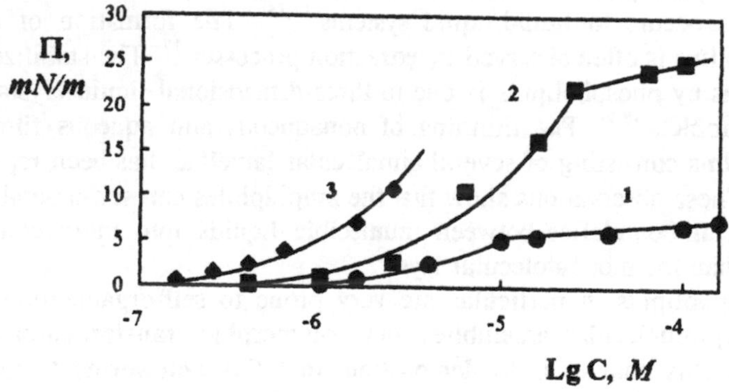

Figure 1. Interfacial tension at the *n*-decane/water interface as a function of the logarithm of egg-yolk lecithin concentration in alkane. Interfacial tensions were measured by: (1) drop volume and (2,3) drop pendant techniques in 3-5 min (1), 30 min (2) and 12-15 h (3) after a water drop was squeezed out into nonaqueous solution. (From Shchipunov, Yu. A. and Kolpakov, A. F., *Adv. Colloid and Interface Sci.*, 35, 31, 1991. With permission from Elsevier Science Publishers, B. V.)

The interfacial pressure at the *n*-heptane/water interface as a function of the logarithm of lecithin concentration in alkane is presented in Fig. 1. The measurements were taken by drop-volume and pendant drop techniques within various time of contact of immiscible liquids. Equilibrium values of the interfacial pressure, represented by curve 3, were obtained within 12-15

h. This could be done using only the pendant drop method (specificity of methods are considered in section V).

The surface excess and an area A occupied by a phospholipid molecule at the oil/water interface ($A = 1/\Gamma N_A$, where N_A is the Avogadro number) determined by the Gibbs equation (1) from the experimental dependence in Fig. 1 suggest that an adsorption layer simulate to a monomolecular film, is formed at egg yolk lecithin concentrations less than 0.002 mM. Even at 0.002 mM, the amount of adsorbed phospholipid appears to be sufficient to create an interfacial film three molecules thick.[14,16]

The results of thermodynamic calculations are borne out by studying the adsorption kinetics. As seen in Fig. 2, the interfacial pressure at the *n*-heptane/water interface is proportional to the square root of time measured since the contact of lecithin solution with water. This temporal dependence, satisfying diffusion kinetics,[2] occurs until equilibrium is nearly attained in the system. The number of adsorbed lecithin molecules, n, may be calculated from the interfacial tension measurements using [2,16]:

$$n = 2\, C\, N_A\, (D\, t/\pi)^{1/2} \qquad (2)$$

where D is the diffusion coefficient ($D = 2.10^{-10}$ m^2/s [14,16]), t is the time measured from the moment the immiscible liquids are brought into contact, π is equal to 3.14. The amount of adsorbed phospholipid has been found to be more than that needed for monomolecular filling of the interfacial boundary. Good agreement has been found with values computed from adsorption measurements under equilibrium conditions.[16]

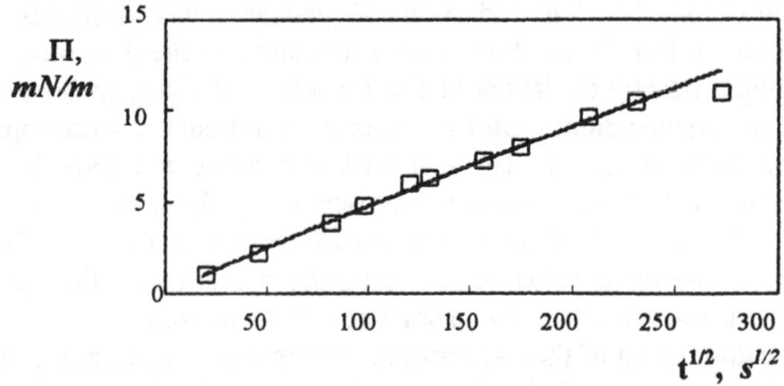

Figure 2. Interfacial tension at the *n*-decane/water interface as a function of the square root of time counted from the water drop formation in nonaqueous solution. Egg-yolk lecithin concentration in alkane was 0.002 mM. (From Shchipunov, Yu. A. and Kolpakov, A. F., *Adv. Colloid Interface Sci.*, 35(1), 31, 1991. With permission from Elsevier Science Publishers, B. V.)

Studies of adsorption from diluted solutions of egg yolk lecithin has revealed that most of the phospholipid in the system is concentrated at the oil/water interface. Reasonable diffusion kinetics over the period of adsorption is possible only when the counterflow of a substance is negligibly small. Since this is observed here (Fig. 2), lecithin appears to bind in the neighborhood of the oil/water interface, presumably because it does not readily desorb.

The observed accumulation of lecithin at the boundary between immiscible liquids has been explained in [14,16] in terms of hydration. When a phospholipid molecule arrives at the interface, it can add 33 to 39 water molecules [38-40] owing to its extensive polar region. The hydration results in nearly 1.5 increase in the molecular volume.[41] Increasing hydrophilicity in turn would bring about a decrease in the solubility of lecithin in nonpolar media and, as a result, its accumulation at the oil/water interface.

Thus, the studying of the adsorption kinetics and adsorption under equilibrium conditions suggests that lecithin is concentrated at the interfacial boundary between immiscible liquids in quantities which exceed those needed for monomolecular filling. This is observed even in very dilute solutions. A decrease in solubility owing to the hydration of the phospholipid appears to be responsible for its accumulation in the vicinity of the oil/water interface.

B. CONCENTRATED SOLUTIONS

Naturally occurring lecithin starts aggregating in alkalis at a concentration 0.01 mM.[37,42] For this reason, the approach used in the previous section cannot be applied to study filling of the oil/water interface by phospholipid at higher concentrations.

The accumulation of lecithin at the boundary between immiscible liquids in dilute solutions suggests that in concentrated mixtures this effect will be enhanced. These expectation is supported by numerous experimental results with emulsions.[18-24] The addition of phospholipids promotes a profound stabilizing effect. The stabilization is attributed to the formation of a three-dimensional adsorption layers at the oil/water interface, possessing liquid-crystalline organization. Under certain conditions, anisotropic interfacial films thick enough to be seen with the naked eye have been observed at the planar boundary between immiscible liquids in the presence of lecithin.[15,16,28] An example of such structures is shown in Fig. 3A. The evidence in [18-24] allows the conclusion that naturally occurring lecithin self-organizes at the oil/water interface into a smectic interfacial film.

Closer examination of the *n*-decane/water has shown that adsorption of soybean lecithin is accompanied by interfacial processes that have not been observed previously. [43] After a lecithin nonaqueous solution is brought into contact with water, separation of a new isotropic phase on the side of the nonpolar solution was observed, but only when the system was examined in transmitted light directed through partially crossed polarizers. With time an interfacial film developed. Its surface, presented to the nonaqueous phase, took on a wavelike profile (Fig. 3B). The amplitude of waves increased, and sometimes a wave "burst" with a stream of fluid, moving up (Fig. 3C). Near the alkane/air interface, the stream spread along the boundary.

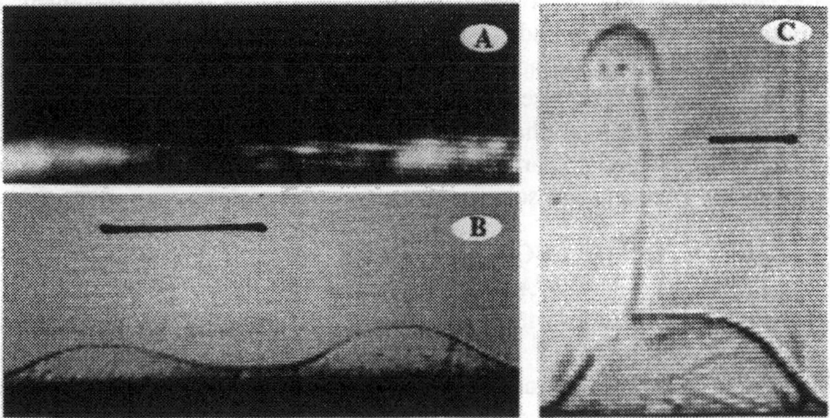

Figure 3. Photographs: (A) anisotropic film at the *n*-decane/water interface; (B) separated interfacial layer with wavelike profile; (C) outgoing stream of fluid (marked with an arrow) in *n*-decane solution. The photographs were taken in transmitted light with completely (A) and partially (B and C) crossed polarizers within 3.0 (B); 3.5 (C) and 5.0 (A) min after immiscible liquids were brought into contact. Soybean lecithin concentration in n-decane was 10 mg/ml. In all the pictures a bar indicate 1 mm.

Samples of the solution were taken at various points for analysis and densities were measured with a precision densitometer. It was established that the liquid phase separated near the boundary between immiscible liquids is the solvent, alkane, or, what is more probable, a very dilute solution. Since the density decreased with dilution, the separated fluid tends to transfer to the top of the solution.

Thus, numerous observations in the literature and our own studies of concentrated nonaqueous solutions of lecithin allow the conclusion that lecithin self-assembles into a thick interfacial film with liquid crystalline organization, resembling a lamellar phase. In addition, a process in the neighborhood of the oil/water interface occurs with the separation of organic solvent. An understanding of this phenomenon was gained when effects of water on the phase behavior of nonaqueous phospholipid solutions were examined. Pertinent data and models for interfacial processes will be considered in the next section.

III. INTERFACIAL STRUCTURES AND TERNARY PHASE DIAGRAMS

The interfacial boundary between immiscible liquids represents an intermediate region where mixing of all the components of a system takes place. Water, for example, can transfer into nonpolar media and attach to the polar region of phospholipids. Their phase state depends on the extent of hydration. Its successive addition promotes various polymorphic transformations.[29-32] It seems reasonable to relate the interfacial processes on the nonaqueous side, described in the previous section to rearrangements of phospholipid structures under the action of water. Because of concentration gradients in the neighborhood of the oil/water interface, observation of the phase transformations presents many difficulties. A useful approach to reveal the nature of interfacial phases and processes is the examination of ternary mixtures which are prepared by addition of specified quantities of polar solvent into a nonaqueous solution.

A. PROPERTIES OF LECITHIN IN THE LECITHIN/ALKANE/WATER SYSTEMS

Naturally occurring lecithin begins to form clusters of 4-5 molecules in alkanes at 0.01 mM.[37,42] In concentrated solutions there are micelles composed of about 100 molecules.[44] When dissolved in nonpolar media, lecithin retains its hygroscopicity and has the ability to absorb water from humid air.[16] The solubilization processes have been studied in solutions prepared with of aromatic and chlorinated solvents.[45] Solubilized water is used at first to fill hydration shells and then for the water pool in the interior of micelles, which transform into swollen reverse micelles with no change of spherical shape.[16]

Solubilization processes in alkane solutions are distinctive in several respects. The addition of water, as first established by Scartazzini and Luisi [46], produces the thickening effect (organogel formation). An important point is that the transformation takes place at quantities of polar solvent at which the filling of the hydration shell is far from complete. With the help of neutron scattering, dynamic light scattering and rheology it has been shown [47-51] that water addition promotes the transformation of spherical reverse micellar aggregates into elongated tubular ones. After reaching a critical length, they become entangled, forming a three-dimensional network. Entanglement of worm-like micelles leads to viscoelastic rheological behavior, similar to that demonstrated by polymers in the semidilute regime in good solvents.

With added water a nonaqueous lecithin solution undergoes several transformations. This can be illustrated by Fig. 4A, which shows the dependence of static storage modulus G_o, characterizing elastic properties on the number, N, of added water molecules per phospholipid molecule. The viscoelastic properties reveal that about one water molecule binds per lecithin molecule. The static storage modulus increased sharply over a very narrow concentration range and then decreased. The curve peaked at N equal to 2. The maximum is consistent with the initial separation of a homogeneous jelly-like phase into a low viscosity solution and a precipitated compact gel. With further increasing N the separated gel solidifies, so that a solid precipitate is found in ternary mixture. The approximate boundaries between various phase states are shown with vertical lines in Fig. 4A.

The separation of concentrated mixtures into low viscosity solution and gel, [52,53] is the most salient characteristic of lecithin jelly-like phases. This is reproducible and can be easily verified by different methods, for example, by observation of a solution placed between crossed polarizers.[52,53] The critical concentration can be useful for defining the existence region of phospholipid organogels, as in the partial ternary phase diagram of egg yolk lecithin in Fig. 4B.

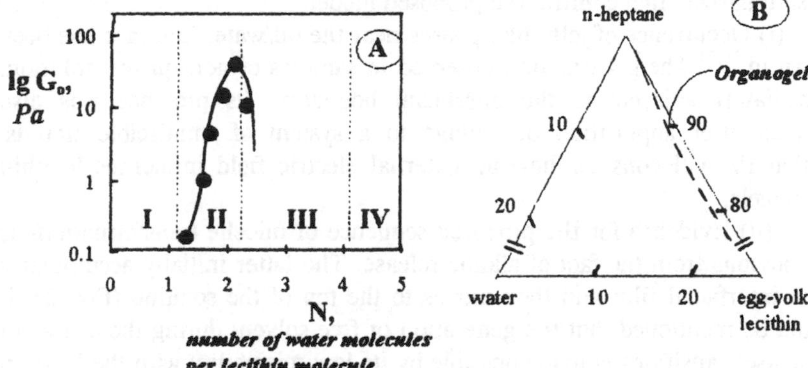

Figure 4. (A) Static storage (elastic) modulus of *n*-decane solution versus number of water molecules per soybean lecithin molecule. The lecithin concentration was 10 mg/ml. The vertical lines indicate approximate boundaries between various phase states: (I) low viscosity solution with Newtonian rheology; (II) organogel; (III) two-phase mixture composed of low viscosity solution and precipitated highly viscous gel; (IV) two-phase mixture with solid precipitate. (B) Ternary phase diagram egg-yolk lecithin-heptane-water. The critical concentrations of the organogel separation into two-phase mixture is shown by a dashed line. Concentrations are given in weight percent.

It should be emphasized that the phase or pseudophase transitions in nonaqueous lecithin solutions occur in a very narrow range of water concentrations. The attachment of only one water molecule to the phospholipid molecule appears to be enough to promote the rearrangement of spherical reverse micelles into elongated tubular aggregates (Fig. 4A), and further solvent molecules induce a phase separation. The latter is accompanied with a release of entrapped alkane from the three-dimensional network of entangled micellar aggregates.

The rearrangements of lecithin structures promoted by water might lead to a better understanding of interfacial processes observed after contact of a phospholipid solution with water (section II B). A plausible model is considered in the next section.

B. MODELS FOR INTERFACIAL PROCESSES

A schematic drawing of micelles and their transformations near the oil/water interface is shown in Fig. 5. The process begins when a spherical micellar aggregate arrives from the nonaqueous solution bulk phase at the interface with the aqueous solution where it can take on water. Even trace amounts of attached polar solvent induce a micelle shape change.[46-53] As a consequence, the initial spherical micelles undergo radical transformation into elongated micellar aggregates. The change of micelle shape is followed by the formation of a jelly-like phase. This phase is an intermediate structure because of its existence within a narrow range of water concentrations (Fig. 3). With further attachment of water the organogel separates into a compact gel and alkane incorporated previously into the three-dimensional network of entangled tubular micelles. The process will be completed with the transfer of separated gel into a solid precipitate. Below some experimental observations are summarized that confirm the proposed model.

(i) Occurrence of jelly-like phases near the oil/water interface has been shown in.[16,54] The gel was first observed in samples of nonaqueous solution, immediately adjacent to the interfacial boundary. Its presence was also revealed after application of voltage to a system of immiscible liquids. Section IV will consider how an external electric field influences lecithin organogels.

(ii) Evidence for the proposed sequence of micelle transformations is also obvious from the fact of alkane release. The latter initially accumulates as an interfacial film and then moves to the top of the solution (Fig. 2). It should be mentioned that the generation of free solvent during the course of the phase transitions is made possible by its low miscibility with the lecithin solution.[43]

(iii) A solid precipitate occurring in parallel with the alkane is always present after some period of contact between the lecithin solution and water.

The case in question shows that examination of ternary phase diagrams may sometimes provide insight into interfacial processes at the boundary between immiscible liquids.

IV. ELECTROINTERFACIAL PHENOMENA

The experimental results discussed above show that lecithin adsorption at the oil/water interface does not lead to monomolecular filling of the interfacial boundary as in the case of common surfactants. The phospholipid is prone to self-organize into different supramolecular assemblies. Their presence has a remarkable effect on the properties of a boundary between immiscible liquids. This is most evident in experiments in which a DC electric field is applied to liquid/liquid systems containing phospholipids. A variety of novel interfacial phenomena occurs[16,54-57] termed "electrointerfacial phenomena".[16]

The effects produced by application of a voltage to the liquid/liquid systems in the presence of naturally occurring lecithin are:

- Accelerated reduction in interfacial tension with time
- Reduced tension at the oil/water interface
- Electrohydrodynamic instability
- Emulsification
- Gel formation

Some of these effects can be observed in the absence of phospholipids as well, but the lecithin addition results in a 50-80 fold decrease in the voltage intensity inducing them.[16,54-57] This fact implies that the added lecithin leads to a pronounced increase in the sensitivity of the boundary between immiscible liquids to the action of an external electric field. Let us consider the electrointerfacial phenomena in greater detail. The diagram in Fig. 6 is illustrative of the topic in question.

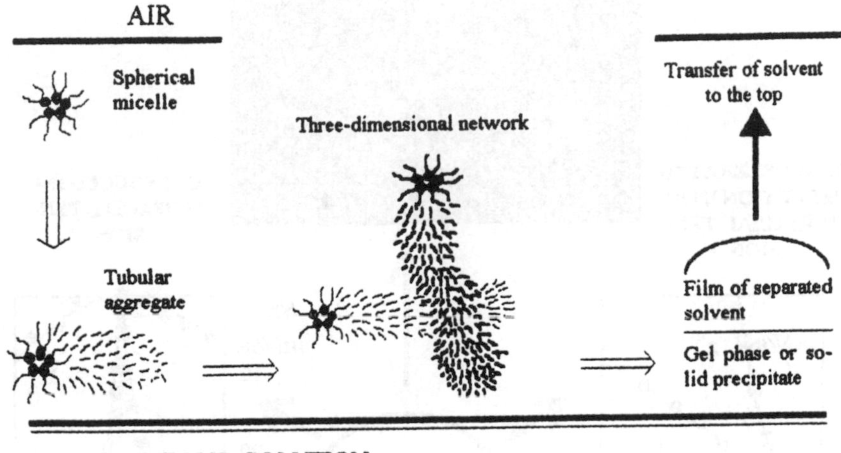

Figure 5. Possible structural changes induced in reverse micellar aggregates due to the hydration of lecithin in the vicinity of interfacial boundary with water.

A. BREAKDOWN PHENOMENON

The phenomenon, added for comparison purposes, is typical of systems composed of a conducting liquid such as water and a nonconducting one in the absence of phospholipids. When reaching a critical value, the electric field triggers the development of electrohydrodynamic instability at a planar interfacial boundary, followed by a spontaneous dispersion of water in the oil in the wake of the dielectric breakdown of a nonconducting liquid layer confined between the aqueous phase and an electrode in the organic media. The photograph in Fig. 6A was taken at the instant a spark occurred in the system. The breakdown in liquid/liquid systems usually occurs at field strengths of 5.105-8.105 V/m.[58] The presence of common surface-active substances does not markedly influence the characteristics of the phenomenon. The behavior is radically changed with introduction of phospholipids[14-16, 54-57] as described below.

10 Immiscible Liquid Interface and Self-Organized Assemblies of Lecithin

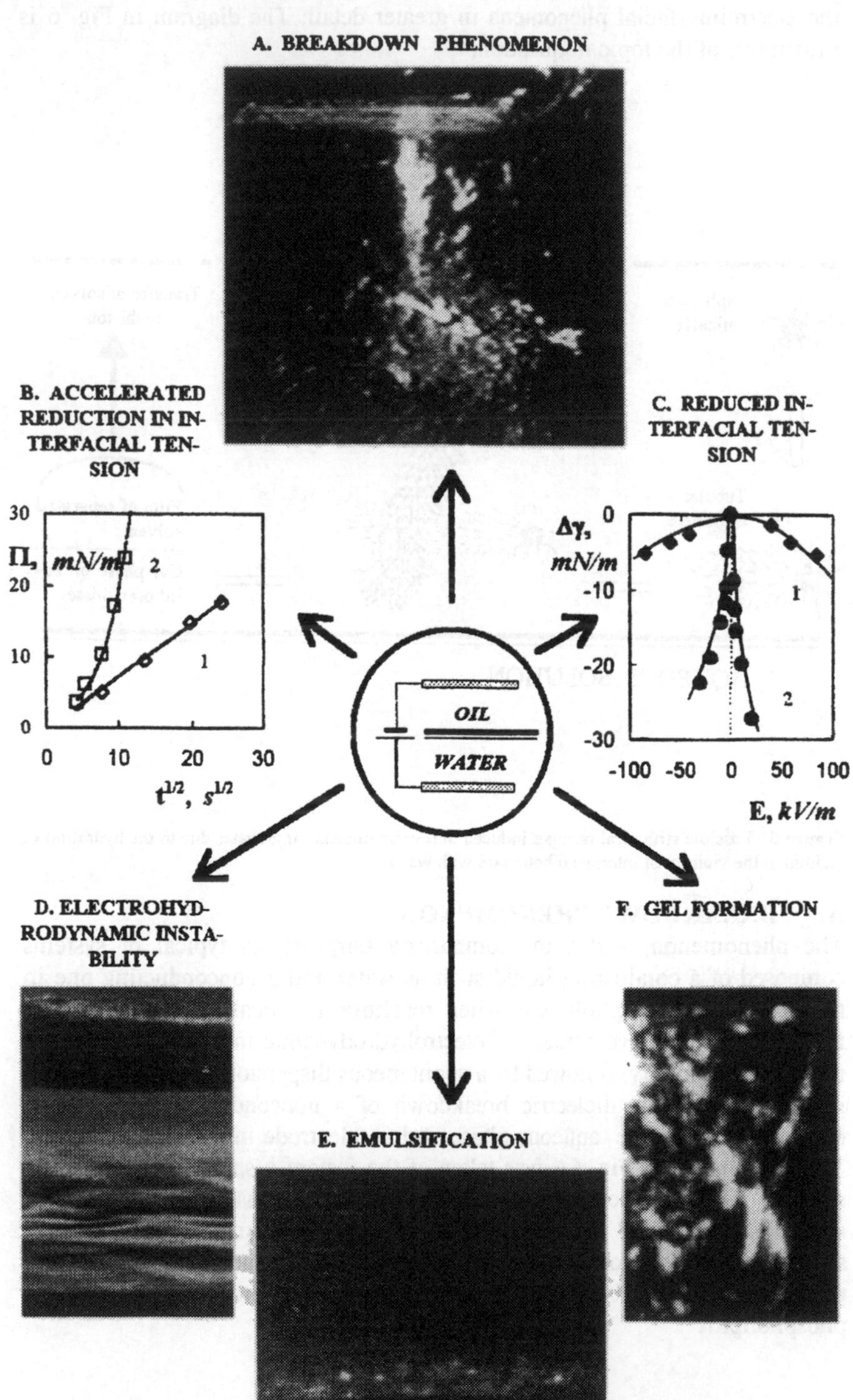

Opposite: **Figure 6.** Interfacial phenomena caused by application of a DC electric field to the oil/water interface. (A) Dielectric breakdown of *n*-decane layer confined between a platinum electrode and aqueous phase. Electric field intensity was 200 kV/m. The phenomenon occurs in the absence of phospholipid. (B) Interfacial pressure at the *n*-decane/water interface as a function of the square root of time. Electric intensities were: (1) 0 and (2) 9 kV/m. Egg-yolk lecithin concentration in alkane was 0.02 mM. Interfacial tension was measured by a pendant drop technique. (C) Difference in interfacial tensions measured in the electric field and without external influences as a function of electric field intensity. The sign of potential is shown for an electrode in the aqueous phase. Egg-yolk lecithin concentration were: (1) 0 and (2) 0.033 mM. (D) Example of wave-like oscillations on the surface between *n*-decane and 1 mM KCl aqueous solution. Electric field intensity was 60 kV/m. Egg-yolk lecithin concentration was 2 mM. Dark band at the top is an electrode in nonaqueous phase. Magnification x10. (E) Water droplets in the neighborhood of *n*-decane/1 mM KCl aqueous solution interface within 15 s after the application of a 20 kV/m electric field. Egg-yolk lecithin concentration was 2 mM. Magnification x10. (F) Electrically induced jelly-like phase confined between water phase and a platinum electrode (dark band at the top) in *n*-decane solution. Egg-yolk lecithin concentration was 2 mM. Electric field intensity was 5 kV/m. Photograph taken under oblique illumination. Magnification x20. (Figures B, C, and D from Shchipunov, Yu. A. and Kolpakov, A. F., *Adv. Colloid Interface Sci.*, 35, 31, 1991. With permission from Elsevier Science Publishers, B. V.)

B. ACCELERATED REDUCTION IN INTERFACIAL TENSION

When water and a nonaqueous solution of lecithin are brought into contact, interfacial tension decrease as a function of $t^{1/2}$ (Figs. 2 and 6 B). A voltage applied perpendicularly to the interfacial boundary strongly influences the adsorption kinetics. The effect is evident from comparison of curves 1 and 2 in Fig. 6 B. The voltage accelerates tension decrease, perhaps by hastening diffusion of molecules to the interface. However, the effect is more likely to be caused by formation of tension-reducing interfacial structures than by changing diffusion kinetics.[16]

C. REDUCED INTERFACIAL TENSION

A result of the accelerated tension decrease with applied voltage is reduced tension at the oil/water interface at steady state (curve 2, Fig. 6 C). This conclusion can be inferred from experimental results of various authors.[16,55,59,60] The effect of the field, shown in comparison with an electrocapillary curve of an alkane/water interface in Fig. 6 C, is dramatic. Its nature is not conclusively established. In [16] it was suggested that the tension decrease is related to formation of swollen reverse micellar aggregates which act as microemulsions.

D. ELECTROHYDRODYNAMIC INSTABILITY

Ripples and waves visible to the naked eye can be seen at the interface between water and nonaqueous lecithin solutions when a voltage is applied, illustrated by a photograph in Fig. 6 D. The generation of electrohydrodynamic instability in alkane/water systems in the absence of phospholipids [58] is observed at field strengths of $5 \cdot 10^5$-$8 \cdot 10^5$ V/m. The lecithin addition lowers the critical value of field intensity down to 102-103 V/m.[16] Analogous wavelike interface oscillations at such the electric intensities occur only in systems consisting of two conducting liquids, e. g., of water and mercury.[61] In that case, the instability is due to the considerable convective flow of liquids near the dividing surface, caused in turn by an electric current. Seeing the currents is negligible in the alkane/water system, the nature of the phenomenon with lecithin is basically different: the electrohydrodynamic instability is governed by field effects.

E. EMULSIFICATION

The reduced interfacial tension and the generation of wavelike oscillations at the oil/water interface under an applied electric field require interfacial dispersion processes to occur.[16,56,57] After application of a voltage, water transfer into the nonaqueous phospholipid solution takes place (Fig. 6 E). The emulsification proceeds when electric field intensity exceeds 10^4 V/m. The dispersion of the interface does not require the electric breakdown which is typical of systems that do not contain lecithin (Fig. 6 A). In the presence of phospholipid the emulsion formation comes about at electric field strengths at which no changes in the free interfacial boundary are detectable. With applied voltage water droplets appear at the oil/water interface on the nonpolar side, then migrate to the electrode. The initial stage of the process can be seen in Fig. 6 E.

The process ultimate in turns the nonaqueous layer between the electrode and water into an emulsified state. If the emulsion is sufficiently dense, secondary processes aggregate the emulsion droplets and order them into chains aligned along the electric field lines.[16,56,57] The chain-forming processes caused by electric fields in nonpolar media containing dispersed particles are well known.[62,63]

F. GEL FORMATION

The emulsion dimensions tend to decrease as the electric field intensity is lowered. If it becomes less than 10^4 V/m, a jelly-like phase has been observed in 1-10 mM lecithin solutions.[16,51,57] The gel is generated in the emulsion in close to the oil/water interface and then fills the space between water and electrode in the nonaqueous phase (Fig. 6 F). The jelly-like phase is viscous, homogeneous, and transparent. If the voltage is switched off, the gel settles to the interface and dissipates with time. The thickening effect may be produced repeatedly.

The gel phases generated by applying voltage to alkane/water systems bear a striking resemblance to lecithin organogels (section IIIA). It is noteworthy that the gel is produced within minutes, while hours are required to dissolve water in a lecithin solution.[52] It appears that the external electric field accelerates the transfer of water into the nonaqueous solution and the redistribution of polar solvent in lecithin structures.[16,57]

Examination of gel phases produced in oil/water systems under the action of external electric field presents difficulties. As shown in [64], their properties and behavior are most conveniently studied in ternary mixtures with specified amounts of substances.

Effects of an external electric field on nonaqueous solutions of lecithin with various amounts of water have been investigated in [64]. It has been established that phospholipid supramolecular assemblies are susceptible to the field action. The observed effects depend on the phase state of a ternary mixture. In the case of a lecithin organogel, the electric field brings about a decrease in viscosity, as shown in Fig. 7 A. At the same time, the applied voltage makes the isotropic organogel birefringent (Fig. 7 B). The field-induced optical effect is similar to flow birefringence. These experimental results suggest that the viscosity decrease and optical anisotropy are related to the orientation of tubular lecithin micelles along the electrical field lines. Their ordered arrangement diminishes the entangled aggregation and thereby changes the rheological properties of ternary mixtures.

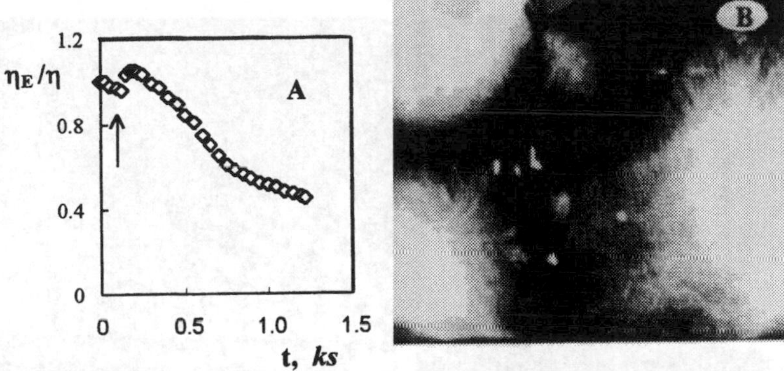

Figure 7. (A) Temporal changes in viscosity represented as a ratio of viscosity measured in electric field to viscosity of initial organogel. Measurement was made at a constant oscillation frequency of 0.1 Hz at 25.0 + 0.1°C. Soybean lecithin concentration in n-decane was 10 mg/ml. Water content was 2.1 molecules per phospholipid molecule. Arrow marks the time when a 10 kV/m electric field was applied. (B) Electrically induced optical anisotropy in the same organogel under the action of a 100 kV/m electric field. The photograph was taken in transmitted light with crossed polarizers. Dark bands at the bottom and the top are platinum electrodes positioned horizontally. Bar indicates 1 mm.

It should be pointed out that the electric field promotes a phase separation in the lecithin organogel in which the gel phase is confined to the interelectrode spacing (Fig. 7 B) and the remaining solution is low viscosity. The field-induced effect resembles the separation of the organogel into a gel phase and nonaqueous solution at high water concentrations (Fig. 4).

Two-phase ternary mixtures containing a solid precipitate under the action of an external electric field demonstrate a response different from that of the homogeneous organogel. By their properties, such mixtures can be related to electrorheological fluids.[64] The resemblance makes itself evident in viscosity increase (Fig. 8 A) and fibril formation from solid particles in the interelectrode spacing (Fig. 8 B). These phenomena, known as electrorheological effects, have been observed previously in nonpolar organic solvents with suspended particles of various materials.[65,66] The fibrous phospholipid structures obtained by applied voltage were first observed in [64].

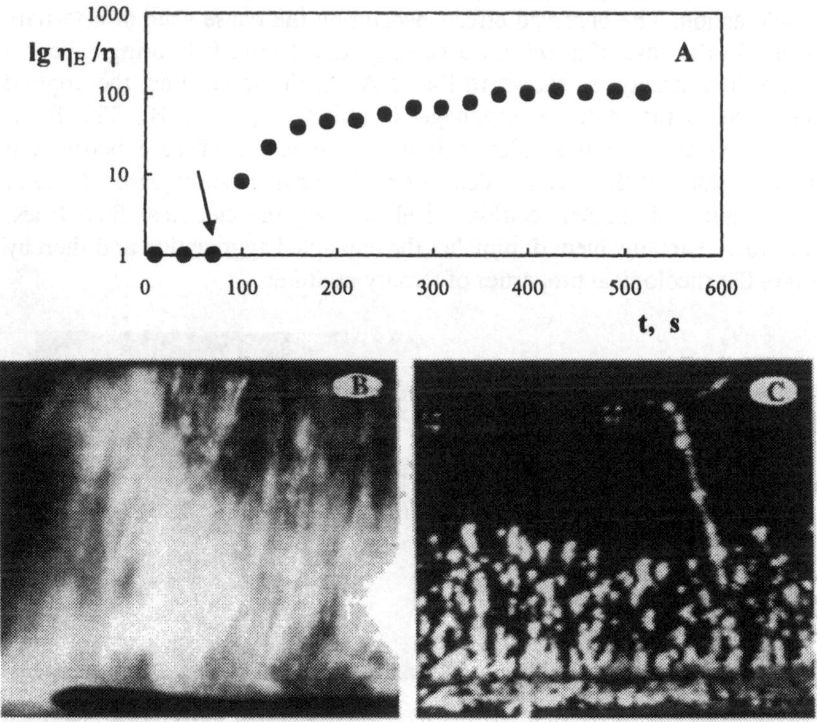

Figure 8. (A) Temporal dependence of viscosity represented as a ratio of viscosity measured in electric field to viscosity of initial two-phase mixture with solid precipitate. Measurement was made at a constant oscillation frequency of 17 Hz at 25.0 + 0.1°C. Soybean lecithin concentration was 10 mg/ml. Water content was 4.6 molecules per phospholipid molecule. Arrow indicates the time when a 80 kV/m electric field was applied. (B) Electrically induced fibrillation in the same two-phase mixturecaused by an 80 kV/m electric field. Dark bands at the top and the bottom are platinum electrodes. The gap between them is 6 mm. The photograph was taken in transmitted light with crossed polarizers within 3 min after a voltage was switched on. (C) Fibril structures in a nonaqueous layer between water phase and platinum electrode (dark band at the top) in n-decane formed by application of a 30 kV/m electric field. Soybean lecithin concentration was 10 mg/ml. Before the experiment, immiscible liquids were brought into contact for 30 min and then voltage was applied for 5 min. The spacing between the electrode and aqueous phase is 2 mm.

At the same time, lecithin-containing mixtures should be differentiated from typical electrorheological fluids. The most marked difference between them is in the transformation of phospholipid structures under the action of an external electric field. It has been ascertained [64] that prolonged applied voltage produces an anisotropic mesophase instead of fibrils and to a sharp decrease in viscosity. The nature of these phase transitions is not yet understood.

The results described here show that supramolecular assemblies of lecithin at immiscible liquid interfaces are highly sensitive to weak electric fields. As a result, applied voltage promotes electrointerfacial phenomena which include a sharp drop in the interfacial tension, dispersion of the interfacial boundary, and generation of a water-in-oil emulsions and a gel phases. In addition, behavior of the emulsion and gel is regulated by the external electric field.

V. METHODS

Measurement of the surface tension at the liquid/liquid interfaces figures prominently in studies of interfacial phenomena.
The corresponding methods are so well known that often they do not receive sufficient emphasis and their full potential is not realized.

When initiating a study involving interfacial tension, considerable attention should be paid to selection of a measuring method. As evident from curves 1 and 3 in Fig. 1, results obtained with various techniques differ significantly. This can be important for determining thermodynamic characteristics of adsorption. Although the Wilhelmy plate technique is in wide use, it is not necessarily the most appropriate method. This technique is most useful in measuring precise surface tension at air/liquid interfaces. Accuracy of measurements is dependent on the wettability of the plate and the contact angle. Surface-active agents, which influence the wetting parameters and cause instability of the contact angle, also give rise to measurement errors.[2,67,68]

Precise and reproducible data on the adsorption of surfactants can be obtained with the drop-volume and pendant drop methods. The former is best applied to high-rate interfacial processes if equilibrium is attained within minutes. Otherwise, the latter should be used, and lecithin-containing systems are one example (see section II A). The drop-volume and pendant drop methods possess many advantages over other methods. For instance, the measurements can be made by using small volumes of solutions and the experimental cell is easily thermostated. Improvements in the measuring setup and the high speed drop profile analysis by means of a computer have been proposed.[69-73]

Studying the effects of an external electric field on interfacial processes adds complexity to an experimental setup because at least two electrodes are introduced into opposite phases. An appropriate solution of the problem was suggested by Popov.[74] The electrode in the aqueous solution can be of arbitrary shape, while the organic phase electrode is shaped like a funnel, designed so that the water drop was spaced equidistantly from the electrode surface at any one point.

The funnel electrode is unusable in the pendant drop technique because the drop becomes unavailable for observation. Fortunately, electrointerfacial phenomena with phospholipids require only a weak external electric field (see section IV) which does not induce noticeable distortion in the drop shape.[16] This enables one to place a plate electrode underneath the water drop.

Experimental data for interfacial tension allow one to determine thermodynamic and kinetic parameters of the liquid/liquid interface and characteristics of aggregation processes in bulk solution. It is worthwhile to outline all possibilities here since it is rare for them to be exploited to the fullest extent.

- Filling of the interfacial boundary. To gain an insight into how a substance fills the liquid/liquid interface, one is faced with the necessity of finding its concentration at the interfacial boundary. The surface excess is determined using the Gibbs equation (1) from a concentration dependence of interfacial tension or pressure (Fig. 1). The G values allow the type of the adsorption isotherm, i. e., the expression relating the concentration of a substance in the bulk to that of the interface to be found.
- Areas of molecules in the adsorption layer. The area A occupied by a molecule at the oil/water interface is related to the surface excess according to:

$$A=1/N_A\,\Gamma \tag{3}$$

- A useful parameter thus evaluated is the minimal area per adsorbed molecule. This can be attributed to the cross-sectional area of a molecule and gives information on its orientation, packing and interactions in the adsorption layer.[2]
- Standard free energy of adsorption. This may be obtained from the initial linear part of a curve plotted on the Π - X coordinates (X is the mole fraction of surfactant in the bulk).[75] The standard free energies of adsorption offer an insight into interactions at the interface.[75] Since it is equal to a difference between the standard chemical potentials of a substance in the bulk solution and at the interface, the most contribution to the adsorption energy for amphiphiles with extended polar region is made by their hydration. Proofs for lecithin have been presented in [16].
- Adsorption kinetics. Examination of a temporal dependence of interfacial tension or pressure provides an inference about the adsorption kinetics regime and the limiting stage of a process.[2] An example of diffusion controlled kinetics described by Eq. (2) is presented in Fig. 2. One may see that the temporal dependence allows the diffusion coefficient to be estimated from the slope of the linear portion in the curve. For surfactants dissolved in nonaqueous solutions this method provides an effective means for determining the diffusion coefficients.
- Micelle formation. It is common practice to find out the critical micelle concentrations from a kink on plots of interfacial tension or pressure versus the logarithm of concentration.[36] Such inflection points are seen

on curves 1 and 2 in Fig. 1. The critical micelle concentrations can be employed for calculating the thermodynamic parameters characterizing the surfactant transfer from solution bulk to the micellar aggregates.[36]

- Premicelle association. Another convenient procedure for examining data is to represent a dependence of interfacial tension or pressure on the concentration in double logarithmic coordinates. A graph usually consists of two linear regions. The initial region refers to the Henry adsorption isotherm, the second region to the Freundlich adsorption isotherm. Change in the slope of curves is caused by the formation of associations composed of a few surfactant molecules.[76,77] Such associations is typical of substances dissolved in nonpolar media.[78] The graph in the bilogarithmic coordinates seems to be best suited to the estimation of both critical association concentration and the number of molecules involved in an associate. The latter parameter is determined from the slope of the linear portion of a curve obeying the Freundlich adsorption isotherm.[76,77]

Concentrated solutions require a different approach. Phospholipids are prone to self-organize into various structures at the interface between immiscible liquids. To investigate such structures, any one of several physico-chemical methods may be implemented. They are also applicable for studying field-induced effects on phospholipid self-organized assemblies. However, complications can occur when it is necessary to apply electric field to the interface. To simplify the experiment and interpretation of results, it may be beneficial in some instances to study ternary mixtures of constituents comprising the liquid/liquid system (see sections III and IVB).

VI. PROSPECTS FOR APPLICATIONS AND FURTHER STUDIES

The ability of lecithin to self-assemble into thick interfacial films gained wide acceptance in stabilization of emulsions long before it was revealed that the interfacial phenomena are caused by lecithin self-organization into three-dimensional assemblies on a two-dimensional surface. Nowadays this phospholipid is a major emulsifying agent among natural amphiphiles and heavily used in food industry, cosmetics, medicine and biotechnology.

Little is known about the behavior of lecithin at the liquid/liquid interface exposed to an external electric field and about electrointerfacial phenomena, which represent an area of considerable promise for chemical and biotechnological industries. An attractive feature lies in the fact that the field-induced effects occur under the action of small voltages. Electric fields have previously been used to prepare emulsions [79,80] but could not be exploited successfully for industrial applications. A 100-fold decrease in the electric strength needed for dispersion of liquid/liquid interfaces in the presence of lecithin offers new opportunities in this field.

To a large extent, fundamental studies must still be done to improve our understanding of the decreased interfacial tension, electrohydrodynamic instability, emulsification, structure of gel phases and their transformation in external fields. The relationship of interfacial phenomena to the macroscopic properties of immiscible liquids is a subject for fruitful research as well.

Of particular importance are interfacial phenomena accompanied by formation of disperse phases in a nonaqueous solution. In recent years, there has been an upsurge of interest in reverse micelles, microemulsions and organogels, and in their possible exploitation in various biotechnological processes ranging from selective amino acid and protein extraction to biocatalyzed synthesis.[45,81-84] The functional activity of biologically active compounds depends strongly on their surroundings, which should be similar to those in living systems. This problem is solved by using phospholipid-based dispersions in which the interfacial films mimic the lipid matrix of biological membranes and membranous organelles. From this standpoint, the lecithin assemblies generated in the oil/water system with the help of an electric field possess considerable potential for pharmaceutical applications.

In summary, there are numerous possible applications of self-organized assemblies of lecithin at the oil/water interface. Such systems have unusual properties and behavior, phenomena and structural organization, and represent a new area for scientific exploration in supramolecular chemistry, nanostructures and biological mimetic chemistry.

VII. ACKNOWLEDGMENTS

I wish to thank my collaborators and postgraduates who are mentioned in the references. Particular appreciation is extended to Prof. H. Hoffmann and Peter Schmiedel at Bayreuth University for discussion and help with rheological measurements. Some of the experimental results were made possible by financial support from the Russian Foundation for Fundamental Studies (grant No. 94-04-11311), the International Science Foundation (grant No. RJL000) and the Sonderforschungsbereich 213 "Topomac".

VIII. REFERENCES

1. **Langmuir, I.**, The constitution and fundamental properties of solids and liquids. II. Liquids, *J. Am. Chem. Soc.*, 39, 1848, 1917.
2. **Davies, J. T. and Rideal, E. K.**, *Interfacial Phenomena*, Academic Press, London, 1663.
3. **Moehwald, H.**, Phospholipid and phospholipid-protein monolayers at the air/water interfaces, *Annu. Rev. Phys. Chem.*, 41, 441, 1990.
4. **Knobler, C. M. and Desai, R. C.**, Phase transitions in monolayers, *Annu. Rev. Phys. Chem.*, 43, 207, 1992.
5. **Larsson, K.**, Lipid multilayers, *Surface Colloid Sci.*, 6, 261, 1973.
6. **Barnes, G. T.**, Insoluble monolayers - Dynamic aspects, in *Colloid Sciences Specialist Periodical Reports*, Vol. 3, Chemical Society, London, 1979, chap. 3.
7. **Ries, H. E., Albrecht, G. and Ter-Minassian-Saraga, L.**, Collapsed monolayers of egg lecithin, *Langmuir*, 1, 135, 1985.
8. **Iwahashi, M., Maehara, N., Kaneko, Y., Seimiya, T., Middleton, S. R., Pallas, N. R. and Pethica, B. A.**, Spreading pressure for fatty-acid crystals at the air/water interface, *J. Chem. Soc. Faraday Trans. I*, 81, 973, 1985.
9. **Harwell, J. H., Hoskins, J. C., Schechter, R. S. and Wade, W. H.**, Pseudophase separation model for surfactant adsorption: isomerically pure surfactants, *Langmuir*, 1, 251, 1985.

10. **Besio, G. J., Prud'homme, R. K. and Benziger, J. B.**, Ellipsometric observation of the adsorption of sodium dodecyl sulfate, *Langmuir*, 4, 140, 1988.
11. **Rupprecht, H. and Gu, T.**, Structure of adsorption layers of ionic surfactants at the solid/liquid interface, *Colloid Polym. Sci.*, 269(5), 506, 1991.
12. **Imae, T., Araki, H. and Ikeda, S.**, The anomalous behavior of surface tension of aqueous solutions of dimethyloleylamine oxide, and its multimolecular adsorption on aqueous surface, *Colloids Surf.*, 17(2), 207, 1986.
13. **Gershfeld, N. L.**, The critical unilamellar lipid state: a perspective for membrane bilayer assembly, *Biochim. Biophys. Acta*, 988, 335, 1989
14. **Shchipunov, Yu. A. and Kolpakov, A. F.**, Kinetics and equilibrium characteristics of adsorption of phosphatidylcholine at the oil/water interface. Influence of an electric field, *Izv. Acad. Sci. Latv. SSR, Ser. Khim.*, No.1, 53, 1988.
15. **Shchipunov, Yu. A. and Kolpakov, A. F.**, Self-assembly of phosphatidylcholine into liquid-crystalline structures at the oil/water interface in the course of adsorption from nonaqueous solution, *Izv. AN SSSR, Ser. Fiz.*, 55, 1844, 1991.
16. **Shchipunov, Yu. A. and Kolpakov, A. F.**, Phospholipids at the oil/water interface: adsorption and interfacial phenomena in an electric field, *Adv. Colloid Interface Sci.*, 35, 31, 1991.
17. **Tarasov, V. V. and Pichugin, A. A.**, Role of interfacial phenomena in processes of ionic transport through liquid membranes, *Usp. Khim.*, 57(6), 990, 1988.
18. **Ogino, K. and Onishi, M.**, Interfacial action of natural surfactants in oil/water systems, *J. Colloid Interface Sci.*, 83(1), 18, 1981.
19. **Davis, S. S. and Hansrani, P.**, The coalescence behavior of oil droplets stabilized by phospholipid emulsifiers, *J. Colloid Interface Sci.*, 108, 285, 1985.
20. **Friberg, S. E. and Solans, C.**, The Kendall Award Address. Surfactant association structures and the stability of emulsions and foams, *Langmuir*, 2, 121, 1986.
21. **Pilpel, M. and Rabbani, M. E.**, Formation of liquid crystals in sunflower oil-in-water emulsions, *J. Colloid Interface Sci.*, 116, 550, 1987.
22. **Pilpel, M. and Rabbani, M. E.**, Interfacial films in the stabilization of sunflower oil-in-water emulsions with nonionics, *J. Colloid Interface Sci.*, 122, 266, 1988.
23. **Yatagai, M., Komaki, M., Nakajima, T. and Hashimoto, T.**, Formation of a liquid crystalline phase between aqueous surfactant solutions and oily substances, *J. Am. Oil Chem. Soc.*, 67, 154, 1990.
24. **Van der Meeren, P., Stastny, M., Vanderdeelen, J. and Baert, L.**, Functional properties of purified soybean phospholipids o/w emulsions, paper presented at *6th Int. Colloquium on Phospholipids*, Hamburg, Germany, October 25-27, 1993.
25. **Kruglijakov, P. M. and Rovin, Yu. G.**, *Physico-Chemistry of Black Hydrocarbon Films*, Khimiaya Publ. House, Moscow, 1978.
26. **Manev, E. D., Sazdanova, S.V. and Wasan, D. T.**, Stratification in emulsion films, *J. Dispersion Sci. Techn.*, 5, 111, 1984.
27. **Exerova, D. and Lalchev, Z.**, Bilayer and multilayer films. Model for study of the alveolar surface and stability., *Langmuir*, 2, 668, 1986.
28. **Shchipunov, Yu. A. and Kolpakov, A. F.**, Structurization at the boundary of immiscible liquids in the presence of phospholipids and the formation of bilayer lipid membranes, *Kolloidn. Zh.*, 50, 1216, 1988.
29. **Hoffmann, H.**, From micellar solutions to liquid crystalline phases, *Ber. Bunsenges. Phys. Chem.*, 88, 1078, 1984.
30. **Small, D. M.**, *Handbook of Lipid Research, The Physical Chemistry of Lipids. From Alkanes to Phospholipids*, Vol. 4, Plenum Press, New York and London, 1986.
31. **Larsson, K.**, Physical properties - structural and physical characteristics, in *The Lipid Handbook*, Gunstone, F. D., Harwood, J. L. and Padday, F. B., Eds., Chapman and Hall, London, 1986, p. 321.
32. **Seddon, J. M.**, Structure of the inverted hexagonal (HII) phases, and non-lamellar phase transitions of lipids, *Biochim. Biophys. Acta*, 1031, 1, 1990.
33. **Yue, B. Y., Jackson, C. M., Taylor, J. A. C., Mingins, B. A. and Pethica, B. A.**, Phospholipid monolayers at non-polar oil/water interfaces. 1. Phase transitions in distearoyllecithin films at the *n*-heptane/aqueous sodium chloride interface, *J. Chem. Soc. Faraday Trans. I*, 72, 2685, 1976.

34. **Taylor, J. A. C., Mingins, B. A., Pethica, B. A.**, Phospholipid monolayers at nonpolar oil/water interfaces. 2. Dilute monolayers of saturated 1,2-diacyl-lecithins and a-cephalines, *J. Chem. Soc. Faraday Trans. I*, 72, 2694, 1976.
35. **Mingins, B. A., Taylor, J. A. C., Pethica, B. A. and Jackson, C. M.**, Phospholipid monolayers at non-polar oil/water interfaces. 3. Effect of chain length on phase transitions in saturated diacyl lecithins at the *n*-heptane/aqueous sodium chloride interface, *J. Chem. Soc. Faraday Trans. I*, 78, 323, 1982.
36. **Tanford, C.**, *The Hydrophobic Effect: Formation of Micelles and Biological Membranes*, Wiley-Interscience, New York, 1980.
37. **Shchipunov, Yu. A. and Drachev, G. Yu.**, Adsorption of choline- and ethanolamine-containing phospholipids at the n-heptane/water interface, *Kolloidn. Zh.*, 45, 1212, 1983.
38. **Ter-Minassian-Saraga, L.**, Hydration in two-dimensional systems, *Pure Appl. Chem.*, 53(11), 2149, 1981.
39. **Sjolund, M., Lindblom, G., Rilfors, L. and Arridson, G.**, Hydrophobic molecules in lecithin systems. 1. Formation of reversed hexagonal phases at high and low water content, *Biophys. J.*, 52(2), 145, 1987.
40. **Gruner, S. M., Tate, M. W., Kirk, G. L., So, P. T. C., Turner, D. C., Keane, D. T., Tilcock, C. P. S. and Cullis, P. R.**, X-Ray diffraction study of the polymorphic behavior of N-methylated dioleylphosphatidylethanolamine, *Biochemistry*, 27(8), 2853, 1988.
41. **White, S. and King, G. I.**, Molecular packing and area compressibility of lipid bilayers, *Proc. Natl. Acad. Sci. USA*, 82, 6532, 1985.
42. **Drachev, G. Yu., Shchipunov, Yu. A. and Kostetsky, E. Ya.**, Some physico-chemical properties of phospholipids with choline and ethanolamine functional groups. Comparative characteristics and possible biological consequence of distinctions, *Biochim .Biophys. Acta*, 813, 243, 1985.
43. **Shchipunov, Yu. A. and Schmiedel, P.**, unpublished results.
44. **Ramakrishnan, V. R., Darszon, A. and Montal, M.**, Small-angle X-ray scattering study of a rhodopsin-lipid complex in hexane, *J. Biol. Chem.*, 258, 4857, 1983.
45. **Walde, P., Giuliani, A. M., Boicelli, C. A. and Luisi, P. L.**, Phospholipid-based reverse micelles, *Chem. Phys. Lipids*, 53(2), 265, 1990.
46. **Scartazzini, R. and Luisi, P. L.**, Organogels from lecithins, *J. Phys. Chem.*, 92, 829, 1988.
47. **Schurtenberger, P., Scartazzini, R. and Luisi, P. L.**, Viscoelastic properties of polymer-like reverse micelles, *Rheol. Acta*, 28, 372, 1988.
48. **Schurtenberger, P., Scartazzini, R., Magid, L., Leser, M. E. and Luisi, P. L.**, Structural and dynamic properties of polymer-like reverse micelles, *J. Phys. Chem.*, 94, 3695, 1990.
49. **Schurtenberger, P., Magid, L. J., Lindner, P. and Luisi, P. L.**, A sphere to flexible coil transition in lecithin reverse micellar solutions, *Prog. Colloid Polym. Sci.*, 89, 274, 1992.
50. **Schurtenberger, P. and Cavano, C.**, Polymer-like lecithin reverse micelles. 1. A light scattering study, *Langmuir*, 10, 100, 1994.
51. **Schurtenberger, P.**, Structure and dynamics of viscoelastic surfactant solutions - an application of concepts from polymer science, *Chimie*, 48, 72, 1994.
52. **Shchipunov, Yu. A.**, Lecithin organogels: rheological properties of polymer-like micelles produced by water addition, *Kolloidn. Zh.*, submitted for publication.
53. **Shchipunov, Yu. A. and Shumilina, E. V.**, Lecithin-bridging by hydrogen bonds in the organogel, *Colloids Surf.*, submitted for publication.
54. **Shchipunov, Yu. A. and Kolpakov, A. F.**, The formation of anisotropic mesophase of phosphatidylcholine in alkane/water system by the action of an electric field, *J. Dispersion Sci. Techn.*, 9, 258, 1988.
55. **Popov, A. N., Drachev, G. Yu. and Shchipunov, Yu. A.**, Electrocapillary phenomena at the *n*-heptane/water interface in the presence of phospholipids, *Zh. Fiz. Khimii*, 57, 2288, 1983.
56. **Shchipunov, Yu. A. and Kolpakov, A. F.**, Formation of emulsion into nonaqueous solution of phosphatidylcholine under the action of an external electric field, *Kolloidn. Zh.*, 46, 1204, 1984.
57. **Shchipunov, Yu. A. and Kolpakov, A. F.**, Unusual processes of phospholipid dispersion formation by the action of an external electric field, *Colloids Surf. A: Physicochem. Eng. Aspects*, 76 15, 1993.
58. **Taylor, G. I. and McEwan, A. D.**, The stability of a horizontal fluid interface in a vertical electric field, *J. Fluid Mech.*, 22, 1, 1965.

59. **Girault, H. H. J. and Schiffrin, D. J.**, Adsorption of phosphatidylcholine and phosphatidylethanolamine at the polarized water/1,2-dichloroethane interface, *J. Electroanal. Chem.*, 179, 277, 1984.
60. **Kakiuchi, T., Nakanishi, M. and Senda, M.**, The electrocapillary curve of the phosphatidylcholine monolayer at the polarized oil-water interface. 1. Measurement of interfacial tension using a computer-aided pendant-drop method, *Bull. Chem. Soc. Jpn.*, 61, 1845, 1988.
61. **Makino, T. and Aogaki, R.**, Occurrence of regular convection at the liquid-liquid interface of two immiscible electrolyte solutions by resonance with a pulsated potential, *J. Electroanal. Chem.*, 198, 209, 1986.
62. **Winslow, W. M.**, Induced fibrillation of suspensions, *J. Appl. Phys.*, 20, 1137, 1949.
63. **Arp, P. A.., Foister, R. T. and Mason, S. G.**, Some electrohydrodynamic effects in fluid dispersion, *Adv. Colloid Interface Sci.*, 12, 295, 1980.
64. **Shchipunov, Yu. A. and Schmiedel, P.**, Electrorheological phenomena in lecithin-decane-water mixtures, *J. Colloid Interface Sci.*, submitted for publication.
65. **Gast, A. P. and Zukoski, C. F.**, Electrorheological fluids as colloidal suspensions, *Adv. Colloid Interface Sci.*, 30, 153, 1989.
66. **Toor, W.**, Structure formation in electrorheological fluids, *J. Colloid Interface Sci.*, 156, 335, 1993.
67. **Padday, J. F.**, Surface tension. 2. The measurement of surface tension, *Surface Colloid Sci.*, 1, 101, 1969.
68. **Princen, H. M., Cazabat, A. M., Stuart, M. A. C., Heslot, F. and Nicolet, S.**, Instabilities during wetting processes: Wetting by tensioactive liquids, *J. Colloid Interface Sci.*, 126, 84, 1988.
69. **Kakiuchi, T., Nakanishi, M. and Senda, M.**, The electrocapillary curves of the phosphatidylcholine monolayer at the polarized oil-water interface. I. Measurement of interfacial tension using a computer-aided pendant-drop method, *Bull. Chem. Soc. Jpn.*, 61, 1845, 1988.
70. **Boyce, J. F., Schurch, S., Rotenberg, Y. and Neumann, A. W.**, The measurement of surface and interfacial tension by the axisymmetric drop technique, *Colloids Surf.*, 9, 307, 1984.
71. **Girault, H. H. J., Schiffrin, D. J. and Smith, B. D. V.**, The measurement of interfacial tension of pendant drops using a video image profile digitizer, *J. Colloid Interface Sci.*, 101, 257, 1984.
72. **Pallas, N. R. and Harrison, Y.**, An automated drop shape apparatus and the surface tension of pure water, *Colloids Surf.*, 43, 169, 1990.
73. **Miller, R., Hofmann, A., Hartmann, R., Schano, K.-H. and Halbig, A.**, Measuring dynamic surface and interfacial tensions, *Adv. Mater.*, 4, 370, 1992.
74. **Popov, A. N.**, Electrocapillary phenomena at the interfacial boundary between aqueous and organic phases, *Elektrokhimiya*, 13, 1393, 1977.
75. **Shchipunov, Yu. A.**, Hydrophobic and electrostatic interactions in adsorption of surface-active substances. Tetraalkylammonium salts, *Adv. Colloid Interface Sci.*, 28, 135, 1988.
76. **Shchipunov, Yu. A.**, Adsorption of surfactants in a case of their association in solution, *Zh. Fiz. Khimii*, 56, 2783, 1982.
77. **Shchipunov, Yu. A.**, Adsorption at the interfaces of two immiscible liquids and association of surface-active substances in bulk phase. 1. Application of the modified Gibbs equation, *J. Colloid Interface Sci.*, 102, 36, 1984.
78. **Kertes, A. S. and Gutmann, H.**, Surfactants in organic solvents: the physical chemistry of aggregation and micellization, *Surface Colloid Sci.*, 8, 193, 1976.
79. **Watanabe, A.**, Electrochemistry of oil-water interfaces, *Surf. Colloid Sci.*, 13, 1, 1984.
80. **Scott, T. C.**, Use of electric field in solvent extraction: a review and prospectus, *Separation Purification Methods*, 18, 65, 1989.
81. **Fendler, J. H.**, *Membrane Mimetic Chemistry*, Wiley, New York, 1982.
82. **Leser, M. E. and Luisi, P. L.**, Application of reverse micelles for the extraction of amino acids and proteins, *Chimia*, 270, 279, 1990.
83. **Scartazzini, R. and Luisi, P. L.**, Reactivity of lipase in an optically transparent lecithin-gel matrix, *Biocatalysis*, 3, 377, 1990.
84. **Rees, G. D. and Robinson, B. H.**, Microemulsions and organogels: Properties and novel applications *Adv. Mat.*, 5, 608, 1993.

Chapter 14

PHOSPHOLIPID MONOLAYERS AND INTERFACIAL ENZYME REACTIONS OF PHOSPHOLIPASES AT ITIES

Takashi Kakiuchi

A monolayer composed of lipids and, in particular, of phospholipids at the interface between two immiscible electrolyte solutions (ITIES) is a useful model system for studying electrical aspects of biological and artificial membranes. The advantage of this system over lipid monolayers at the air-water or at the nonpolar oil/water interfaces is that the accurate control of the potential drop across the monolayer is easily achieved at ITIES. This controllability enables us to apply various electrochemical techniques for characterizing interfacial processes, such as the change in state of monolayers in response to the potential across the monolayer, ion and electron transfer across the monolayer, and electrical-state dependent enzymatic reaction at the lipid-solution interface.

The usefulness of interfaces between polar oil and water as well as those between nonpolar oil and water as a model of biological membranes was recognized at the beginning of this century.[1] Although some pioneering work on electrocapillarity at the liquid-liquid interface had been reported in the 60's and early 70's,[2,3] electrochemically well-defined data on the phospholipid monolayers at ITIES have become available only during the last two decades,[4-6] after the establishment of the polarized liquid-liquid interface both theoretically and experimentally.[7,8]

This chapter first summarizes the fundamental properties of phospholipid monolayers at ITIES and then describes interfacial enzymatic reactions of phospholipases using phospholipid monolayers at ITIES.

I. PROPERTIES OF PHOSPHOLIPID MONOLAYERS AT ITIES

Phospholipids in general are highly soluble in both nitrobenzene (NB) and 1,2-dichloroethane (DCE), the two most frequently used solvents for the studies at ITIES. The monolayer is therefore formed by adsorption of phospholipids from the organic phase to the interface. When the monolayer is in the liquid-expanded state, the formation of the monolayer is limited by the diffusion of phospholipid molecules from the organic phase.[9,10] However, monolayers in the liquid-condensed phase or solid phase need several hours or even days to reaching a stable state.[11] The method in which a certain amount of phospholipid solution is spread at the liquid-liquid interface has been used for certain purposes, taking account of the escape of the spread molecules from the interface to the organic phase.[9,10] Phospholipid monolayers typically become saturated at concentrations above 20 μmol dm^{-3} in the organic phase. The formation of multilayers at the interface is unlikely

0-8493-7694-7/96/$0.00+$.50

below this concentration, as indicated by experiments using the spread method.[9,10]

Double layer capacitance at ITIES, C_{dl}, is very sensitive to adsorbed phospholipids and also changes in the state of the monolayer. The simplicity of the measurement also merits using this technique. Interfacial tension is a particularly useful measure for determining the thermodynamic surface excess of phospholipids. Video-image processing technique has been conveniently utilized for measuring interfacial tension with high precision.[12-14] Other methods frequently used for characterizing the properties of phospholipid assemblies, such as fluorescence technique, have not yet been applied at ITIES.

A. PHOSPHATIDYLCHOLINE MONOLAYERS

By using synthetic phospholipids with definite hydrocarbon chain length, Kakiuchi et al. studied the phase behavior of phosphatidylcholine (PC),[9,11] phosphatidylethanolamine (PE)[10] and phosphatidylserine (PS)[15] monolayers at the NB/W interface through differential capacitance and interfacial tension measurements. Dilauroylphosphatidylcholine (DLPC) forms a stable saturated monolayer in the liquid-expanded state at the interface. The value of adsorption Gibbs energy is 31 kJ mol-1 at 25° C and at $\Delta^{W}{}_{O}\phi = -0.1$ V, where $\Delta^{W}{}_{O}\phi$ is the rational potential, a measure of the inner potential of the aqueous phase with respect to that of the organic phase. The area occupied by a DLPC (12 carbon chains) monolayer at saturation is 0.7 - 0.9 nm^2 per molecule, suggesting that the lateral attractive interaction between DLPC molecules is considerably weakened by penetrated NB molecules between hydrocarbon chain part of the monolayer.[9,16] This saturated monolayer is stable against the variation of the potential in the negative branch where $\Delta^{W}{}_{O}\phi < 0$.[16] In the positive branch where $\Delta^{W}{}_{O}\phi > 0$, adsorbed DLPC molecules partially desorb from the interface and the monolayer becomes unstable.[16]

The phase transition causes a drastic change in C_{dl}. The elongation of the hydrocarbon chain of phosphatidylcholine leads to the phase transition of the monolayer from the liquid-expanded state, $C_{dl} \cong 10$ μF cm^{-2}, to the liquid-condensed state, $C_{dl} \cong 2$ μF cm^{-2}.[11] When the hydrocarbon residue is longer than 18 carbons, the monolayer takes the liquid-condensed state, while dimyristoylphosphatidylcholine (14 carbons) is in the liquid-expanded state at 25°C.

Figure 1 illustrates the C_{dl} in the presence of DLPC, the dipalmitoyl-phosphatidylcholine (DPPC), or dibehenoylphosphatidylcholine (DBPC) at the minimum of each C_{dl} vs. the applied potential (E) curve.[17] The change in temperature induces a phase transition of DPPC monolayer (Fig. 1). The phase of the monolayer also depends on the electrical potential: DPPC monolayer is in liquid-expanded phase in the positive branch, while it is in the liquid-condensed phase in the negative branch.[11]

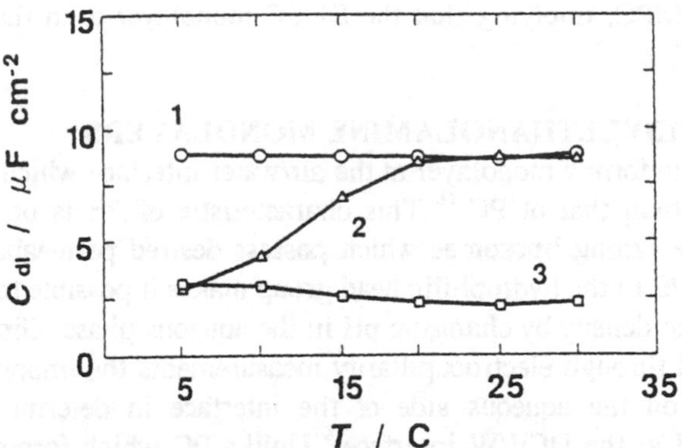

Figure 1. Temperature dependence of the double-layer capacitance in the presence of a saturated monolayer of DLPC (1), DPPC (2) and DBPC (3) at the NB/W interface. (From T. Kakiuchi, J. Noguchi and M. Senda, unpublished result, 1988. With permission.)

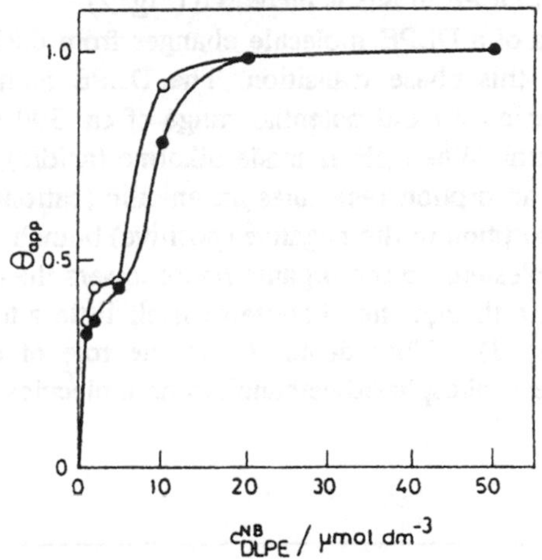

Figure 2. Apparent surface coverage Θ_{app} vs. concentration of DLPE in NB at E = 0.38 (o) and 0.455 (•) V. (From T. Kakiuchi, T. Kondo, M. Kotani and M. Senda, Langmuir, 8, 169, 1992. With permission.)

The transition temperature, T_c, is about 13°C (Fig. 1), which is 29°C lower than the T_c at the air/water interface. This lowering of T_c reflects the reduced attraction between adsorbed DPPC molecules, as has been observed for PC monolayers at the nonpolar oil/water interface.[18]

Wandlowski et al. confirmed the weak lateral interaction between adsorbed DLPC, dimyristoylphosphatidylcholine, and DPPC from detailed analysis of differential capacitance data.[19] Little is known about the monolayer properties of PC having unsaturated hydrocarbon chains. The C_{dl} of the monolayer of dioleoylphosphatidylcholine at NB/W is similar to those of DLPC and DMPC, implying that the DOPC monolayer is in the liquid-expanded state.[20]

B. PHOSPHATIDYLETHANOLAMINE MONOLAYERS

PE is known to form a monolayer at the air/water interface which is more densely packed than that of PC.[18] This characteristic of PE is of decisive importance in designing liposomes which possess desired permeability. An amino group of PE in the hydrophilic head group makes it possible to change the surface charge density by changing pH in the aqueous phase. Girault and Schiffrin showed through electrocapillarity measurements the importance of the surface pH on the aqueous side of the interface in determining the adsorption of PE at the DCE/W interface.[6] Unlike PC which forms liquid-expanded monolayers, dilauroylphosphatidylethanolamine (DLPE) has an adsorption isotherm with a characteristic kink, which is associated with the phase transition from liquid expanded phase to the liquid condensed phase as the concentration of DLPE in NB is increased (Fig. 2).[10]

The occupied area of a DLPE molecule changes from 0.83 nm^2 to 0.50 nm^2 accompanied by this phase transition. The DLPE monolayer at the NB/W interface is stable over the potential range of ca. 300 mV when the aqueous phase is neutral. When pH is made alkaline (acidic), the potential dependence of DLPE adsorption resembles an anionic (cationic) surfactant, showing a marked desorption in the negative (positive) branch.

The addition of cholesterol to the organic phase lowers the capacitance of the DLPE monolayer, although the cholesterol itself little alters the double layer capacitance (Fig. 3).[21] This demonstrates the role of cholesterol in filling the space between phosphatidylethanolamine molecules in the liquid-expanded monolayer.

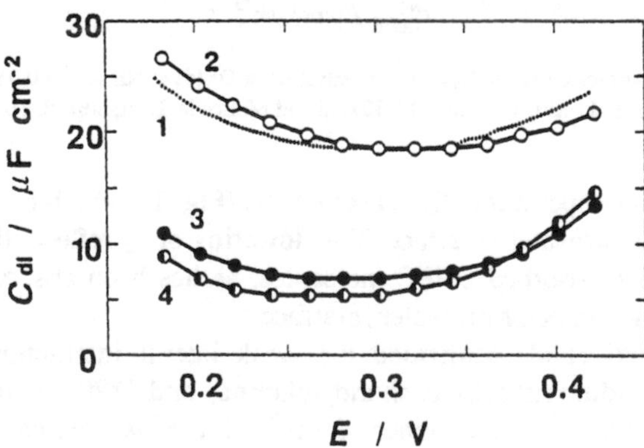

Figure 3. Double-layer capacitance vs. potential curves at the NB/W interface: (1) base solution; (2) 10 μmol dm^{-3} cholesterol in NB; (3) 10 μmol dm^{-3} DLPE in NB; (4) 10 μmol dm^{-3} DLPE + 10 μmol dm^{-3} cholesterol in NB. (From T. Kakiuchi, M. Kotani and M. Senda, unpublished result, 1987. With permission.).

C. PHOSPHATIDYLSERINE MONOLAYERS

Dipalmitoylphosphatidylserine (DPPS) forms a saturated monolayer at the NB/W interface when the concentration of DPPS is greater than 20 μmol dm^{-3}. When a saturated DPPS monolayer is in contact with an aqueous phase containing 0.1 mol dm^{-3} LiCl, the value of C_{dl} is 9.5 μF cm^{-2}, showing that the monolayer is in a liquid-expanded state similar to PC monolayers with shorter hydrocarbon chains. The presence of Ca^{2+} at a concentration greater than 2 μmol dm^{-3} in the aqueous phase induces a striking decrease in C_{dl} down to 1.5 μF cm^{-2}.[15] This change corresponds to the phase transition of DPPS monolayer from the liquid-expanded phase to the condensed phase which may be characterized as a solid monolayer.[18] The condensed DPPS monolayer is stable against the change in the applied potential across the interface between $\Delta^{W}{}_{O}\phi$ = -0.14 and 0.10V. The presence of the Mg^{2+} in the aqueous phase exerts the same effect as Ca^{2+} ion on the phase behavior of the monolayer.[15]

This indicates that the condensation of DPPS monolayers caused by the interaction with divalent cations is of pure electrostatic nature, though it has been reported that PS assemblies more strongly interact with Ca^{2+} ions than with Mg^{2+} ion.[22] The results at the NB/W interface are in harmony with the observation that Mg^{2+}-DPPS and Ca^{2+}-DPPS complexes form similar bilayer structures.[23] The threshold level of divalent cation concentration for the phase transition is 2 mmol dm^{-3} for both Ca^{2+} and Mg^{2+}.

The stability of the condensed DPPS monolayer against the applied potential suggests that the negative charges on DPPS molecules are effectively neutralized by the adsorbed divalent cations by forming a 2:1 (DPPS:ion) complex.

D. PHOSPHATIDIC ACID MONOLAYERS

Phosphatidic acid monolayers at the NB/W interface show phase behavior similar to PS monolayers described above. PA forms a liquid-expanded monolayer at the NB/W interface when the aqueous phase contains no divalent ions.[24] The presence of Ca^{2+} or Mg^{2+} in the aqueous phase solidifies the monolayer to give a liquid-condensed or a solid-condensed monolayer. Dilauroylphosphatidic acid monolayers also shows similar characteristics.[25] This property of PA monolayers is distinct from PC monolayers having the same hydrocarbon chains, and has been utilized to detect hydrolysis of PC at the interface by phospholipase D (*vide infra*).

II. CHARGE TRANSFER ACROSS THE PHOSPHOLIPID MONOLAYER AT ITIES

The transfer of lipophilic ions across a lipid membrane has been studied mainly by using bilayer lipid membranes. However, the presence of the two interfaces on both sides of the membrane complicates interpretation of experimental data related to the mechanism of ion transfer. The difficulty arises from the fact that the potential drop across each interface cannot be controlled separately. On the other hand, lipid monolayers at the polarized oil/water interface, though less relevant to biological membranes, have advantages in that the potential drop across the single membrane/solution interface may be controlled externally and standard electrochemical methodology is easily applied for studying the mechanism of charge transfer across the interface.

A. EFFECT OF PHOSPHOLIPID MONOLAYERS ON THE RATE OF ION TRANSFER ACROSS ITIES

Koryta et al. observed retardation of the transfer of Cs^+ and tetramethylammonium ion (TMA^+) ions and also of the facilitated transfer of Na^+ ion by dibenzo-18-crown-6, when lecithin of unspecified composition and concentration was added to the NB phase.[4] The increasing irreversibility of these ion transfer processes at lower temperatures was ascribed to the gradual change in the state of the monolayer. Girault and Schiffrin's preliminary work on the effect of egg yolk lecithin on tetraethylammonium ion, TEA^+, transfer across the DCE/W interface also indicated that the addition of lecithin made the transfer completely irreversible.[5]

Cunnane et al. focused on the effect on TEA^+ transfer of egg lecithin in a concentration range higher than that corresponding to a saturated monolayer.[26] The observed linear correlation between the logarithm of the rate constant of TEA^+ ion transfer with the surface pressure was utilized to deduce the radius of pore to be formed in the monolayer for the TEA^+ ion transfer. The radius of the pore is estimated to be between 0.39 and 0.53 nm, which is greater than the radius of unhydrated TEA^+ ion of 0.31 nm.

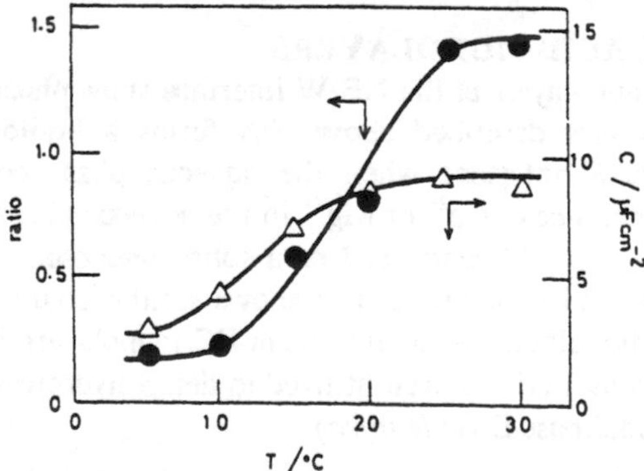

Figure 4. Temperature dependence of the double-layer capacitance (Δ) and the ratio of the apparent standard rate constant of TEA^+ in the presence of a DPPC monolayer to that in the absence of a PC monolayer (o). (From T. Kakiuchi, M. Kotani, J. Noguchi, M. Nakanishi and M. Senda, J. Colloid Interface Sci., 149, 279, 1992. With permission.)

Using an ac impedance method, Kakiuchi et al. measured the rate of TMA^+ and TEA^+ ions across the PC monolayer in the liquid-expanded or liquid-condensed state.[11] The monolayers in the liquid-condensed state reduce the rate of the transfer of both TMA^+ and TEA^+ ions. In contrast, monolayers in the liquid-expanded state do not alter the transfer of both ions. The apparent acceleration with the liquid-expanded monolayer has been interpreted in terms of double layer effect. The change in the standard rate constant of TEA^+ ion with the temperature-induced phase transition of DPPC monolayers is illustrated in Fig. 4.[11]

A phosphatidylcholine monolayer in the liquid-condensed state exerts a hydrodynamic friction on transferring ions, whereas a monolayer in the liquid-expanded state does not apparently hinder ion transfer. In PC monolayers in the liquid-expanded state where the packing density is of the order of 0.7 nm^2, NB molecules fill the space between the adsorbed PC molecules. Since the cross-sectional area of a PC molecule in a crystalline state is 0.41 nm^2, the NB molecules occupy one-third of the interfacial area. Transferring ions can then pass through a part of the monolayer filled with NB molecules without significantly interacting with PC molecules. The absence of hindrance by an adsorbed monolayer has been observed also for the transfer of TEA+ ion in the presence of sorbitan fatty acid esters which form fluid monolayers at the NB/W interface.[27]

When the monolayer is in the liquid-condensed state, there is little room between hydrocarbon chains to accommodate solvent NB molecules. The transferring ions should then partition into the layer of hydrocarbon chains which are tightly packed to form a liquid-condensed monolayer. In this migration process, the hydrodynamic friction of transferring ions with the hydrocarbon chains becomes significant.

The PE monolayer in the liquid-condensed state also decelerates the transfer of TEA^+ ion, but slightly accelerates the transfer of ClO_4^- ion.[10] In this case, the double layer structure in the presence of the monolayer should be further elucidated for understanding the mechanism of ion transfer. A decrease in the rate of ion transfer has been observed for a PS monolayer tightly packed through the interaction with divalent cations. It is noted that even this solid-like PS monolayer cannot completely block the transfer of TEA^+ ion across the monolayer. The degree of the decrease in the rate constant is of one order of magnitude, i.e. $\approx 10^{-3}$ cm s^{-1} for both densely packed PS and PC monolayers.

B. EFFECT OF PHOSPHOLIPID MONOLAYER ON ELECTRON TRANSFER ACROSS ITIES.

Phospholipid monolayers at ITIES also affect the rate of electron transfer across ITIES. Cheng and Schiffrin have shown that the addition of egg lecithin-cholesterol mixture completely inhibits the interfacial electron transfer between lutetium bisphthalocyanine ($Lu(PC)_2$) in DCE and hexacyanoferrate (II/III).[28] The electron transfer between bis(pyridine) *meso*-tetraphenylporphyrinato ruthenium(II) complex ($Ru(TPP)(py)_2$) in DCE and $Fe(CN)_6^{3-/4-}$ is also completely inhibited. However, the ET between 7,7,8,8-tetracyanoquinodimethane (TCNQ) and $Fe(CN)_6^{3-/4-}$ is not completely blocked; the apparent standard rate constant of electron transfer is reduced from $5.4 \bullet 10^{-3}$ cm s^{-1} to $1.8 \bullet 10^{-3}$ cm s^{-1}. Cheng and Schiffrin interpreted this difference in terms of the distance of closest approach between two redox active species, one in W and the other in DCE. TCNQ molecules having smaller size easily penetrate into the monolayer and undergo electron transfer with hexacyanoferrate. TCNQ also functions as a mediator of electron transfer between $Lu(PC)_2$ or $Ru(TPP)(py)_2$ in DCE and hexacyanoferrate across the monolayer.

The barrier introduced by a phospholipid monolayer against ion transfer is only important kinetically for the transfer of moderately lipophobic ions. This is probably characteristic of fluid monolayers in general. This is not the case, however, for interfacial electron transfer, in which the electron transfer across the interface is totally blocked when the size of reactants is large. This reflects the fact that the probability of electron transfer decays exponentially with the distance between the reactants. The electrostatic interactions plays a decisive role in determining the affinity of enzyme with the substrate.

III. INTERFACIAL ENZYMATIC REACTIONS AT ITIES

The activity of lipolytic enzymes such as phospholipases and lipases at organized lipid/water interfaces is markedly dependent on the physicochemical properties of the interface. One of the variables which decisively influences the enzyme activity is the electrical state of the interface. The use of phospholipid monolayers at ITIES has been proposed for measuring enzyme activity under the precise control of the electrical state of the monolayer.[24,29]

A. HYDROLYSIS OF PHOSPHATIDYLCHOLINE BY PHOSPHOLIPASE D.

Kondo et al. studied the hydrolytic activity of phospholipase D (PLD) at ITIES by making use of a large difference in C_{dl} before and after the hydrolysis.[24,25] The liquid-expanded state of a PC monolayer turns into the liquid-condensed state of a corresponding PA monolayer, giving distinctively lower value of C_{dl} in the presence of Ca^{2+} ions in W. The measuring cell is illustrated in Fig. 5[25]

The polarized NB/W interface was formed at the upper end of the inner glass tube in the middle of the cell. A lipid monolayer is formed at the interface through adsorption from the NB side of the interface. To start the enzyme reaction, the aqueous phase is replaced with a solution containing PLD. A typical time course of the capacitance at $\Delta^W_O\phi = 10$ mV is shown in Fig. 6[25]

Two PLDs from *streptomyces* spp. (SC-PLD and SS-PLD) hydrolyze the monolayer completely, whereas peanut and cabbage PLDs (PN-PLD and CB-PLD) hydrolyze only 75 % and 60 % of the monolayer, respectively. The

initial slope of these plots can be correlated with the initial rate of hydrolysis, $v_{t=0} = -d\Gamma_s/dt$, at t = 0, where Γ_s is the adsorbed amount of substrate.[24]

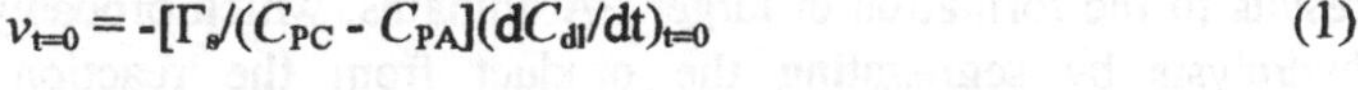

$$v_{t=0} = -[\Gamma_s/(C_{PC} - C_{PA}](dC_{dl}/dt)_{t=0} \quad (1)$$

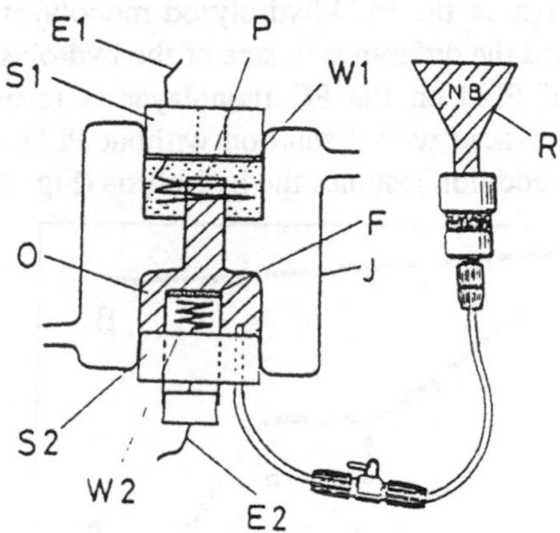

Figure 5. Cell design for impedance measurement: W1: aqueous solution; W2: aqueous solution of 50 mmol dm^{-3} tetrabutylammonium chloride; O: nitrobenzene solution of 0.1 mol dm^{-3} tetrapentylammonium tetraphenilborate; E1 and E2: Ag/AgCl electrodes; F: glass frit; S1 and S2: silicone rubber stoppers; J: water jacket; R: nitrobenzene solution reservoir; P: polarized NB/W interface. (From T. Kondo, T. Kakiuchi and M. Senda, Bioelectrochem. Bioenerg., 34, 93, 1994. With permission.)

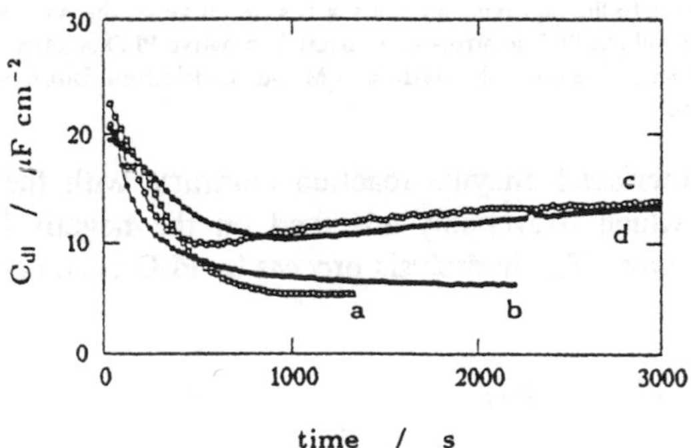

Figure 6. Time dependence of C_{dl} at $\Delta^W_O\phi$ =10 mV during the hydrolysis of DLPC monolayers by (a) 3.6 nmol dm^{-3} SC-PLD, (b) 1.1 nmol dm^{-3} SS-PLD, (c) 25 nmol dm^{-3} PN-PLD and (d) 46 nmol dm^{-3} CB-PLD in aqueous solution at 30°C. The aqueous solution contains 50 mmol dm^{-3} acetate buffer and 50 mmol dm^{-3} $CaCl_2$ (pH 5.2). (From T. Kondo, T. Kakiuchi and M. Senda, Bioelectrochem. Bioenerg., 34, 93, 1994. With permission.)

Here C_{PC} and C_{PA} are the capacitance of PC and PA monolayers, respectively, at the full coverage. The implied assumption is that the C_{dl} at a given coverage of PC, Θ, is given by

$$C_{dl} = \Theta\, C_{PC} - (1 - \Theta)\, C_{PA} \quad (2)$$

The gradual increase observed for PN-PLD and CB-PLD at longer times in Fig. 6 reflects the formation of small domains (< μm) of PA in the monolayer. On the other hand, the hydrolysis by SC-PLD and SS-PLD results in the formation of larger PA domains, which probably facilitate the hydrolysis by segregating the product from the reaction system. The fluorescence microscopy of the PLD-hydrolyzed monolayer at the air/water interface has confirmed the difference in size of the hydrolysis products.[30]

The adsorption of PLD on the PC monolayer is reversible; when the aqueous solution is replaced with a solution without PLD, the hydrolysis is suspended and the re-addition resumes the hydrolysis (Fig. 7).[24]

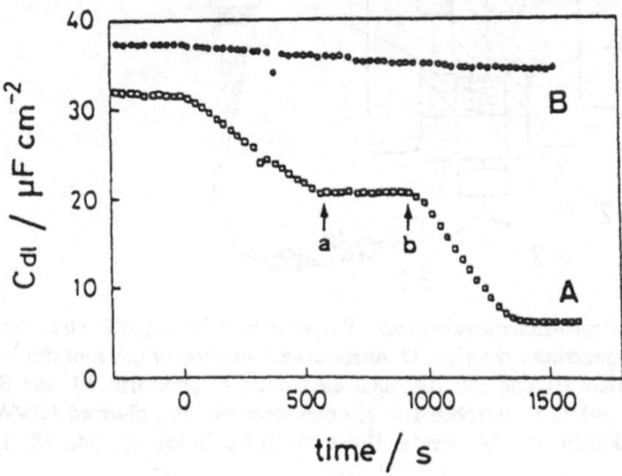

Figure 7. Time dependence of C_{dl} at $\Delta^{W}{}_{O}\phi$ =60 mV after adding native (□) and thermally denatured peanut PLD (o) into the aqueous phase at t = 0 s. In curve A, the aqueous phase was replaced with the solution without PLD at arrow a. At arrow b, a native PLD solution was re-added to the aqueous phase. (From T. Kondo, T. Kakiuchi and M. Senda, Biochim. Biophys. Acta, 1124, 91, 1992. With permission.)

This mode of interfacial enzyme reaction contrasts with the action of phospholipase A_2, which irreversibly adsorbed on the negatively charged lipid surfaces (*vide infra*). The hydrolysis process by PLD is composed of the following steps:

$$E(bulk) \xrightarrow{Diffusion} E(x=+0) \tag{3}$$

$$E(x=+0) \underset{\longleftarrow}{\xrightarrow{fast}} E(ads) \tag{4}$$

$$E(ads) + S \underset{k_{-1}}{\overset{k_1}{\Leftrightarrow}} ES(ads) \tag{5}$$

$$ES(ads) \xrightarrow{k_2} E(x=+0) + P(ads) \tag{6}$$

where E is the enzyme, S is the substrate, ES is the ES complex, and P is the product and E(x = +0) is the E right at the solution side of the lipid-solution interface. Figure 8 schematically represents this model. Theoretical C_{dl} vs. t

curves are predicted based on this model by combining mass transport, adsorption isotherm and an enzymatic reaction and the Eq.(2). Using the diffusion equation and the Langmuir isotherm, Kondo et al. calculated C_{dl} vs. t curves shown in Fig. 9, without assuming the steady state with respect to ES complex.[31] These curves at different enzyme concentrations well reproduce the experimentally observed time courses for the hydrolysis by peanut and *Streptomyces* PLDs as illustrated in Fig. 6.

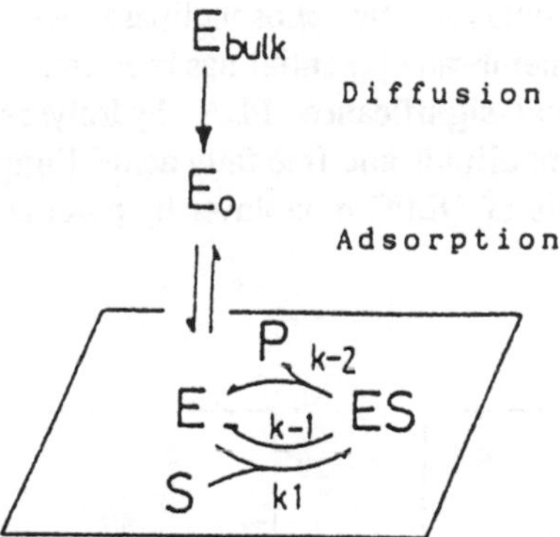

Figure 8. Schematic representation of the interfacial enzyme reaction which takes account of the transport process of enzyme E. E_{bulk}, E_0 and E denote the enzymes in the bulk, in the solution side of the interface, and on the surface, respectively. S, P and ES denote the substrate, product and enzyme-substrate complex, respectively. (From T. Kondo, T. Kakiuchi and M. Senda, Anal. Sci. (Supplement), 1725, 1991. With permission.)

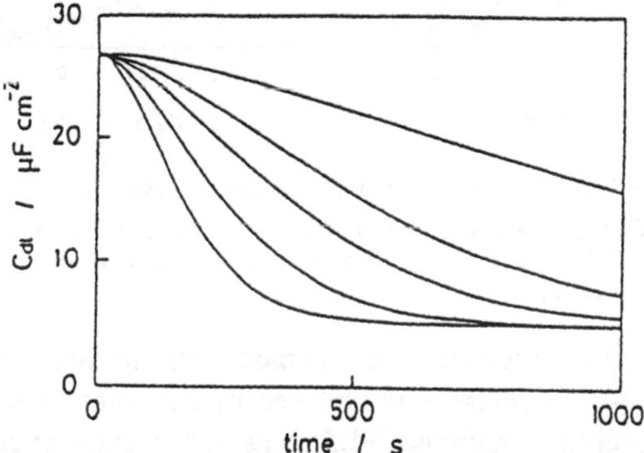

Figure 9. Theoretical curves for the time course of C_{dl} at different concentrations of PLD in the bulk when $k_1 = 5.0 \cdot 10^9$ mol^{-1}cm^{2}s^{-1}, $k_{-1} = 0.1$ s^{-1}, $k_2 = 10.0$ s^{-1}, and $\beta = 1.0 \cdot 10^{11}$ mol^{-1}cm^3, where β is the adsorption coefficient. The concentration of the enzyme is $1.0 \cdot 10^{-11}$, $3.0 \cdot 10^{-11}$, $5.0 \cdot 10^{-11}$, $1.0 \cdot 10^{-10}$ and $2.0 \cdot 10^{-10}$ mol cm^{-3} from top to the bottom. (From T. Kondo, T. Kakiuchi and M. Senda, Anal. Sci. (Supplement), 1725, 1991. With permission.)

The rate of hydrolysis by PLDs from plants is little dependent on interfacial potential, while the rate by *Streptomyces* spp. shows a marked dependence on the potential (Fig. 10). Kondo et al. has shown that this dependence is explained by taking account of the difference in the potential dependence of adsorption Gibbs energy of PLDs, which was assumed to be described by the Frumkin's two parallel condenser model.[25] This means that average adsorbed amount of PLD, rather than the hydrolytic activity of PLD itself, primarily determines the observed overall rate of interfacial hydrolysis.

B. HYDROLYSIS OF PHOSPHATIDYLCHOLINE BY PHOSPHOLIPASE A

The above method of monitoring C_{dl} has been extended to measure the rate of hydrolysis of PC monolayers by phospholipase A_2 (PLA_2), whose dependence of activity on membrane potential has been intensively studied in view of varied physiological significance. PLA_2 hydrolyses 3-*sn*-phosphoglycerides to give lysophospholipids and free fatty acids. Figure 11 shows the relative degree of hydrolysis of DLPC monolayer by porcine pancreas PLA_2 as a function of time

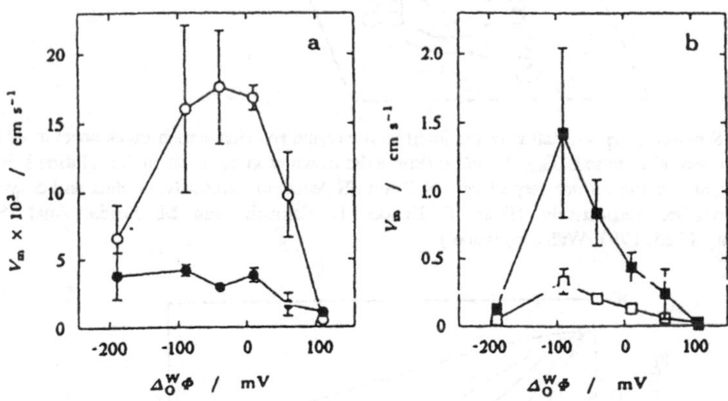

Figure 10. Effect of $\Delta^W{}_O\phi$ on V_m: (a) PN-PLD (o) and CB-PLD (●), (b) (SC-PLD (□) and SS-PLD (■). V_m is defined by v_m/c_E, where c_E is the bulk concentration of PLD. Experimental conditions are the same as in Fig. 7.(From T. Kondo, T. Kakiuchi and M. Senda, Bioelectrochem. Bioenerg., 34, 93, 1994. With permission.)

The adsorption of PLA_2 molecules on the monolayer surface is irreversible.[29] At point **a**, the aqueous phase was replaced by the solution with no PLA_2. However, the hydrolysis continued. PLA_2 was added again at point **b**, which only slightly increased the rate of hydrolysis. This irreversible adsorption supports the scooting model of the action of PLA_2 on phospholipid surfaces.[32]

Both the rate of hydrolysis and the degree of hydrolysis depends on the value of $\Delta^W{}_O\phi$ as shown in Fig. 11. The activities of both porcine PLA_2 and it *Naja naja* PLA_2 show peaks around $\Delta^W{}_O\phi = 60$ mV. This clearly shows the importance of local electrostatic interactions between the positively charged domain of PLA_2, the recognition site, and the negatively charged substrate side of the interface.[29] PLA_2 has a net negative charge at this pH.

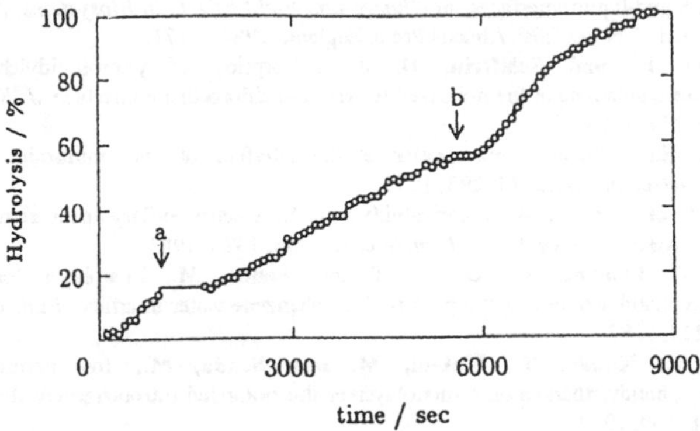

Figure 11. Time-course of hydrolysis of DLPC monolayer by porcine pancreas PLA_2 at $\Delta^{W}{}_{O}\phi$ = 60 mV. The aqueous phase was replaced with the solution without PLA_2 at arrow **a**. At arrow **b**, PLA_2 was re-added to the aqueous phase. (From T. Kondo and T. Kakiuchi, Bioelectrochem. Bioenerg., 36, 53, 1995. With permission.)

IV. CONCLUSIONS.

Phospholipid monolayers at ITIES have revealed new aspects of surface phenomena, especially in relation to the effect of electrical variables on interfacial properties of the monolayers, ranging from potential-dependent phase transition to interfacial enzyme reactions. Further development in this direction is promising in both physicochemical studies of membranes and applications, e.g. assay of the activities of interface - specific enzymes.

Experimental methods so far employed are limited to classical electrochemical techniques with intrinsically low temporal and spatial resolutions. The application of new techniques seems to be promising for elucidating dynamic and molecular aspects of phospholipids and also of enzyme reactions at ITIES.

REFERENCES

1. **Nernst, W. and Riesenfeld, E. H.,** Über electrolytische Erscheinungen an der Grenzfläche zweier Lösiingsmittel, *Z. Phys. Chem.*, 8, 600, 1902.
2. **Watanabe, A., Matsumoto, M., Tamai, H. and Gotoh, R.,** Electrocapillary phenomena at oil-water interfaces. Part III: The behaviour of lecithin at oil-water interfaces, *Kolloid Z. Z. Polym.*, 228, 58, 1968.
3. **Watanabe, A., Fujii, A., Sakamori, Y., Higashituji, K. and Tamai, H.,** Studies on the behaviour of phospholipids at oil-water interfaces. (1) The isoelectric points of phospholipids, *Kolloid Z. Z. Polym.*, 243, 42, 1971.

4. **Koryta, J., Hung, L. Q. and Hofmanova, A.,** Biomembrane transport processes at the interface of two immiscible electrolyte solutions with an adsorbed phospholipid monolayer, *Studia Biophys.*, 90, 25, 1982.
5. **Girault, H. H. and Schiffrin, D. J.,** Charge transfer through phospholipid monolayers adsorbed at liquid-liquid interfaces, in *Charge and Field Effects in Biosystems*, Allen, M. J. and Usherwood, P. N. R., Eds., Abacus Press, England, 1984, p.171.
6. **Girault, H. H. and Schiffrin, D. J.,** Adsorption of phosphatidylcholine and phosphatidylethanolamine at the polarized water/1,2-dichloroethane interface. *J. Electroanal. Chem.*, 179, 277, 1984.
7. **Koryta, J.,** Electrochemical polarization at the interface of two immiscible electrolyte solutions, *Electrochim. Acta*, 24, 293, 1979.
8. **Kakiuchi, T. and Senda, M.,** Polarizability and the electrocapillary measurements of the nitrobenzene-water interface. *Bull. Chem. Soc. Jpn.*, 56, 1322, 1983.
9. **Kakiuchi, T., Yamane, M., Osakai, T. and Senda, M.,** Monolayer formation of dilauroylphosphatidylcholine at the polarized nitrobenzene-water interface, *Bull. Chem. Soc. Jpn.*, 60, 4223, 1987.
10. **Kakiuchi, T., Kondo, T., Kotani, M. and Senda, M.,** Ion permeability of dilauroylphosphatidylethanolamine monolayer at the polarized nitrobenzene/water interface, *Langmuir*, 8, 169, 1992.
11. **Kakiuchi, T., Kotani, M., Noguchi, J., Nakanishi, M. and Senda, M.,** Phase transition and ion permeability of phosphaitidylcholine monolayers at the polarized oil/water interface, *J. Colloid Interface Sci.*, 149, 279, 1992.
12. **Girault, H. H., Schiffrin, D. J. and Smith, B. V. D.,** Drop image processing for surface and interfacial tension measurements, *J. Electroanal. Chem.*, 37, 207, 1982.
13. **Girault, H. H., Schiffrin, D. J. and Smith, B. V. D.,** The measurement of interfacial tension of pendant drops using a video image profile digitizer, *J. Colloid Interface Sci.*, 101, 257, 1984.
14. **Kakiuchi, T., Nakanishi, M. and Senda, M.,** The electrocapillary curves of the phosphatidylcholine monolayer at the polarized oil-water interface. Measurement of interfacial tension using a computer-aided pendant-drop method, *Bull. Chem. Soc. Jpn*, 61, 1845, 1988.
15. **Kakiuchi, T., Kondo, T., and Senda, M.,** Divalent cation-induced phase transition of phosphatidylserine monolayer at the polarized oil-water interface and its influence on the ion-transfer processes, *Bull Chem. Soc. Jpn.*, 63, 3270, 1990.
16. **Kakiuchi, T., Nakanishi, M. and Senda, M.** The electrocapillary curves of the phosphatidylcholine monolayer at the polarized oil-water interface. 11. Double layer structure of dilauroylphosphatidylcholine monolayer at the nitrobenzene-water interface. *Bull. Chem. Soc. Jpn.*, 62, 403, 1989.
17. **Kakiuchi, T., Noguchi, J. and Senda, M.,** unpublished result, 1988.
18. **Mingins, J., Llerenas, E. and Pethica, B. A.,** The role of interfacial charges in the phase behaviour of lipid monolayers and bilayers, in *Ions in Macromolecular and Biological Systems*, Everett, D. H. and Vincent, V., Eds., Scientechnica, Bristol, 1978, p.41.
19. **Wandlowski, T., Račinský, S., Mareček, V. and Samec, Z.,** Adsorption of phospholipids at the interface between two immiscible electrolyte solutions, *J. Electroanal. Chem.*, 227, 281, 1987.
20. **Kotani, M.,** Master's thesis, Kyoto University, 1988.
21. **Kakiuchi, T., Kotani, M. and Senda, M.**, unpublished result, 1987.
22. **McLaughlin, S., Mulrine, N., Gresalfi, T., Vaio, G. and McLaughlin, A.,** Adsorption of divalent cations to bilayer membranes containing phosphatidylserine, *J. Gen. Physiol.*, 77, 445, 1981.
23. **Hauser, H. and Shipley, G. G.,.** Interactions of divalent cations with phosphatidylserine bilayer membranes, *Biochemistry*, 23, 34, 1984.
24. **Kondo, T., Kakiuchi, T. and Senda, M.,** Hydrolysis of phospholipid monolayers by phospholipase D at the oil/water interface under the control of the potential drop across the monolayer, *Biochim. Biophys. Acta*, 1124, 1, 1992.
25. **Kondo, T., Kakiuchi, T. and Senda, M.**, Hydrolytic activity of phospholipase D from plants and *streptomyces* spp. against a phosphatidylcholine monolayer at a polarized oil/water interface, *Bioelectrochem. Bioenerg.*, 34, 93, 1994.

26. **Cunnane, V. J., Schiffrin, D. J., Fleischmann, M., Geblewicz, G. and Williams, D.**, The kinetics of ionic transfer across adsorbed phospholipid layers, *J. Electroanal. Chem.*, 243, 455, 1988.
27. **Kakiuchi, T., Teranishi, Y. and Niki, K.**, Adsorption of sorbitan fatty acid esters and a sucrose monoalkanoate at the nitrobenzene-water interface and its effect on the rate of ion transfer across the interface, *Electrochim. Acta*, in Press, 1995.
28. **Cheng, Y. and Schiffrin, D. J.**,. Redox electrocatalysis by tetracyanoquinodimethane in phospholipid monolayers adsorbed at a liquid/liquid interface, *J. Chem. Soc. Faraday Trans.*, 90, 2517, 1994.
29. **Kondo, T. and Kakiuchi, T.**, Effect of electrostatic interaction on hydrolytic activity of phospholipase A2 at the, polarized oil-water interface, *Bioelectrochem. Bioenerg.*, 36, 53, 1995.
30. **Kondo, T., Kakiuchi, T. and Simomura, M.**, Fluorescence microscopic imaging of hydrolysis of phospholipid monolayers by phospholipase D at air-water interface, *Thin Solid Films*, 244, 887, 1994.
31. **Kondo, T., Kakiuchi, T. and Senda, M.**, Kinetics of the hydrolysis of phospholipid monolayers by phospholipase D at the oil/water interface, *Anal. Sci.*, 300, 1725, 1991.
32. **Jain, M. K. and Berg, O.**, The kinetics of interfacial catalysis by phospholipase A_2 and regulation of interfacial activation: Hopping versus scooting, *Biochim. Biophys. Acta*, 1002, 127, 1989.

Chapter 15

ELECTRODIALYSIS THROUGH LIQUID ION-EXCHANGE MEMBRANES AND THE OIL-WATER INTERFACE

Alexander Popov

I. INTRODUCTION

A. LIQUID MEMBRANES IN GENERAL

A liquid membrane is a layer of an organic solvent separating two aqueous solutions. Compounds that promote the transport of ions from one aqueous solution to another may be dissolved in the organic phase. The transfer of ions through the membrane can then take place down the gradient of chemical (electrochemical) potential. During this process the ions successively cross the water/oil and oil/water interfaces. The structure of these interfaces is the main factor controlling ion transport through the membrane.

Although investigations of the physical chemistry of membranes have been carried out for more than a century, the practical importance of liquid membranes, if compared with that of solid ion-exchange membranes, is not consistent with their potential. Instead,[1-7] liquid membranes were more often considered only as a convenient laboratory model of biomembranes.[8-10] For instance, liquid membranes are commonly used to investigate transport abilities of newly synthesized ionophores.[11-13] Liquid membranes are also used in ionometry, and applications in analytical chemistry are also common.[14-17]

A high rate of the ion transfer through the membrane is possible only if the membrane is sufficiently thin, and the interface between the aqueous solutions and the membrane is highly developed.[18] This is possible if the membranes are supported on porous hydrophobic matrices such as hollow fibers.[19] Such membranes are convenient both for research and industrial applications,[15,17,20,21] but are limited by the fact that the organic phase is sometimes forced out of the porous matrix by the aqueous phase.[22]

Another method for creating useful liquid membranes was developed by N. Li,[23] who used water/oil/water double-emulsions. The double emulsion membranes, both in terms of their production and number of parameters, are similar to liquid extractions.[a] A comparative analysis of various types of liquid membranes shows that each has advantages and, consequently, specific applications.[25]

In membrane systems the concentration of a given ion can increase against its concentration gradient. The coupled flow of a second ion such as

---

[a] To signify the transmembrane transfer of various substances, S. Schlosser and E. Kosatsky [24] have proposed the term "pertraction", in analogy with "extraction".

0-8493-7694-7/96/$0.00+$.50

H^+ along the gradient of chemical potential is the driving force of the process. The coupled flows may be in the same (symport) or the opposite (antiport) direction as the ions under extraction.[26-28] The coupled flows of ions may be generated by means of two types of carriers, spatially separated, in the same membrane.[29] Formally, it is possible to promote the transfer of electrons through liquid membranes, although in fact it is achieved via the transfer of oxidized or reduced forms of the extracted substance or carrier. Transition from the one to the other form is caused by a chemical reaction, electrolysis or photolysis at the interface of the phases.[30,31]

Most liquid extraction characteristics, such as interface film formation, and catalysis or inhibition of ion mass transfer with charged adsorption layers, remain preserved during liquid membrane function[32]. A spontaneous interphase convection, considerably influencing the rate of the transmembrane transfer, is also possible.[33,34] A method for delivering energy directly to the water/oil interface has been developed, allowing interface mass transfer to be accelerated many times. In this case, in the opinion of the author [35], the interface becomes an analogue of the wave-carrier. This method may be applied also to liquid membranes, but details remain to be published.

B. LIQUID MEMBRANES IN ELECTRODIALYSIS

To accelerate ion transfer through liquid ion-exchange membranes, an electric current may be used. If compared with solid ion-exchange membranes, liquid membranes provide broader control of selectivity, limited principally by the variety of membrane-active agents. By application of diverse complexing agents, it is possible to accumulate impurities in the membrane. A pioneer in this field was B. Purin,[36] who used electrodialysis through bulk liquid membranes to concentrate Rhenium from industrial solutions. The ReO_4^- carrier was a trioctylamine salt. Subsequent work in this field has largely been directed to systems having practical interest, see references [37-42].

In contrast to solid ion-exchange membranes, liquid membranes tend to accumulate water during electrodialysis. Water accumulation is due to the transfer of the ionic hydration-solvation sheath as well as to electroosmosis.[43] Since the majority of membrane-active substances are surfactants,[44] water accumulation normally leads to the formation of reverse micelles. In the process of further electrodialysis, an emulsion occurs in the membrane. Water droplets containing salts may form channels across the membrane followed by electrical breakdown.[45] The presence of water in the membrane leads to substantial changes in selectivity, which vanishes entirely after breakdown.[46] The rate of water accumulation increases with the density of the current passing though the membrane. The presence of water in the membrane leads also to electric instability, which can have periodicity.[47] In the electrodialysis of acidocomplexes of metals through the membrane made of tributhylphosphate, most of the water enters the organic phase with Cl^- ions.[48,49] Analysis suggests that the maximum density of the current passing through the liquid membrane may be determined by inter- and extra-diffusion mechanisms.[50,51] However, the inter-diffusion mechanism, due to the substantial changes of the membrane electric conductivity caused by the water accumulation, often cannot be realized in practice.

Currents higher than those maximally possible cause water dissociation on the surface of the solid ion-exchange membrane and the transfer of H^+ and OH^- ions.[1] In this case transfer through the membrane becomes non-selective. Under similar conditions, either the organic ions come from the liquid membrane into the water solutions, or the complexes of macrocyclic ionophores with cations begin to break up.[52,53]

Electrodialysis is used to study the mechanisms of ion transport in plasticized membranes of ion-selective electrodes. Such experiments enabled W. Morf to develop a cyclic model for a neutral carrier in the membrane.[14,b] Electrochemistry of such plasticized membranes is thoroughly described by R. Buck.[55-57] In such materials loss of selectivity with relatively high current values has also been observed. This phenomenon is related to Donnan exclusion failure in membranes.[58]

A method for concentrating gases by means of liquid membranes containing redox pairs has considerable interest. The most detailed studies have been made in the case of the Fe^{2+}/Fe^{3+} system used for NO transport and of the Cu^+/Cu^{2+} system for CO transport.[59-61] The mesh electrodes are placed in the membrane (a solution of the corresponding salt in formamide) at the interface. Through the application of an electric current, the concentration of these gases can be increased more than a hundredfold.

The use of electric fields for creating and destroying emulsions is useful in liquid extraction and double-emulsion membranes[62]. Alternating electric fields of various intensities, which change the hydrodynamic conditions in the membrane phase, can accelerate mass transfer.[63,64] Such phenomena are known both for immobilized and spatial liquid membranes.[65,66] However, significant acceleration of mass transfer through the water/oil interface under the influence of low-frequency electric field has not been observed.

II. REGULARITIES IN THE ELECTRODIALYSIS THROUGH LIQUID MEMBRANES

The thickness of liquid membranes used in electrodialysis is normally within the range of 0.1-1 cm, and the volume of the membrane is at least 10 times less than the volume of an adjacent aqueous phase. Both

---

[b] A similar scheme of carrier diffusion (larger and smaller cycles) is described in detail in reference [52].

characteristics - the volume limit and the thickness - strongly influence the electrochemistry of liquid membranes. The current passing through a liquid ion-exchange membrane is in practice totally determined by its ohmic resistance: The overpotential of ion transport through an interface in the presence of ionophores or ion-exchangers is at least 50-100 times less than the membrane potential drop.[40, 67-69] Depending on the ratio of the ion current from the aqueous phase to the membrane and its conductance, the composition and concentration of the electrolyte in the non-aqueous phase may undergo significant changes. That is why, despite the fact that the dependence between the current and the membrane voltage is determined by Ohm's law, the voltammogram may be far from linear.[c]

The problem of obtaining voltammograms of such systems amounts to the determination of the ion concentration in the membrane, calculated by means of Ohm's law:

$$i(t) = l^{-1} vt \sum \Lambda_i C_i(t) \qquad (1)$$

where $i(t)$ is the current density, l is the membrane thickness, v is the voltage sweeping rate, Λ_i and $C_i(t)$ are the molar conductivity and the i-th ion concentration. To simplify this calculation, it may be assumed that the concentration of ions at any moment is equal at all points in the membrane. The numeric value of the concentration is equal to its mean value within the membrane cross-section, and is identical to that determined experimentally. This agrees with the assumption that ions in membranes exist mainly in pairs.[70] To establish simultaneous differential equations describing changes in the concentration of ions, we assume organic phase electrical neutrality and equal currents passing through the interface and the membrane volume. A more complicated interpretation of voltammograms recorded under linear voltage sweeping, if compared with chronopotentiometry, is compensated by higher repeatability and accuracy of such experiments.

A. ION-EXCHANGE MEMBRANES

1. Anion-Exchange Membranes

Solutions of *n*-trioctylamine salts (Oct_3NHX, X^- - anion) in organic solvents are widely used as membranes when metal-containing anions are being separated or concentrated.[18] The electric conductivity of n-trioctylamine salt solutions in *1,2*-dichloroethane or *o*-dichlorobenzene depends on the nature of anions. Solutions with more lipophilic anion salts (ClO_4^-, $Au(CN)_2^-$) show 4-8 times higher conductivity compared with chlorides. That is why changes in the concentration and nature of the

---

[c] Current-voltage dependence at a sweep rate of 400 V/s in reverse at any point in the voltammogram is seen as a straight line emanating from the origin of coordinates. This fact confirms the ohmic nature of the membrane resistance.

anions in the membrane, occurring during the electric current transfer, are visually reflected in the voltammograms.

In the simplest case, all current through interface 1 is transported by anions Y^- contained in the water chamber C (t_y=1), and through the membrane and interface 2 - by both anions: X^- and Y^-. After all the X^- anions, initially contained in the organic phase, undergo transfer to the chamber A, only the Y^- anions will transport the current in the system. Changes in the concentration of X^- ions in the membrane are described by the following equation:

$$\frac{dC_x(t)}{dt} = -\frac{i(t)}{lF}\left[\frac{C_x(t)\Lambda_x}{C_x(t)\Lambda_x + C_y(t)\Lambda_y}\right] - k_1 C_x(t) + k_{-1}\left(C_0 - C_x(t)\right) \quad (2)$$

where F is Faraday's number, k_1 and k_{-1} are conventional constants of the ion exchange rates of the reaction involving pairs of ions and taking place at interface 1:

$$Y_w^- + (R^+ \cdot X^-)_o \underset{k_{-1}}{\overset{k_1}{\leftrightarrow}} (R^+ \cdot Y^-)_o + X_w^- \quad (3)$$

A member in the rectangular brackets (Equation 2) denotes the transport number for the anion X^- through interface 2 .

Neglecting the contribution of the alkylamine salt cation into the conductivity of the organic phase and the possibility of the inverse reaction of ion exchange (3), we may simplify equation (2). Substituting its solution into Ohm's law (Equation 1), it follows that

$$i(t) = vtC_0 l^{-1}\left\{(\Lambda_x - \Lambda_y)\exp\left(-\frac{v\Lambda_x}{2l^2F}t^2 - k_1 t\right) + \Lambda_y\right\} \quad (4)$$

The following initial conditions were used: $C_x(O)=C_o$, $C_y(O)=0$, $C_R(t) \equiv Co$;

The slope of the voltammograms at the initial point is determined by the molar conductivity of ions initially contained in the non-aqueous phase, and at the end point by the conductivity of ions introduced into the membrane as a result of the electric current transfer. During electrodialysis, the system undergoes transition from one level of electric conductivity to another, this transition being reflected in the voltammograms.[71]

Selectivity within the transmembrane transfer of anions is determined by Hofmeister's lyotropic series. Substantial flows of ions with a low hydration energy (ClO_4^-, $AuCl_4^-$, $Au(CN)_2^-$, $PtCl_6^{2-}$) through the interphase boundary, arising in the process of electrodialysis, lead to a decrease in the concentration of extractable anions in the solution layer adjacent to the membrane since these anions are usually present in negligible quantities. In such a situation, the electric current passing through the solution/membrane interface is partially transporting anions from the background electrolyte. As a result, the process of extraction loses selectivity. When the concentration of extracted ions is less than 10^{-3}M, the current efficiency drops to less than one percent.[39, 72, 73] Since alkylamine salts of lipophilic anions are much weaker surfactants than chlorides,[44] such changes in the anion composition in the layer adjacent to the membrane have been observed experimentally.[72]

In its initial part, voltammogram 1 (Figure 1) has an S-like shape due to the appearance of the ClO_4^- ions with a higher conductivity in the membrane. The corresponding part of curve 2 is a straight line, since the anion composition in the membrane remains unchanged. With the onset of polarization during the concentration stage, the Cl^- ions begin to take part in the interfacial ion transfer. The peak of curve 2 reflects essentially a complete exchange of the ClO_4^- ions against the Cl^- ions in the membrane. ClO_4^- content in the membrane, beginning at the merging point of curves 1 and 3, never exceeds 3%. Equation (4) describes the corresponding voltammograms.

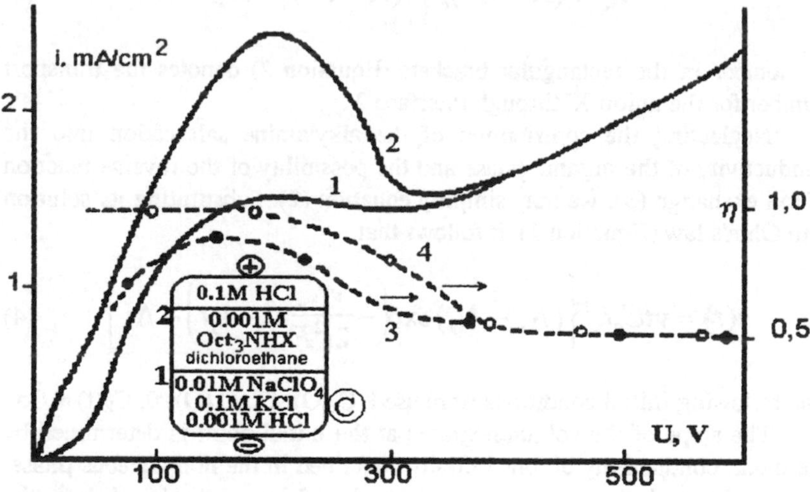

Figure 1. Voltammograms of the liquid membranes - 1,2, and current efficiency for ClO_4^- ions transfer - 3,4. Organic phase: 1,3 - Oct_3NHCl, 2,4 - Oct_3NHClO_4. Rate of potential sweep - 6 V/s.

Alkylamine cations may also participate in the electric current transfer through the interface. The value of the current transferred by the cations is equal to the difference between the current passing through the membrane and that transferred by the anions through interface I. If the alkylamine cations participate in the electric current transfer through the interface I, they move from the organic to the aqueous phase. Sometimes this process is accompanied by formation of an emulsion in the aqueous solution [73,74]. The alkylamine cations formed by combination of protons with amines other than quaternary amines, may participate in the H^+ ion transfer through the interface. An estimation made in reference 71 (see also ref. 74) shows that at pH>3 dissociation of Oct_3NH^+ take place in the aqueous layers adjacent to the interface. The quantity of trioctylamine in its deprotonized Oct_3N form, which begins to accumulate in the membrane, corresponds to the changes of pH in the aqueous phase. In solutions with pH $\leq$ 3 the deprotonization of alkylamine cations is suppressed, and the differences between quaternary and ternary alkylamine salts cease to exist.

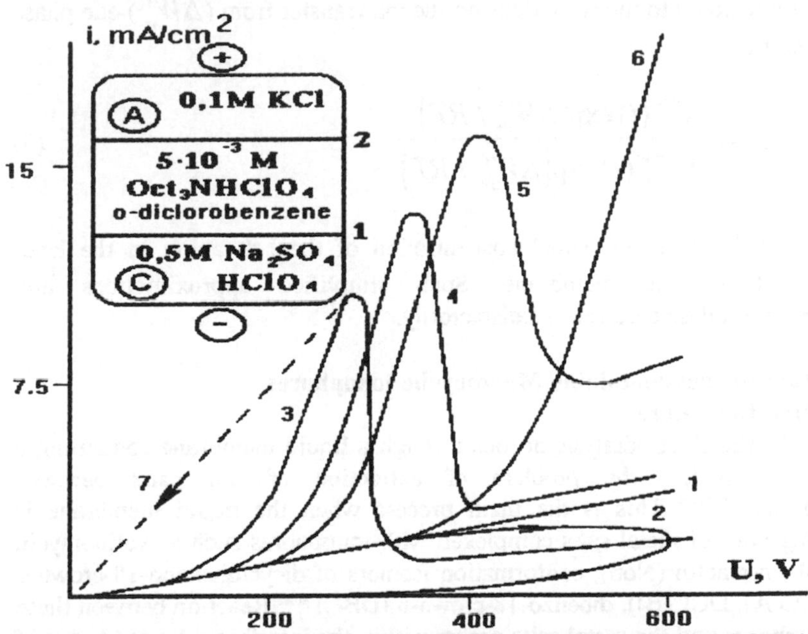

Figure 2. Voltammograms of the liquid membrane. $HClO_4$ concentration (M):1 - 1.0; 2,3 -0.01; 4 - 0.033; 5 - 0.066; 6 - 0.1. Curves 1,2 were registered in back-ground electrolyte absence. Rate of potential sweep: 6 V/s. 7 (—) - reversal of potential (400v/s).

The conductivity of an equimolar mixture of trioctylamine sulphate and perchlorate in *o*-chlorobenzene is 5-7 times higher than that of Oct_3NHClO_4 or $(Oct_3NH)_2SO_4$ solutions of the same concentration. The SO_4^{2-} ions begin to take part in the current transfer to the membrane only after a decrease of the ClO_4^- concentration in the layers adjacent to the membrane is reached (Figure 2). The accumulation of SO_4^{2-} ions in the membrane is accompanied by an abrupt increase of the current, partly transferred through the interface by the alkylamine cations. After the initial voltage sweep cycle, peaks of current are never observed, although the membrane conductivity, due to the organic phase heating and water accumulation in the membrane, increases as compared with the initial value. If the concentration of $HClO_4$ is low and the background electrolyte is absent, the voltammograms show a characteristic hysteresis caused by partial transfer of alkylamine cations into the aqueous solution. When the concentration of $HClO_4$ increases, the hysteresis is not observed (curves 1 and 2, Figure 2).

To calculate the parameters of the process, it is necessary to solve a set of differential equations describing the changes in the concentration of ions in the organic phase and in the aqueous layers adjacent to the membrane. To do so, a number of simplifying assumptions have been made.[70,72] The transport number from the aqueous phase to the organic one is assumed to be proportional to the work done on the ion transfer from (ΔW_w^o) one phase to another

$$t_i = \frac{C_i^w(t)\exp\left(\Delta W_{iw}^o / RT\right)}{\sum C_j^w(t)\exp\left(\Delta W_{jw}^o / RT\right)} \tag{5}$$

where $C_i^w(t)$ is the actual concentration of the i-th anion in the layer adjacent to the membrane. Such simplified approximations and experimental data correlate satisfactorily.

2. Membranes containing Macrocyclic Ionophores

a. Free Ionophores

In the electrodialysis of ions through a liquid membrane containing a neutral carrier, the problem of extraction of ion pairs becomes important.[57,77-79] This is the main process when the liquid membrane is filling with of metal salts complexed with ionophores such as valinomycin (Val), nonactin (Non), conformation isomers of dicyclohexano-18-crown-6 (DCC(A), DCC(B)), dibenzo-18-crown-6 (DBC).[80,81] Reaction between these ionophores and the metal salts occurs within the interface-adjacent layers of an aqueous phase.[82,83,44] The rate constant of complex formation between the ionophores and the cations is of the order 10^7-$10^9 s^{-1}$. Therefore, the rate of this reaction as well as that of ion pair formation[70] never influence the kinetics of electrodialysis. The $L^*(M^+X^-)$ complexes are extracted into the membrane, and since this ionic pair is neutral, there is no electrical current. The current through an interface is transferred by the ions extracted into the membrane, in which cations and anions move further into the corresponding aqueous solutions. In the liquid membrane where the ionophore complexes with cations occur, the anions are transferred by ion exchange. For the cations, such an opportunity exists only in the presence of free ionophores in the layers adjacent to interface 1. If only an indifferent electrolyte is contained in one of the water chambers , then the changes in the concentration of the ionophore complexes in the membrane, in the case of a cation current, are described as follows:

$$\frac{dC(t)}{dt} = -\frac{i(t)}{lF} + k_1(C_0 - C(t)) - 2k_{-1}C(t) \tag{6}$$

where k_1 and k_{-1} are the conventional rate constants of the direct and reverse reactions of extraction of ion pairs, and C_o is the initial concentration of ionophore in the membrane.

The concentration of ions in the chamber A is constant. By substitution of the solution of (6) into (1), we derive an expression for the voltammogram:

$$i(t) = vt\Lambda l^{-1}k_1C_0 \exp\left(-Bt^2/2 - At\right)\int_0^t \exp(B\xi^2/2 + A\xi)d\xi \tag{7}$$

where $A=(k_1 - 2k_{-1})$, and $B= v\Lambda / l^2F$.

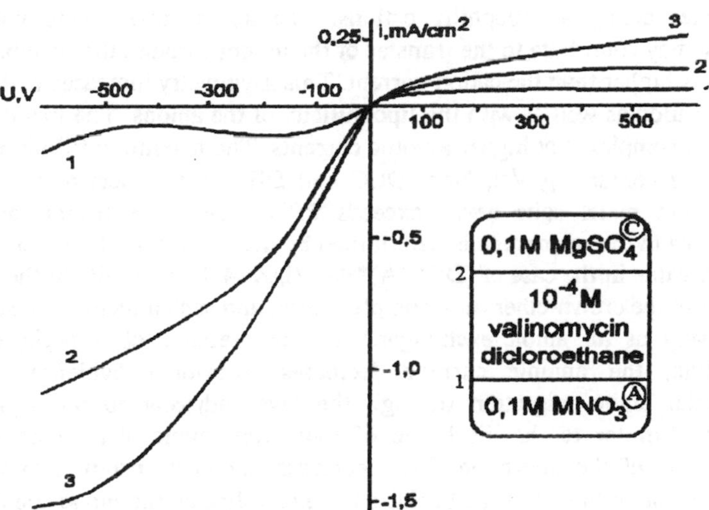

Figure 3. Voltammograms of the liquid membrane. Aqueous chamber A: 1 - $LiNO_3$; 2 - $CsNO_3$; 3 - KNO_3. Rate of potential sweep: 6 V/s.

Equation (7) satisfactorily describes ion transfer through the membrane containing a neutral carrier [80] (Figure 3). As follows from (7), the concentration of a complex reaches a maximum, then decreases, while the voltammograms are either passing through their maximum or changing slope. A linear dependence between the current and the initial concentration of the crown ether is true for all ionophores studied. In the case of DCC (A) it is valid at concentrations up to $5 \cdot 10^{-2}$M. The proportionality between the current value and the complex formation constant has also been observed.

Existence of such dependence is most obvious in the electrodialysis of Rb^+ and Tl^+ ions through the membranes containing various conformation isomers of DCC - A (cis-sin-cis) and B (cis-anti-cis). The complex formation constants of these ions referring to various isomers have different values.

The nature of anions in the aqueous phase "A" strongly influences the transfer of cations through the membrane: The transfer rate increases with the lipophilicity of anions. The presence of a background electrolyte practically never changes the value of the cation current. These facts reveal the mechanism of ion transfer through the membrane, which is related to extraction of ion pairs of $L^*(M^+X^-)$. The LM^+ complexes provide a substantial contribution to current transfer through an interface in the electrodialysis of ions having low complex formation constants ($\lg K \leq 1.5$) from solutions of chlorides or sulfates. At concentrations of these cations 0.005 M and lower, the presence of a background electrolyte in an aqueous solution decreases the current by 25-50%. The anions could be transferred through the membrane by means of ion exchange, in this case the LM^+ complexes acting as lipophilic cations. The anion current (the voltage polarity may contribute to the transfer of the anions through the membrane) usually is higher than the cation current. This asymmetry increases with salt concentration as well as with the lipophilicity of the anions. The membrane fills with complexes at higher anionic currents. The maximum filling of the membrane containing Val, Non, DCC and DBC in the electrodialysis of monovalent metal salts never exceeds 25%. The concentration of the complexes in the membrane is determined by the L^*M^+ formation constant. Its high value in the case of (DCC(A)*Pb^{2+} ($\lg K$=4.95 [82]) results in the total binding of the crown-ether in a complex form, and such a membrane serves exclusively as an anion exchanger.[85] In the presence of a background electrolyte, the anionic current decreases, providing evidence of a substantial anion migration through the layer adjacent to the aqueous solution. Similar to the discharge of ions from monovalent electrolyte, suppression of the migration flow decreases the total current two-fold.[86] However, the influence of the background electrolyte on the monovalent ion transfer through the membrane is usually lower. By suppression of the migration current, it is possible to evaluate the share of various processes in the membrane transfer.[80] In a quantitative analysis, it is necessary to supplement Equation 6 with a term reflecting the process of ion exchange, as was done in A.1. The flow of X^- in the membrane may approximately be represented as follows:

$$i_{x^-}(t) = i_d \frac{C(t)}{C_o}\left[1 - \exp\left(\frac{i(t)C_0}{i_d C(t)}\right)\right] \tag{8}$$

where i_d is an limiting diffusion current at the concentration C_o of the complex, and C(t) is the actual concentration of the complex[85].

The asymmetry in the conductivity observed is similar to the phenomenon of reversion of cation electrode function into anion electrode function in ion-selective electrodes with a liquid membrane containing macrocyclic ionophore.[14,80]

b. Complexes of Macrocyclic Ionophores with Metal Salts

Electrodialysis of ions through a membrane containing a complex of ionophore (L) with a metal salt (LM^+X^-) is characterized by a number of special features. If the ions from aqueous solutions never penetrate into the membrane (t_i=0), then the interface current transfer is produced by the ions of the organic phase alone. In this case, the only effect of the electric current transfer through the membrane is destruction of the ionophore*(metal salt) complex. After such destruction, the anions and the cations move to corresponding chambers, but ionophore remains in the membrane (Figure 4a, curve 1). The concentration of the complexes in the membrane is determined by equation

$$\frac{dC(t)}{dt} = -\frac{i(t)}{lF} - 2k_{-1}C(t) \qquad (9)$$

where k_{-1} is the salt re-extraction rate constant. Substituting a solution of (9) into (1), we derive the following voltammogram formula:

$$i(t) = v\Lambda l^{-1}C_0 \exp\left(-v\Lambda t^2 / 2 - 2k_{-1}t\right) \qquad (10)$$

where the exponent reflects a decrease in the concentration of the ionophore complex in the membrane. Equation (10) gives a maximum where the value of the current is proportional to the concentration of the complex in the organic phase and to the square root of the voltage sweeping rate, and is independent of membrane thickness. The current passing through the membrane is proportional to the product of the linear voltage increase and the concentration of the complex in the membrane, the latter being reduced during the process from the initial value C_o to zero. Thus, the maximum in the voltammogram has a clear physical meaning. Voltammograms, calculated in accordance with Kohlrausch's equation and taking into account the molar conductivity dependence of the concentration, render the shape of experimental curves with an accuracy of 3-5%.[87]

If the liquid membrane is composed of solutions of ion associates such as tetraphenylphosphonium salts or dyes of the triphenylmethane series, then the process of electrodialysis is similar to that described above[52]. In this case, however, the organic ions also leave the membrane, where only a pure solvent remains after electrodialysis. In such membranes, electrodialysis has much in common with the process of demineralization[1]: The water/oil interfaces serve as solid ion-exchange membranes, and the liquid membrane itself replaces the solution under demineralization. The high efficiency of the process is due to a fortunate choice of the indifferent electrolyte in the aqueous phase: $MgSO_4$ practically never comes into contact with oxygen-containing crown-ethers, valinomycin and nonactines.[82]

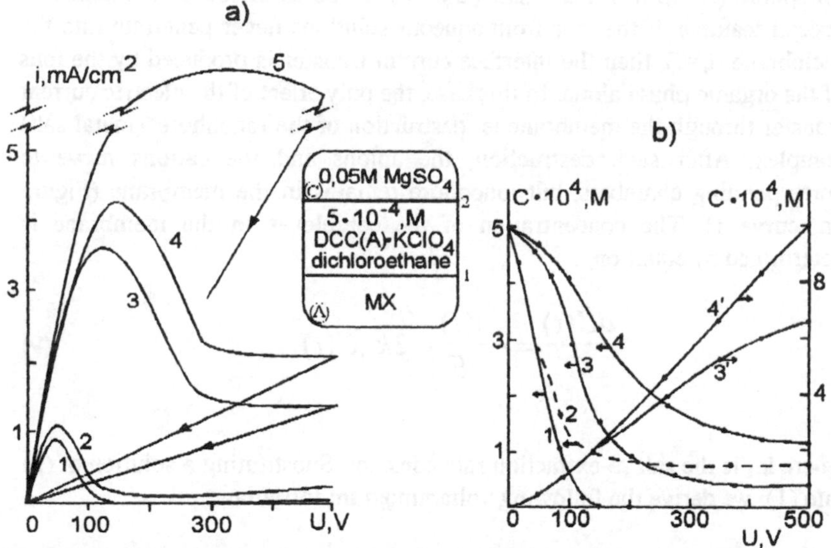

Figure 4. a) Voltammograms of the liquid membrane. **b)**The change of the concentration of the crown ether complex in the non-aqueous phase and ClO_4^- ions in chamber C. Aqueous chamber A: 1 - 0.05M $MgSO_4$; 2 - 0.1M $KClO_4$; 3 - 0.1M HCl_{O4} + 1M $MgSO_4$; 4 - 0.1M HCl_{O4}; 5 - 0.5M $HClO_4$; 3 ,4, 5 - anion current; 2 - cation current; 3' and 4' concentration of the ClO_4^- ions in chamber C.

The high stability of the DCC*Pb^{2+} complex causes difficulties during Pb^{2+} ion re-extraction from the membrane, for instance, in the presence of acetate ions in an aqueous solution[85]. The mechanism of re-extraction is associated with formation of a DCK(A)*$PbAc^+$ complex in the membrane. The stability constant of these complexes is low (lgK~2).

The cations M^+ and the anions X^- in aqueous solutions ($t_i > 0$) can also participate in the transfer of current through the membrane, and voltammograms of such systems also have a bell shape (Figure 4, curves 2-5); however, the current values at the maximum point are higher. After free ionophore appears in the membrane, the main features of the electrodialysis become similar to those described in section 2a.

3. Cation Exchange Membranes

Tetraphenylborate (Ph_4B^-) and dicarbollide (DC^-) salts are commonly used cation exchangers. The voltammograms of membranes containing these agents reveal a characteristic hysteresis caused by departure of ions from the organic phase into corresponding aqueous solutions (Figure 5). Within a membrane containing CsDC or $NaPhB_4$, cation transfer falls into the Hofmeister's series. Li^+ ions are transferable through the membrane containing DC^- anions but in the presence of the less lipophilic PhB_4^- ions, there is no transport of Li^+. In the case of Cs^+, the voltammograms reveal some peculiarities.[80,81] Quite surprising are periodical changes of the current values during cation transfer through membranes containing CsDC.[88] The quantitative description of ion transfer through cation exchange membranes is the same as for anions (A.1). The model of cation transport through a non-steering liquid membrane proposed in reference [89], is difficult to reproduce experimentally.

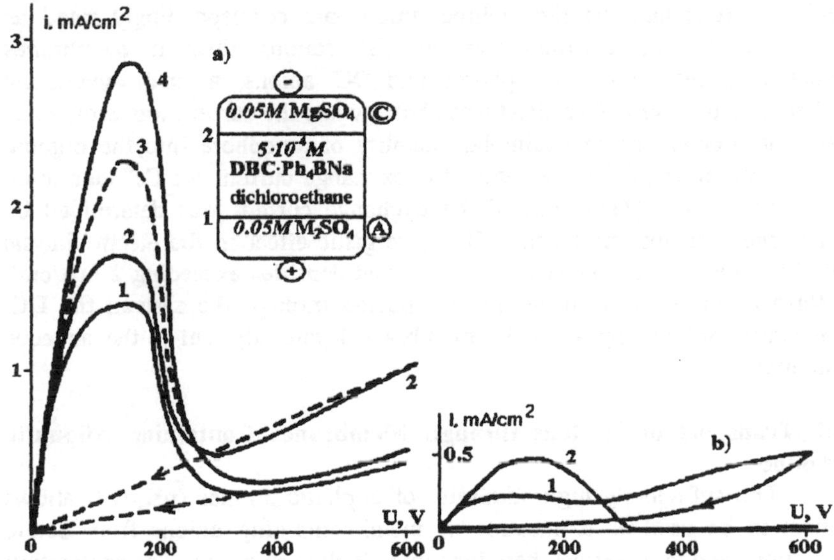

Figure 5. Voltammograms of the liquid membrane. Aqueous chamber A: **a)** 1 - K_2SO_4; 2 - 0.01M K_2SO_4 + 0.05M Li_2SO_4; 3 - Cs_2SO_4; 3 - 0.001M K_2SO_4 + 0.05M Li_2SO_4; 4 - Li_2SO_4; **b)** 1 - 0.05M Cs_2SO_4; 2 - 0.05M Li_2SO_4; Organic phase: 10^{-4}M Ph_4BNa. Rate of potential sweep: 1.2 V/s.

In the presence of the DBK*Ph_4BNa complex, the Li^+ ions are transferred through the membrane (Figure 5a), demonstrating a synergistic effect if both crown ether and Ph_4BNa are present. When compared to the effectiveness of the electrodialysis through such a membrane, the cations could be placed in the following sequence: $Li^+ > Na^+ > Cs^+ > K^+ > Rb^+$. Such an arrangement is related to a higher conductivity of lithium or sodium complexes with the crown ether being compared to cesium or potassium. However, the membrane selectivity relative to metal ions is determined by the value of the crown ether complex stability constant. For example, a fivefold excess of the Li^+ ions relative to the K^+ ions exerts no influence on voltammogram (Figure 5a, curve 1). A decrease in the concentration of K^+ ions down to 0.005M results in a loss of selectivity related to concentration polarization.

Contrary to the Ph_4B^- salts, the selectivity of ion transfer in membranes containing macrocyclic ions and CsDC is determined by the energy of the specific interaction of dicarbollide ions with ions of alkaline metals.[88] This interaction may be quantitatively evaluated by the adsorption energy of corresponding salts from dichloroethane through an interface to aqueous solutions and by the method described in reference 44. The cations, compared by surface activity of their dicarbollide salts, can be arranged in the sequence $Li^+ > Na^+ > K^+ > Rb^+ > Cs^+$, which is a mirror image of Hofmeister's lyotropic series. The constants of interaction between the Li^+, K^+, Cs^+ ions and the dicarbollide anions are correspondingly rated as 1:6.5:52. In the electrodialysis of Cs^+ cations through membranes containing macrocyclic ionophores and DC^- anions, a small synergistic effect was observed. This effect was absent when the current was zero, since the introduction of an equimolar quantity of ionophore into the organic phase containing CsDC decreases the exchange current for Cs^+ ions more than two times. (The value of the exchange current was determined by radiochemical measurements). The synergistic effect in the electrodialysis of Cs^+ cations was observed only at current densities exceeding 2 mA/cm^2. When a current of such density has passed through the system, the DC^- lipophilic anions appear in the membrane layers adjacent to the aqueous solution.

B. Transport of H^+ Ions through Membranes Containing Aliphatic Amines

The sufficiently high alkalinity of aliphatic amines ($pK_a > 10$) allows them to be used as extractants of metal-containing anions from acidic solutions and to re-extract these ions into alkaline solutions. The application of these compounds as carriers through impregnated liquid membranes with possible coupled flows is based on the same property.[4,5] For re-extraction of anions from solutions of aliphatic amine salts, electrodialysis could be used.[73,90] The current through interface 2 is due to neutralization of the Oct_3NH^+ cations by hydroxyl ions, and the current through interface 1 uses the re-extracted X^- anions. The process of re-extraction with alkali is spatially separated by a liquid membrane; the anions are re-extracted into the chamber A, where H^+ ions are absent. The only effect of the current passing through the liquid membrane is a decrease in the concentration of ions in the non-aqueous phase. That is why Equations (8) and (9), obtained after studying the re-extraction of complexes formed by macrocyclic ionophores with metal salts (A2b) are applicable to this process as well.

During re-extraction, the Oct_3N molecules appear in the membrane. These molecules further react with the acid available in chamber A (Figure 6). This reaction at the interface is accompanied by formation of ion pairs of $Oct_3N^+{*}X^-$, which afterwards are extracted into the organic phase. There is no transfer of electricity through the interface. The current through interface 1 is transferred by the X^- anions, which are present in the organic phase as a result of the re-extraction of ion pairs, so that this process may be formally described as a charge transfer through the interface by H^+ ions. At the initial stages of this process, there is practically no transfer of the H^+ ions through the interface. The process becomes noticeable only after the deprotonization of an amine salt (~80%). This moment corresponds to the point "a" in voltammograms 1 and 2 (Figure 6). Position of this point is determined only by the quantity of electricity passed through, and does not depend on the rate of the voltage sweep. Further, the current in the membrane is carried by H^+ ions only.

Linearity in the voltammograms implies that the concentration of ions in the membrane remains constant, and the quantity of the Oct_3NH^+ ions participating in the reaction of neutralization at interface 2 is equal to the quantity of these ions appearing at interface 1.

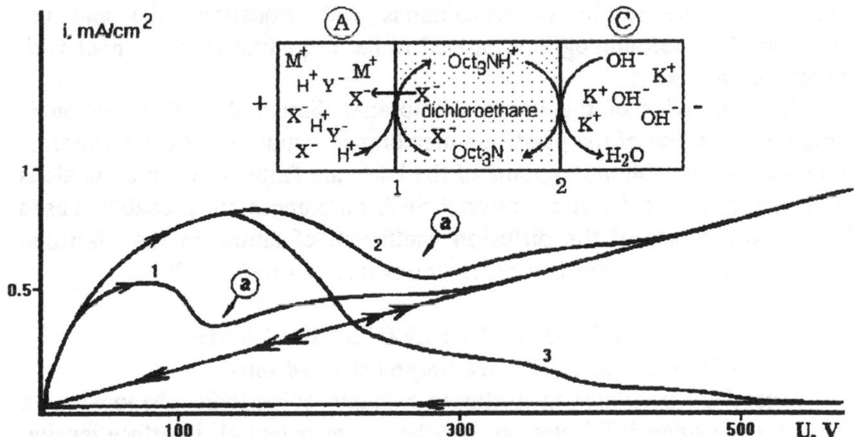

Figure 6. Voltammograms of the liquid membrane. Aqueous chamber A: 1,2 - HCl; 3 - KCl. Rate of potential sweep (V/s): 1 - 1; 2, 3 - 6.

The rate of the voltage sweep never influences linear parts in the voltammograms; that is why the limiting stage of the process is connected with the transfer of neutral particles, but not of ions. Since the stirring in the organic phase never exerts any substantial influence on the process, the transfer of the Oct_3N molecules through the membrane is based on convective diffusion. The rate of proton transfer is determined by diffusion of the trioctylamine molecules through the layers of the organic phase being not stirred. The changes in the concentration of a trioctylamine salt in the membrane while separating the solutions of acid and alkali are described by the equation:

$$\frac{dC(t)}{dt} = -\frac{i(t)}{lF} + \frac{D\left(C_0 - C(t)\right)}{l\delta} \tag{11}$$

where D is a coefficient of diffusion of the Oct_3N molecules in the organic phase, and C_o implies the initial salt concentration in the membrane. In (11), the concentration of Oct_3N was considered to be equal to zero: All the trioctylamine molecules passing through the diffusion layer had to instantly react with an acid. As a further simplification, the thickness of the diffusion layer (δ) was supposed to be constant. A solution of (11) is the following equation:

$$C(t) = AC_0 \exp\left(-Bt^2/2 - At\right)\int_0^t \exp\left(B\xi^2/2 + A\xi\right)d\xi + C_0 \exp(-Bt^2/2 - At) \tag{12}$$

where $A = D/\delta l$, and $B = \nu\Lambda/l^2F$

Comparison of (12) with (10) and (7) reveals that (12) is a sum of the two terms reflecting decrease and formation of an amine salt in the membrane. The results of calculations with Equation (12) and the corresponding voltammograms proved to be in qualitative agreement with experimental data.[90]

The behavior of the liquid membranes discussed in this section is different from that of the plastified membranes containing tridodecylamine. The steady-state voltammograms of the latter are featured by an anomalous influence of the acid concentration.[91] Such differences are probably caused by the low values of the diffusion coefficient of amine in the plastified matrix, which are at least two orders lower than in dichloroethane.

C. PERIODIC PHENOMENA IN ELECTRODIALYSIS

1. Current Oscillations in Electrodialysis of Lead Ions

Teorella's oscillator is a classic example of periodic phenomena in membrane systems.[54, 92] Later on, oscillations of potential, interface tension and other phenomena occurring at the interfaces of immiscible liquids, including those at the electrolyte/liquid membrane interfaces, have been found.[74, 93-97] In some membrane systems, voltage oscillations caused by changes of the membrane resistance during current flow have been observed.[98,99] The transfer of electricity by cesium or tetramethylamine cations through the water/nitrobenzene (or 1,2-dichloroethane) interface in the presence of tetraphenylborate ions in the organic phase is sometimes accompanied by abrupt periodic changes in the interface voltage.[100]

In some instances (Figure 7), periodic current variations during linear sweeps of the polarizing voltage as well as voltage variations in the galvanostatic regime occur in the system.[101,102] The frequency and amplitude of these oscillations depend on the concentration of $Pb(NO_3)_2$, magnesium acetate ($Mg(Ac)_2$) and crown ether. An increase in the membrane thickness decreases their frequency and amplitude; an increase in the voltage sweep rate decreases the frequency, and increases the amplitude of the oscillations.

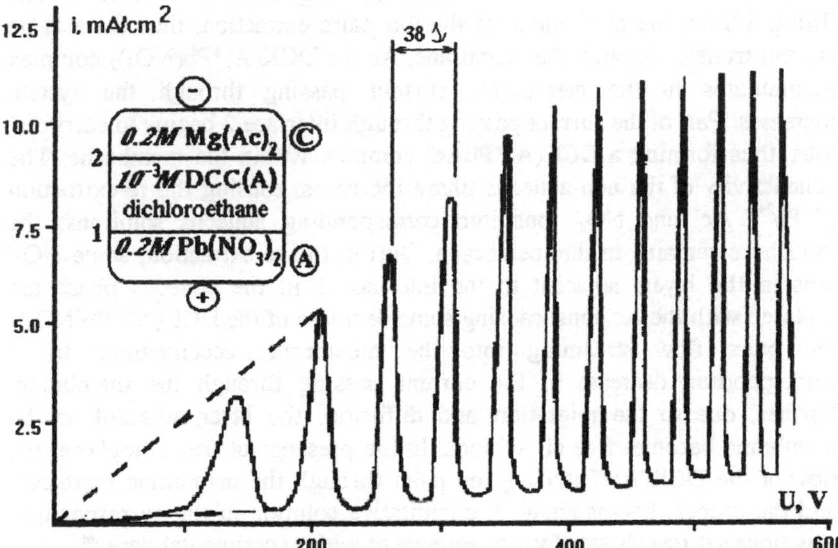

Figure 7. Voltammograms of the liquid membrane. Rate of potential sweep: 1.2 V/s. (—)Reversal of potential (400v/s) (From Author, J. *Electroanal. Chem.*, 280, 61, 1990. Elsevier Sequoia S.A. With permission).

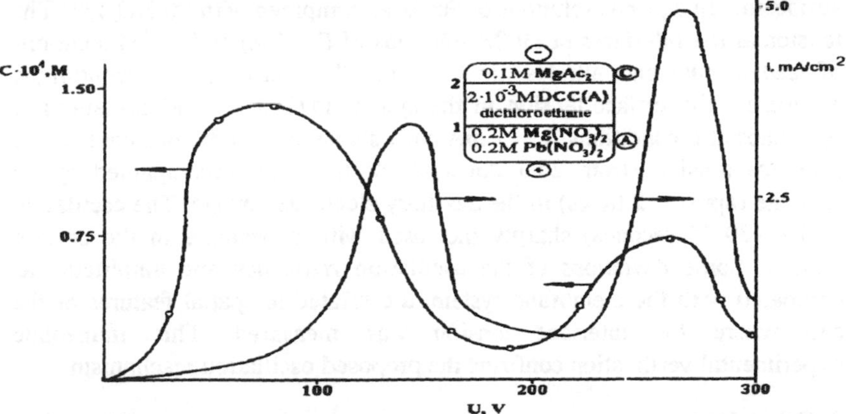

Figure 8. Voltammogram of the liquid membrane and the change of the concentration of the crown ether complex in the non-aqueous phase. Rate of potential sweep: 1.2 V/s. (From Author, *J. Electroanal. Chem.*, 280, 61, 1990. Elsevier Sequoia S.A. With permission).

The concentration of the DCK(A)*Pb^{2+} complex in the membrane also experiences periodic changes; at the beginning of the process, the changes in concentration precede current changes (Figure 8). The proposed mechanism of the current variations is based on the periodic occurrence of the DCK(A)*$PbAc^+$ complex in the membrane, which has a lower formation constant value and higher conductivity than DCK(A)*Pb^{2+}. At initial stages of the process, the membrane fills with the DCK(A)*$Pb(NO_3)_2$ complex that is formed in the water layers adjacent to interface 1. The filling follows the mechanism of the ion pairs extraction, thus there is no current transfer through the membrane. As the DCK(A)*$Pb(NO_3)_2$ complex accumulates in the membrane, current passing through the system increases. Part of the current passing through interface 2 begins to carry Ac^- ions, thus forming a DCK(A)*$PbAc^+$ complex within the membrane. The conductivity of the non-aqueous phase increases, causing the re-extraction of Pb^{2+}, Ac^- and NO_3^- ions into corresponding aqueous solutions; the ionophore remains in the membrane. During the re-extraction, some NO_3^- ions in the layers adjacent to the interface 1 in the aqueous phase are replaced with the Ac^- ions, causing some decrease of the DCK(A)*$Pb(NO_3)_2$ ion pairs flow streaming into the membrane, accompanied by a corresponding decrease of the current passing through the membrane. Further, due to the migration and diffusion, the layer adjacent to the membrane becomes free of Ac^- ions. In the presence of free ionophore, the flow of the DCK(A)*$Pb(NO_3)_2$ ion pairs through the membrane increases, and the process begins anew. A quantitative solution of the corresponding equations set reveals satisfactory agreement with experimental data.[101]

As a significant parameter of the proposed mechanism, the periodic replacement of NO_3^- ions with acetate anions at the interface should be mentioned. The DCC(A) solutions in dichloroethane are stronger surfactants in aqueous solutions of $Pb(Ac)_2$, compared with $Pb(NO_3)_2$[103]. The tension at the interfaces of 10^{-3}M solutions of DCC(A) and 10^{-1}M solutions of lead acetate and nitrates are 21.9 and 26.6 mN/m, correspondingly. Measuring the surface tension in the system $Pb(NO_3)_2$ solution/membrane (galvanostatic conditions, I = 3 mA/cm^2) shows a periodic decrease in the interface tension (from 26.5 down to 22 mN/m)[102] accompanied by an increase (approx. 2 times) in the auxiliary electrode voltage. The oscillation period (20-35 seconds) sharply increased with a decrease in the current density. Some deviations of the oscillation frequency and amplitude, as compared with the membrane system, are related to spatial features of the cell where the interface tension was measured. This immediate experimental verification confirms the proposed oscillation mechanism.

2. Other Ions

In order to produce oscillations based on the mechanism described above, it is necessary that the formation constant of the ionophore *metal

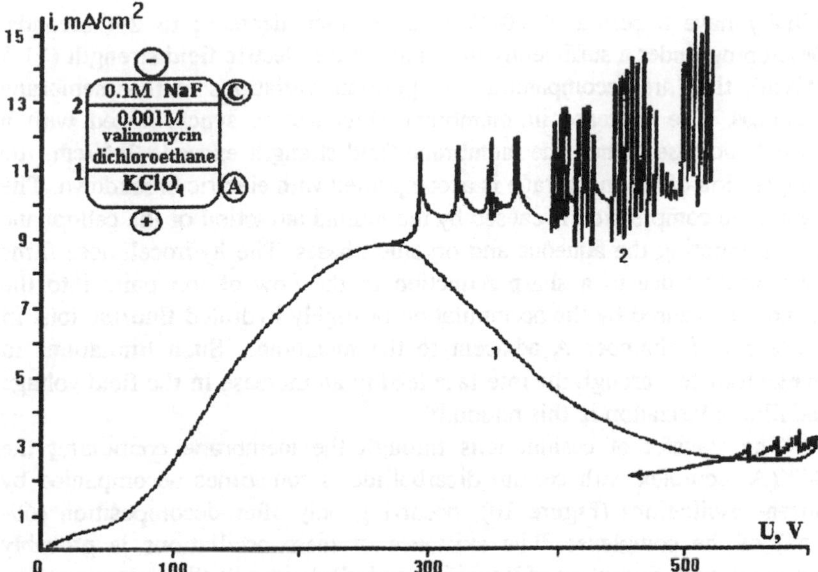

Figure 9. Voltammograms of the liquid membrane. $KClO_4$ concentration (M):1 - 0.01; 2 - 0.1. Rate of potential sweep: 1.2 V/s.

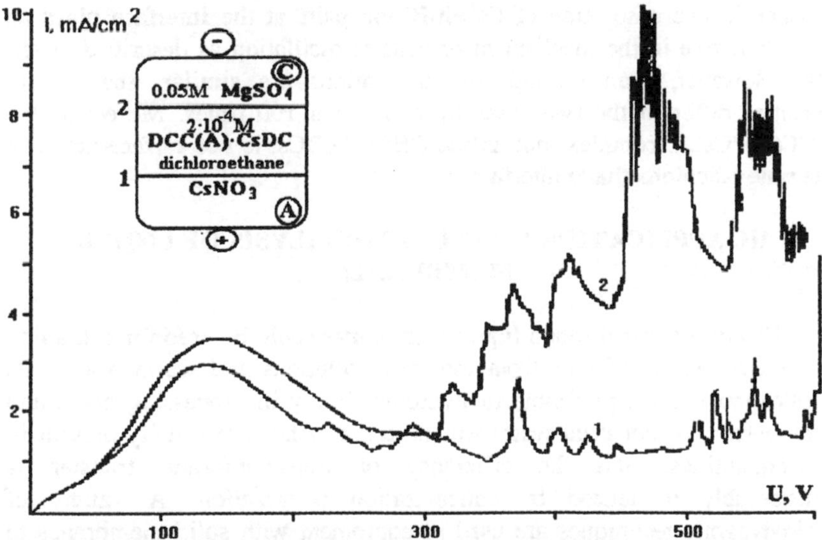

Figure 10. Voltammograms of the liquid membrane. Aqueous chamber A: 1 -0.05M Cs_2SO_4; 2 - 0.1M $CsNO_3$. Rate of potential sweep: 1.2 V/s.

salt complex should be sufficiently high (logK> 4). In this case, the flow of L*MX ion pairs provides an adequate rate of membrane filling with such complexes. If this condition is not satisfied, no oscillations occur. However, characteristic current fluctuations are possible (Figure 9). These oscillations initially have a period of 20-25 seconds, then decrease to 2-4 seconds. Developing under a sufficiently high membrane electric field strength (>1.5 kV/cm), they are accompanied with periodic variations of the membrane thickness. The decrease in membrane thickness is synchronized with a current increase. When the membrane field strength exceeds 2kV/cm, the compression of the membrane is accompanied with electric breakdown. The membrane compression is caused by the mutual attraction of the cellophane films separating the aqueous and organic phases. The hydrocellulose films are polarized due to a sharp reduction in the flow of ion pairs into the membrane, caused by the accumulation of highly hydrated fluorine ions in the layers of chamber A adjacent to the membrane. Such limitations in charge transfer through the interface lead to an increase in the field voltage and film polarization in this region.[102]

The transfer of cesium ions through the membrane containing the DCK(A) complex with cesium dicarbollide is sometimes accompanied by current oscillations (Figure 10), occurring only after decomposition (60-80%) of the complexes. The existence of these oscillations is probably connected with formation of lipophilic carbollide ions in the aqueous phase. The Cs^+DC^- ion pairs formed are further extracted into the membrane, and the process begins anew. Such a scheme is similar to catalytic ion transfer[104]. The adsorption of $Cs^+Ph_4B^-$ ion pairs at the interface plays an important role in the mechanism of voltage oscillation as described in ref. 100. However, even through the oscillations are similar, the current densities differ in the two cases by more than 100 times. Moreover, the DCC(A)*CsDC complex, not unlike DBC*Ph_4BCs, is not surface-active at the water/dichloroethane interface.[81]

III. APPLICATION OF ELECTRODIALYSIS OF LIQUID MEMBRANES

Electrodialysis through liquid membranes could be used for extraction and concentration of ions from industrial solutions and waste waters. Its application is most profitable in hydrometallurgy in processing noble and rare metals. In industrial waste waters, these metals are usually present in microquantities, and the efficiency of transmembrane transfer is considerably influenced by concentration polarization. A variety of hydrodynamic techniques are used in equipment with solid membranes to decrease this polarization effect.[105]

A highly effective concentration is achievable at saturating diffusion current densities for the ions under extraction. The re-extraction of lipophilic ions from membranes is normally carried out with higher current densities. Therefore it is expedient to use an asymmetric cell for concentration, where the area of the interface source solution/membrane is larger than the surface of the opposite interface.[72]

The problem of concentration polarization never arises during the re-extraction of ions from the membrane. Here, the organic phase serves as a membrane, the former containing an extractable compound transferred previously into the latter by liquid extraction. One example of such a process is the re-extraction of ions from membranes containing ionophore complexes of amine salts. The re-extraction is also accomplished by exchange of counter-ions in the membrane.

In analytical practice, electrodialysis can be used for measuring the concentration of ionophore complexes, ionic associates and amine salts in the organic phase.[85,87,90] Such measurements are based upon the proportionality of the current at linear voltage sweep and maximum concentration of the complex. The lower sensitivity level is of the order 3-$5*10^{-7}$M for ionophore complexes and 10^{-6}M for ionic associates and amine salts. When measuring the concentration of the complexes and amine salts dissolved in solvents with a low dielectric constant, such as toluene, the membrane should be diluted with a polar aprotonic solvent (dichloroethane, nitrobenzene) in the ratio of 1:1.

Electrodialysis can also be applied to the purification of neutral ionophores to remove ionic impurities, with an ionophore solution in dichloroethane used as a membrane and with a flow-through technique when purifying large quantities. The aqueous phase should contain a practically non-extractable electrolyte. For most macrocyclic polyesters, valinomycin and nonactin, magnesium sulphate is suitable as a background electrolyte. The process should be carried out in a galvanostatic regime until a sharp increase of the polarizing voltage is reached.

IV. EXPERIMENTAL APPARATUS

A. Electrodialysis through Liquid Membranes

A schematic of the experimental setup for the electrodialysis in liquid membranes by linear voltage sweep is shown in Figure 11a. As a voltage source, a controlling generator and a power amplifier (500 W), providing linear voltage sweep with a rate up to 400 V/s within the range up to 400 V, are necessary. The liquid membrane (thickness 0.2 cm, surface 7 cm^2) was separated from aqueous solutions with hydrocellulose films commonly used for hemodialysis. Such films provide a reproducible hydrodynamic interface but represent an additional hydrodynamic resistance[53]. The water chambers (volume 20 cm^3) were separated from the electrode chambers with solid ion-exchange membranes. The block-designed cell was made of Teflon. Luggin's capillaries for the indicator electrodes were formed as passages in Teflon (ca. 0.2 cm), reaching the membrane from both sides. A rough Teflon rod (ca. 0.13 cm) reinforced with a steel needle was used for membrane stirring. The lower end of the rod had a support in the membrane frame made of Teflon.

In a cell with vertical open interfaces, the organic phase could be held in the Teflon due to adhesion (Figure 11b) [53]. Before the experiment, the chamber was filled with a background electrolyte, then an organic phase was added through an opening (5). The optimal dimensions of the membrane were as follows: diameter - 0.25 cm, diameter of the opening - 0.8 cm, volume - 0.2 ml. Organic solutions containing tether salts, did not adhere to the Teflon due to their high surface activity. The most suitable objects for such a cell were ionophores, since their surface activity was rather low.

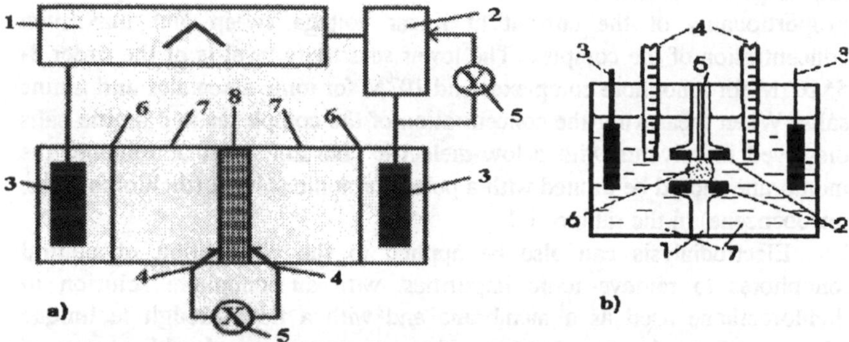

Figure 11. a). Block diagram of experimental set-up: 1 - generator and power amplifier; 2 - variable resistance; 3 - auxiliary electrodes; 4 reference electrodes; 5 - X,Y recorder 6 - solid ion- exchange membranes; 7 - water chambers; 8 - liquid membrane.
b). Membrane cell. 1 - Teflon partition; 2 - glass rings; 3 - auxiliary electrodes; 4 - reference electrodes; 5 - canal for membrane forming; 6 - liquid membrane; 7 - water chambers;

In the setup shown in Figure 12a, an organic phase with a density higher than that of the water may be used as a membrane. One of the interfaces coincides with a boundary of the porous glass filter (2). The level of the water phase in the lower chamber is controlled by a piston (3). The glass cylinder (4) with a highly polished end is pressed against the base of Teflon. The electrode chambers are separated by solid ion-exchange membranes, the higher membrane being welded as a cylinder. The indicator electrodes have been made by soldering a platinum wire ca. 0.05 cm into a glass piece, the end of electrode then being polished. The glass surface (excluding the flat end) was made hydrophobic by means of trimethylchlorosilicane followed by heating up to 200°C. Such a cell, in combination with an electrode-probe, could be used to measure the voltage drop in the membrane body. In all the membranes studied (complexes of macrocyclic ionophores, alkylamine salts, dicarbollide salts), this distribution proved to be linear. The measurement errors (+-5%) are compatible with the measurement accuracy of the probe positioning and with the end effects.

Of all the procedures, that of a neutral ionophore purification (extraction of ionic impurities) is quite important. It is practical to perform it shortly before the measurement, after which the magnesium sulphate solution is replaced with the working solution. The possibility of the dichloroethane interaction with alkylamines should also be taken into account.[71] To obtain reproducible results in this case, it is necessary to use fresh solutions of the alkylamine salts.

B. MEASUREMENT OF INTERFACIAL TENSION AT THE WATER/MEMBRANE INTERFACE IN THE ELECTRIC FIELD.

The interfacial tension at the water/membrane interface can be measured by means of the drop-volume method (Figure 12b). A drop of the $Pb(NO_3)_2$ aqueous solution was formed at an end of the glass capillary (external ∅ 2.45 and 5.2 mm) pressed into a Teflon piece. The drop volume during the measurements was about 40% of the maximal volume. The use of larger capillaries was preferred since the errors connected with drop polarization became less.[106] The picture of the drop on a monitor screen was recorded by a VCR or photographic camera. The error of the interfacial tension measurements never exceeded 5%. The gap width between the top of the drop and the planar water/dichloroethane interface was chosen experimentally and was usually about 2-3 mm. The gap width was controlled by vertical movements of the cell with a micrometer system. The rectangular cell was made of Teflon; the three cell walls (15 mm thick) had pressed-in optic glass windows. The drop was illuminated through a fiber light guide and a diffusing opal glass. In the upper part of the cuvette, in a special cavity, an auxiliary AgCl rode shaped as a rectangular frame (wire ∅2 mm) was placed. In some cases, a platinum electrode having the same

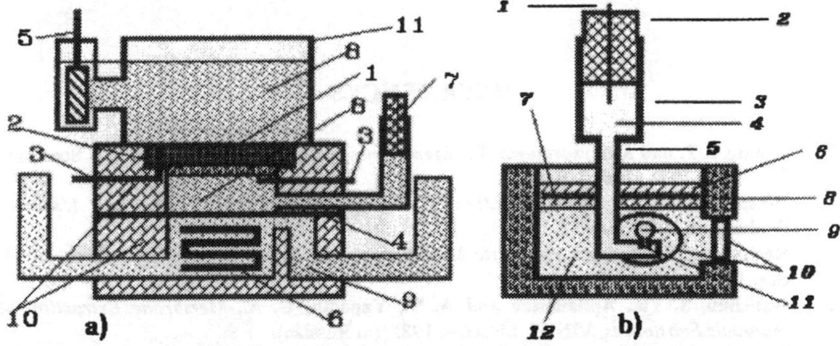

Figure 12. a). Membrane cell. 1 - liquid membrane; 2 - glass filter; 3 - reference electrodes; 4 - solid ion-exchange membrane; 5,6 - auxiliary electrodes; 7 - plunger; 8,9 - water chambers; 10 - Teflon body; 11 - glass cylinder.

b). Cell for measurement interfacial tension of water/membrane interface. 1 - Ag wire; 2 -Teflon plunger; 3- glass cylinder; 4 - 0.1M $Pb(NO_3)_2$ solution; 5 - Teflon part of capillary; 6 - 0.2M $Mg(Ac)_2$ solution; 7 - auxiliary electrode; 8- Teflon body; 9 - drop of 0.1M $Pb(NO_3)_2$ solution; 10 - optical windows; 11 - glass capillary; 12 - 10^{-3}M DCC(A) solution in dichloroethane.

shape was used. This electrode was normally used as a cathode; the anode was made of a silver wire pressed into one end of the Teflon piston, a design which prevented gas excretion in the cylinder. The silver ions corresponding to the quantity of electricity passed during the experiment, exerted no influence on the measurement results. Magnesium acetate (0.2 M solution) was used as the upper aqueous solution, and DCK(A) - 10^{-3} M solution in dichloroethane was used as the organic phase. A solution of the DCK(A)*$Pb(NO_3)_2$ complex in a corresponding concentration, previously obtained by extraction, could be used to increase the conductivity of the organic phase.

V. CONCLUSION

The processes of electrodialysis discussed here are mostly irreversible: the densities of the interfacial currents are at least an order of magnitude higher than the current of the quasi-reversible ion transfer. The parameters of electrodialysis depend on the relationship between the current passing through the membrane determined by its ohmic resistance, and the ion flows through the aqueous solution/membrane interface. When the aqueous phase loses extractable ions, first the ions of the background electrolyte, and then the lipophilic ions of the membrane begin to participate in current transfer through the solution/ membrane interface. The ionic exchange reactions at the interfaces, and ion pairs extraction as well, play an important role in the transmembrane ion transfer. The features discussed here show that electrodialysis through liquid membranes remains an interesting subject of inquiry.

REFERENCES

1. **Hwang, S-T. and Kammermeyer, K.**, *Membranes in Separations*, John Wiley & Sons Inc., New York, 1975, chap. 3, 9.
2. **Brock, T. D.**, *Membrane Filtration*, A publication of Science Tech., Inc. Madison, Washington, 1983, chap.13.
3. **Kesting, R. E,** *Synthetic Polymeric Membranes*, John Wiley & Sons, New York, 1985, chap.1.
4. **Ivanchno, S. Yu., Aphanasiev and A. V., Yagodin, G. A.,** *Membrane Extraction of Inorganic Substances*, VINITI, Moscow, 1985, (in Russian).
5. *Liquid Membranes. Theory and Application.* Noble, R. D., Way, J. D. Eds., ACS Symp. Ser., No 347, Am. Chem. Soc., Washington, 1987.
6. **Schlosser, S.,** Liquid Membranes- Theory and Practice, in *Advances in Membrane Phenomena and Processes*, Mika, A. M., Winnicki, T. Z. Eds., Wroclaw Technical University Press, Wroclaw, 1989, 163.
7. **McDonnell, M. B. and Vadgama, P. M.,** Membranes: separation principles and sensing, *Selective Electrode Rev.*, 11, 17, 1989.

8. **Lev, A. A.,** *Modeling of Ionic Selectivity of Cell Membranes*, Nauka, Leningrad, 1976, chap.2, 3, 7 (in Russian).
9. **Kocherginsky, N. M., Osak, I. S., Demochkin and V. V., Rubaylo, V. L.,** Physico-chemical mechanism of ionophoric activity of fatty acids as stimulants of transmembrane momovalent cations exchange, *Biol. Membranes*, 4, 838, 1987.
10. **Ovchinnikov, Yu. A., Ivanov, V. T. and Shcrob, A. M.,** *Membrane Active Complexons*, Nauka, Moscow, 1974, chap. 5 (in Russian).
11. **Izatt, R. M., Lindh, G. C, Bruening, R. L., Brandshaw, J. S., Lamb, J. D. and Christensen, J. J.,** Design of cation selectivity into liquid membrane systems using macrocyclic carriers, *Pure Appl. Chem.*, 58, 1453, 1986.
12. **Kobuce, Y., Tabushi, I., Oh, K. and Aoki, T.,** Transport of uranil ions through liquid membrane mediated by macrocyclic policarbocsilate in combinations with hydrophobic quaternary ammonium cations, *J. Org. Chem.*, 53, 5933, 1989.
13. **Lindoy, L. F. and Baldwin, D. S.,** Ligand design for selective metal-ions transport through liquid membranes, *Pure Appl. Chem.*, 61, 909, 1989.
14. **Morf, W. E.,** *The Principles of Ion-Selective Electrodes and of Membrane Transport*, Akademiai Kiado, Budapest, 1981, chap. 7, 11, 12.
15. **Yatsimirskii, K. B. and Talanova, G. G.,** Liquid membranes with macrocyclic ionophores and perspectives of their application in analytical chemistry, *Zur. Anal. Chem.*, 45, 1686, 1990.
16. **Jonson, J. and Mathianson, L.,** Supported liquid membranes techniques for sample preparation in environmental and biological analysis, *Trac. Trends Anal. Chem.*, 11, 106, 1992.
17. **Parthasathy, N. and Buffle, J.,** Supported liquid membrane for analytical separation of transition metal ions, *Anal. Chim. Acta*, 254, 9, 1991.
18. **Danessi, P. R.,** Separation of metal species by supported liquid membranes, *Sep. Sci. Technol.*, 19, 857, 1984-85.
19. **Danessi, P. R.,** A simplified model for the coupled transport of metal ions through hollow-fiber supported liquid membranes, *J. Membrane Sci.*, 20, 231, 1984.
20. **Chiarizia, R.** Application of supported liquid membranes for removal of nitrate, technetium and chromium from ground water, *J. Membrane Sci.*, 55, 39, 1991.
21. **Ruppert, M., Draxler, R. and Marr, R.,** Liquid membrane-permeation and its experience in pilot-plant and industrial scale, *Sep. Sci. Technol.*, 21, 1659, 1988.
22. **Dannesi, P. R., Reichley-Yinger, L. and Rickert, P. G.,** Lifetime of supported liquid membranes: influence of interfacial properties, chemical composition and water transport on the long-term stability of the membranes, *J. Membrane Sci.*, 31, 117, 1987.
23. **Ho, W. S. and Li, N. N.,** Modeling of liquid - membrane extraction processes, *Hydrometallurgical Process Fundamentals*, Proc. NATO Adv. Res. Int. Cambridge, 555, 1984.
24. **Schlosser, S. and Kossaczky, E.,** Comparison of pertraction through liquid membranes and double liquid-liquid extraction, *J. Membrane Sci.*, 6, 83, 1980.
25. **Izzat, R. M., Lamb, J. D. and Bruening, R. L.,** Comparison of bulk, emulsion, thin sheet supported, and hollow fiber supported membranes in macrocycle-mediater separations, *Sep. Sci. Technol.*, 23, 1645, 1988.
26. **Cussler, E. L.,** *Multicomponent Diffusion*, Elsivier Scientific Publishing Company, Amsterdam, 1976, chap.8.
27. **Cussler, E. L.,** Membranes which pump, *AIChE J.*, 17, 1309, 1971.
28. **Cussler, E. L.,** *Diffusion*, Cambridge University Press, New York, 1984, chap.1.
29. **Sugawara, M., Omoto, M., Yoshida, H. and Umezawa, Y.,** Enchanament of uphill transport by a double carrier membrane system, *Anal. Chem.*, 60, 2301, 1988.
30. **Santis, G. D., Fabbrizzi, L., Poggi, A. and Seghi, B.,** Metal complexes that transport electrons across liquid membranes, *J. Chem. Soc. Dalton Trans*, 87, 33, 1991.
31. **Yau, S.-L., Rullema, D. P., Jackman, D. C. and Daignault, L. G.,** Electron transport reactions in immobilized liquid membranes: a comparison of the carriers vitamin K and 2-tetra- butylanthraquinone, *J. Membrane Sci.*, 37, 27, 1988.

32. **Tarasov, V. V. and Yagodin, G. A.**, Interfacial phenomena in solvent extraction, in *Ion Exchange and Solvent Extraction,* Marinsky, J.A. and Marcus, Y. Eds., Marcel Dekker, Inc., New York, vol. 10, 1988. chap.4.
33. **Tarasov, V. V. and Pichugin, A. A.**, Interfacial phenomena and ions transport through liquid membranes, *Advances in Chemistry (USSR)*, 57, 990, 1988.
34. **Chaara, M. and Noble, R. D.**, Effect of convective flow across a film on facilitated transport, *Sep. Sci. Technol.*, 24, 893, 1989.
35. **Tarasov, V. V.**, Dissipative structures at the oil/water interface, *Papers of X Russian Solvent Extraction Conference*, Russian Academy of Science, Moscow, 82, 1994, (in Russian).
36. **Purin, B. A.**, Electrochemical extraction as the method of the purification of metals using liquid membranes, *Izv. Akad. Nauk LatvSSR*, N5, 31, 1971, (in Russian).
37. **Moore, J. H. and Schechter, R.S .**, Liquid ion-exchange membranes, *AIChE J.*, 19, 741, 1973.
38. **Moskvin, L. N., Krasnoperov, V. M., Grigorjev, G. L. and Kartuzov, A. H.**, Selectivity of the liquid membranes during electrodyalisis, *Soviet J. Appl. Chem.*, 54, 563, 1981.
39. **Moskvin, L. N., Shmatko, A. G. and Krasnoperov, V. M.**, Mechanism of ions transfer by electrodialysis across a liquid extraction membrane, *Elektrokhimiya*, 22, 1109, 1986.
40. **Gokalp, M., Hodgson, K. T. and Cussler, E. L.**, Selective electrorefining with liquid membranes, *AIChE J.*, 29, 144, 1983.
41. **Timofeyeva, S. K., Popov, A. N. and Purin, B. A.**, Kinetics of electrodialysis of dicianoaurate ions by liquid membranes - tetraphenylphosphonium chloride chloroform solutions, *Izv. Akad. Nauk LatvSSR, Ser.Khim.*, 4, 402, 1983 (in Russian).
42. **Igawa, M., Saitou, K., Kasai, H., Tanaka, M. and Yamabe T.**, Electrodialysis with liquid membranes containing dibenzo-18-crown-6 as carrier, *Chem. Letters*, 861, 1985.
43. **Golybev, V. N. and Purin, B. A.**, Investigation of the electrical breakdown of the liquid membranes during anions transfer, *Doklady Akad. Nauk SSSR*, 232, 1340, 1977.
44. **Popov, A. N.**, Counterions and adsorption of ion-exchange extractants at the water/oil interface, in *The Interface Structure and Electrochemical Processes at the Boundary Between Two Immisible Liquid*, Kazarinov, V.A. Eds, Springer-Verlag, Berlin, Heidelberg, 1987, 179.
45. **Golubev, V. N., Popov, A. N. and Purin, B. A.**, About electrical break- down of liquid membrane, *Elektrokhimiya*, 12, 1478, 1976.
46. **Golubev, V. N. and Kontush, A. S.**, Cotransfer of water during transport of cations across liquid membranes modified by a macrocyclic carriers, *Elektrokhimiya*, 23, 105, 1987.
47. **Golubev, V. N. and Kontush, A. S.**, Electrochemical instability of liquid membranes during cation transfer by electrodialysis, *Elektrokhimiya*, 23, 249, 1987.
48. **Shmatko, A. G. and Moskvin, L. N.**, Solvatation model of water transport into impregnated membrane during electrodialysis, *Elektrokhimiya*, 27, 38, 1991.
49. **Shmatko, A. G. and Moskvin, L. N., Krasnoperov, V. M.**, Water oversaturation of an tributilphosphate impregnated membrane during the electrodialysis ion transfer from hydrochloric acid solutions, *Elektrokhimiya*, 27, 1092, 1991.
50. **Sandblom, J. and Eisenman, G., Walker, J. L**, Electrical phenomena associated with the transport of ions and ion pairs in liquid ion-exchange membranes. II. Non-zero current properties, *J. Phys. Chem.*, 71, 3871, 1967.
51. **Gnusin, N., Nikonenko, V. and Zabolotsky,** V., On the mechanism of beginning of limiting state in system liquid ion-exchange membrane - solution, *Izv. Akad. Nauk LatvSSR, Ser. Khim.*, 6, 717, 1983 (in Russian).
52. **Popov, A. N. and Timofeyeva, S. K**, Voltammetry of liquid membranes. II. Solution of tetraphenylphosphonium and malachite green salts in 1,2-dichloroethane, *Izv. Akad. Nauk LatvSSR*, Ser. Khim. , 4, 410, 1983 (in Russian).
53. **Popov, A., Timofeyeva, S. and Purin, B. A.**, Voltammetry of liquid membranes. IV. Cellophane on water/oil interfaces, *Izv. Akad. Nauk LatvSSR, Ser. Khim.*, 6, 676, 1986 (in Russian).
54. **Markin, V. S. and Chizmadzhev, Yu. A.**, *Induced Ion Transport,* Nauka, Moscow, 1974 (in Russian).

55. **Strover, F. S. and Buck, R. P.**, Electrical properties of mobile site ion exchange membranes with interfacial permselectivity breakdown: Non-zero current properties, *J. Electroanal. Chem.*, 107, 165, 1980.
56. **Nahir, T. M. and Buck, R. P.**, Transport processes in membranes containing neutral ion carriers, positive ion complexes, negative mobile sites, and ion pairs, *J. Phys. Chem.*, 97, 12363, 1993.
57. **Nahir, T. M. and Buck, R. P.**, Transport properties of H^+-selective membranes containing amine-derivative ionophores and mobile sites, *Helvetica Chimica Acta*, 76, 407, 1993.
58. **Buck, R. P., Toth, K., Graf, E., Horvai, G. and Pungor, E.**, Donnan exclusion failure in low anions site density membranes containing valinomycicin, *J. Electroanal .Chem.*, 223, 51, 1987.
59. **Ward, W, J, III**, Electrically induced carrier transport, *Nature*, 227, 162, 1970.
60. **Athayde, A. L. and Ivory, C. F.**, Electric pumping in carrier-mediator membrane transport, *J. Membrane Sci.*, 24, 309, 1985.
61. **Gallagher, P. M., Athayde, A. L. and Ivory, C. F.**, Electrochemical coupling in carrier-mediator membrane transport, *J. Membrane Sci.*, 29, 49, 1986.
62. **Hsu, E. C. and Li, N. N.**, Membranes recovery in liquid membrane separation processes, *Separ. Sci. Technol.*, 20, 115, 1985.
63. **Ptasinski, K. L. and Kerkhof, P. J. A. M.**, Electric field driven separations phenomena and applications, *Separ. Sci Technol.*, 27, 995, 1992.
64. **Leiber, J. P., Noble, R. D., Way, J. D. and Bateman, B. R.**, Mathematical modeling of facilitated liquid membrane transport esters containing ionically charged species, *Separ. Sci Technol.*, 20, 231, 1985.
65. **Plonski, J. W., Hoburg, J. F., Evans, D. F. and Cussler, E. L.**, Mixing liquid membranes with electric fields, *J. Membrane Sci.*, 5, 371, 1979.
66. **Popov, A. N. and Timofeyeva, S. K.**, Effect of an alternating electric field on the transfer of dicyanoaurate ions across a liquid ion-exchange membrane by direct current, *Izv. Akad. Nauk LatvSSR, Ser. Khim.*, 1, 100, 1982 (in Russian).
67. **Koryta, J., Du, G., Ruth, W. and Vanysek, P.**, Transfer of alkali-metal and hydrogen ions liquid/liquid interfaces mediated by monensin, *Faraday Discuss. Chem. Soc.*, 77, 209, 1984.
68. **Kihara, S., Suzuki, M., Maeda, K., Ogura, K. and Matsui, M.**, The transfer of anions at the aqueous/organic solutions interface studied by current-scan polarography with electrolyte dropping electrode, *J. Electroanal .Chem.*, 210, 147, 1986.
69. **Kontturi, A.-K., Konturri, K. and Schiffrin, D. J.**, Kinetics of K ion transfer at the water/1,2-dichloroethane interface, *J. Electroanal .Chem.*, 255, 331, 1988.
70. **Gordon, J. E.**, *The Organic Chemistry of Electrolyte Solutions*, John Wiley & Sons Inc., New York, 1975, chap.3.
71. **Popov, A. and Timofeyeva, S.**, Voltammetry of liquid membranes. 8. *n*-Trioctylamine salt solutions in 1,2-dichloroethane. Peculiarities of anion transfer, *Izv. Akad. Nauk LatvSSR, Ser. Khim.*, 6, 707, 1990 (in Russian).
72. **Popov, A., Timofeyeva, S. and Serga, V.**, Voltammetry of liquid membranes. 9. *n*-trioctylamine salt solutions in 1,2-dichloroethane. Influence of nonintermixing layers on the selectivity of anion transfer, *Izv. Akad. Nauk LatvSSR, Ser. Khim.*, 6, 675, 1991 (in Russian).
73. **Popov, A. and Timofeyeva, S.**, Ion Exchange between aqueous and organic phases in electrodialysis of liquid membranes - solutions of trioctylamine salts in halocarbons, in *Conference Papers International Solvent Extraction Conference*, USSR, Nauka, Moscow, 3, 38, 1988.
74. **Popov, A. and Licis, J.**, Changes in concentration of ions at the oil/water interface under action of electric current, *Izv. Akad. Nauk LatvSSR, Ser. Khim.*, 2, 192, 1975 (in Russian).
75. **Watanabe, A., Higashitsuji, K. and Nishizawa, K.**, Studies of electrocapillary emulsification, *J. Colloid Inter. Sci.*, 64, 278, 1978.
76. **Homolka, D., Marezek, V., Samec, Z., Bale, K. and Wendt, H.**, The partion of amines between water and organic solvent phase, *J. Electroanal. Chem.*, 163, 159, 1984.
77. **Malev, V. V.**, The electrode function of thick liquid membranes, *Elektrokhimiya*, 12, 710, 1976.

78. **Karlin, Yu. V. and Panteleev, V. I.**, Mathematical model of mass transfer across a liquid membrane a neutral carrier upon application an external constant electric field, *Elektrokhimiya*, 24, 43, 1988.
79. **Shmatko, A. G., Moskvin, L. N. and Krasnoperov, V. M.**, Influence of the rate of formation of the compound being extracted on the electrodialysis transport across a liquid membrane, *Elektrokhimiya*, 23, 30, 1987.
80. **Poop, A., Gutsol, A. and Timofeyeva, S.**, Voltammetry of liquid membranes. 5. Solutions of macrocyclic ionophore in polar solvents, *Izv. Akad. Nauk LatvSSR, Ser. Khim.*, 3, 302, 1988(in Russian).
81. **Popov, A. and Timofeyeva, S.**, Voltammetry of liquid membrane. 11. Ion transfer through membranes containing complexes of macrocyclic ionophores with metal salts, *Izv. Akad. Nauk LatvSSR, Ser. Khim.*, 3, 291, 1993 (in Russian).
82. **Izatt, R. M., Pawlak, K, Bradshaw, J. S. and Bruening, R. L.**, Thermodynamic and kinetic data for macrocyclic interaction with cations and anions, *Chem. Rev.*, 91, 1721, 1991.
83. **Sinru, L., Zaofan, Z. and Freizer, H.**, Potassium ion transport processes across the interface of an immiscible liquid pair in the presence of crown ethers, *J. Electroanal. Chem.*, 210, 137, 1986.
84. **Yoshida. Z. and Freizer, H.**, Mechanism of the carrier-mediated transport of potassium ion across water-nitrobenzene interface by valinomycin, *J. Electroanal. Chem.*, 179, 31, 1984.
85. **Popov, A., Yevlanova, T. and Timofeyeva, S.**, Voltammetry of liquid membranes. 7. Re-extraction of lead (II) ions from 1,2-dichloroethane solutions of dicyclohexano-18-crown-6 complexes, *Izv. Akad. Nauk LatvSSR, Ser. Khim.*, 1, 44, 1990(in Russian).
86. **Vetter, K. J.**, *Electrochemische Kinetik*, Springer-Verlag, Berlin, Heidelberg, 1961, chap.2.
87. **Popov, A. and Timofeyeva, S.**, Voltammetry of liquid membranes. 6. Determination of macrocyclic ionophore - Metal salt complex concentrations and re-extraction of salts from organic solvents, *Izv. Akad. Nauk LatvSSR, Ser. Khim.*, 3, 313, 1988 (in Russian).
88. **Gehrig, P., Morf, W.E., Welti, M., Pretsch, E. and Simon, W.**, Catalysis of ion transfer by tetraphenylborates in neutral carrier-based ion-selective electrodes, *Helvetica Chim. Acta*, 73, 203, 1990.
89. **Popov, A., Timofeyeva, S. and Borisova, T.**, Voltammetry of liquid membranes. 12. Synergism in membranes containing macrocyclic ionophores and cesium dicarbollide, *Izv. Akad. Nauk LatvSSR, Ser. Khim.*, 3 ,292, 1993 (in Russian).
90. **Popov, A. and Timofeyeva, S.**, Voltammetry of liquid membranes. 10. Neutralization of *n*-trioctylamine salts, *Izv. Akad. Nauk LatvSSR, Ser. Khim.*, 1 ,73, 1992 (in Russian).
91. **Beruge, T., Buck, R., Graf, E., Horvai, G., Iglehart, M., Linder, E., Niegreisz, Z., Pungor, E., Sandifer, J. and Toth, K.**, Electrochemistry of passive membranes with neutral crriers, in *5th Symposium on Ion-Selective Electrodes*, Matrafured, Pergamon Press, Oxford, Akademiai Kiado, Budapest, 1989, 3.
92. **Teorell, T.**, Electrokinetical considerations of mechanoelectrical transduction, *Ann. N.Y. Acad. Sci.*, 137, 950, 1966.
93. **Nakache, E. and Dupeyrat, M.**, The contribution of chemistry to new Marangoni mass-transfer instabilities at the oil/water interface, *Faraday Discuss. Chem. Soc.*, 77, 189, 1984.
94. **Yamaguchi, T. and Shinbo, B.**, A Novel interfacial engine between two immiscible liquid, *Chem. Letters*, 935, 1989.
95. **Arai, K., Kusu, F. and Takamura, K.**, A Novel explanation for the mechanism of electrical oscillation across a liquid membrane, *Chem. Letters*, 1517, 1990.
96. **Motoaki, S., Hidehiro, N., Hideo, A. and Toshimitsu, M.**, Model study of spontaneous discharge fluctuations of a membrane potential, *Jap. J. Appl. Phys.*, Pt.1, 29, 2186, 1990.
97. **Miyamura, K., Morooka, H., Hirai, K. and Gohshi, Y.**, A conveniet apparatus for the study of the electric pulse generation in the liquid membrane system, *Chem. Letters*, 1883, 1990.
98. **Arisawa, J. and Misawa, K.**, Structural changes and oscillation of electrical resistance in a millipore DOPH model membrane, *J. Membrane Sci.*, 42, 57, 1989.
99. **Urbane, K. and Sakaguchi, H.**, Electric current induced self-sustained oscillation of electric potential across a membrane filter impregnated with triolein, *Chem. Phys. Letters*, 176, 361, 1991.

100. **Maeda, K., Kihara, S., Suzuki, M. and Matsui, M.**, Voltammetric study on the oscillation at a liquid/liquid or liquid/membrane interface accompanied by ion transfer, *J. Electroanal. Chem.*, 295, 183, 1990.
101. **Popov, A., Timofeyeva, S. and Yevlanova, T.**, Current oscillations in electrodialysis of lead ions through liquid membranes, *J. Electroanal. Chem.*, 280, 61, 1990.
102. **Popov, A., Timofeyeva, S. and Borisova, T.**, Voltammetry of liquid membranes. 13. Periodical phenomena at the ion transfer through membranes containing macrocyclic ionophores, *Latvian J. Chem.*, 5 ,564, 1993 (in Russian).
103. **Yevlanova, T. and Popov, A.**, Adsorption of dicyclohexano-18-crown-6 from non-aqueous phase on water/toluene and water/dichloroethane interface in presence of lead ions, *Izv. Akad. Nauk LatvSSR, Ser. Khim.*, 1, 43, 1989 (in Russian).
104. **Gehrig, P., Morf, W.E., Welti, M., Pretsch, E. and Simon, W.**, Catalysis of ion transfer by tetraphenylborates in neutral carrier-based ion-selective electrodes, *Helvetica Chimica. Acta*, 73, 203, 1990.
105. **Shmatko, A. G., Krasnoperov, V. M. and Moskvin, L. N.**, Influence of a condition electrodialysis process on the separation efficiency of a liquid extraction membrane, *Elektrokhimiya,* 24, 54, 1988.
106. **Harris, M. T. and Basaran, O. A.**, Capillary electrohydrostatics of conducting drops hanging from a nozzle in an electric field, *J. Colloid Inter. Sci.*, 161, 389, 1993.

Chapter 16

OIL/WATER INTERFACES AND THE ORIGIN OF LIFE.

David W. Deamer and Alexander G. Volkov

I. LIQUID-LIQUID INTERFACES AND CHEMICAL EVOLUTION ON THE EARLY EARTH.

Liquid-liquid interfaces have not previously been considered in terms of their possible relationship to the origin of life. However, it is clear that the first living cells necessarily utilized lipid-like hydrocarbon derivatives as component of their functioning membrane structure. Such hydrocarbons were presumably available on the primitive Earth, and would have taken the form of oil-water interfaces in early lakes and oceans. What was the primary source and chemical nature of such compounds? Did the chemical and physical properties of oil-water interfaces contribute to mechanisms by which energy could be captured from the environment? And how did hydrocarbons chemically evolve into amphiphilic compounds that could self-assemble into the first membranous structures? Although there are no simple answers to these questions, progress in prebiotic chemistry has recently pointed to some useful research directions. We will first describe current advances in our knowledge of the early Earth environment, particularly as related to non-polar and amphiphilic organic compounds that were potentially available to participate in the chemical evolution leading to the first forms of life.

II. ENVIRONMENTAL CONDITIONS ON THE PREBIOTIC EARTH

In earlier research, the problem of life's origin was largely confined to chemical approaches involving synthetic pathways leading to the monomeric compounds common to the major macromolecules of the living state. Miller et al.[1,2] first demonstrated that amino acids were synthesized when a mixture of reduced gases was exposed to electrical discharges, a result that has now been repeated with a variety of energy inputs. The reduced gas mixture was assumed to simulate the early terrestrial atmosphere which, by analogy with the outer planets, would have contained gases such as hydrogen, methane, ammonia and water vapor. Other organic compounds relevant to biological process could also be synthesized under simulated primitive Earth conditions. For instance, Oro[3] showed that adenine, a basic molecular component of nucleotides and nucleic acids, could be synthesized through hydrogen cyanide pentamerization. It was also found that a variety of sugars, including ribose, resulted when formaldehyde participated in the formose reaction[4]. Furthermore, Fischer-Tropsch syntheses[5,6] involving carbon monoxide and water condensation on a metal catalyst such as hot metallic

0-8493-7694-7/96/$0.00+$.50

iron could potentially produce long-chain hydrocarbons and their oxidized derivatives such as fatty acids.

The presumed synthesis of organic compounds in prebiotic conditions was confirmed when it was found that carbonaceous meteorites contain up to several percent of their mass as a organic carbon, including amino acids, hydrocarbons, and even traces of purines. Assuming that such meteorites represent samples of the primitive solar system, it is not difficult to imagine that similar reactions occurred on the Earth's surface. These results, taken together, led early workers to assume that the prebiotic oceans were rich in all the organics required for life, and that self-assembly processes would readily lead to the origin of life over the billion or so years available after the Earth's primary accretion.

The assumptions underlying this scenario began to be challenged in the late 1970s, when a consensus was reached that the Earth's early atmosphere was volcanic in origin and composition, containing largely carbon dioxide and nitrogen, rather than the mixture of reducing gases assumed by the Miller-Urey model [7, 8, 9]. Because carbon dioxide does not support the array of synthetic pathways leading to possible monomers, other primary sources of organics began to be considered, particularly delivery of preformed organic substances by cometary and meteoritic infall[10 - 14].

Planetary scientists then determined that the origin of the Earth-moon system resulted when a Mars-sized object collided with the Earth over 4.4 billion years ago [15, 16]. The energy released by such a collision would degrade any organic compounds that were present previous to this event. Furthermore, as our knowledge of the lunar surface increased, it became generally recognized that the early Earth-moon system underwent a late bombardment of asteroid-sized objects. Impacts similar to those producing the larger craters on the moon would have been sufficient to vaporize the ocean, suggesting that life may have arisen on several occasions, only to be lost to global sterilization[17, 18]. This point was made abundantly clear by the immense energies released by the Shoemaker-Levy comet collision with Jupiter in July, 1994.

Given these environmental conditions on the primitive Earth, we can now go on to discuss primary sources of organic compounds, with a particular focus on hydrocarbons and their derivatives. We will show how photochemical processes could synthesize amphiphilic molecules from hydrocarbons at liquid-liquid interfaces, then discuss possible ways that primitive pigment systems could have been involved in the capture of light energy at liquid-liquid interfaces in the prebiotic environment.

III. SOURCES OF PREBIOTIC ORGANIC COMPOUNDS

Because all planets in the solar system accreted from a nebular disk of dust and gas around the early sun, it follows that all carbon on the Earth had an extraterrestrial origin. The only question is how much processing the carbon went through before being incorporated into primitive forms of life. As noted earlier, Miller[1] showed that organic compounds could have been synthesized at the Earth's surface from atmospheric gases that were activated by light or electrical discharge to more reactive compounds such as formaldehyde and hydrogen cyanide. It is reasonable to think that some amount of organic material was synthesized by the Miller-Urey pathway, but because a carbon dioxide atmosphere would markedly reduce the yield, other sources are now being considered. One possibility is that extraterrestrial delivery of pre-existing organic material also played a significant role. This was first proposed by Oro[10] and Delsemme[11] then more recently elaborated by Anders[12] and Chyba et al.[13,14]. Conservative calculations suggest that total organic carbon added by extraterrestrial infall over several hundred million years post-accretion would be in the range of 10^{16} - 10^{18} kgs , mostly as micrometeorites and to a lesser extent as comets. This figure is several orders of magnitude greater than the total organic carbon in the biosphere, estimated to be 6 x 10^{14} kg, and it follows that extraterrestrial infall may have been a significant source of organic carbon in the prebiotic environment.

Assuming an extraterrestrial source, what kinds of molecules may have been present in the prebiotic environment? Carbonaceous meteorites provide important guidelines to this question, in that they contain pristine samples of abiotically synthesized organic compounds. The Murchison meteorite, a carbonaceous chondrite which fell near Murchison, Australia in 1969, has been extensively investigated. A complex polymer composed of linked polycyclic aromatic hydrocarbons represents the most abundant organic material in such meteorites (~90% of total organic content) followed by a variety of organic acids. Aliphatic and aromatic hydrocarbons, amino acids, ureas, ketones, alcohols, aldehydes and perhaps purines are present in smaller quantities. (For review, see Cronin et al.[19]). If cometary and meteoritic infall can survive atmospheric entry and impact processes, most of the mass would presumably have fallen into early oceans and released organic components over long intervals of time. Water soluble compounds would dissolve, while hydrocarbons and their derivatives would accumulate at the ocean surface, forming a kind of prebiotic oil slick only a few monolayers thick. Wind and tide would presumably concentrate the films at intertidal zones, just as occurs today. It follows that likely sites for the origin of cellular life are cycling environments such as tide pools that are associated with intertidal zones.

Organic compounds are reactive under such conditions, and photochemical reactions combined with hydrolysis would markedly affect the concentrations of organics accumulating in the oceans. Even under the most favorable conditions of Miller-Urey synthesis, amino acid concentrations would reach little more than millimolar ranges in the global oceans[20] and actual concentrations were more likely in the micromolar range. Concentration of organic compounds was therefore essential to the origin of cellular life, including hydration-dehydration cycles in tide pools and adsorption to mineral surfaces. Significantly, hydrocarbons derivatives are often surface active, providing a natural concentrating mechanism at air-water interfaces or by aggregation into micelles, bilayers and emulsions.

IV. MEMBRANES AND LIQUID-LIQUID INTERFACES.

Boundary membranes play a key role in the cells of all contemporary organisms, and simple models of membrane function are therefore of considerable interest. The interface of two immiscible liquids has been widely used for this purpose. For example, the fundamental processes of photosynthesis, biocatalysis, membrane fusion, ion pumping and electron transport have all been investigated in such interfacial systems.

Each of the above processes requires an input of energy. The quantum yield of the photocatalytic reaction depends first of all on the efficiency of the photochemical charge separation. The most effective system should be a heterogeneous system in which the oxidant and the reductant are either in different phases or sterically separated. The difference in solubility of the substrates and reaction products in both phases of such heterogeneous structure as the octane/water interface can shift the reaction equilibrium. The redox potential scale is thereby altered, making it possible to carry out reactions that cannot be performed in a homogeneous phase.

The interface between two immiscible liquids with dissolved non-polar pigments can serve as a simple model of a biological membrane which is convenient for investigating photoprocesses that are accompanied by spatial separation of charges. It is also a model for hydrocarbons on the prebiotic Earth, and we are currently studying relatively simple pigment systems that could act at the liquid-liquid interface, with a particular focus on polycyclic aromatic hydrocarbons (PAH). As noted earlier, PAH and their derivatives are abundant components of the organic material present in carbonaceous meteorites[21] and were presumably available in the prebiotic environment. Significantly, most PAH derivatives absorb light in the near UV and blue region, which suggests that they represent potential pigment systems available to participate in chemical evolution leading up to the first forms of cellular life. If they are partitioned into the liquid-liquid interface or membranes, PAH can capture light energy, either by donating electrons to produce molecules with higher chemical potential, or by generation of ionic gradients. Several examples of PAH-mediated reactions will now be described.

V. PHOTOCHEMISTRY IN THE PREBIOTIC ENVIRONMENT: SYNTHESIS OF AMPHIPHILES

Polycyclic aromatic hydrocarbons absorb near-UV and far blue light energy. If PAH are partitioned into liquid-liquid interfaces or lipid bilayer membranes, they can capture light energy by donating electrons to produce molecules with higher chemical potential[22]. They also release protons during photochemical reactions, and photosensitize the photooxidation of alkanes[23, 24, 25]. Because light is the most abundant energy source in the contemporary biosphere, and presumably was equally abundant on the early Earth, it is interesting to ask whether photochemical synthesis of amphiphiles could occur under simulated prebiotic conditions. To this end, we will describe a recent series of experiments in some detail.

Carbonaceous chondrites contain cyclic alkanes and polycyclic aromatic hydrocarbons that have the potential to form amphiphiles if oxidized to more polar compounds. In earlier studies, Folsome and Morowitz[26] and Seleznev[27] showed that ultraviolet illumination of hydrocarbons in aqueous environments could produce oxidized derivatives with amphiphilic properties. Klein and Pilpel[25] demonstrated that amphiphiles can be synthesized by a light-dependent reaction using polycyclic aromatic hydrocarbons as photosensitizers. However, illumination in these experiments was carried out in air, so that 0.2 bars of oxygen was available as a potential reactant. Because molecular oxygen would have been present only in trace amounts in the prebiotic environment, it seemed worth determining whether amphiphilic molecules can be synthesized by photochemical mechanisms under essentially anaerobic conditions. To address this question, we have illuminated hydrocarbons as aqueous dispersions and at aqueous interfaces in carbon dioxide and argon atmospheres with varying contents of oxygen. We also investigated the possibility that polycyclic aromatic hydrocarbons might serve as photosensitizers for such reactions.

Illumination of a hexadecane - PAH mixture deposited on an aqueous subphase causes the hydrocarbon droplet to spread, a process that can readily be followed by the fluorescence of the PAH. This phenomenon was first described in detail by Hatchard and Pilpel [28]. When the spreading film fills the surface of the container, marked changes in the surface tension can be measured by the Wilhelmy plate method, reaching a surface pressure in the range of 15 mN/m, at which point a solid film was present. A barrier filter with band pass of 380-460 nm permits the reaction to continue at about half the original rate, but other filters completely inhibit the reaction. In the dark, or in the absence of PAH, no reaction occurs.

We have extended this approach to a variety of PAH, looking for the most reactive compounds and optimal conditions. Results of this survey are shown in Figure 1. It is clear that some PAH derivatives show little reactivity, while others efficiently capture light energy and produce surface active material. In particular, we found that substituted anthracenes are highly reactive pigment systems, and have chosen these for further experimentation.

Thin layer chromatography of the products showed a consistent pattern of polar photochemical products, several of which were fluorescent and produced spots against a streak of unresolved material. Analysis by gc-ms indicated that 1-hexadecanol and 2-hexadecanone were major products (Figure 2). These amphiphilic compounds would account for the surface activity observed during the course of the reaction.

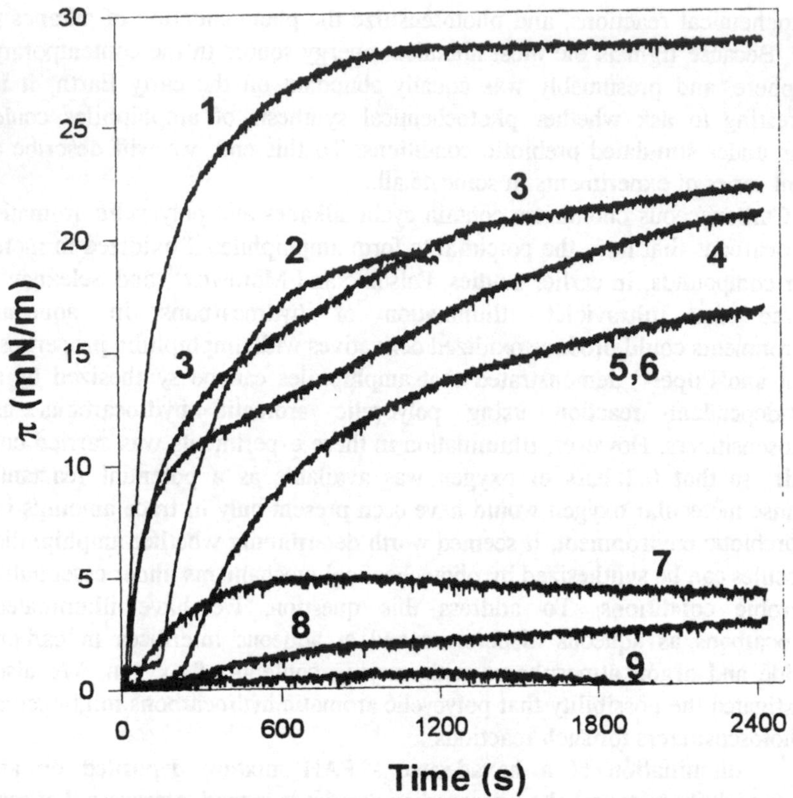

Figure 1. Dependencies of surface pressure at air/water interface on time of illumination. Aliquots (10μL) of hexadecane (9) or hexadecane:PAH mixtures (98:2) were placed on water surfaces and illuminated with a 50 W mercury arc lamp. PAH were 2 methyl-1,4-naphthoquinone (1), 9-methylanthracene (2), 2-methyl-anthracene (3), 2-methylanthroquinone (4), fluoranthene (5), 2-ethyl-anthracene (6), 9-fluorenone (7), anthracene (8).

A general mechanism for such processes was proposed by Gesser et al. [29] and is outlined below:

1. X + hν --> X*
2. X* + RH --> XH + R*
3. XH + O_2 --> X + HO_2
4. R* + O_2 ---> RO_2*
5. RO_2* + RH --> ROOH + R*
6. RO_2* + XH --> ROOH + X*
7. ROOH --> RO* + *OH
8. RO* + RH --> ROH + R*
9. ROOH + R* --> RO* + ROH

where X is an aromatic compound such as xanthone and RH is an aliphatic hydrocarbon. Note that the primary products are alcohols (ROH).

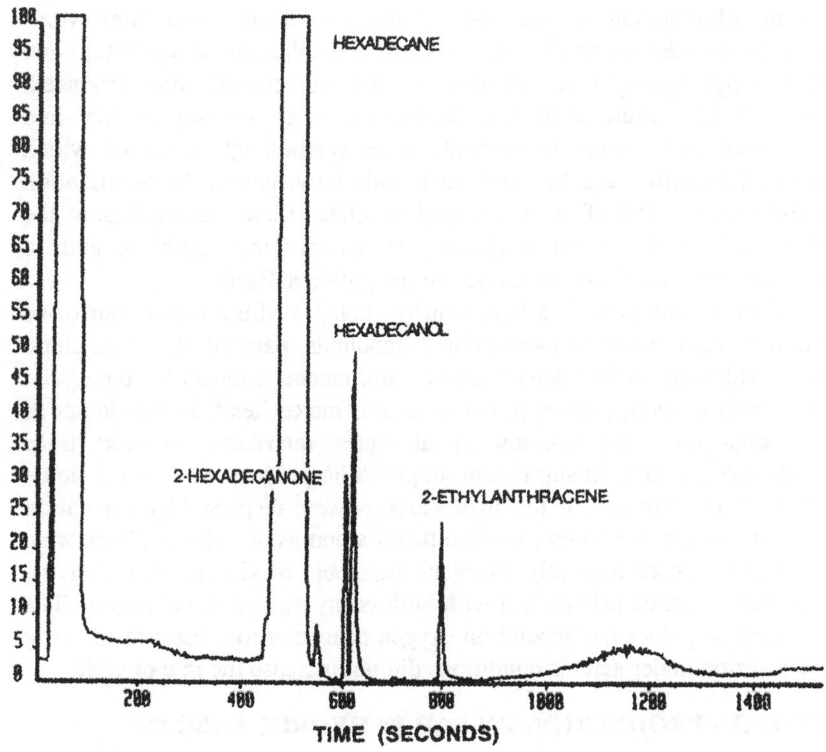

Figure 2. Gas chromatography - mass spectrum of polar products after illumination of emulsion (4 ml of aqueous solution of 1 M LiCl and 0.2 ml of 2% solution of 2-ethyl-anthracene in hexadecane). Products of photoreaction were extracted in 4 ml of hexane. The pH of the emulsion before illumination was 3.7 and the reaction was carried out in CO_2 atmosphere. The gas chromatogram of underivatized products showed unreacted hexadecane together with 1-hexadecanol and 2-hexadecanone peaks.

Photooxidation of hexadecane can be driven by singlet oxygen. It is generally assumed that singlet oxygen is formed in different dye-sensitized reactions via energy transfer between the excited triplet state of the dye and molecular oxygen in its ground triplet state. The involvement of singlet oxygen can be tested by carrying out control experiments in the present of β-carotene, which effectively quenches singlet oxygen [30]. For example, Larson and Hunt [31] found that β-carotene inhibits oxidation of mixed petroleum oil exposed to UV radiation. We found that β-carotene at 0.1 mM concentrations markedly inhibited the hexadecane photooxidation to amphiphilic reaction products described earlier. It follows that singlet oxygen is likely to be involved in the reaction pathway.

Although PAH clearly act as photosensitizers in such systems, they do not appear to be absolute requirements, particularly under conditions of long-term illumination in air. For example, Folsome and Morowitz[26] illuminated hexadecane in air over concentrated solutions of phosphate and found that aggregates of phosphate-containing compounds were produced. Seleznev et al.[27] illuminated hexadecane-sea water systems in air, and reported that amphiphilic compounds were synthesized, some of which formed multilamellar liquid crystals that could be visualized by polarization light microscopy. Both of the above studies related their observations to the possible synthesis of membrane-forming compounds that might be able to serve as primitive lipid-like molecules on the prebiotic Earth.

The results described here confirm that UV illumination can drive oxidation of hexadecane to more polar compounds, particularly long chain alcohols, which are surface active. 2-Ethyl anthracene, a model for polycyclic aromatic hydrocarbons present in carbonaceous meteorites[32], is able to act as a photosensitizer. The reaction at air-water interfaces required trace molecular oxygen to yield significant amphiphilic products within 1-2 hours of illumination. However, if the hydrocarbons were dispersed by sonication before illumination, we found that significant amounts of polar products were produced even under relatively stringent anaerobic conditions in which the samples were continuously purged with high purity deoxygenated argon. The rate limiting step does not depend on oxygen concentration, because carrying out the reaction under aerobic conditions did not increase the rate or yield.

VI. PROTON PRODUCTION BY PAH IN HYDROCARBONS

Upon illumination of an anaerobic alkane/water system containing a PAH derivative, marked acid pH shifts are readily observed. For instance, 2-ethyl anthracene dissolved in hexadecane and dispersed by sonication in 1 M LiCl, produced pH shifts corresponding to the release of 4 mM protons upon illumination with a Zeiss 50 watt filtered mercury arc lamp (Figure 3).

The quantity of protons released during illumination depends on concentration of inorganic electrolyte and initial pH of the emulsion. The reaction is favored by high electrolyte concentrations, and the inorganic cation also had a modest effect, in the sequence: $Li^+ > Na^+ > K^+ > Rb^+$.

The production of protons in an anaerobic aqueous system of dispersed hydrocarbons was unexpected, and we do not yet understand the underlying mechanism. Nonetheless, it is clear that PAH dissolved in hydrocarbon environments can absorb light energy, then react to release protons. Proton production in this case must reflect a more basic photochemical process, most likely involving oxidation-reduction reactions in the components of the system. Since molecular oxygen is not present at the start of the reaction, it is possible that a source of the electrons is water itself, in which case one might expect molecular oxygen to be a product of the reaction. We therefore employed an oxygen electrode to determine whether oxygen appeared in the medium, with negative results. However, if the reaction was carried out in an air-saturated emulsion we found that oxygen was entirely consumed within 50-70 seconds upon illumination. This suggests that even if oxygen was produced at the oil/water interface, secondary reactions would remove it from the medium before it could be detected by the oxygen electrode. Further investigation of this interesting reaction will be required to understand it fully.

VII. CARBON DIOXIDE REACTIVITY IN PAH-ALKANE SYSTEMS

In the presence of saturating carbon dioxide, we noted the formation of a water-soluble organic product with an absorption maximum at 206 nm (Figure 4). The UV and infrared spectra coincide with that of simple monocarboxylic acids (Figure 5). The absorption maximum at 206 nm was not observed if argon was substituted for CO_2. It is highly dependent on lower pH ranges. For instance, no products were observed if the reaction was carried out at pH 7 in 1.0 M $NaHCO_3$. If the reaction was carried out with oxygen present, an oxygen electrode indicated that molecular oxygen was rapidly used, but there was no increase in the absorption at 206 nm. This showed that formation of the organic product did not depend on aerobic oxidation of one of the reactants present, for instance, hexadecane or ethylanthracene.

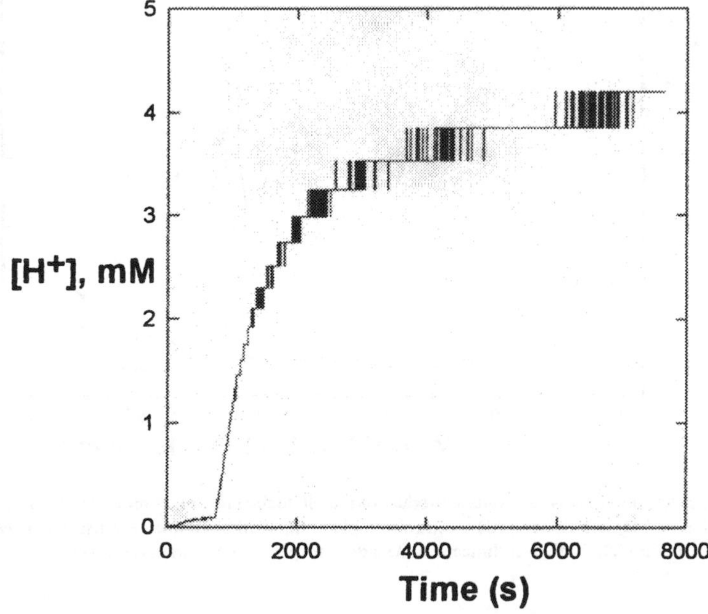

Figure 3. Kinetics of proton release during illumination of a hexadecane-ethylanthracene emulsion in the presence of saturating carbon dioxide. Medium: 4 ml 1 M LiCl, 0.2 ml 2% 2-ethyl-anthracene in hexadecane. The initial pH of the emulsion was 3.7, and dropped to 2.5 during illumination.

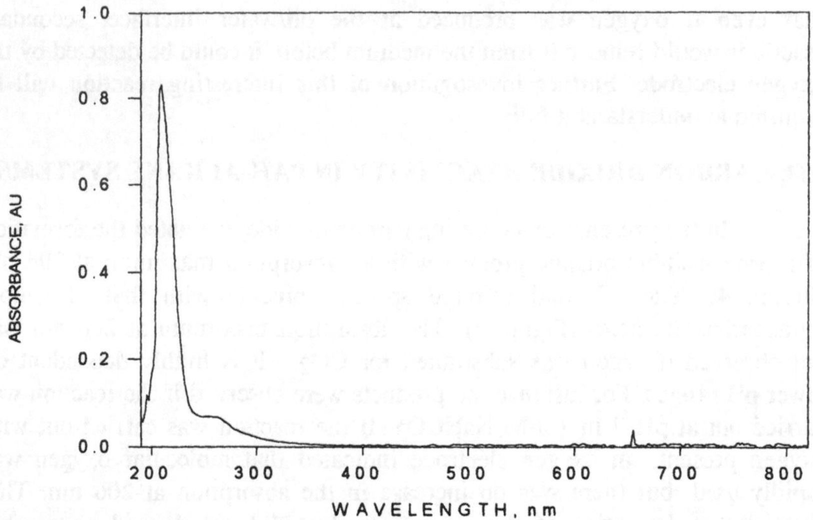

Figure 4. Absorption spectrum of the emulsion after 10 min illumination. Medium: 4 ml 1 M LiCl, pH=3.7, 0.2 ml 2% 2-ethyl-anthracene in hexadecane. Reference - emulsion before illumination, 1 cm pathlength.

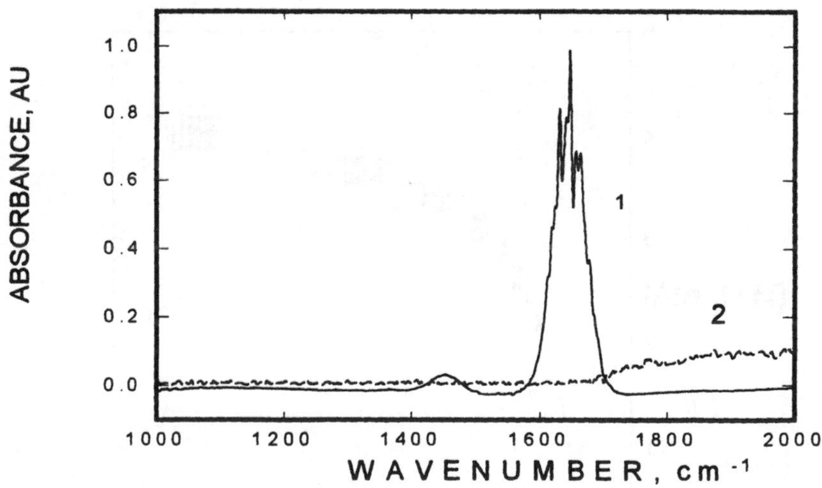

Figure 5. FTIR spectrum of the water soluble product of the photochemical reaction in emulsion: (1) -after illumination in CO_2 atmosphere, (2) - control sample without illumination. Emulsion consists of 4 ml 1 M LiCl, 0.2 ml 2% 2-ethyl-anthracene in hexadecane. pH before illumination was 3.7.

The photosynthesis of an organic acid from carbon dioxide at liquid-liquid interfaces would be very exciting, particularly in regard to primitive photosynthetic systems on the early Earth. One possible reaction pathway that accounts for our data is shown below:

$$CO_2 + H_2O + \text{hexadecane} \rightarrow RCOO^- + H^+ + \text{hexadecanol}$$

Taking this reaction as a working hypothesis, we are now exploring possible ways to directly demonstrate water soluble organic acid synthesis from carbon dioxide.

VII. CONCLUSIONS

The interface between two immiscible liquids has unexpected properties that follow from thermodynamic and kinetic principles controlling reactions in biphasic environments. We have shown in this chapter that photochemical reactions in particular have remarkable characteristics when carried out at interfaces. Early photochemical processes that may have permitted light harvesting by primitive cells can be studied at liquid-liquid interfaces of emulsified alkanes and polycyclic aromatic hydrocarbons. The photoproducts of such reactions - amphiphiles, protons and perhaps fixed CO_2 - are all relevant to the chemical and energetic requirements of early life.

IX. REFERENCES

1. **Miller, S.**, A production of amino acids under possible primitive Earth conditions, *Science*, 117, 528, 1953.
2. **Miller, S., Urey, H. and Oro, J.**, Origin of organic compounds on the primitive Earth and in meteorites, *J. Mol. Evol.*, 9, 59, 1976.
3. **Oro, J.**, Synthesis of adenine from ammonium cyanide, *Biochem. Biophys. Res. Commun.*, 2, 407, 1960.
4. **Schwartz, A. W. and Graaf, R. M. de**, The prebiotic synthesis of carbohydrates. - A reassessment. *J. Mol. Evol.*, 36, 101, 1993.
5. **Hayatsu, R. and Anders, E.**, Organic compounds in meteorites and their origins, *Topics Curr. Chem.*, 99, 1, 1977.
6. **Nooner, D. R. and Oro, J.**, Hydrocarbon synthesis from carbon monooxide and hydrogen, *Adv. Chem. Series*, Vol. 178, American Chemical Society, Washington D.C., 1979.
7. **Holland, H. D.**, *The Chemical Evolution of the Atmosphere and Oceans*, Princeton University Press, Princeton, 1984.
8. **Walker, J. C. G.**, Possible limits on the composition of the Archaean ocean, *Nature*, 302, 518, 1983.
9. **Kasting, J. and Ackerman, T. F.**, Climatic consequences of very high carbon dioxide levels in the Earth's early atmosphere, *Science*, 234, 1383, 1986.
10. **Oro, J.**, Comets and the formation of biochemical compounds on the primitive Earth, *Nature*, 190, 389, 1961.
11. **Delsemme, A.**, The cometary connection with prebiotic chemistry, *Origins of Life*, 14, 51, 1984.

12. **Anders, E.**, Prebiotic organic matter from comets and asteroids, *Nature*, 342, 255, 1989.
13. **Chyba, C. F., Thomas, P. J., Brookshaw, L. and Sagan, C.**, Cometary delivery of organic molecules to the early Earth, *Science*, 249, 366, 1990.
14. **Chyba, C. F. and Sagan, C.**, Endogenous production, exogenous delivery and impact-shock synthesis of organic molecules: An inventory for the origin of life, *Nature*, 355, 125, 1992.
15. **Hartman, W. K. and Davis, D. R.**, Satellite-sized planetesimals and lunar origins, *Icarus*, 24, 504, 1975.
16. **Boss, A. P.**, The origin of the moon, *Science*, 231, 341, 1986.
17. **Maher, K. A. and Stevenson, J. D.**, Impact frustration of the origin of life, *Nature*, 331, 612, 1988.
18. **Sleep, N. H., Zahnle, K. J., Kasting, J. F. and Morowitz, H.**, Annihilation of ecosystems by large asteroid impacts on the early Earth, *Nature*, 342, 139, 1989.
19. **Cronin, J. R., Pizzarello, S. and Cruickshank, D. P.**, Organic matter in carbonaceous chondrites, planetary satellites, asteroids and comets, in *Meteorites and the Early Solar System*, Kerridge, J. F. and Matthews, M. S., Eds., University of Arizona Press, Tucson, p. 819, 1988.
20. **Stribling, R. and Miller, S.**, Energy yields for hydrogen cyanide and formaldehyde: The HCN and amino acid concentration in the primitive ocean, *Orig. Life Evol. Biosphere*, 17, 261, 1987.
21. **Basile, B. P., Middleditch, B. S. and Oro, J.**, Polycyclic aromatic hydrocarbons in the Murchison meteorite, *Org. Geochem.*, 5, 211, 1978.
22. **Escabi-Perez, J. P., Romero, A., Lukak, S. and Fendler, J. H.**, Aspects of artificial photosynthesis. Photoionization and electron transfer in dihexadecyl phosphate vesicles, *J. Am. Chem. Soc.*, 101, 2231, 1979.
23. **Harris, C. M. and Selinger, B. K.**, Excited state processes of naphthols in aqueous surfactant solution, *Z. Physikal. Chem.*, 134, 65, 1983.
24. **Deamer, D. W.**, Polycyclic hydrocarbons: primitive pigment systems in the prebiotic environment, *Adv. Space Res.*, 12, 183, 1992.
25. **Klein, A. E. and Pilpel, N.**, Oxidation of *n*-alkanes photosensitized by 1-naphthol, *J. Chem. Soc. Faraday I.*, 69, 1729, 1973.
26. **Folsome, C. E. and Morowitz, H. J.**, Prebiological membranes: Synthesis and properties. *Space Life Sci.*, 1, 53, 8, 1969.
27. **Seleznev, S. A., Fedorov, L. M., Kuzina, S. I . and Mikhailov, A. I.**, UV-synthesis of amphiphilic molecules from *n*-alkanes and its biological significance, *Rev. Franc. Corps Gras*, 24, 191, 1977.
28. **Hatchard, C. G. and Pilpel, N.**, The effect of artificial sunlight upon floating oils, *J. Chem. Soc. Faraday I*, 69, 1729, 1974.
29. **Gesser, H. D., Wildman, T. A. and Tewari, Y. B.**, Photooxidation of *n*-hexadecane by xanthone, *Env. Sci. Technol.*, 11, 605, 1977.
30. **Telfer, A., Dhami, S., Bishop, S. M., Phillips, D. and Barber, J.**, β-Carotene quenches singlet oxygen formed by isolated photosystem II reaction centers, *Biochemistry*, 33, 14469, 1994.
31. **Larson, R. A. and Hunt, L. L.**, Photooxidation of a refined petroleum oil: inhibition by β-carotene and role of singlet oxygen, *Photochem. Photobiol.*, 28, 553, 1978.
32. **Krishnamurthy, R. V., Epstein, S., Cronin, J. R., Pizzarello, S. and Yuen, G. U.**, Isotopic and molecular analyses of hydrocarbons and monocarboxylic acids of the Murchison meteorite, *Geochim. Geophys. Acta*, 56, 4045, 1992.

Chapter 17

ELECTROCHEMICAL BEHAVIOR OF DRUGS AT OIL/WATER INTERFACES

Kensuke Arai, Fumiyo Kusu, and Kiyoko Takamura

I. INTRODUCTION

Drug behavior at biomembranes is an important determining factor of pharmacological activity[1]. However, the structures of biomembranes are complicated so that artificial models of biomembranes with simple structure become desirable. Immiscible oil/water interfaces may serve in this regard.

Bioelectrochemistry of drugs can be studied on polarizable and non-polarizable interfaces. Ion-transfer voltammetry at the polarized oil/water interface was established by Gavach *et al.*[2] in 1968, and has been used to examine transport of various drugs. For instance, Vanysek and Behrendt[3] determined the standard potential for the transfer of choline and acetylcholine by cyclic voltammetry. Homolka *et al.*[4] investigated the partition of amines, including biogenic amines, by cyclic voltammetry and differential pulse stripping voltammetry. Shao *et al.*[5,6] examined the kinetics of acetylcholine transfer at the interface. Ohkouchi *et al.*[7] studied the ion transfer of uncouplers of phosphorylation in mitochondria by potential step chronoamperometry and cyclic voltammetry. Ion-transfer voltammetry has been applied to the determination of acetylcholine (Marecek and Samec[8]) and tetracycline antibiotics (Kozlov and Koryta[9]). To clarify transport of drugs at the interface, ion-transfer voltammetry of a number of drugs exemplified by hypnotic, anesthetic, cholinergic, anti-cholinergic, adrenergic and anti-adrenergic drugs[10], belonging to various pharmaceutical groups, was conducted.

Nonpolarizable oil/water interfaces have physical properties similar close to biological systems[11], and electrochemistry at such interfaces has been investigated by a number of workers. This type of interface has been used as a model of drug delivery[12,13], biological systems such as skin[14], nerve[15], and biomembranes related to taste[16] and olfaction[17]. Spontaneous oscillating phenomena have been observed which produce electric signals. Such systems may be a promising model for converting chemical information into electric signals in a manner similar to biological systems.

In 1978, Dupeyrat *et al.*[18] discovered irregular dynamic movement of an oil/water interface in the presence of a surfactant. Yoshikawa and Matsubara[19] expanded the system to a liquid membrane of water/nitrobenzene/water with a surfactant and demonstrated spontaneous oscillation of electrical potential between the aqueous phases. It was possible to recognize sugars[20], amine chirality[21] and taste[22] based on measurement of potential oscillation. Nakajo *et al.*[23] reported the frequency and amplitude of oscillation across the liquid membrane to be affected by diethyl ether, a volatile anesthetic drug. Our research group[24] studied potential oscillation across a liquid membrane of water/octanol/water with a surfactant, and oscillation was shown to be affected by hypnotic and local anesthetic drugs present in the system. This effect on the oscillation mode probably arises from interactions between such drugs and the surfactant layer adsorbed at one of the oil/water interfaces, so that the surfactant layer appears to behave essentially as a biomembrane.

0-8493-7694-7/96/$0.00+$.50

This review includes our recent research on ion-transfer voltammetry of drugs and electrical potential oscillation across a liquid membrane of water/octanol/water in the presence of drugs. Characteristic parameters, such as half-wave potential and the mode of oscillation were clarified and compared with the pharmacological activity of drugs. The relationship between pharmacological activity and a drug parameter differed for each drug. This is of interest from pharmaceutical as well as bioelectrochemical viewpoints.

II. ION-TRANSFER VOLTAMMETRY AT THE OIL/WATER INTERFACE

A. ION-TRANSFER VOLTAMMETRY

1. Experimental Techniques

Various methods such as cyclic voltammetry, differential pulse voltammetry, differential pulse stripping voltammetry, chronoamperometry and potential step chronoamperometry have been used to study the ion transfer of drugs at the oil/–water interface. Polarography at an ascending water electrode[25,26] should prove useful since the continuous renewal of the electrode greatly lessens the chance of the contamination of the electrode surface, which is a major difficulty in voltammetry[26]. Potential-scan or current-scan polarography at an ascending water electrode was conducted in the present study. Figure 1 shows the electrolytic cell setup used for ion-transfer voltammetry of drugs[10,27]. A drop of aqueous solution was introduced into a nitrobenzene solution from the tip of a Teflon capillary inserted so that the flow rate of the aqueous solution could be maintained at a certain value. A three-electrode system was used for potential-scan polarography, and four-electrode system, for current-scan polarography. Reference electrodes in the nitrobenzene and aqueous phases were Ag/AgCl electrodes, and auxiliary electrodes in both phases were Ag/AgCl or platinum electrodes.

The cells for ion-transfer voltammetry of drugs are shown below:

Ag/AgCl	0.5 M TBACl (W1)	0.1 M TBATPhB (NB)	buffer (0.1–0.5 M) + drug (W2)	3.0 M LiCl (W3)	Ag/AgCl	(1)

or

Ag/AgCl	0.1 M TPACl (W1)	0.1 M TPATPhB (NB)	0.1 M LiCl + buffer (0.1 M) + drug (W2)	0.1 M LiCl (W3)	Ag/AgCl	(2)

where TBACl, TPACl, TBATPhB and TPATPhB are tetrabutylammonium chloride, tetrapentylammonium chloride, tetrabutylammonium tetraphenylborate and tetrapentylammonium tetraphenylborate, respectively. Cell (1) was used for potential-scan polarography[10], and cell (2), for current-scan polarography[27]. Each drug was added to aqueous phase W2 containing a pH buffer solution.

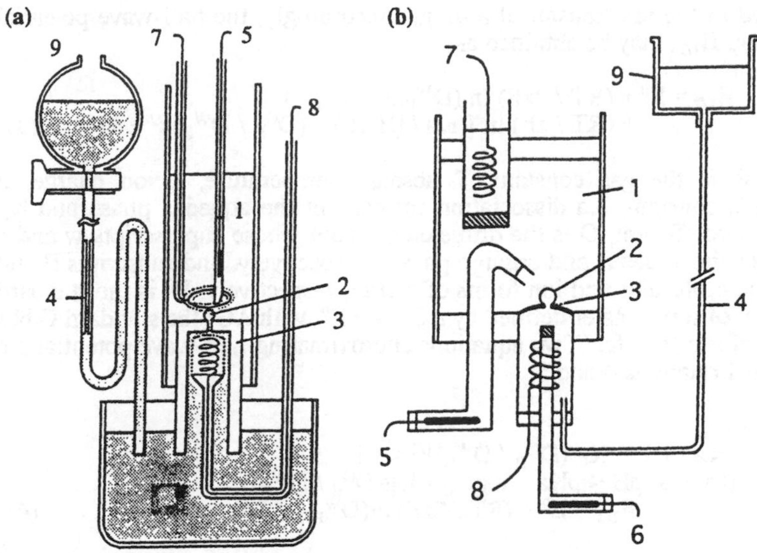

Figure 1. Apparatus for (a) potentiostatic and (b) galvanostatic measurements of ion-transfer voltammograms: (1) nitrobenzene phase, (2) water drop, (3), (4) Teflon capillaries, (5) reference electrode for aqueous phase, (6) reference electrode for nitrobenzene phase, (7) counter electrode for nitrobenzene phase, (8) counter electrode for aqueous phase, (9) reservoir. (From Arai, K., Ohsawa, M., Kusu, F. and Takamura, K., *Bioelectrochem. Bioenerg.*, 31(1), 65, 1993; From Arai, K., Kusu, F., Tsuchiya, N., Fukuyama, S. and Takamura, K., *Denki Kagaku*, 62(9), 840, 1994. With permission.)

2. Ion Transfer at the Nitrobenzene/–Water Interface

Yoshida and Freiser[28] and Doe *et al.*[29] noted the dissociation of 1,10-phenanthroline, a weak base, in the aqueous phase and partition of the molecular form of the compound between the organic and aqueous phases. Ion transfer and half-wave potential of the compound were found to depend on the pH of the aqueous phase and dissociation constant of the compound. Ohkouchi *et al.*[7] reported pH dependence of the half-wave potential even in the case of weak acids. Matsuda *et al.*[30] investigated the transfer of metal ions facilitated by crown ethers, in which the half-wave potential of polarographic waves is a logarithmic function of metal concentration. The same situation is encountered by replacing metal ions and crown ethers with protons and the molecular form of the basic compound, respectively. Since most drugs are weak electrolytes, assessment should be made of pH dependence on the half-wave potential.

Subsequent examination was made assuming the following:

(1) The dissociation of a drug in the organic phase and ion pair formation with supporting electrolyte ions are negligible.

(2) The aqueous phase is well buffered so that protons at the interface are readily made available in abundance relative to ion transfer.

(3) Equilibrium reaction rates are much higher than that of the ion transfer.

It follows that dissociation in the aqueous phase and partition of the molecular form of a drug between the organic and aqueous phases should be included in the ion transfer of a drug. Accordingly, the half-wave potential of a drug, $E_{1/2}$, may be obtained as,

$$E_{1/2} = E^0 + (RT / 2zF) \ln (D^W_{BH^+} / D^O_{BH^+}) + (RT / zF) \ln [(Ka / [H^+]) K_D (D^O_B / D^W_B)^{1/2} + 1] \quad (3)$$

where R is the gas constant, T absolute temperature, z ion charge, F Faraday's constant, Ka dissociation constant in the aqueous phase and K_D partition coefficient. D is the diffusion constant whose superscripts w and o stand for the aqueous and organic phases, respectively, and subscripts B and BH^+, the molecular and ion forms of a drug, respectively. E^0 is the standard potential of ion transfer defined by $\Delta G^0 = -zFE^0$, with ΔG^0 the standard Gibbs energy of ion transfer. Two equations approximating half-wave potential are given as Equations 4 and 5:

Case I:

$(Ka / [H^+]) K_D (D^O_B / D^W_B)^{1/2} << 1$

(that is, $pH < pKa - \log K_D - \log(D^O_B / D^W_B)$)

$$E_{1/2} = E^0 + (RT / 2zF) \ln(D^W_{BH^+} / D^O_{BH^+}) \quad (4)$$

Case II:

$(Ka / [H^+]) K_D (D^O_B / D^W_B)^{1/2} >> 1$

(that is, $pH > pKa - \log K_D - \log((D^O_B / D^W_B))$)

$$E_{1/2} = E^0 + (RT / 2zF) \ln(D^W_{BH^+} / D^O_{BH^+}) + (RT / zF) \ln Ka + (RT / zF) \ln K_D - (RT / zF) \ln [H^+] \quad (5)$$

From these equations, it would appear possible to predict pH dependence on the half-wave potential of a drug. The half-wave potential of a drug should become more positive by as much as 0.059 V per unit pH at $pH > pKa - \log K_D - \log (D^O_B / D^W_B)$, whereas at $pH < pKa - \log K_D - \log (D^O_B / D^W_B)$, this parameter should remain constant.

Equations 4 and 5 were validated by measurement of the voltammograms of weak electrolyte drugs at various pH[27]. Figure 2 shows voltammograms obtained in the presence of 2.0×10^{-4} M (solid line) and 0 M (dotted line) scopolamine in aqueous phase W2 at various pH. In the voltammograms, the anodic current (positive current) corresponds to transfer of cations from W2 to NB or anions from NB to W2. At each pH, an anodic wave was observed when scopolamine was present in W2. Figure 3 shows the pH dependence of the half-wave potential of scopolamine. This potential become more positive by 0.059 V per unit pH at pH>7, whereas at pH<7, it remained constant. The pKa of scopolamine was obtained from the literature, $\log K_D$ was obtained by potentiometric titration and $\log(D^O_{BH^+} / D^W_{BH^+})$ was determined from the peak height ratio of anodic and cathodic waves in the cyclic voltammogram. $\{pKa - \log K_D - \log(D^O_B / D^W_B)\}$ was found to be 7, showing the potential at the point of the intersection of the two lines shown in Figure 3 to be consistent with this value. Voltammograms of lidocaine were also measured (Figure 4) and the half-wave potential of lidocaine linearly increased by 0.059 V per unit pH at pH>5.5, whereas at pH<5.5, this parameter remained constant, as shown in Figure 5. $\{pKa - \log K_D -$

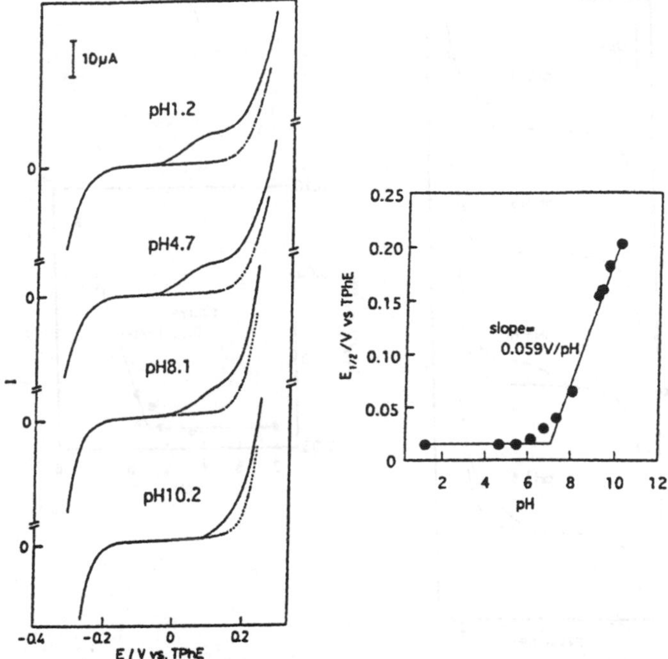

Figure 2. Ion-transfer voltammograms of 0 M (·····) and 2x10^{-4} M (—) scopolamine at various pH. (From Arai, K., Kusu, F., Tsuchiya, N., Fukuyama, S. and Takamura, K., Ion transfer of weak electrolytes across the oil/water interface. Ion transfer of scopolamine and lidocaine, *Denki Kagaku*, 62(9), 840, 1994. With permission.)

Figure 3. Relationship between pH and half-wave potential of scopolamine. (From Arai, K., Kusu, F., Tsuchiya, N., Fukuyama, S. and Takamura, K., Ion transfer of weak electrolytes across the oil/water interface. Ion transfer of scopolamine and lidocaine, *Denki Kagaku*, 62(9), 840, 1994. With permission.)

$\log(D^O_B / D^W_B)\}$ was 5.5, and even for this drug, the potential at the point of intersection was consistent with this value. The equations approximating half-wave potentials for ion transfer of drugs could thus be established. In *case I*, the half-wave potential is independent of pH, whose potential corresponds to the half-wave potential of a drug itself. Drug voltammograms were therefore measured under the condition, pH < pKa – $\log K_D - \log(D^O_B / D^W_B)$. Variation in the second term on the right in Equation 4 is small relative to the first term and may be regarded constant, and the half-wave potential accordingly may be considered proportional to the standard potential of the drug. The latter parameter is related to standard Gibbs energy of ion transfer, and consequently the half-wave potential may be taken as an index of drug hydrophobicity[10].

B. DRUG VOLTAMMOGRAMS

Depending upon the degree to which chemical structure affects biological action, the drugs can be classified as *structurally specific* and

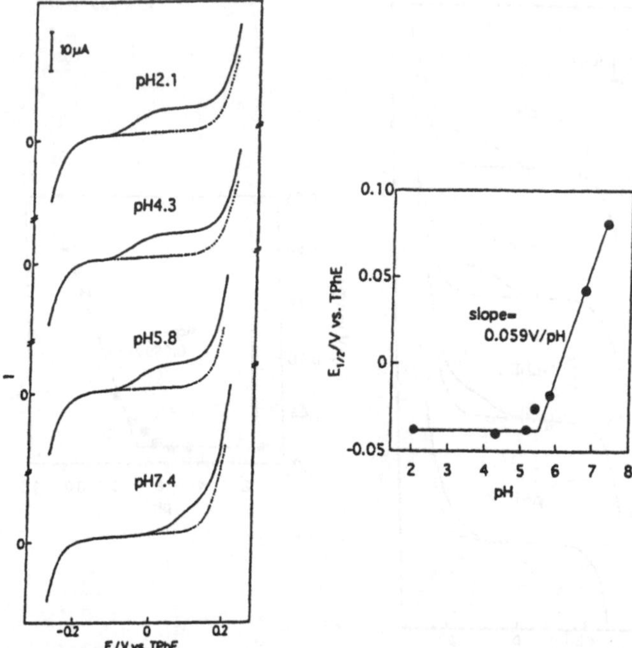

Figure 4. Ion-transfer voltammograms of 0 M (·····) and 2×10^{-4} M (—) lidocaine at various pH. (From Arai, K., Kusu, F., Tsuchiya, N., Fukuyama, S. and Takamura, K., *Denki Kagaku*, 62(9), 840, 1994. With permission.)

Figure 5. Relationship between pH and half-wave potential of lidocaine. (From Arai, K., Kusu, F., Tsuchiya, N., Fukuyama, S. and Takamura, K., *Denki Kagaku*, 62(9), 840, 1994. With permission.)

nonspecific[1]. The former includes hypnotic and anesthetic drugs, whose pharmacological activities are affected by their physical properties of the molecules, while the latter includes cholinergic, anti-cholinergic, adrenergic and anti-adrenergic drugs, whose activities are affected by the chemical structures. Comparison between electrochemical behavior of two types of drug groups is a matter of interest from a pharmaceutical point of view.

1. Hypnotic Drugs

As hypnotic drugs, barbiturate derivatives were used in our study[9]. They depress the synaptic transmission of the central nervous system and then produce hypnotic activity[31].

Figure 6 shows voltammograms of (a) pentobarbital, (b) amobarbital, (c) phenobarbital, (d) allobarbital and (e) barbital. A cathodic wave appeared in the voltammogram of each drug. The hypnotic drugs being weak acids, the transfer of drug ions was recorded as the cathodic wave. The half-wave potential became more positive with pharmacological activity:

$$\log(1 / ID_{50}) = 3.16 (E_{1/2})^2 - 4.26 E_{1/2} + 35.43 \qquad (s=0.008, n=5) \qquad (6)$$

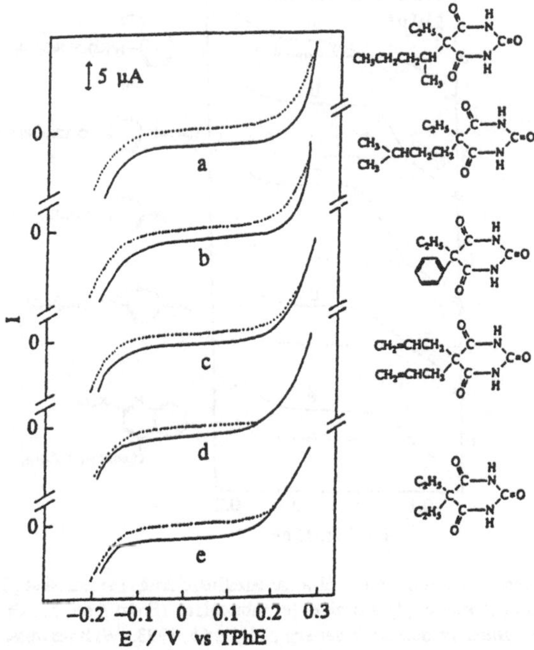

Figure 6. Ion-transfer voltammograms of hypnotic drugs measured at pH 11.0: (a) pentobarbital, (b) amobarbital, (c) phenobarbital, (d) allobarbital, (e) barbital. (From Arai, K., Ohsawa, M., Kusu, F. and Takamura, K., *Bioelectrochem. Bioenerg.*, 31(1), 65, 1993. With permission.)

The index of pharmacological activity of a drug is expressed as the median inhibiting concentration, ID_{50}. ID_{50} values were taken from the literature[32]. Since the drugs are transferred across the interface as anions, half-wave potential became more positive with an increase in drug hydrophobicity. Increased hydrophobicity of barbiturate derivatives results in greater pharmacological activity[31] and this is reflected in the present data.

2. Local Anesthetic Drugs

Most local anesthetic drugs are amphiphilic compounds having a tertiary amine. They penetrate excitable membranes of nerve cells to prevent the generation and conduction of nerve impulses[33]. Figure 7 shows voltammograms of (a) lidocaine, (b) tetracaine, (c) benzocaine, (d) procaine and (e) dibucaine. An anodic wave was seen in the voltammogram of each drug. The drugs are weak bases and thus, the transfer of their ions was recorded as cathodic waves. A comparison of half-wave potentials was made with ID_{50}[34]. As shown in Figure 12, b, this parameter became more positive with an increase in pharmacological activity

$$\log(1 / ID_{50}) = -42.34\, E_{1/2} - 0.16 \quad (r=0.855,\ n=5) \tag{7}$$

Since the drugs transferred across the interface as cations, the half-wave potential became more negative with higher hydrophobicity. The pharmacological activity of local anesthetic drugs increases in direct proportion to hydrophobicity[35], consistent with the result demonstrated here.

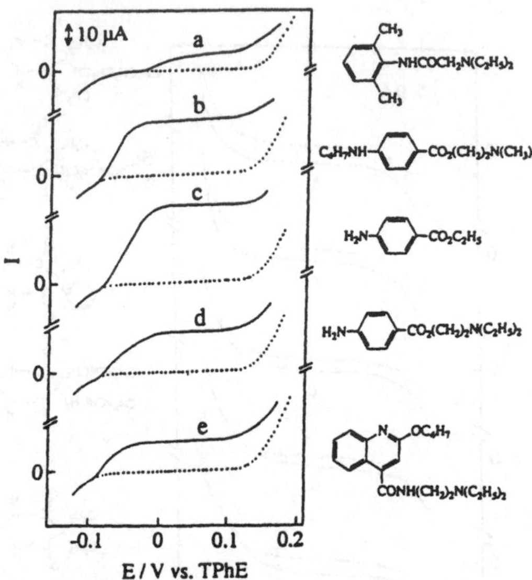

Figure 7. Ion-transfer voltammograms of local anesthetic drugs measured at pH 3.0: (a) lidocaine, (b) tetracaine, (c) benzocaine, (d) procaine, (e) dibucaine. (From Arai, K., Ohsawa, M., Kusu, F. and Takamura, K., *Bioelectrochem. Bioenerg.*, 31(1), 65, 1993. With permission.)

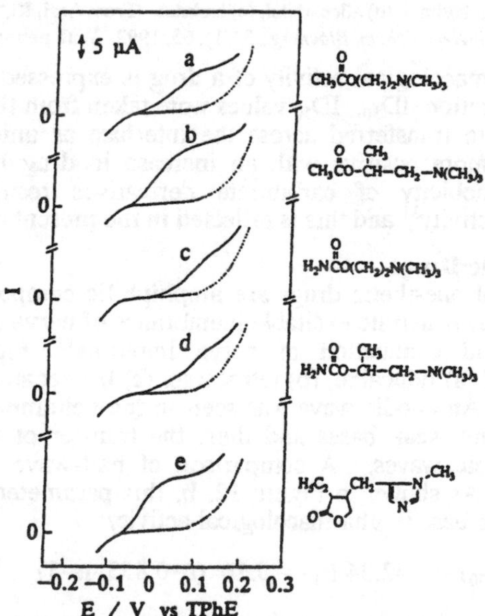

Figure 8. Ion-transfer voltammograms of cholinergic drugs measured at pH 6.8: (a) acetylcholine, (b) acetyl-*b*-methylcholine, (c) carbamylcholine, (d) carbamyl-*b*-methylcholine, (e) pilocarpine. (From Arai, K., Ohsawa, M., Kusu, F. and Takamura, K., *Bioelectrochem. Bioenerg.*, 31(1), 65, 1993. With permission.)

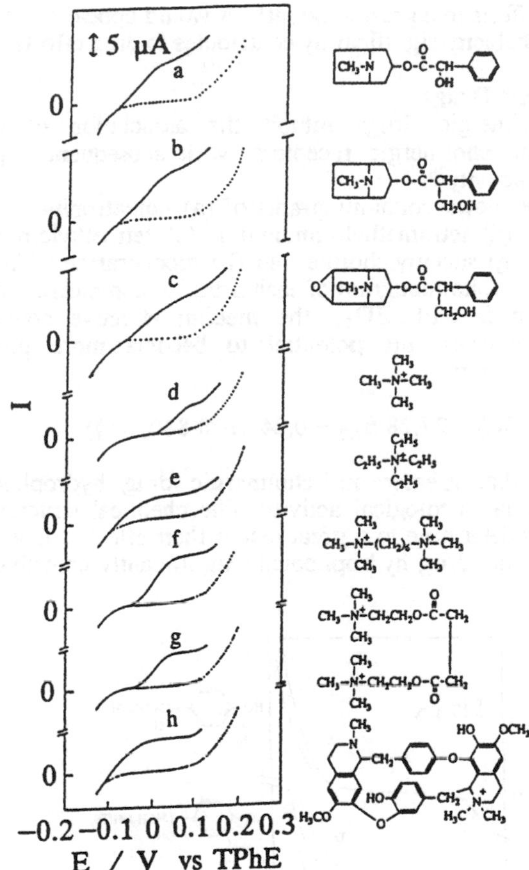

Figure 9. Ion-transfer voltammograms of anti-cholinergic drugs measured at pH 6.8: (a) homatropine, (b) atropine, (c) scopolamine, (d) tetramethylammonium, (e) tetraethyl-ammonium, (f) hexamethonium, (g) succinylcholine, (h) tubocurarine. (From Arai, K., Ohsawa, M., Kusu, F. and Takamura, K., *Bioelectrochem. Bioenerg.*, 31(1), 65, 1993. With permission.)

3. Cholinergic Drugs

Cholinergic drugs excite autonomic effector cells that are innervated by all preganglionic autonomic and postganglionic parasympathetic nerves. They associate with cholinergic receptors on membranes of effector cells in the same manner as endogenous acetylcholine, with consequent expression of parasympathetic activity[36].

Figure 8 shows voltammograms of (a) acetylcholine, (b) acetyl-*b*-methylcholine, (c) carbamylcholine, (d) carbamyl-*b*-methylcholine and (e) pilocarpine. An anodic wave appeared in the voltammogram of each drug. A comparison of half-wave potentials was made with ID_{50}[37]. Figure 12, c shows this parameter to become more positive with pharmacological activity:

$$\log(1 / ID_{50}) = -14.14\, E_{1/2} - 5.63 \quad (r=0.990,\ n=4) \qquad (8)$$

Greater hydrophobicity of cholinergic drugs would thus appear to lessen pharmacological activity. The chemical structures of cholinergic drugs determine their effects to a greater extent[1]. It would appear from Equation 8 that drug hydrophobicity significantly contributes to drug effects.

4. Anti-cholinergic Drugs

Anti-cholinergic drugs inhibit the association of endogenous acetylcholine with cholinergic receptors, with subsequent expression of pharmacological activity[38].

Figure 9 shows voltammograms of (a) homatropine, (b) atropine, (c) scopolamine, (d) tetramethylammonium, (e) tetraethylammonium, (f) hexamethonium, (g) succinylcholine and (h) tubocurarine. There was an anodic wave in the voltammogram of each drug. A comparison of half-wave potentials was made with ED_{50}, the median effective concentration[39]. Figure 12, d indicates this potential to become more positive with pharmacological activity:

$$\log(1 / ED_{50}) = 27.28\, E_{1/2} + 0.24 \quad (r{=}0.880, n{=}4) \tag{9}$$

It thus follows that greater anti-cholinergic drug hydrophobicity may possibly reduce pharmacological activity. The chemical structures of anti-cholinergic drugs determine to a great extent their effects[1]. It would appear from Equation 9 that drug hydrophobicity significantly contributes to drug efficacy.

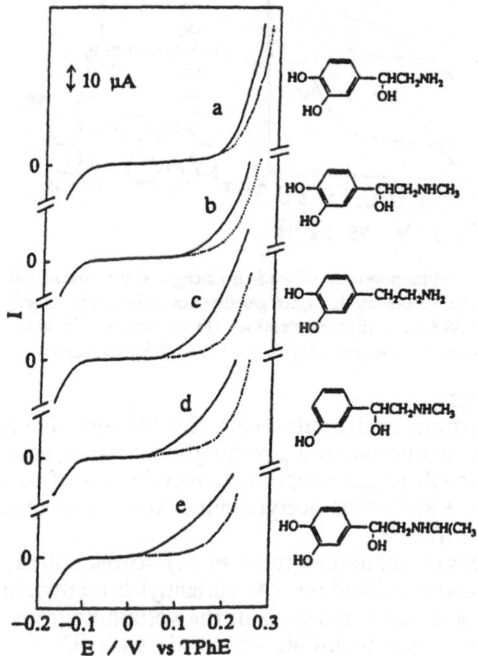

Figure 10. Ion-transfer voltammograms of adrenergic drugs measured at pH 3.0: (a) epinephrine, (b) norepinephrine, (c) dopamine, (d) phenylephrine, (e) isoproterenol. (From Arai, K., Ohsawa, M., Kusu, F. and Takamura, K., *Bioelectrochem. Bioenerg.*, 31(1), 65, 1993. With permission.)

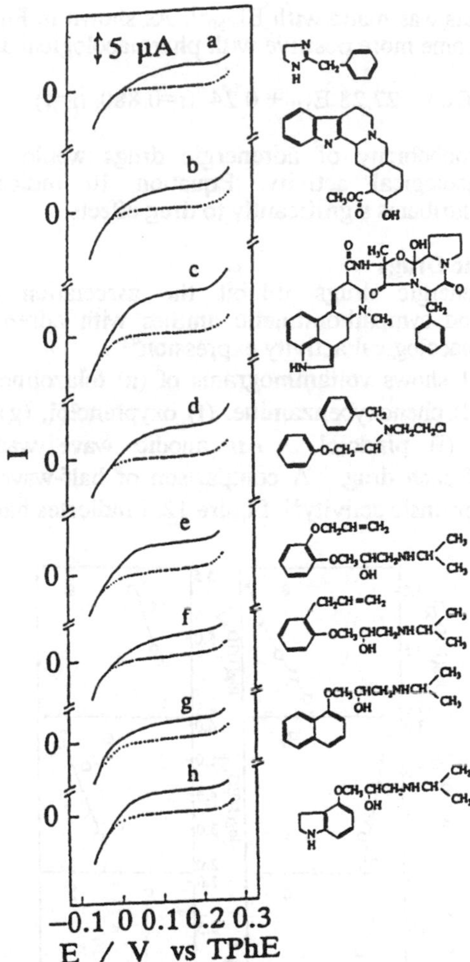

Figure 11. Ion-transfer voltammograms of anti-adrenergic drugs measured at pH 3.0: (a) tolazoline, (b) yohimbin, (c) ergotamine, (d) phenoxybenzamine, (f) oxyprenolol, (g) alprenolol, (h) propranolol, (i) pindolol. (From Arai, K., Ohsawa, M., Kusu, F. and Takamura, K., *Bioelectrochem. Bioenerg.*, 31(1), 65, 1993. With permission.)

5. Adrenergic Drugs

Adrenergic drugs excite autonomic effector cells that are innervated by postganglionic sympathetic nerves. They associate with adrenergic receptors on membranes of effector cells in the same manner as endogenous norepinephrine (noradrenaline, levaterol), followed by the expression of sympathetic activity[40].

Figure 10 shows voltammograms of (a) epinephrine, (b) norepinephrine, (c) dopamine, (d) phenylephrine and (e) isoproterenol. An anodic wave appeared in the voltammogram of each drug. A comparison of half-wave potentials was made with ED_{50}[41]. As shown in Figure 12, e, half-wave potential became more positive with pharmacological activity:

$$\log(1 / ED_{50}) = 27.28\ E_{1/2} + 0.24 \quad (r=0.880, n=4) \tag{10}$$

Increase in hydrophobicity of adrenergic drugs would thus appear to decrease pharmacological activity. Equation 10 indicates that drug hydrophobicity contributes significantly to drug effects.

6. Anti-adrenergic Drugs

Anti-adrenergic drugs inhibit the association of endogenous norepinephrine and sympathomimetic amines with adrenergic receptors, followed by pharmacological activity expression[42].

Figure 11 shows voltammograms of (a) tolazoline, (b) yohimbin, (c) ergotamine, (d) phenoxybenzamine, (f) oxyprenolol, (g) alprenolol, (h) propranolol and (i) pindolol. An anodic wave was seen in the voltammogram of each drug. A comparison of half-wave potentials was made with *I*, the intrinsic activity[42]. Figure 12, f indicates half-wave

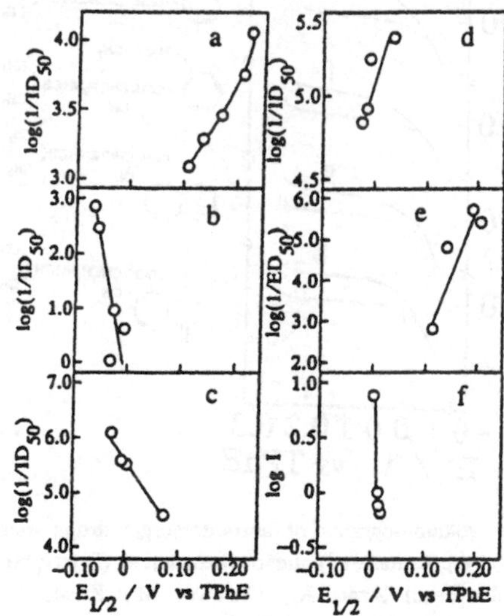

Figure 12. Relationships between half-wave potential and pharmacological activity: (a) hypnotic drugs, (b) local anesthetic drugs, (c) cholinergic drugs, (d) anti-cholinergic drugs, (e) adrenergic drugs, (f) anti-adrenergic drugs. Values of ID_{50}, ED_{50} and *I* are cited from the literature[32,34,37,39,41,42]. (From Arai, K., Ohsawa, M., Kusu, F. and Takamura, K., *Bioelectrochem. Bioenerg.*, 31(1), 65, 1993. With permission.)

potentials to be essentially the same even though pharmacological activity differs considerably. It thus follows that hydrophobicity contributes little to pharmacological activity.

7. General View on Half-Wave Potentials

Table 1 shows half-wave potentials of the voltammograms and the values in each drug group to be essentially the same. In certain cases, they

Table 1. Half-wave Potential of Drugs

	Drug	Half-wave potential / V vs. TPhE
Hypnotic drugs	Pentobarbital	0.225
	Amobarbital	0.210
	Phenobarbital	0.170
	Allobarbital	0.135
	Barbital	0.110
Local anesthetic drugs	Lidocaine	-0.005
	Tetracaine	-0.057
	Benzocaine	-0.030
	Procaine	-0.025
	Dibucaine	-0.065
Cholinergic drugs	Acetylcholine	0.005
	Acetyl-*b*-methylcholine	-0.005
	Carbamylcholine	0.075
	Carbamyl-*b*-methylcholine	0.065
	Pilocarpine	-0.025
Anti-cholinergic drugs	Homatropine	-0.030
	Atropine	-0.025
	Scopolamine	0.025
	Tetramethylammonium	0.035
	Tetraethylammonium	-0.060
	Hexamethonium	-0.015
	Succinylcholine	-0.010
	Tubocurarine	-0.087
Adrenergic drugs	Epinephrine	0.190
	Norepinephrine	0.205
	Dopamine	0.185
	Phenylephrine	0.140
	Isoproterenol	0.115
Anti-adrenergic drugs	Tolazoline	0.050
	Yohimbin	0.035
	Ergotamine	0.035
	Phenoxybenzamine	0.030
	Oxyprenolol	0.018
	Alprenolol	0.015
	Propranolol	0.013
	Pindolol	0.004

(From Arai, K., Ohsawa, M., Kusu, F. and Takamura, K., *Bioelectrochem. Bioenerg.*, 31(1), 65, 1993. With permission.)

correspond to considerable pharmacological activity. This parameter in the antagonist group was more negative than in the agonist group; that is, anti-adrenergic and anti-cholinergic drugs showed more negative values than adrenergic and cholinergic drugs, respectively. It follows that antagonists block cholinergic or adrenergic receptors, thereby inhibiting the association of agonists with receptors by hydrophobicity greater than that of agonists.

All the drugs in this study could interact with biomembranes for the expression of pharmacological activity. Hydrophobicity is essential to such interaction and thus is a major determinant of pharmacological activity[1]. Ion-transfer voltammetry reflects the transfer energy corresponding to the half-wave potential, an index of drug hydrophobicity, and thus may serve as a means for assessing pharmacological activity.

III. ELECTRICAL POTENTIAL OSCILLATION ACROSS A LIQUID MEMBRANE

A. ELECTRICAL POTENTIAL OSCILLATION

1. Experimental Technique

Yoshikawa *et al.*[19] first observed the spontaneous oscillation of an electrical potential across a liquid membrane consisting of water/nitrobenzene/water containing a surfactant. However, there has always been some difficulty in establishing a reproducible potential oscillation across the membrane due to both aqueous phases floating on the organic phase and the oil/water interface situated at the bend of the U-shaped glass tube. The former causes instability of the oil/water interface and the latter, low reproducibility of the shape and area of the interface. Miyamura *et al.*[43] solved the latter problem by replacing the U-shaped glass cell with a hollow glass tube inserted into a glass beaker. Taking into account that an organic solvent with specific gravity with less that of water is essential for creating potential oscillation with high reproducibility, the present authors[44] developed an apparatus by which potential oscillations across the liquid membrane of water/1-octanol/water (octanol membrane) could be measured Figure 13. Water (a1) and aqueous solution containing a surfactant and 5 M ethanol (a2), were introduced, each in the amount of 1 ml, into an inverted U-shaped cell made of Kel-F (g). 2 ml octanol solution containing 5 mM tetrabutylammonium chloride or 3 mM picric acid (b) were carefully placed on top the aqueous solutions without stirring. Potential difference between phases a1 and a2 was measured with a potentiometer (c), using a pair of Ag/AgCl electrodes (d). This cell was indispensable for attaining reproducible oscillation. With a glass cell instead of the Kel-F cell the edge of the oil/water interface would creep up the inner surface of the cell, causing slight mixing of the two aqueous solutions and, accordingly, less reproducibility.

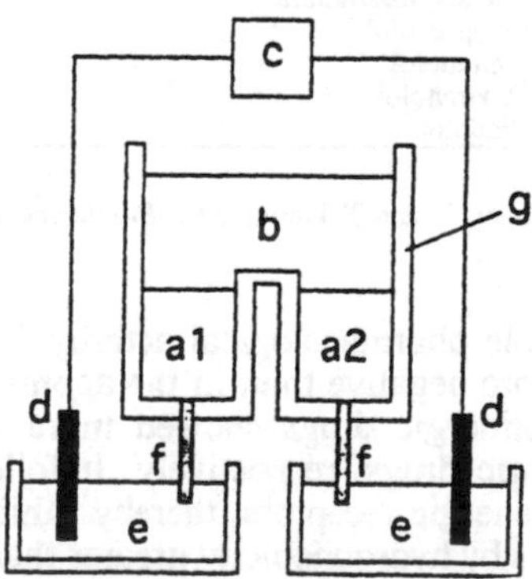

Figure 13. Apparatus for measuring electrical potential oscillation across the liquid membrane of water–octanol–water (an octanol membrane): (a1), (a2) aqueous phases, (b) octanol phase, (c) potentiometer, (d) Ag/AgCl electrode, (e) saturated KCl, (f) KCl salt bridge, (g) Kel-F cell. (From Arai, K., Fukuyama, S., Kusu, F. and Takamura, K., *Bioelectrochem. Bioenerg.*, 33(2), 159, 1994. With permission.)

2. Mechanisms of Oscillation

Figure 14, a shows typical potential oscillations across the octanol membrane with sodium dodecyl sulfate (SDS) as the surfactant in phase a2. The potential in phase a2 was measured relative to phase a1. Spontaneous oscillation started about 10 min after the octanol solution had come in contact with the aqueous solutions. The amplitude of the first oscillation was ca. 150 mV and oscillatory period, ca. 1 min. Potential oscillation gradually ceased and could no longer be detected after 1 day. With hexadecyltrimethyl-ammonium bromide (CTAB) as the surfactant, pulse direction became opposite that when using SDS, whereas other characteristics such as amplitude, oscillatory period and induction period remained essentially the same as those with SDS (Figure 14, b). SDS is an anionic surfactant, and CTAB, a cationic surfactant, and thus, according to which is added to phase b2, the direction of the pulse will be determined.

The rapid potential change observed across a liquid membrane is due to changes in the oil–water interface[45]. Potential oscillation across a liquid membrane was previously shown to be induced at the oil–water interface between the organic and aqueous phases to which no surfactant had been added, but not at the other oil–water interface[46,47]. For the octanol membrane, such an interface corresponds to that between phases b and a1 (interface b/a1). The upper and lower potentials of oscillation at this interface were determined in part according to the electrolytes in phase a1[47]. This effect on upper and lower potentials was basically the same as that on potentials at the interface of an octanol–water system in the absence or presence of a surfactant. The surfactant may thus be concluded to cause oscillation across a liquid membrane through the repetitive formation and destruction of the surfactant ion layer adsorbed on interface b/a1.

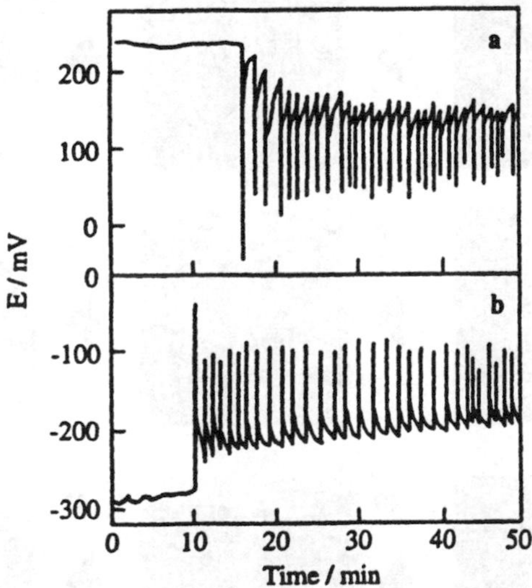

Figure 14. Electrical potential oscillation across the octanol membrane: (a) 8 mM SDS and 5 M ethanol in phase a2 and 5 mM tetrabutylammonium chloride in phase b, (b) 2 mM hexadecyl-trimethylammonium bromide and 5 M ethanol in phase a2 and 3 mM picric acid in phase b.

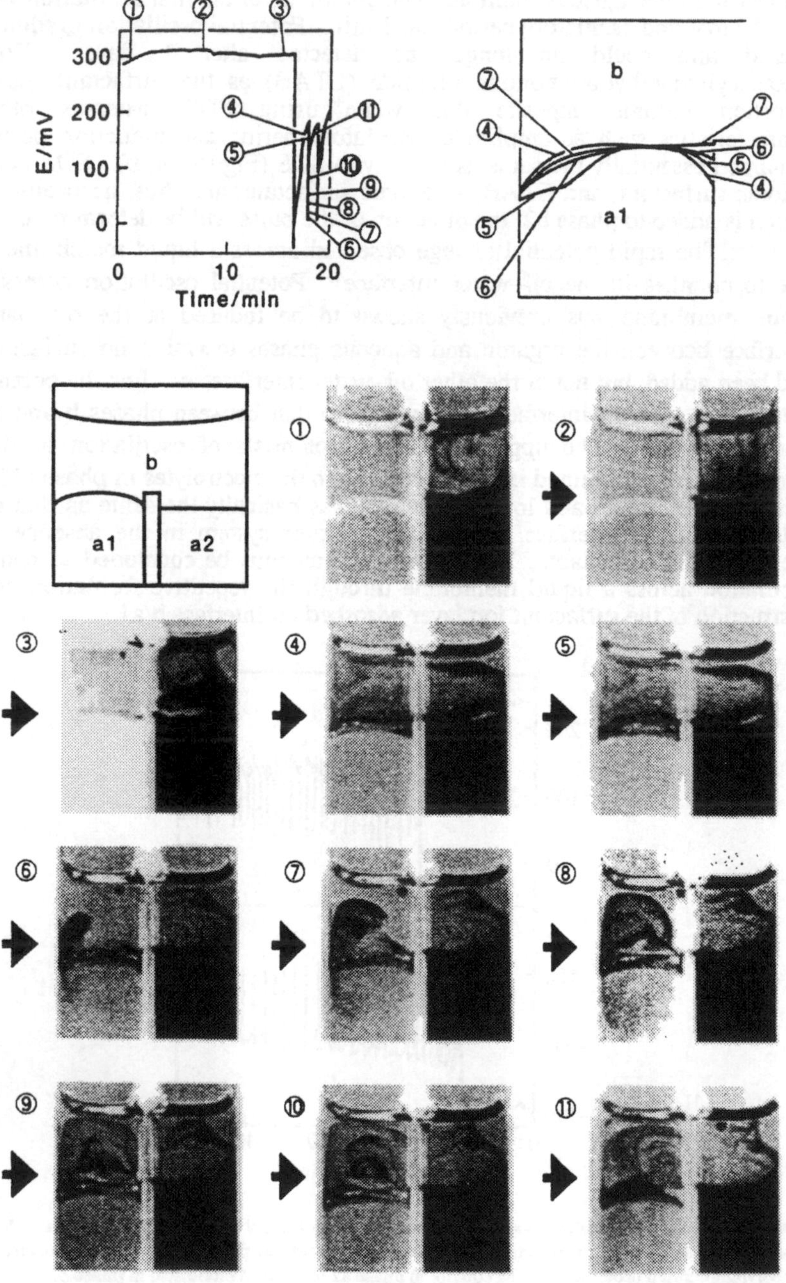

Figure 15. Fluctuation of the oil–water interface between phases b and a1 and movement of eriochrome black T added to phase a2.

Electrical potential oscillation across the octanol membrane using eriochrome black T (EBT) instead of SDS or CTAB in phase a2 was measured[48]. The movement of EBT in the liquid membrane is shown in Figure 15. Its migration from the interface between phases b and a2 (interface b/a2) toward the bulk of phase b could be seen during the induction period of oscillation (1–3 in Figure 15). Oscillation was started after EBT had reached interface b/a1. Considerable convection was then seen to occur synchronously with potential oscillation in phase b (4–11). Interface b/a1 fluctuating synchronously with potential oscillation was also evident. The behavior of EBT being the same as that of SDS or CTAB, potential oscillation should most likely start after the surfactant has reached the interface b/a1, and convection in phase b should occur synchronously with potential oscillations.

The most probable mechanism for electrical potential oscillation across the octanol membrane with SDS is shown in Figure 16. Dodecyl sulfate (DS) ions in phase a2 form a complex with tetrabutylammonium ions at interface b/a2 (State I), diffuse into phase b (State II) and reach interface b/a1 (State III). When DS ion concentration at this interface attains a critical value, a DS ion layer forms at the interface (State IV) and at which time, potential at the interface suddenly becomes more negative values. Surface pressure at the interface increases due to this formation, causing destruction of the layer and DS ions proceed to phase a1 (State V). Accordingly, potential at the interface slowly becomes more positive again. Potential oscillation is induced by the repetitive formation and destruction of this layer (States IV and V). A similar mechanism should be applicable to oscillation with CTAB; that is, potential oscillation across the octanol membrane with CTAB is induced by the repetitive formation and destruction of the hexadecyl-trimethylammonium ion layer adsorbed on interface b/a1.

Since biomembrane surfaces, interposed between phospholipid and water in a biological system, are negatively charged, a liquid membrane with an anionic surfactant should be used for determining drug characteristics. Thus, in this study, SDS was used as surfactant in phase a2 though electrical potential oscillation could also be detected with CTAB.

B. EFFECTS OF DRUGS ON OSCILLATION MODE

1. Hypnotic Drugs

Figure 17 shows potential oscillation measured in the presence of (1) barbital, (2) allobarbital, (3) phenobarbital and (4) amobarbital in phase a1[24]. Amplitude, induction and oscillatory periods are shown in Table 2. The values of an amplitude and oscillatory period are the mean values obtained from the initial five pulses of potential oscillation. Amplitude decreased in the order, barbital > allobarbital > phenobarbital > amobarbital. Induction period decreased in the order, barbital < allobarbital < phenobarbital < amobarbital. The oscillatory period decreased in the order, barbital < allobarbital < phenobarbital < amobarbital. These parameters were also determined in part by drug concentration. Increase in drug concentration resulted in less amplitude and longer induction and oscillatory periods.

Organic ions with high hydrophobicity caused the mode of oscillation to change considerably[44,49,50]. Structural change in the DS ion layer adsorbed at the interface may have been the reason for this. Hypnotic drugs in phase a1 may dissolve in the DS ion layer or were adsorbed on the oil–water interface, causing the DS ion layer to take on a tightly knit

18 Electrochemical Behavior of Drugs at Oil–Water Interfaces

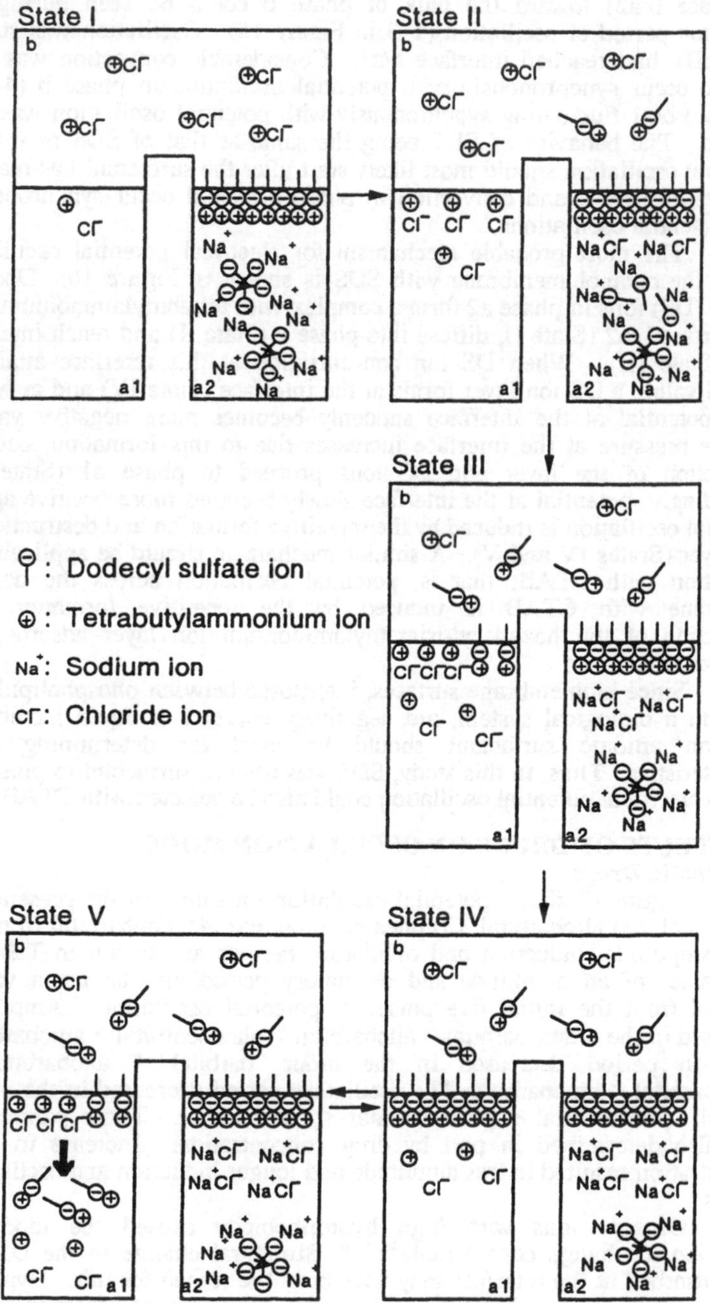

Figure 16. Mechanism for potential oscillation across the octanol membrane with SDS as surfactant. States I, II, III and IV: induction period, State V: occurrence of pulse, State V ⇄ IV: potential oscillation.

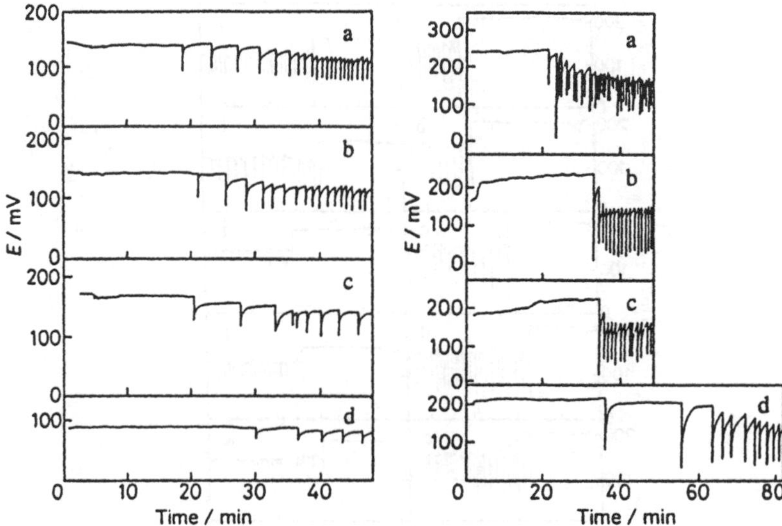

Figure 17. Electrical potential oscillation in the presence of hypnotic drugs in phase a1: (a) barbital, (b) allobarbital, (c) phenobarbital, (d) amobarbital. Concentrations: 100 mM. (From Arai, K., Fukuyama, S., Kusu, F. and Takamura, K., *Bioelectrochem. Bioenerg.*, 33(2), 159, 1994. With permission.)

Figure 18. Electrical potential oscillation in the presence of hypnotic drugs in phase a1: (a) procaine, (b) lidocaine, (c) tetracaine, (d) dibucaine. Concentrations: 0.5 mM. (From Arai, K., Fukuyama, S., Kusu, F. and Takamura, K., *Bioelectrochem. Bioenerg.*, 33(2), 159, 1994. With permission.)

structure. The formation and destruction of this layer are thus inhibited, so that there is lower amplitude and longer induction and oscillatory periods.

Mode change reflects interactions between chemical substances and the DS ion layer. This layer may be considered a biomembrane model in consideration of the hydrophobic phase interposed between the aqueous phases. This result is of interest from a pharmaceutical point of view. Figure 21 a shows relationships between pharmacological activity[32] and amplitude,oscillatory and induction periods. Pharmacological activity increased with lower amplitude and longer oscillatory and induction periods. The pharmacological activity of barbiturates increases within the hydrophobic compartment in a biological system[31] thus showing mode change to be correlated with pharmacological activity.

2. Local Anesthetic Drugs

Figure 18 shows potential oscillation measured in the presence of (a) procaine, (b) lidocaine, (c) tetracaine and (d) dibucaine in phase a1[24]. Amplitude decreased in the order, procaine > lidocaine > tetracaine > dibucaine. Induction period decreased in the order, dibucaine > tetracaine _ lidocaine > procaine. The oscillatory period decreased in the order, dibucaine > tetracaine > lidocaine > procaine. Amplitude and oscillatory and induction periods were also determined in part by drug concentration. Increase in drug concentration resulted in less amplitude and longer induction and oscillatory periods.

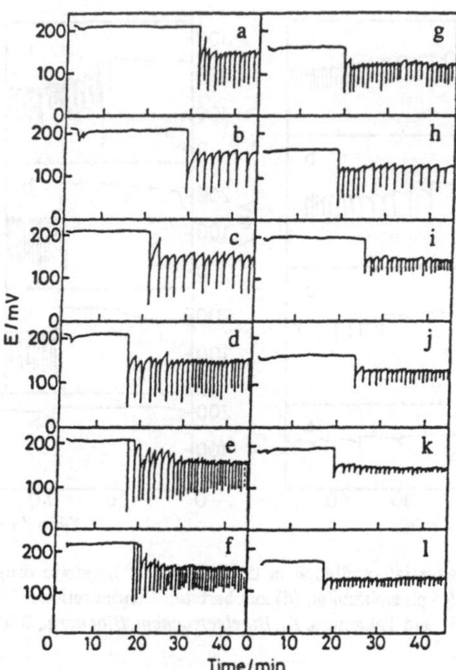

Figure 19. Electrical potential oscillation in the presence of cholinergic and anti-cholinergic drugs in phase a1: (a) acetylcholine, (b) acetyl-*b*-methylcholine, (c) carbamylcholine, (d) carbamyl-*b*-methylcholine, (e) tetramethylammonium, (f) tetraethylammonium, (g) hexamethonium, (h) succinylcholine, (i) scopolamine, (j) homatropine, (k) atropine, (l) tubocurarine. Concentrations: 20 mM. (From Reference 51.)

Figure 21 b shows relationships between pharmacological activity[34] and amplitude and oscillatory and induction periods. Pharmacological activity increased with lower amplitude and longer oscillatory and induction periods. Local anesthetic drugs interact with biomembranes for the expression of their pharmacological activity. The pharmacological activity of local anesthetic drugs becomes more intense with solubility in the hydrophobic compartment of a biological system[35], demonstrating mode change in potential oscillation to be correlated to pharmacological activity.

3. Cholinergic and Anti-cholinergic Drugs

Figure 19 shows potential oscillation measured in the presence of (a) acetylcholine, (b) acetyl-*b*-methylcholine, (c) carbamylcholine, (d) carbamyl-*b*-methylcholine, (e) tetramethylammonium, (f) tetraethylammonium, (g) hexamethonium, (h) succinylcholine, (i) scopolamine, (j) homatropine, (k) atropine and (l) tubocurarine in phase a1[51]. Amplitude decreased in the order, acetylcholine > carbamylcholine > carbamyl-*b*-methylcholine > acetyl-*b*-methylcholine > tetramethyl-ammonium > succinylcholine > tetraethyl-ammonium > hexamethonium > scopolamine > atropine = homatropine > tubocurarine. Amplitude was affected in part by drug concentration. Increase in drug concentration

Table 2. Amplitude, Oscillatory and Induction Periods of Electrical Potential Oscillation in the Presence of Drugs

	Drug	Amplitude / mV	Oscillatory period / min	Induction period / min
Hypnotic drugs [a]	Barbital	30	3.0	16
	Allobarbital	30	4.5	19
	Phenobarbital	20	5.5	21
	Amobarbital	16	6.5	30
Local anesthetic drugs [b]	Procaine	245	1.2	17
	Lidocaine	232	1.1	31
	Tetracaine	208	1.0	35
	Dibucaine	174	6.9	35
Cholinergic drugs [c]	Acetylcholine	186	-	-
	Acetyl-β-methylcholine	150	-	-
	Carbamylcholine	170	-	-
	Carbamyl-β-methylcholine	165	-	-
Anti-cholinergic drugs [c]	Tetramethylammonium	165	-	-
	Tetraethylammonium	138	-	-
	Hexamethonium	129	-	-
	Succinylcholine	160	-	-
	Scopolamine	100	-	-
	Atropine	86	-	-
	Homatropine	86	-	-
	Tubocurarine	80	-	-
Adrenergic drugs [c]	Epinephrine	133	-	-
	Isoproterenol	109	-	-
	Dopamine	114	-	-
	Phenylephrine	98	-	-
Anti-adrenergic drugs [c]	Tolazoline	54	-	-
	Oxyprenolol	42	-	-
	Alprenolol	32	-	-
	Propranolol	8	-	-

[a,b] From Reference 24.
[c] From Reference 51.
[a] Concentrations: 100 mM.
[b] Concentrations: 0.5 mM.
[c] Concentrations: 20 mM.

resulted in lower amplitude. Large variation in induction and oscillatory periods was observed in each measurement for cholinergic, anti-cholinergic, adrenergic and anti-adrenergic drugs and thus no examination was made of change in these parameters.

Table 2 shows that amplitude of anti-cholinergic drugs (tetramethyl-ammonium, succinylcholine, tetraethylammonium, hexamethonium, scopolamine, atropine, homatropine and tubocurarine) to be less than that of cholinergic drugs (acetylcholine, carbamylcholine, carbamyl-*b*-methylcholine and acetyl-*b*-methylcholine). The mode change reflects interactions between drugs and the DS ion layer, indicating the affinity of anti-cholinergic drugs toward the DS ion layer to possibly exceed that of cholinergic drugs. Figure 21 c shows the relationship between the pharmacological activity[37,40] of cholinergic and anti-cholinergic drugs and amplitude. Pharmacological activity increased with lower amplitude. Thus, anti-cholinergic drugs may associate with their receptors to block the association of cholinergic drugs with their receptors owing to their greater affinity toward membranes.

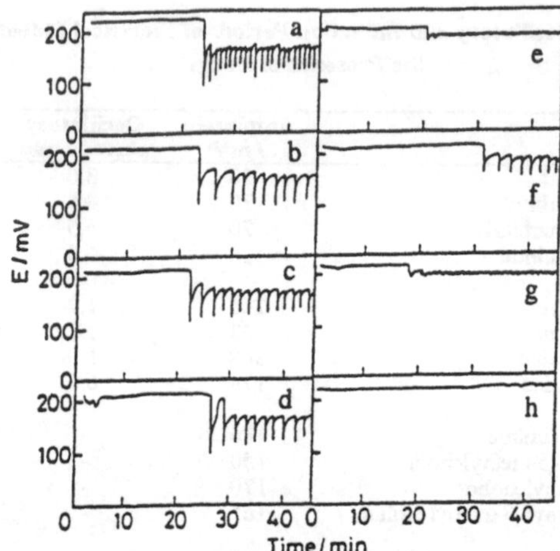

Figure 20. Electrical potential oscillation in the presence of adrenergic and anti-adrenergic drugs in phase a1: (a) epinephrine, (b) isoproterenol, (c) phenylephrine, (d) dopamine, (e) alprenolol, (f) tolazoline, (g) oxyprenolol, (h) propranolol. Concentrations: 20 mM. (From Reference 51.)

4 Adrenergic and Anti-adrenergic Drugs

Figure 20 shows potential oscillation measured in the presence of (a) epinephrine, (b) isoproterenol, (c) phenylephrine, (d) dopamine, (e) alprenolol, (f) tolazoline, (g) oxyprenolol and (h) propranolol in phase a1[51]. Amplitude decreased in the order, epinephrine > dopamine > isoproterenol > phenylephrine > tolazoline > oxyprenolol > alprenolol > propranolol. Amplitude was determined in part by drug concentration. Increase in drug concentration resulted in lower amplitude. The amplitude of anti-adrenergic drugs (tolazoline, oxyprenolol, alprenolol and propranolol) was less than that of adrenergic drugs (epinephrine, dopamine, isoproterenol and phenylephrine). The mode change reflects interactions between drugs and the DS ion layer, indicating the affinity of anti-adrenergic drugs toward the DS ion layer to be greater than that of adrenergic agents. Figure 21, d shows the relationship between pharmacological activity[41,42] of adrenergic and anti-adrenergic drugs and amplitude. Pharmacological activity increased with lower amplitude. Anti-adrenergic drugs may associate with their receptors to block the association of adrenergic drugs with their receptors owing to their greater affinity toward membranes.

IV. CONCLUSION

The present review describes recent research on ion-transfer voltammetry of drugs and electrical potential oscillation across the liquid membrane of water/octanol/water in the presence of drugs. Half-wave potential and oscillation mode were found to directly reflect drug behavior at oil/water interfaces; that is, the former reflects drug hydrophobicity, and the latter, affinity of a drug for the surfactant ion layer adsorbed at an oil/water interface. Relationships between drugs pharmacological activity and these

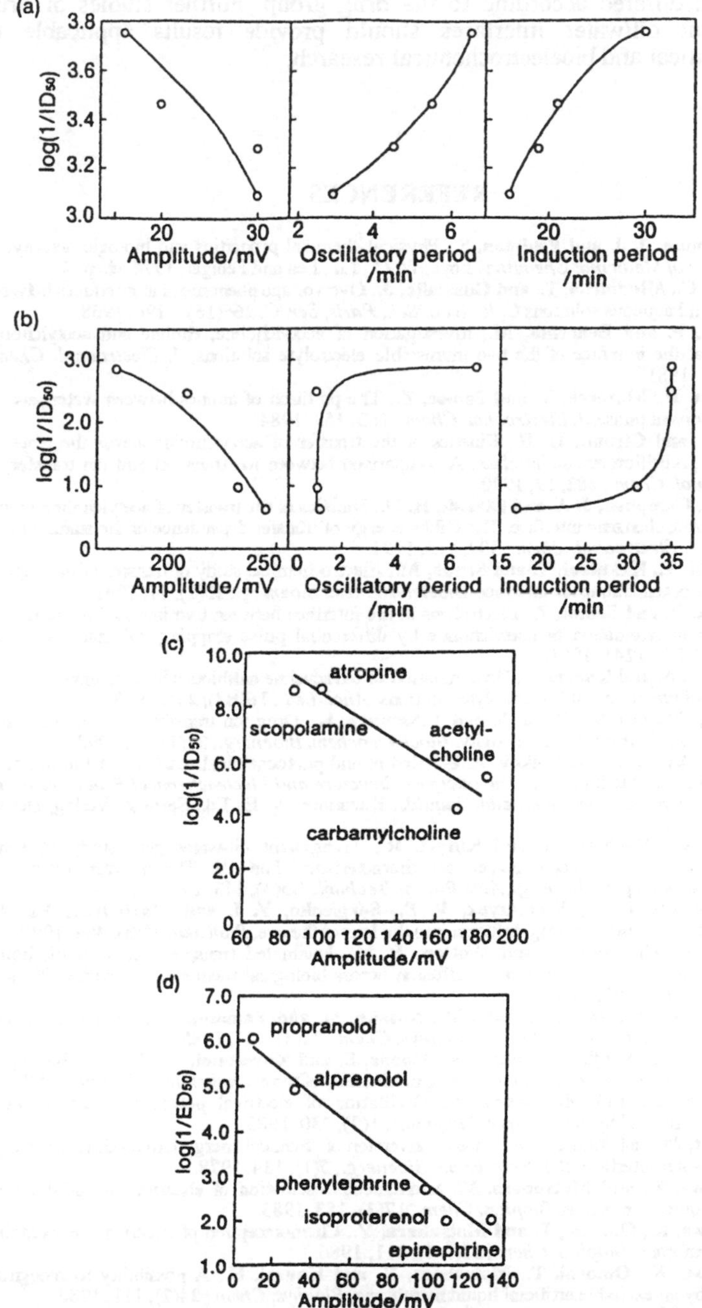

Figure 21. Relationships between pharmacological activity and amplitude, oscillatory period and induction period of oscillation in the presence of drugs in phase a1: (a) hypnotic drugs, (b) anesthetic drugs (c) cholinergic and anti-cholinergic drugs, (d) adrenergic and anti-adrenergic drugs. Values of ID_{50} and ED_{50} are cited from the literature[32,34,37,40-42]. ((a) and (b), From Arai, K., Fukuyama, S., Kusu, F. and Takamura, K., ***Bioelectrochem. Bioenerg.***, 33(2), 159, 1994. With permission.)

parameters differed according to the drug group. Further studies of drug behavior at oil/water interfaces should provide results applicable to pharmaceutical and bioelectrochemical research.

REFERENCES

1. **Zimmerman, J. J. and Feldman, S.**, Physical-chemical properties and biologic activity, in *Principles of Medicinal Chemistry*, Foye, W. O., Ed., Lea and Febiger, 1974, chap. 2.
2. **Gavach, C., Mlodnicka, T., and Guastalla, J.**, Overvoltage phenomena at interfaces between organic and aqueous solutions *C. R. Acad. Sci., Paris, Ser. C*, 266(16), 1196, 1968.
3. **Vanysek, P. and Behrendt, M.**, Investigation of acetylcholine, choline and acetylcholinesterase at the interface of the two immiscible electrolyte solutions, *J. Electroanal. Chem.*, 130, 287, 1981.
4. **Homolka, D., Marecek, V. and Samec, Z.**, The partition of amines between water and an organic solvent phase, *J. Electroanal. Chem.*, 163, 159, 1984.
5. **Shao, Y. and Girault, H. H.**, Kinetics of the transfer of acetylcholine across the water + sucrose/1,2-dichloroethane interface. A comparison between ion transport and ion transfer, *J. Electroanal. Chem.*, 282, 59, 1990.
6. **Shao, Y., Campbell, J. A. and Girault, H. H.**, Kinetics of the transfer of acetylcholine across the water/nitrobenzene interface. The Gibbs energy of transfer dependence of the standard rate constant, *J. Electroanal. Chem.*, 300, 415, 1991.
7. **Ohkouchi, T., Kakutani, T. and Senda, M.**, Electrochemical study of transfer of uncouplers across the organic/aqueous interface, *Bioelectrochem. Bioenerg.*, 25(1), 71, 1991.
8. **Marecek, V. and Samec, Z.**, Electrolysis at the interface between two immiscible electrolyte solutions: determination of acetylcholine by differential pulse stripping voltammetry, *Anal. Lett.*, 14(B15), 1241, 1981.
9. **Kozlov, Y. N. and Koryta, J.**, Determination of tetracycline antibiotics by voltammetry at the interface of two immiscible electrolyte solutions, *Anal. Lett.*, 16(B3), 255, 1983.
10. **Arai, K., Ohsawa, M., Kusu, F. and Takamura, K.**, Drug ion transfer across an oil-water interface and pharmacological activity, *Bioelectrochem. Bioenerg.*, 31(1), 65, 1993.
11 **Boguslavsky, L. I. and Volkov, A. G.**, Redox and photochemical reactions at the interface between immiscible liquids, in *The Interface Structure and Electrochemical Processes at the Boundary Between Two Immiscible Liquids*, Kazarinov, V. E., Ed., Springer Verlag, Berlin, 1987, pp. 143-178.
12. **Provost, C., Herbots, H. and Kinget, R.**, Transparent oil-water gels. study of some physicochemical and biopharmaceutical characteristics. Part IV: The in vitro release of hydrophilic and lipophilic drugs, *Acta Pharm. Technol.*, 35(3), 143, 1989.
13. **Chasovnicova, L. V., Formazyuk, V. E., Sergienko, V. I. and Vladimirov, Yu. A.**, Modeling of anticataract drug diffusion into the lens of the eye, *Biofizika*, 35(3), 464, 1990.
14. **Barker, N., Hadgraft, J. and Wotton, P. K.**, Facilitated transport across liquid/liquid interfaces and its relevance to drug diffusion across biological membrane, *Faraday Discuss. Chem. Soc.*, (77), 97, 1984.
15. **Toko, K., Yoshikawa, K., Tsukiji, M., Nosaka, M. and Yamafuji, K.**, On the oscillatory phenomena in an oil/water interface, *Biophys. Chem.*, 22(3), 151, 1985.
16. **Yoshikawa, K., Shoji, M., Nakata, S., Maeda, S. and Kawakami, H.**, An excitable liquid membrane possibly mimicking the sensing mechanism of taste, *Langmuir*, 4(3), 759, 1988.
17. **Yoshikawa, K. and Matsubara, Y.**, Oscillation of electrical potential across a liquid membrane induced by amine vapor, *Langmuir*, 1(2), 230, 1985.
18. **Dupeyrat, M. and Nakache, E.**, Direct conversion of chemical energy into mechanical energy at an oil water interface, *Bioelectrochem. Bioenerg.*, 5(1), 134, 1978.
19. **Yoshikawa, K. and Matsubara, Y.**, Spontaneous oscillation of electrical potential across organic liquid membranes, *Biophys. Chem.*, 17(3), 183, 1983.
20. **Yoshikawa, K., Omochi, T. and Matsubara, Y.**, Chemoreception of sugars by an excitable liquid membrane, *Biophys. Chem.*, 23(3-4), 211, 1986.
21. **Yoshikawa, K., Omochi, T., Matsubara, Y. and Kourai, H.**, A possibility to recognize chirality by an excitable artificial liquid membrane, *Biophys. Chem.*, 24(2), 111, 1986.
22. **Yoshikawa, K., Shoji, M., Nakata, S., Maeda, S. and Kawakami, H.**, An excitable liquid membrane possibly mimicking the sensing mechanism of taste, *Langmuir*, 4(3), 759, 1988.
23. **Nakajo, N., Yoshikawa, K., Shoji, M. and Ueda, I.**, Spontaneous oscillation of artificial membrane: equivalence in effects of temperature and volatile anesthetic, *Biochem. Biophys. Res. Commun.*, 167(2), 450, 1990.

24. **Arai, K., Fukuyama, S., Kusu, F. and Takamura, K.**, Effects of biologically important substances on spontaneous electrical potential oscillation across a liquid membrane of a water/octanol/water system, *Bioelectrochem. Bioenerg.*, 33(2), 159, 1994.
25. **Koryta, J., Vanysek, P. and Brezina, M.**, Electrolysis with an electrolyte dropping electrode, *J. Electroanal. Chem.* 67(2), 263, 1976.
26. **Kihara, S., Yoshida, Z. and Fujinaga, T.**, Current-scan polarography at the aqueous/organic solutions interface, *Bunseki Kagaku*, 31(9), E297, 1982.
27. **Arai, K., Kusu, F., Tsuchiya, N., Fukuyama, S. and Takamura, K.**, Ion transfer of weak electrolytes across the oil/water interface. Ion transfer of scopolamine and lidocaine, *Denki Kagaku*, 62(9), 840, 1994.
28. **Yoshida, Z. and Freiser, H.**, Ascending water electrode studies of metal extractants. Faradaic ion transfer of protonated 1,10-phenanthroline and its derivatives across an aqueous 1,2-dichloroethane interface, *J. Electroanal. Chem.*, 162, 307, 1984.
29. **Doe, H., Yoshioka, K. and Kitagawa, T.**, Voltammetric study of protonated 1,10-phenanthroline cation transfer across the water/nitrobenzene interface, *J. Electroanal. Chem.*, 324, 69, 1992.
30. **Matsuda, H., Yamada, Y., Kanamori, K., Kudo, Y and Takeda, Y**, On the facilitation effect of neutral macrocyclic ligands on the ion transfer across the interface between aqueous and organic solutions. I. Theoretical equation of ion-transfer-polarographic current-potential curves and its experimental verification, *Bull. Chem. Soc. Jpn.*, 64(5), 1497, 1991.
31. **Rall, T. W.**, Hypnotics and sedatives; ethanol, in *The Pharmacological Basis of Therapeutics*, 8th edition, Gilman, A. G., Rall, T. W., Nies, A. S. and Taylor, P., Eds., Pergamon Press, New York, 1990, chap. 17.
32. **Hansch, C., Steward, A. R., Anderson, S. M. and Bentley, D.**, The structure-activity relation in barbiturates and its similarity to that in other narcotics, *J. Med. Chem.*, 10(5), 745, 1967.
33. **Ritchie, J. M. and Greene, N. M.**, Local anesthetics, in *The Pharmacological Basis of Therapeutics*, 8th edition, Gilman, A. G., Rall, T. W., Nies, A. S. and Taylor, P., Eds., Pergamon Press, New York, 1990, chap. 15.
34. **McNeal, E. T., Lewandowski, G. A., Daly, J. W. and Creveling, C. R.**, [^{3}H] Bactrachotoxinin A 20a-benzoate binding to voltage-sensitive sodium channels: a rapid and quantitative assay for local anesthetic activity in a variety of drugs, *J. Med. Chem.*, 28(3), 381, 1985.
35. **Takman, B. H., Boyes, R. N. and Vassallo, H. G.**, Local anesthetics, in *Principles of Medicinal Chemistry*, W. O. Foye, Eds., Lea and Febiger, 1974, chap. 14.
36. **Taylor, P.**, Cholinergic agonists, in *The Pharmacological Basis of Therapeutics*, 8th edition, Gilman, A. G., Rall, T. W., Nies, A. S. and Taylor, P., Eds., Pergamon Press, New York, 1990, chap. 6
37. **Yamamura, H. I. and Snyder, S. H.**, Muscarinic cholinergic receptor binding in the longitudinal muscle of the guinea pig ileum with tritium-labeled quinuclidinyl benzilate, *Mol. Pharmacol.*, 10(6), 861, 1974.
38. **Brown, J. H.**, Atropine, scopolamine, and related antimuscarinic drugs, in *The Pharmacological Basis of Therapeutics*, 8th edition, Gilman, A. G., Rall, T. W., Nies, A. S. and Taylor, P., Eds., Pergamon Press, 1990, chap. 8.
39. **Liang, C. C. and Quatel, J. H.**, Effects of drugs on the uptake of acetylcholine in rat brain cortex slices, *Biochem. Pharmacol.*, 18(5), 1187, 1969.
40. **Hoffman, B. B. and Lefkowitz, R. J.**, Catecholamines and sympathomimetic drugs, in *The Pharmacological Basis of Therapeutics*, 8th edition, Gilman, A. G., Rall, T. W., Nies, A. S. and Taylor, P., Eds., Pergamon Press, 1990, chap. 10.
41. **van den Brink, F. G.**, Molecular basis for the activity of drugs. III. Substances with multiple effects,, *Artneim-Forsch.*, 16(11), 1403, 1966.
42. **Hoffman, B. B. and Lefkowitz, R. J.**, Adrenergic receptor antagonist, in *The Pharmacological Basis of Therapeutics*, 8th edition, Gilman, A. G., Rall, T. W., Nies, A. S. and Taylor, P., Eds., Pergamon Press, 1990, chap. 11.
43. **Miyamura, K., Morooka, H., Hirai, K. and Gohshi, Y.**, A convenient apparatus for the study of the electric pulse generation in the liquid membrane system. Critical behavior of the voltage generation, *Chem. Lett.*, 1990(10), 1833.
44. **Arai, K., Kusu, F. and Takamura, K.**, Electrical potential oscillation across a water-octanol-water liquid membrane with an anionic surfactant, *Bunseki Kagaku*, 40(11), 775, 1991.
45. **Yoshikawa, K. and Matsubara, Y.**, Chemoreception by an excitable liquid membrane: characteristic effects of alcohols on the frequency of electrical oscillation, *J. Am. Chem. Soc.*, 106(16), 4423, 1984.
46. **Arai, K., Kusu, F. and Takamura, K.**, A novel explanation for the mechanism of electrical oscillation across a liquid membrane, *Chem. Lett.*, 1990(9), 1517.
47. **Arai, K., Fukuyama S., Kusu, F. and Takamura, K.**, Role of a surfactant in the electrical potential oscillation across a liquid membrane, *Electrochim. Acta*, in press.
48. **Fukuyama, S., Arai, K., Kusu, F. and Takamura, K.**, Comparison between electrical potential oscillation across a liquid membrane of a water/oil/water system and interfacial

potential at an oil/water system, paper presented at 43rd Ann. Meet. Jpn. Soc. Anal. Chem., Fukuoka, October 13 to 15, 1994, 14.

49. **Arai, K., Kusu, F. and Takamura, K.**, Electrical potential oscillation across a liquid membrane of water-octanol-water system, *Anal. Sci.*, 7(supplement), 599, 1991.
50. **Arai, K., Fukuyama, S., Kusu, F. and Takamura, K.**, Effects of chemical substances on electrical potential oscillation across an octanol liquid membrane, in *Proc. the Fifth Int. Symp. Redox Mechanisms and Interfacial Properties of Molecules of Biological Importance*, Schultz, F. A. and Taniguchi, I., Eds., The Electrochemical Society, Inc., Pennington, 1993, 333.
51. **Arai, K.**, *Electroanalytical Study of the Electrical Potential Oscillation Across a Liquid Membrane and Drug Transfer at an Oil/Water Interface*, Ph.D. thesis, Tokyo College of Pharmacy, Tokyo, 1994.

Chapter 18

ELECTRON TRANSFER REACTIONS AT THE POLARIZED LIQUID/LIQUID INTERFACE

Vincent J Cunnane and Lasse Murtomäki

I. INTRODUCTION

A. OVERVIEW

Let us consider a system where an aqueous redox couple O_1/R_1 is in contact with a redox couple O_2/R_2 in an organic phase; the organic solvent and water are assumed to be mutually immiscible. The net reaction of electron transfer at the liquid/liquid interface can formally be presented as

$$n_2 O_1^w + n_1 R_2^o \Leftrightarrow n_2 R_1^w + n_1 O_2^o \qquad (1)$$

The superscripts 'w' and 'o' denote the aqueous and organic phases hereafter. The Nernst equation of reaction (1) is

$$\phi^w - \phi^o = \Delta_o^w \phi = \Delta_o^w \phi_{O_1/R_2}^0 + \frac{RT}{n_1 n_2 F} \ln\left(\frac{a_{R_1}^{n_2} a_{O_2}^{n_1}}{a_{O_1}^{n_2} a_{R_2}^{n_1}}\right) \qquad (2)$$

where n_1 and n_2 are the number of electrons related to the redox couples 1 and 2, and a refers to the activities of the species. The standard potential of the reaction is equal to

$$\Delta_o^w \phi_{O_1/R_2}^0 = E_{O_2/R_2}^{0,o} - E_{O_1/R_1}^{0,w} \qquad (3)$$

i.e., the difference between the standard potentials of the redox couples in the appropriate phases. Standard potentials are usually known only in the aqueous phase, but the first term of Eq. (3) can be corrected for the solvent as

$$E_{O_2/R_2}^{0,o} = E_{O_2/R_2}^{0,w} + \frac{\Delta G_{t,O_2}^{0,w\to o} - \Delta G_{t,R_2}^{0,w\to o}}{n_2 F} \qquad (4)$$

0-8493-7694-7/96/$0.00+$.50

where $\Delta G_t^{0,w\rightarrow o}$ is the free energy of transfer from water to oil. Equation (3) thus describes a process in which R_2 is transferred from oil to water, where it reacts producing O_2, and the product is then transferred back to the organic phase. Alternatively, the standard transfer potentials can easily be measured by, for example, cyclic voltammetry using an ultramicroelectrode in the organic phase.

When the aqueous redox couple is added in excess compared to the organic redox couple, the aqueous phase can be considered as an extension of metal, since there are minimal changes in the concentrations of the aqueous redox components due to the reaction, and hence its Fermi level remains constant during an experiment. Still, there is a fundamental difference between solid/liquid and liquid/liquid redox systems. In a solid/liquid system the degree of freedom is equal to one: there are three quantities fully characterizing the system, the concentrations of the species O and R and the electrode potential, and two restricting conditions, the mass balance between the species and the Nernst equation.

In a liquid/liquid system there are five parameters, the concentrations of the four species and the Galvani potential difference. The number of restricting conditions is three, two mass balances in the two phases and the Nernst equation. The degree of freedom thus is two, provided that none of the species involved can partition to the opposite phase. If one of the species can partition between the phases, it brings an additional restricting condition, the partition equilibrium, and the degree of freedom is reduced to one.

In the absence of partitioning, it is possible to vary independently two parameters, contrary to the homogeneous reaction. This has interesting practical consequences. If two immiscible solutions, both containing a redox couple, are brought in contact, a reaction need not necessarily take place, regardless of how strong the oxidizing or reducing agents present are; however, a Galvani potential difference (Eq. (2)) will be established.

The interface between two immiscible liquids (ITIES) is one of the simplest systems to model and study electron transfer reactions occurring in non-homogeneous environments, since the interfacial electrical potential can be easily controlled externally. Despite its obvious analogy to, *e.g.*, biological systems where heterogeneous electron transfer has enormous importance, very few experimental studies of electron transfer at the liquid/liquid interface have been reported. One of the main reasons for their absence is the difficulty in finding a system where none of the reactants depicted in reaction (I) is transferring across the interface, thereby causing simultaneous ion and electron transfer, which complicates the evaluation of the reaction mechanism and/or kinetic parameters. Also, the organic supporting electrolyte may react in the bulk organic phase with R_2 or O_2, or at the interface with O_1 or R_1.

B. REVIEW OF LITERATURE

The history of electron transfer at polarized liquid/liquid interfaces is only 20 years old. The very first work was by Guainazzi *et al.*[1] who applied a constant current to the system $CuSO_4(w)$, tetrabutylammonium hexacarbonyl-vanadate in 1,2-dichloroethane, obtaining a layer of metallic copper at the interface. The next contribution was due to Samec's group in Prague which published a series of papers[2-5] about oxidation of ferrocene in nitrobenzene using ferricyanide in the aqueous phase. Samec also presented the first theory for a reaction of type (1)[6], based on the classical Marcus theory of electron transfer. Their studies suffered, however, from the chemical instability and partitioning of the ferricenium cation yielded in the oxidation, although the peaks due to ion and electron transfer were clearly separable in cyclic voltammograms (see section III. A).

Geblewicz and Schiffrin[7] studied the system where aqueous $[Fe(CN)_6]^{3-/4-}$ redox couple was in contact with lutetium biphthalocyanine in 1,2-dichloroethane. This system has the distinct advantage that the reactants are not crossing the interface. The observed rate constant of electron transfer was ca. 10^{-3} cm s^{-1}, one order of magnitude lower than at a gold electrode. The authors concluded that this low value was because of the large distance between the redox centers on the different sides of the interface. It was clearly shown that the half-wave potential was the same as at the gold electrode.

Cunnane *et al.*[8] replaced lutetium with tin in a biphthalocyanine complex, and demonstrated how the Galvani potential difference could be adjusted, by use of an external voltage source, or by the use of a common partitioning ion (tetraethyl or tetrapropyl ammonium) in each phase. In the latter case, after equilibrium had been reached, the concentrations of the different tin constituents were spectroscopically analyzed, and the results agreed well with the voltammetric data.

Kihara *et al.*[9] greatly increased the number of systems studied utilizing current-scan polarography at the electrolyte dropping electrode. Aqueous redox couples employed were hydroquinone/quinone, OH^-/HO_2^-, MnO_4^-/Mn^{2+}, $Ce^{3+/4+}$ and $Fe^{2+/3+}$ in a hexacyanate, sulphate or chloride environment. Organic redox couples included tetracyanoquinodimethane (TCNQ), ferrocene and tetrathiafulvalene (TTF). Different combinations of these couples were examined and half-wave potentials calculated, based on the steady-state current-voltage relationship derived by Samec[10]. Many of the systems showed reversible behavior during the scan. Perhaps the most interesting was the observation that permanganate obviously oxidized tetraphenylborate (Ph_4B^-) which was used as an anion of the base electrolyte. This can have serious implications when choosing the base electrolyte in electron transfer experiments (see section III. A).

Later the same group investigated electron transfer coupled with ion transfer[11,12]. Their experiments were supported by the cyclic voltammetry simulations of Stewart *et al.*[13] in which mass transfer of all four species involved in reaction (I) was considered. They ended up with a quadratic expression for the convoluted current[14], $I(t)$:

$$AI(t)^2 + BI(t) + C = 0 \tag{5}$$

where the coefficients A, B and C are

$$A = \frac{\theta S(t)}{\sqrt{D_{R_1} D_{O_2}}} - \frac{1}{\sqrt{D_{O_1} D_{R_2}}} \tag{5a}$$

$$B = \theta S(t)\left[\frac{C_{R_1}}{\sqrt{D_{O_2}}} + \frac{C_{O_2}}{\sqrt{D_{R_1}}}\right] + \frac{C_{O_1}}{\sqrt{D_{R_2}}} + \frac{C_{R_2}}{\sqrt{D_{O_1}}} \tag{5b}$$

$$C = C_{R_1} C_{O_2} \theta S(t) - C_{O_1} C_{R_2} \tag{5c}$$

and $\theta = \exp[nF/RT(E_i - E^{0'})]$ and $S(t) = \exp[-\sigma t + 2\sigma(t-\lambda)H(t-\lambda)]$; H is the Heaviside function, and the other quantities have been quoted as in ref. 14. It appeared that reaction (1) could be considered as a pseudo-first-order reaction only when the concentrations of O_1 and R_1 are equal and much higher than the concentrations of O_2 and R_2.

Experimental techniques were almost entirely restricted to cyclic voltammetry until Chen *et al.*[15] and Cheng and Schiffrin[16] employed *ac* impedance techniques at the equilibrium potential. The former group investigated 'classical' oxidation of ferrocene with $Fe(CN)_6^{3-/4-}$ and found that the effective exchange current density increased linearly as a function of the $K_3Fe(CN)_6$ concentration, but the corresponding increase due to the addition of ferrocene was saturated at a relatively low concentration, ca. 0.1 mM.

Cheng and Schiffrin[16] completed previous experiments[7,8,17] in a more detailed analysis of the impedance data, and a comparison with the recent theoretical developments by Marcus[18-20] was made. The agreement with his theory was at least reasonable.

Later Cheng and Schiffrin[21] observed a mediated electron transfer reaction. In this they deposited a phospholipid monolayer at the water/1,2-dichloroethane interface, inhibiting the transfer between lutetium[8] or ruthenium[17] redox couples and $Fe(CN)_6^{3-/4-}$. Using TCNQ/TCNQ$^{\cdot -}$ as the organic redox couple, electron transfer continued, although retarded, due to the ability of TCNQ to accommodate itself within the adsorbed phospholipid layer. When both ruthenium complex and TCNQ were present in the organic phase, two voltammetric waves were observed, the first corresponding to the oxidation of the ruthenium complex and the second to the TCNQ couple. Hence, TCNQ mediated an electron to the ruthenium complex, but this did not happen with the lutetium complex. These phenomena were discussed in terms of the Marcus theory.

Quite recently Cunnane *et al.*[22] reported their investigations about the mechanism of the coupled ion and electron transfer in the ferrocene - hexaferrocyanate system[5], using substituted ferrocene derivatives in order to increase the hydrophobicity of the ferricenium cation, and to emphasize the effect of the distance between redox centers. Unexpectedly, it appears that rather than separating the transfer potentials for ion and electron transfer, in the case of dimethyl ferrocene the separation was decreased. It is also evident from this work that the mechanism of the ferrocenium transfer involved a catalytic cycle with tetraphenylborate.

Before the theory by Marcus mentioned above[18-20], Girault and Schiffrin[23] modeled the electron transfer reaction using a precursor-successor formalism originally developed by Sutin[24]. They concluded that the measurement of the electron transfer kinetics at the potential of zero charge would be very convenient for the comparison of measured values with electron transfer theories. Lately, Benjamin has widened his molecular dynamic simulations of ion transfer to electron transfer[25]. A more detailed description of the theoretical developments is given in the next section, and of the molecular dynamic simulations in Chapter 10.

II. THEORY OF THE TWO PHASE ELECTRON TRANSFER

A. KINETICS OF ELECTRON TRANSFER

As mentioned earlier, Samec[6] was the first to discuss the theory of reaction (I), considering an activated barrier to electron transfer according to the classical Marcus theory[26]. The activation energy, ΔG^{act}, is then given by

$$\Delta G^{act} = \frac{(\lambda + \Delta G_{et})^2}{4\lambda} \tag{6}$$

where λ is the reorganization energy, and ΔG_{et} is the free energy of reaction (1), including several work terms inherent to the interfacial model.

Girault and Schiffrin[23] proposed a model which involves the formation of a reactive precursor complex followed by the rate determining electron transfer, according to reaction (7):

$$O_1 + R_2 \leftrightarrow O_1|R_2 \leftrightarrow \{O_1R_2\} \xleftrightarrow{V_{eff}} \{R_1O_2\} \leftrightarrow R_1|O_2 \leftrightarrow R_1 + O_2 \tag{7}$$

where $O_1|R_2$ and $R_1|O_2$ represent the precursor and the successor complexes respectively. $\{O_1R_2\}$ is the precursor complex reorganized to a configuration appropriate for electron transfer and $\{R_1O_2\}$ is the reorganized successor before relaxation to the state of the successor complex[23]; ν_{eff} is the effective electron hopping frequency. Now, it can be shown that the observed rate constant, k_{obs}, can be expressed as

$$k_{obs} = Z\exp\left(-w_p / RT\right)k_{et} \tag{8}$$

where Z is a preexponential factor, and k_{et} is the rate constant associated with the reaction between the precursor $O_1|R_2$ and the successor $R_1|O_2$. From the Marcus theory[18] k_{et} is found as

$$k_{et} = \nu_{eff}\exp\left(-\frac{(\lambda + \Delta G^{o'} + w_p - w_s)^2}{4\lambda RT}\right) \tag{9}$$

In Eqs. (8) and (9) w_p is the work to bring the reactants from the bulk to a distance r, to form a precursor, and w_s the work to separate the products from the successor. $\Delta G^{0'}$ is the concentration independent part of the Gibbs energy for the reaction (n is the number of electrons transferred in reaction (1)):

$$\Delta G^{o'} = nF\left(\Delta_o^w \phi - \Delta_o^w \phi^{o'}_{O_1/R_2}\right) \tag{10}$$

The work terms w_p and w_s are not easily found but qualitatively they consist of the following contributions[23]:

(a) change in the standard chemical potential of the reactants associated with the change of their solvation energies between the bulk and the interfacial region

(b) change in the activity coefficient of the reactants due to the change in their ionic atmosphere between the interfacial region and the bulk; provided that the interfacial region is a mixed solvent layer, it has a different relative permittivity from the bulk values

(c) electrical work associated with the Galvani potential distribution across the two phases.

For the first contribution (a) Marcus[18] has given an expression of the form

$$w_p = -\left[\frac{(z_{O_1})^2}{4d_1\varepsilon_{st}^w} - \frac{(z_{R_2})^2}{4d_2\varepsilon_{st}^o}\right]\left[\frac{\varepsilon_{st}^o - \varepsilon_{st}^w}{\varepsilon_{st}^o + \varepsilon_{st}^w}\right] + \frac{2}{R}\frac{z_{O_1}z_{R_2}}{\varepsilon_{st}^w + \varepsilon_{st}^o} \tag{11}$$

where $d_{1,2}$ refer to the distance of the reactants to the interface, ϵ_{st} is the static relative permittivities of the two phases, and R is the distance between the reactants. w_s is obtained from Eq. (10) by changing the appropriate quantities for the reactants to the values of the products. The contribution (b) is very difficult to calculate, though it might not be negligible. The third contribution (c) perhaps is the most important, and is readily found as

$$\begin{aligned} w_p &= z_{O_1} F \Delta_w^a \phi + z_{R_2} F \Delta_o^b \phi \\ w_s &= z_{R_1} F \Delta_w^a \phi + z_{O_2} F \Delta_o^b \phi \end{aligned} \tag{12}$$

where a and b represent the positions of the species relative to the interface, *i.e.*, $\Delta^{\alpha}{}_{w}\phi$ and $\Delta^{\beta}{}_{o}\phi$ are the potential drops in the two diffusion double layers. At the potential of zero charge these two terms are practically zero, which enables a convenient way to compare k_{obs} with k_{et}.

The reorganization energy λ consists of the inner, λ_i, and outer, λ_o, contributions. λ_o has been given by Kharkats and Volkov[27], and by Marcus[19] as:

$$\begin{aligned} \lambda_o = {} & \frac{(ne)^2}{2a_1}\left(\frac{1}{\varepsilon_{op}^w} - \frac{1}{\varepsilon_{st}^w}\right) + \frac{(ne)^2}{2a_2}\left(\frac{1}{\varepsilon_{op}^o} - \frac{1}{\varepsilon_{st}^o}\right) \\ & - \frac{(ne)^2}{4d_1}\left(\frac{\varepsilon_{op}^o - \varepsilon_{op}^w}{\varepsilon_{op}^w(\varepsilon_{op}^w + \varepsilon_{op}^o)} - \frac{\varepsilon_{st}^w - \varepsilon_{st}^o}{\varepsilon_{st}^o(\varepsilon_{st}^w + \varepsilon_{st}^o)}\right) \\ & - \frac{(ne)^2}{4d_2}\left(\frac{\varepsilon_{op}^w - \varepsilon_{op}^o}{\varepsilon_{op}^o(\varepsilon_{op}^w + \varepsilon_{op}^o)} - \frac{\varepsilon_{st}^w - \varepsilon_{st}^o}{\varepsilon_{st}^o(\varepsilon_{st}^w + \varepsilon_{st}^o)}\right) \\ & - \frac{2(ne)^2}{a_1 + a_2}\left(\frac{1}{\varepsilon_{op}^w + \varepsilon_{op}^o} - \frac{1}{\varepsilon_{st}^w + \varepsilon_{st}^o}\right) \end{aligned} \tag{13}$$

where a_1 and a_2 are the radii of the reactants, and ϵ_{op} denotes the optical relative permittivity of the phases. The inner contribution λ_i may be available from spectroscopic data[16,20]

The preexponential factor Z appearing in Eq. (8) has also been given by Marcus[20] for a sharp boundary interface as:

$$Z = 2\pi N_A(a_1 + a_2)\kappa(\Delta R)^3 \quad (14)$$

and for the mixed solvent layer as:

$$Z = 4\pi N_A(a_1 + a_2)^2 \kappa \Delta R L \quad (15)$$

where κ is a transmission coefficient, equal to 1 for adiabatic reactions, and ΔR is a parameter relating the rate of reaction to separation distance and is typically 0.1 nm[18]; L is the thickness of the mixed solvent layer.
Finally, Marcus[20] has given simple and useful 'mixing rules' for the estimation of the heterogeneous rate constant from the homogeneous and metal-liquid rate constants. If the rate constants of the couples 1 and 2 are taken at the metal-liquid interface **at the equilibrium potential**, where the forward and reverse rates are equal, as k_{m1} and k_{m2} (cm s^{-1}), then our second order rate constant, k_{obs}, (mol^{-1} cm^4 s^{-1}) can be approximated at the sharp boundary interface as

$$k_{obs} = \left[2\pi N_A(a_1 + a_2)\ \Delta R / \kappa\, \nu_{eff}\right] k_{m1}\, k_{m2}\ ;\ \Delta\phi_o^w = \Delta_o^w \phi_{O_1/R_2}^{0'} \quad (16)$$

and at the mixed solvent interface as:

$$k_{obs} = \left[4\pi N_A(a_1 + a_2)^2 L / \Delta R \kappa\, \nu_{eff}\right] k_{m1}\, k_{m2}\ ;\ \Delta\phi_o^w = \Delta_o^w \phi_{O_1/R_2}^{0'} \quad (17)$$

Further, when the homogeneous self-exchange rate constants are k_{h1} and k_{h2} (cm^3 s^{-1}), again at the equilibrium potential, then at the sharp boundary interface

$$k_{obs} = \left[N_A(\Delta R)^2 / 2(a_1 + a_2)\right] \sqrt{k_{h1}\, k_{h2}}\ ;\ \Delta_o^w \phi = \Delta_o^w \phi_{O_1/R_2}^{0'} \quad (18)$$

and at the mixed solvent interface

$$k_{obs} = N_A L \sqrt{k_{h1} k_{h2}}\,; \quad \Delta_o^w \phi = \Delta_o^w \phi_{O_1/R_2}^{0'} \tag{19}$$

From Eqs. (16) - (19) the clear value of measurements at the equilibrium potential (or zero charge potential) is apparent.

B. MATCHING POTENTIALS

One of the interesting consequences of Eqs.(1) and (2) is that the position of equilibrium of a two phase electron transfer reaction is determined by the differences in their standard potentials (Eq. (2)) and on the interfacial Galvani potential difference $\Delta_o^w \phi$. As such electron transfers between redox couples across the interface can be investigated within the potential window normally available at the ITIES, irrespective of the value of the standard potentials of the couple in each phase, provided that these standard potentials have been closely matched, and the distance between the respective couples allows for the transfer.

As an example let us consider the case of lutetium biphthalocyanine. The linear sweep voltammogram of lutetium biphthalocyanine at a platinum micro-electrode in 1,2-dichloroethane in the presence of base electrolyte shows two reversible one electron transfer processes (see figure 1), one corresponding to the oxidation and the other to the reduction of the lutetium biphthalocyanine. The separation between the two processes is of the order of 0.51 volts. **Both** the oxidation and reduction electron transfer reactions can be investigated at the ITIES with the **same** organic base electrolyte system. The difference lies in the choice of a redox couple in the aqueous phase. In both cases a fast aqueous couple is required which should be present in excess over the organic couple in order that the reaction is limited by diffusion of the organic couple to the interface region. In the case of lutetium biphthalocyanine the oxidation can be studied by utilising the ferro/ferricyanide couple (CN) and the reduction with ferro/ferrioxalate couple (Ox). The difference in formal potentials between these aqueous couples is ca. 0.59 V, E_{CN}^0 = 0.565 V[7] and E_{Ox}^0 = - 0.025 V *vs.* SHE[28].

In the liquid-liquid case quasireversible electron transfer peaks can be seen by cyclic voltammetry for both the oxidation[7] and reduction[28] of the biphthalocyanine. The cause of the slower kinetics in the liquid-liquid case over the metal/solution case is due to the increased distances between the redox couples in the former case[7,22]. This example illustrates that the polarized liquid-liquid interface is an extremely powerful tool for the elucidation of electron transfer processes of widely varying standard potentials. This has important implications for the range of heterogeneous processes in general.

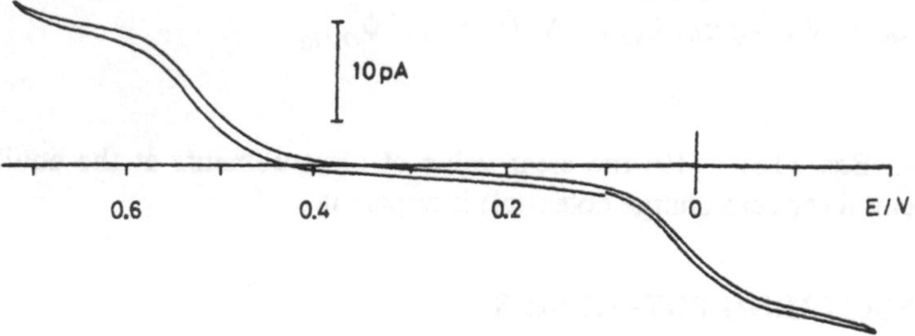

Figure 1. Linear sweep voltammetry of $5{\cdot}10^{-5}$ M $Lu(PC)_2$ + 10^{-3} M $TPAsPh_4BCl$ in 1,2-DCE at a Pt microelectrode[7]. (By kind permission of Elsevier Publishing Company.)

III MODEL SYSTEMS

As stated previously, while the study of ion transfer reactions at polarized liquid-liquid interfaces has received a great deal of attention from both a theoretical and practical viewpoint, the study of electron transfers has until recently been dealt with largely from a theoretical rather than practical approach. The reason for this has been the lack of suitable model systems to study pure heterogeneous transfer across the interface in the absence of associated ion transfer from either redox component in each phase. This coupled ion transfer has mainly been associated with transfer of one of the redox components from the organic phase. The following section will deal with some of the model systems investigated to date.

A. FERROCENES

Samec, in a series of papers[2-4], first studied the ferro/ferricyanide(*w*) in contact with ferrocene(*o*, nitrobenzene). While a reversible electron transfer reaction was noted from cyclic voltammetric data this discussion was complicated by virtue of the partitioning of ferrocene (Fc) and its oxidation product ferricenium from the following reaction:

$$Fc(o) + [Fe(CN)_6]^{3-}(w) \rightleftharpoons Fc^{+}(o) + [Fe(CN)_6]^{4-}(w)$$

In a later paper[5] this group showed that the ion and electron transfer reactions are separated by some 0.120 V in the system studied. However, they also noted that the mechanism of the above reaction is voltammetrically indistinguishable from the following involving ion transfer as one of the steps:

$$Fc(o) \rightleftharpoons Fc(w)$$
$$Fc(w) + [Fe(CN)_6]^{3-}(w) \rightleftharpoons Fc^{+}(w) + [Fe(CN)_6]^{4-}(w)$$

$$Fc^+(w) \rightleftharpoons Fc^+(o)$$

This system has very recently been revisited in connection with other derivatised ferrocenes, dimethyl (DMFc) and decamethylferrocene (DCMFc)[22].

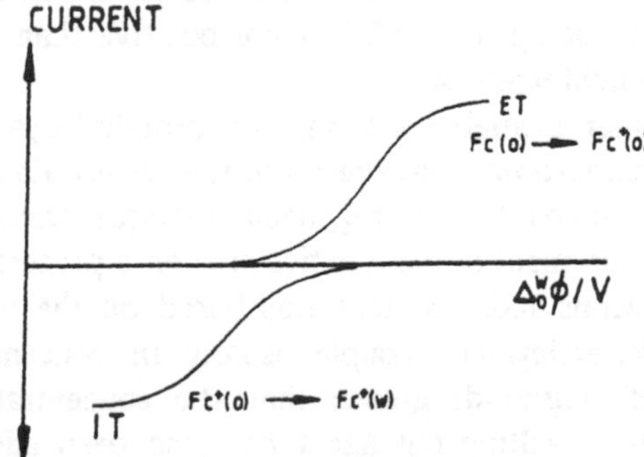

Figure 2. Schematic diagram showing the coupling of electron and ion transfer[22]. (By kind permission of Pergamon Press.)

In this study a comparison was made between the electron transfer potentials and the corresponding ionic transfer potentials of the oxidized organic compounds (see figure 2 above for the ferrocene case). It had been hoped that by the methyl substitution of the cyclopentadienyl rings of ferrocene, uncoupled electron transfer reactions between such species and suitable aqueous redox couples could be brought about uninfluenced by the ion transfer of the formed ferricenium. However, this was not the case and the ferrocene/$Fe(CN)_6^{3-/4-}$ system was also complicated by the rapid interaction of the product ferricenium and the anion of the organic electrolyte, tetraphenylborate, Ph_4B^-:

$$Fc(o) + Fe(CN)_6^{3-}(w) \rightarrow Fc^+(o) + Fe(CN)_6^{4-}(w)$$
$$2\,Fc^+(o) + Ph_4B^-(o) \rightarrow Ph_2(o) + Ph_2B^+(o) + 2\,Fc(o)$$
$$Ph_2B^+(o) + H_2O(w) \rightarrow Ph_2BO^-(w) + 2\,H^+(w)$$

From this it is clear that ferrocene acts as a redox catalyst for the oxidation of Ph_4B^-. Therefore the overall interfacial reaction will also include the two electron oxidation of the anion of the organic base electrolyte in parallel with simple electron transfer, followed by diffusion of the ferricenium species.

The separation in potential between the ion and electron transfer for the DMFc case is of the order of 0.095 V, approximately 0.05 V closer than the above case, and is again complicated by interaction with the organic base electrolyte. The DCMFc is complicated by slow electron transfer kinetics and coupled ion transfer reactions. Certainly the use of salting out agents[29] in the aqueous phase makes the transfer of the ferricenium much less favored. However, it is clear from the above discussion that in terms of electron transfer the ferrocene system is far from simple.

B. OTHER SYSTEMS

Of the other systems investigated to date tetraphenyl porphyrins[16,17] and TCNQ[11,12,16,21] are worth further investigation. In the case of the reduction of TCNQ an associated ion transfer of the radical anion is possible, this has been reported as being over 0.2 V more positive than that of the electron transfer in 1,2-dichloroethane[16].

Of the other available systems the biphthalocyanines, in particular lutetium biphthalocyanine, have received the widest attention in terms of an example of an uncoupled heterogeneous electron transfer process[7,8,16,17,21] and in the measurement of the kinetics of such a process. In all of the these studies the aqueous redox system was based on the well defined, highly reversible ferro/ferricyanide couple usually in concentrations more than three orders of magnitude greater than the concentration of the organic couple. Latterly, a salting out agent has also been added to the aqueous phase to limit the solubility of components of the organic couple. It has also been demonstrated for such systems that the half-wave potential obtained via voltammetric experiments is the same as when the aqueous couple is replaced by a metallic microelectrode. This is an important observation as it allows for the separate evaluation of the possible electron transfer reactions and formal redox potential of the aqueous and organic redox couples prior to their being brought together in a two phase system.

IV. ELECTROCATALYSIS AND ELECTRODEPOSITION

A. ELECTROCATALYSIS

1. Mediated Electron Transfer

Recently Cheng and Schiffrin[21] presented an example of a redox electrocatalytic process in a two phase system. Previously studied electron transfers from ferro/ferricyanide couple to lutetium biphthalocyanine, bis(pyridine)-*meso*-tetraphenylporphyrinato-ruthenium(II) complex and TCNQ were investigated in the presence of an adsorbed layer of phospholipid, formed from a mixture of egg lecithin and cholesterol. The reactions of the lutetium biphthalocyanine, and the bis(pyridine)*meso*-tetraphenylporphyrinato-ruthenium(II) complex were completely inhibited with the adsorbed layer present. However, the reaction with TCNQ was only partially inhibited indicating that TCNQ was incorporated into the monolayer; this latter result is not unexpected as TCNQ is a well known mediator of electron transfer reactions between redox couples separated by a bilayer membrane[30]. Interestingly, when TCNQ was added to the organic solution containing the ruthenium(II) complex the reaction between this couple and the aqueous couple was catalyzed. The proposed reaction scheme is as follows:

$$\mathrm{TCNQ}^{\cdot -}(m) \rightarrow \mathrm{TCNQ}(m) + e^-$$

$$\mathrm{TCNQ}(m) + \mathrm{RuTPP(py)_2}(o) \rightarrow \mathrm{TCNQ}^{\cdot -}(m) + \mathrm{RuTPP(py)2}$$

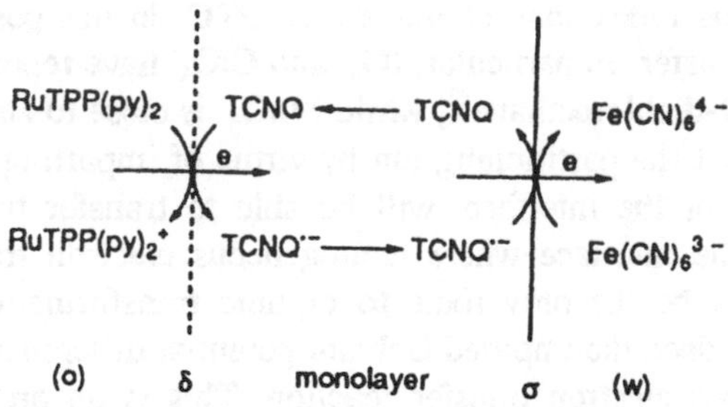

Figure 3. Schematic representation of the mediated electron-transfer reaction at an adsorbed lipid monolayer at the water/1,2-DCE interface, σ denotes an immiscible interface and δ is an imaginary phase of closest approach of $RuTPP(py)_2$[21]. (By kind permission of the Royal Society of Chemistry.)

In the case of the lutetium biphthalocyanine no evidence was found for a mediated electron transfer reaction. This may be due to the large difference in formal redox potentials between these couples.

2. Phase Transfer Catalysis

In the study of the electron transfer reaction between tin biphthalocyanine (in 1,2-dichloroethane) and the aqueous ferro/ferricyanide[8] couple it was shown that the reaction could be controlled either by the use of an externally applied Galvani potential difference delivered via a potentiostat or by the use of a partitioning ion. The role of the partitioning ion is to fix the interfacial Galvani potential difference and as such to determine the position of equilibrium. In the latter case the electron transfer is controlled by an ion partitioning reaction. This result may have important consequences for phase transfer catalysis (PTC).

PTC[31,32] has been extensively utilized in organic synthesis to carry out reactions in organic media when some of the reactants are present in the aqueous phase. In the case of oxidations and reductions it has usually been considered that the role of the PT catalyst is to physically transfer the aqueous redox species to the organic phase where homogeneous electron transfer occurs. While this may well be the case in organic media of low relative permittivity, a different mechanism is possible in media of somewhat higher permittivity.

PT catalysts which are noted for their efficiency in the case of oxidations and reductions are generally tetraalkyl ammonium salts[31]. However, these ions are by their nature capable of partitioning between two immiscible phases thereby setting up a Galvani potential difference at the interface governed by:

$$\Delta_o^w\phi = \Delta_o^w\phi_i^0 + \frac{RT}{z_iF}\ln\frac{a_i^0}{a_i^w} \qquad (20)$$

Many of the aqueous redox ions of interest in PTC do not possess large Gibbs energies of transfer. In particular, IO_4^- and ClO_4^- have reported values of 16 kJ mol^{-1} in 1,2-dichloroethane[33], while MnO_4^- is close to zero volts. It is therefore likely that the partitioning ion by virtue of imparting a Galvani potential difference at the interface, will be able to transfer the aqueous redox ions across the interface where homogeneous electron transfer can occur. This may not be the only route to organic transformations in the organic phase and indeed the imposed Galvani potential difference may well drive a heterogeneous electron transfer reaction. This is an area of study which is expected to receive a great deal more attention over the coming years.

B. ELECTRODEPOSITION

Guainazzi *et al.*[1] successfully deposited copper and silver at a polarized liquid-liquid interface from a variety of aqueous solutions in contact with $Bu_4NV(CO)_6$ as the organic electrolyte in 1,2-dichloroethane or dichloromethane. $V(CO)_6^-$ acts as the reducing agent for the heterogeneous electron transfer. The current efficiency for Cu^{2+} reduction is subject to experimental conditions but is lower than the efficiency of ordinary cathodic deposition for copper. The copper film is usually broken up by evolved CO bubbles formed in the underlying 1,2-dichloroethane phase. However, depending again on the conditions, continuous coherent layers of copper have been recovered.

Much more recently Brust *et al.*[34] described a one step method for the preparation of an unusual new metallic material of alkane thiol derivatised gold particles. A two phase (water-toluene) system was used in which $AuCl_4^-$ was transferred from aqueous solution to organic where it was reduced by sodium borohydride in the aqueous phase and in the presence of dodecanethiol in the organic phase. These new hydrophobic metal clusters have an unusual property in that they can be handled and characterized as a simple chemical compound.

V. SUMMARY AND FUTURE DEVELOPMENTS

While we have stated that theoretical studies have outweighed the experimental studies in electron transfer reactions at polarized liquid-liquid interfaces, this situation is now being addressed and the coming years should see a great deal more studies devoted to the experimental side of this area of heterogeneous reactions. Of particular interest is the area of bioenergetics with particular emphasis on the electron transport chain in mitochondria and photosynthesis. Other areas for which these systems are of relevance include redox liquid extraction, extraction processes, catalysis including phase transfer catalysis, electroanalysis and electrodeposition and phase formation to name but a few.

VI. REFERENCES

1. **Guainazzi, M., Silvestri, G. and Serravalle, G.**, Electrochemical metallization at the liquid-liquid interfaces of non-miscible electrolyte solutions, *J. Chem. Soc. Chem. Commun.*, 200, 1975.
2. **Samec, Z., Mareček, V. and Weber, J.**, Detection of an electron transfer across the interface between two immiscible electrolyte solutions by cyclic voltammetry with four-electrode system, *J. Electroanal. Chem.*, 96, 245, 1977.
3. **Samec, Z., Mareček, V. and Weber, J.**, Electron transfer between hexacyanoferrate(III) in water and ferrocene in nitrobenzene investigated by cyclic voltammetry with four-electrode system, *J. Electroanal. Chem.*, 103, 11, 1979.
4. **Samec, Z., Mareček, V., Weber, J. and Homolka, D.**, Convolution potential sweep voltammetry of Cs^+ ion transfer and of electron transfer between ferrocene and hexacyanoferrate(III) ion across the water/nitrobenzene interface, *J. Electroanal. Chem.*, 126, 105, 1981.
5. **Hanzlík, J., Samec, Z. and Hovorka, J.**, Transfer of ferricenium cation across water/organic solvent interfaces, *J. Electroanal. Chem.*, 216, 303, 1987.
6. **Samec, Z.**, *J. Electroanal. Chem.*, Basic equation for the rate of the charge transfer across the interface, 99, 197, 1979.
7. **Geblewicz, G. and Schiffrin, D. J.**, Electron transfer between immiscible solutions, the hexacyanoferrate-lutetium biphthalocyanine system, *J. Electroanal. Chem.*, 244, 27, 1988.
8. **Cunnane, V. J., Schiffrin, D. J., Beltran, C., Geblewicz, G. and Solomon, T.**, The role of phase transfer catalysts in two phase redox reactions, *J. Electroanal. Chem.*, 247, 203, 1988.
9. **Kihara, S., Suzuki, M., Maeda, K., Ogura, K., Matsui, M. and Yoshida, Z.**, The electron transfer at a liquid/liquid interface studied by current-scan polarography at the electrolyte dropping electrode, *J. Electroanal. Chem.*, 271, 107, 1989.
10. **Samec, Z.**, *J. Electroanal. Chem.*, Stationary curve of current vs. potential of electron transfer across interface, 103, 1, 1979.
11. **Maeda, K., Kihara, S., Suzuki, M. and Matsui, M.**, Voltammetric inter- pretation of ion transfer coupled with electron transfer at a liquid/liquid interface, *J. Electroanal. Chem.*, 303, 171, 1991.
12. **Kihara, S., Maeda, K., Suzuki, M., Sohrin, Y., Shirai, O. and Matsui, M.**, Voltammetric analysis of chemical reactions at liquid/liquid or liquid/membrane interfaces, *Anal. Sci.*, 7, 1415, 1991.
13. **Stewart, A. A., Campbell, J. A., Girault, H. H. and Eddowes, M.**, Cyclic voltammetry for electron transfer reactions at liquid/liquid interfaces, *Ber. Bunsenges. Phys. Chem.*, 94, 83, 1990.
14. **Bard, A. J. and Faulkner, L. R.**, *Electrochemical Methods*, John Wiley & Sons, New York, 1980, chap. 6.
15. **Chen, Q.-Z., Iwamoto, K. and Senō, M.**, Kinetic analysis of electron transfer between hexacyanoferrate(III) in water and ferrocene in nitrobenzene by *ac* impedance measurements, *Electrochim. Acta*, 36(2), 291, 1991.
16. **Cheng, Y. and Schiffrin D. J.**, A.C. impedance study of rate constants for two-phase electron-transfer reactions, *J. Chem. Soc. Faraday Trans.*, 89(2), 199, 1993.
17. **Cheng, Y. and Schiffrin D. J.**, Electron transfer between bis(pyridine) *meso*-tetraphenyl-porphyrinato iron(II) and ruthenium(III) and the hexacyanoferrate couple at the 1,2-dichloroethane/water interface, *J. Electroanal. Chem.*, 314, 153, 1991.
18. **Marcus, R. A.**, Reorganization free energy for electron-transfers at liquid-liquid and dielectric semiconductor-liquid interfaces, *J. Phys. Chem.*, 94(3), 1050, 1990.
19. **Marcus, R. A.**, Theory of electron-transfer rates across liquid-liquid interfaces, *J. Phys. Chem.*, 94(10), 4152, 1990.
20. **Marcus, R. A.**, Theory of electron-transfer rates across liquid-liquid interfaces. 2. Relationships and application, *J. Phys. Chem.*, 95(5), 2010, 1991.
21. **Cheng, Y. and Schiffrin, D. J.**, Redox electrocatalysis by tetracyanoquinodimethane in phospholipid monolayers adsorbed at a liquid/liquid interface, *J. Chem. Soc.*, 90(17), 2517, 1994.
22. **Cunnane, V. J., Geblewicz, G. and Schiffrin, D. J.**, Electron and ion transfer potentials of ferrocene and derivatives at a liquid-liquid interface, *Electrochim. Acta*, 40, 3005, 1995.

23. **Girault, H. H. and Schiffrin, D. J.,** Electron transfer reactions at the interface between two immiscible electrolyte solutions, *J. Electroanal. Chem.*, 244, 15, 1988.
24. **Newton, M. D. and Sutin, N.,** Electron transfer reactions in condensed phases, *Annu. Rev. Phys. Chem.*, 35, 437, 1984.
25. **Benjamin, I.,** Molecular dynamics study of the free energy functions for electron-transfer reactions at the liquid-liquid interface, *J. Phys. Chem.*, 95(17), 6675, 1991.
26. **Marcus, R. A.,** On the theory of electron-transfer reactions. VI. Unified treatment for homogeneous and electrode reactions, *J. Chem. Phys.*, 43(2), 679, 1965.
27. **Kharkats, Y. I. and Volkov, A. G.,** Interfacial catalysis: multielectron reactions at the liquid-liquid interface, *J. Electroanal. Chem.*, 184, 435, 1985.
28. **Cunnane, V. J. and Schiffrin, D. J.,** unpublished results.
29. **Kontturi, K., Murtomäki, L. and Schiffrin, D. J.,** Anion effect on single ionic salting-out coefficients of hydrophobic electrolytes, *Acta Chem. Scand.*, 46, 25, 1992.
30. **Tien, H. T.,** Redox reactions in lipid bilayers and membrane bioenergetics, *Bioelectrochem. Bioenerg.*, 15, 19, 1986.
31. **Starks, C. M. and Liotta, C.,** *Phase Transfer Catalysis*, Academic Press, London, 1978.
32. **Demlow, E.V. and Demlov, S.S.,** *Phase Transfer Catalysis*, 2nd revised edition, Verlag Chemie, Weinheim, 1983.
33. **Kihara, S., Suzuki, M., Maeda, K., Ogura, K., Matsui, M. and Yoshida, Z.,** The transfer of anions at the aqueous/organic solutions interface studied by current-scan polarography with the electrolyte dropping electrode, *J. Electroanal. Chem.*, 210, 147, 1986.
34. **Brust, M., Walker, M., Bethell, D., Schiffrin, D. J. and Whyman, R.,** Synthesis of thiol-derivatised gold nanoparticles in a two-phase liquid-liquid systems, *J. Chem. Soc. Chem. Commun.*, 801, 1994

INDEX

Milton Keynes UK
Ingram Content Group UK Ltd.
UKHW021840071024
449327UK00021B/1522